WITHDRAWN
CARROLL UNIVERSITY LIBRARY

ENCYCLOPEDIA OF SPORTS SCIENCE

Volume 2

EDITOR

John Zumerchik

TECHNICAL EDITORS

David E. Harris
Lewiston-Auburn College
University of Southern Maine

Don C. Hopkins
Department of Physics
Hamline University

David H. Janda
Institute for Preventative Sports Medicine
Ann Arbor, Michigan

David A. Lind
Department of Physics
University of Colorado

Arjun Tan
Department of Physics
Alabama A&M University

Ellen J. Zeman
Department of Molecular Physiology and Biophysics
University of Vermont College of Medicine

SPECIAL MEDICAL ADVISER

John P. Furia
Sun Orthopaedics and Sports Medicine
Lewisburg, Pennsylvania

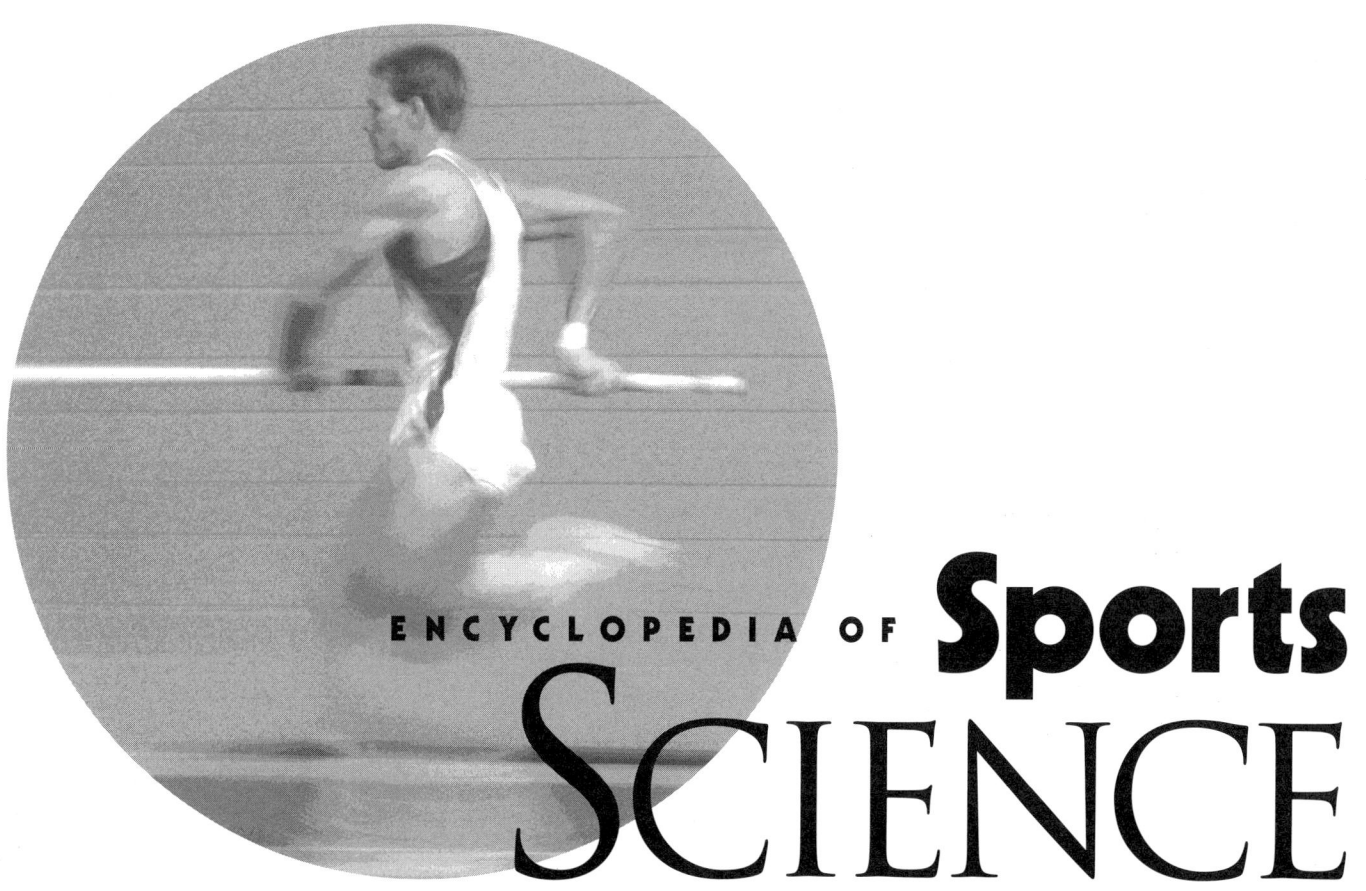

ENCYCLOPEDIA OF Sports SCIENCE

Volume 2

John Zumerchik
EDITOR

MACMILLAN LIBRARY REFERENCE USA
Simon & Schuster Macmillan
NEW YORK

Simon & Schuster and Prentice Hall International
LONDON · MEXICO CITY · NEW DELHI · SINGAPORE · SYDNEY · TORONTO

Copyright © 1997 by John Zumerchik

All rights reserved. No part of this book may be reproduced or transmitted in any form or by any means, electronic or mechanical, including photocopying, recording, or by any information storage and retrieval system, without permission in writing from the Publisher.

Simon & Schuster Macmillan
1633 Broadway, New York, NY 10019

Printed in the United States of America

printing number

10 9 8 7 6 5 4 3 2 1

LIBRARY OF CONGRESS CATALOGING-IN-PUBLICATION DATA
Encyclopedia of sports science / John Zumerchik, editor.
       p. cm.
       Includes bibliographical references and index.
       ISBN 0-02-897506-5 (set : alk. paper). — ISBN 0-02-864665-7 (v. 1 : alk. paper). — ISBN 0-02-864666-5 (v. 2 : alk. paper)
       1. Sports sciences—Encyclopedias. 2. Sports—Physiological aspects—Encyclopedias. I. Zumerchik, John.
GV558.E53 1997
613.7' 1—dc21   96-47502
                                                                                                         CIP

The paper used in this publication meets the minimum requirements of American National Standard for Information Sciences—Permanence of Paper for Printed Library Materials, ANSI Z39.48-1984.

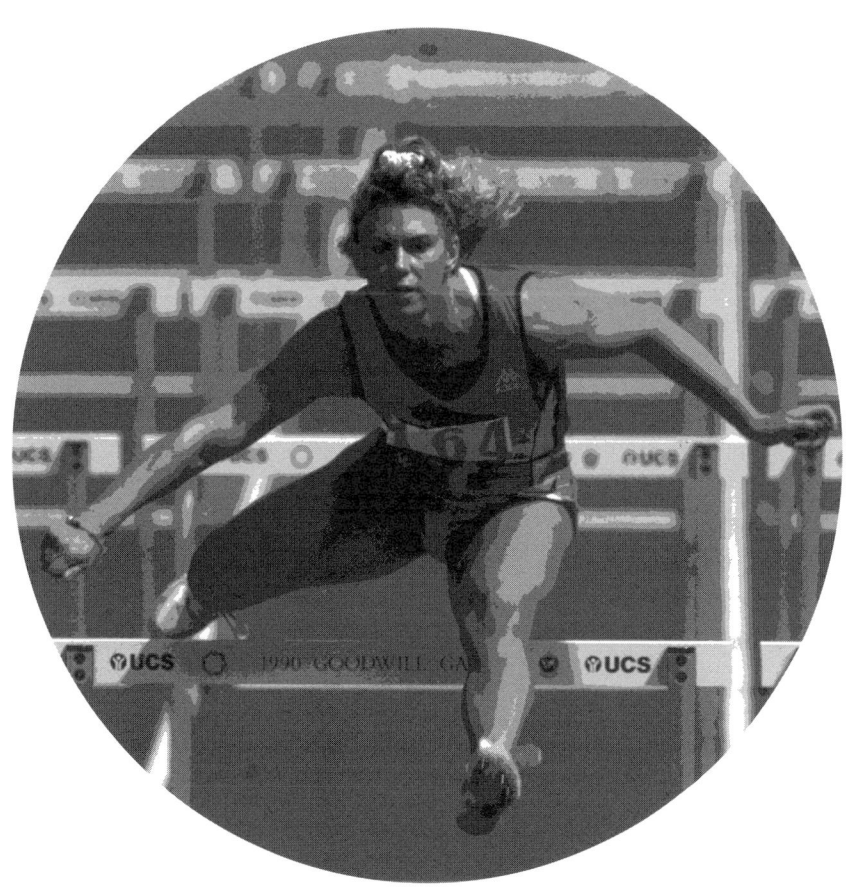

Part One Continued

Sports

Strength Training

MODERN TECHNOLOGY, by making us more sedentary, has taken its toll on all aspects of physical fitness, including muscular strength. Today few people in the affluent industrialized nations work their muscles doing hard manual labor, and even many household and outdoor chores take little effort. The washboard was replaced by the washing machine; the laborious chore of kneading dough can now be done by an electric mixer with a dough hook, or even by an electric breadmaking machine; the manual push mower was replaced by the power mower and then by the riding mower; and the snow shovel has been replaced by the snow blower. With remote controls for stereos, television sets, and video recorders, some people can spend entire weekends rarely leaving the couch. In short, technology has made it easier to be inactive than active. But it is through activity that the body maintains itself, and thus technology is, in a sense, robbing us of one means of self-preservation. As a result of inactivity, muscles that are important for walking, bending, twisting, and lifting heavy objects are unused or underused, and so they start to atrophy (decrease in size) and become weaker. In July 1996, the surgeon general released a landmark report stating that physical inactivity is a major health concern in the United States.

Research involving exercise, and specifically strength training, has shown that regular exercise can prevent atrophy from disuse and help maintain muscle strength. However, there is a problem: in some respects the technology that lets us do things faster and more easily has also made us busier, so that one reason why people do not exercise regularly is a lack of leisure time. Thus a major change is needed in the way Americans think about exercise. Exercise should be thought of not as a leisure acitivity but as a high-priority daily commitment.

Regular exercise should include not only cardiorespiratory activities like running, walking, and swimming but also muscle strengthening. Everyone has muscles, regardless of how active or inactive he or she may be; bodybuilders with bulging, chiseled physiques have no more muscles than anyone else—they simply increase the size of their muscles by doing a lot more training than everyone else. It is a complete misconception to assume that only athletes need strong muscles: the fact is that muscular strength affects almost all daily activities. Strong muscles not only improve performance but also reduce susceptibility to injury; and this helps prevent work-related disabilities, periods of immobility, and acute and chronic pain. A lifelong strength training program is part of a sensible, healthful lifestyle—an important contribution to everyday well-being.

Background

Strength training, as the term implies, increases muscular strength. It includes any type of training program designed to improve the capacity of the muscles to generate force.

Of the various components of physical fitness, muscle strength is perhaps the least appreciated. Almost everyone is aware of the primary function of the muscles: to generate the forces needed for physical activities. But the muscles also have concurrent functions that are less well known. One of these concurrent functions is to make the joints more stable. Muscles increase the integrity (stability) of a joint by holding the bones of the joint together. Typically, muscles and their tendons surround a joint and—along with ligaments and cartilage—make it stronger. A second concurrent function of the muscles is that they serve as the body's shock absorbers. For example, muscles reduce the impact forces encountered during walking, running, and other activities; thus they protect the joints from the repetitive pounding that can cause damage. If everyone of every age kept the muscles strong, millions of dollars in orthopedic care could be saved every year.

Myth—"The decline in strength with age is a consequence of the aging process and thus is inevitable." *Fact*—Inactivity, not aging, is mostly responsible for loss of strength.

Muscle strength is the ability of a muscle or group of muscles to generate force; it is measured in terms of how much weight a person can lift. This is expressed as "repetitions maximum": xRM, where x equals the maximum number of complete lifts a person can perform with a given weight. For example, 1RM is the weight a person can lift only once; 5RM is the weight the person can lift five times but not six. RM can be used to determine what is known as absolute strength. If person A has a 1RM arm curl of 100 pounds (45.5 kg) and person B has a 1RM of 70 pounds (31.8 kg), A has greater absolute strength than B. However, in comparisons among individuals, absolute strength always gives an advantage to larger people. A better way to compare individuals is in terms of relative strength. This involves determining absolute strength and then dividing it by body weight. If person A weighs 200 pounds (91 kg) and B weighs 100 pounds (45.5 kg), even though A is considered absolutely stronger, B is relatively stronger: B lifts 70 percent of body weight; A lifts only 50 percent of body weight.

Myth—"Strength training impairs sports performance because it makes people muscle-bound." In other words, large, bulky muscles are believed to slow down the arms and legs and also to impinge on each other, reducing flexibility. *Fact*—If muscle building is overdone, it can have this effect; but a properly designed and executed strength training program will increase speed and flexibility. It can also improve strength, muscular endurance, and jumping. Many of the world's fastest athletes use strength training to enhance their performance; yet they maintain excellent flexibility.

Whatever one's initial strength, a properly designed and administered training program can increase it. A strength training program must involve resistance exercises—exercises that challenge the muscles to lift or work against loads that are heavier than normal. The most common form of resistance exercise is weight lifting using barbells and dumbbells. However, resistance exercises also can involve lifting other types of heavy objects, lifting one's own body weight, pulling against elastic bands, and pushing or pulling against immovable objects. Strength training programs often use a combination of

Myth—"Muscle turns to fat when resistance training stops." *Fact*—Muscle and fat are two different body tissues, so it is impossible for one to turn into the other. What can happen, however, is that one can be traded for the other. If training is stopped and daily caloric intake is not lowered to compensate for this, the extra calories will be stored as body fat. At the same time, the muscles begin to atrophy because they are not being used to the same extent. The increased fat and decreased muscle give the false impression that muscle is "turning into fat."

Myth—"Strength training is safe and effective only for young, athletic males." *Fact*—If the appropriate guidelines are followed, strength training is safe and effective for nearly everyone. Research has found that such training increased strength significantly for people ranging in age from 6 to 90. In fact, some of the largest increases have been reported in studies of elderly people. It is never too late to start strength training.

different types of resistance exercises to challenge the muscles and make them stronger.

Over weeks, months, or years of resistance training, the muscles respond by becoming larger and stronger. In progressive resistance training, as muscular strength increases, so does the resistance used. Progressive resistance exercise ensures that the muscles continue to be challenged, so that further and further gains will be made. Bodybuilding, Olympic lifting, and power lifting are three sports that depend primarily on progressive resistance training, though their goals are quite different (*see also* WEIGHT LIFTING).

Progressive resistance exercise may have originated as long ago as the sixth century B.C.E.: Milon of Croton is often said to have been its first practitioner. According to legend, Milon had a bull calf which he picked up every day. As the calf grew older and heavier, Milon's muscles became stronger. By the time the calf was mature, this progressive training had enabled Milon to lift the full-grown bull.

"Formal" strength training, however, was virtually nonexistent until the early 1900s, when gymnasiums with weight equipment began to appear in YMCAs. Even then, strength training was mainly limited to a few athletes and "muscle men." "Big muscles" were an oddity, and strength training was not seen as something the general population would participate in. Except for word of mouth among true believers at gymnasiums, relatively little information about it was available. Thus most of the information we now have regarding strength training has been obtained during the past 30 years, as this kind of exercise has become more popular and public awareness has increased. Today the number of men and women who participate in strength training continues to grow. It would be hard to find a health facility that did not have a wide assortment of resistance training equipment, and even many hotels now offer strength training facilities. Despite its popularity, though, there is still a lack of sound information about strength training. Many training techniques and routines remain untested by scientific methodology; they are followed simply because they have stood the test of time. Each generation tends to assume that because a recommended training program is still in use, it must work. Much reliable advice is offered, of course; unfortunately, many myths also continue to be perpetuated.

Principles of Strength Training

Strength training programs should be designed with certain basic principles in mind: these are discussed here as principles 1 through 5. The actual number of principles may vary from source to source, but the same essential concepts are always included.

Principle 1: Stress (Overload)

The first principle is that to increase strength—to bring about muscular change or adaptation—training must overload, or "stress," the muscles beyond what they normally encounter. This can be accomplished by altering three factors associated with training: (1) frequency, (2) intensity, and (3) duration. *Frequency* refers to how often a muscle is trained; this is expressed as frequency per week. *Intensity* refers to the difficulty of a workout: how much resistance (weight) is lifted during the workout. *Duration* refers to both the amount of time spent actually lifting a weight and the length of a workout. Stress on a muscle can be increased by increasing one or any combination of these factors.

Frequency. Frequency is limited by the need for adequate rest between workouts, to enable the body to recover before the next training session. Generally, a rest of 48 hours between workouts is recommended. This would allow three training sessions per week, and research shows that three sessions can significantly increase muscle strength, especially in untrained individuals. Interestingly, highly trained athletes should train the same muscle group only two times per week; this is because their training is more intense and thus requires a longer recovery time—approximately 72 hours between workouts.

Intensity. Intensity is based primarily on the resistance or weight being lifted, generally quantified either as xRM or as a percentage of individual maximal strength. Research has shown that strength training at a weight load of 5RM to 10RM (which is comparable to 80 percent to 90 percent of maximal strength) will increase strength substantially. In other words, this involves using a weight which the individual can lift a maximum of 5 to 10 times.

Duration. The length of time spent working a muscle group depends on the number of repetitions and sets being performed. A set is a series of repetitions performed with no rest in between. The more sets performed, the greater the duration of the load on the muscle. Research has shown that consistent, significant increases in strength are achieved by performing three to five sets with weight loads at 5RM to 10RM.

Research has not established a single "ideal" length for a workout. How much time should be spent depends on how many muscle groups are being trained, how many repetitions and sets are being performed, and how much rest is taken between sets. For average people, a workout may last 45 minutes; for trained athletes, it may last 90 minutes. Rest time between sets is a particularly important factor in the length of a workout. Rest time should be long enough to produce a feeling of recovery; most people feel ready for another set in about 3 to 5 minutes, but some may wait a bit longer.

Principle 2: Progression

The second principle is that in order for gains from strength training to progess steadily, the frequency, intensity, or duration of stress—or any combination of these—must be increased. In other words, once the muscles adapt to a training load, that load must be increased; otherwise, no further gains will be made—the muscles will only maintain their current strength. This second principle is reflected in the term *progressive resistance training*.

Principle 3: Specificity

According to the third principle, strength training must involve resistance exercises that specifically work the muscles in which gains are sought. If, say, the goal is stronger biceps, the training should include exercises that force the biceps muscle to contract against resistance, such as biceps curls. An important aspect of this third principle is that the more an exercise movement is like an actual movement in a given activity or sport, the greater the improvement in performance will be. This is known as biomechanical specificity (*see Figure 1*).

Principle 4: Individuality

The fourth principle is that strength training should be tailored to fit each person's needs, taking into account the individual's initial fitness level, strengths, weaknesses, and limitations. This fourth principle implies that it would be unrealistic, for instance, to offer the same program to a football lineman and to a paraplegic who uses a wheelchair. The best programs are those that are designed specifically for the individual.

Principle 5: Reversibility

The fifth principle is based on the fact that when strength training stops, any gains made up to that point will begin to disappear: declines can occur in as short a time as 2 weeks. How much strength is lost depends on the length of the layoff. In other words, gains in strength are reversible. Therefore, to maintain strength, muscles

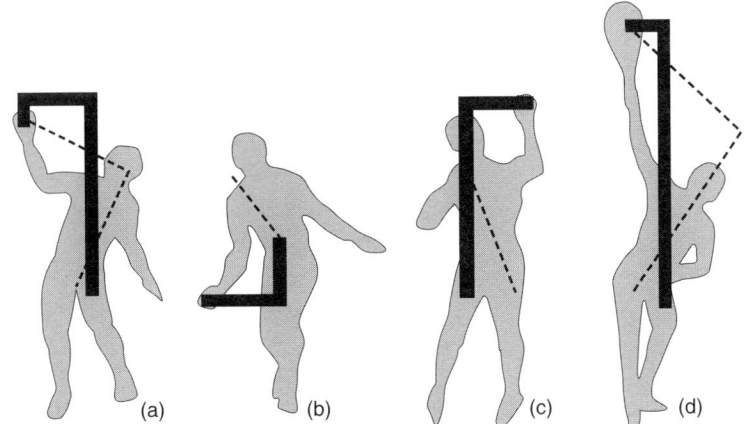

Figure 1. *Biomechanical specificity is a principle of strength training. Because not all throwing is the same, not all strength programs should be the same. Shown here is the length of the movement arm in four patterns of joint action: (a) football pass, (b) underarm throw, (c) shot put, (d) tennis serve; the dotted line indicates angular rotation about the hips, and the solid line indicates angular rotation about the spine. An individual strength training program should simulate the range of motion in these different sports.*

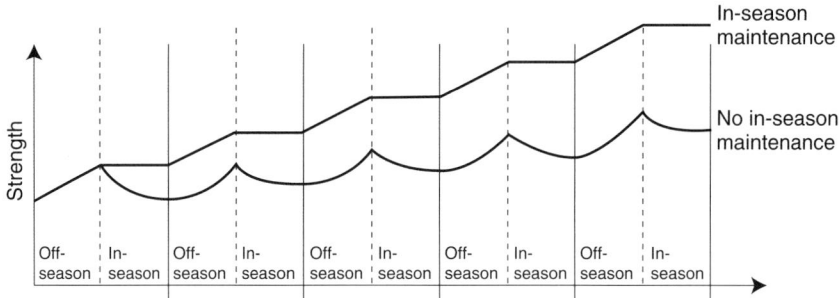

Figure 2. *Difference in strength with both off-season and in-season training (upper curve) as opposed to only off-season training (lower curve). When there is only an off-season program, much of it accomplishes no more than to match the gains of the previous off-season.*

must continue to be stressed at the level to which they have become accustomed. That is, resistance training should never be stopped; like many other forms of physical activity, it should be lifelong. This does not mean that training for improvement—progressive training—must be lifelong; but it does mean that even if the reason for or focus of training has changed, resistance exercises should continue.

When a satisfactory level of strength has been achieved through progressive resistance training, the program can be changed from progressive exercise to maintenance exercise. Actually, the only differences between the two are how often training takes place (frequency) and how long each session lasts (duration). Provided that the weight load (intensity) is unchanged, a maintenance program can involve shorter and less frequent sessions. For example, sessions might last 30 minutes instead of 45 to 60 minutes, and may take place twice a week instead of three times a week. In fact, there is evidence to suggest that even one training session per week is enough to maintain strength.

Maintaining muscle strength is especially important for athletes during the competitive season; thus most strength and conditioning coaches now stress in-season strength training as the only way for athletes to maintain strength gains from their off-season and preseason training. Furthermore, in-season training lets athletes start the next off-season with a higher level of strength than they had the previous year; in other words, they develop strength throughout their careers (*see Figure 2*).

It is worth repeating that for everyone, not only athletes, maintenance should be lifelong. Maintenance can greatly slow, if not stop, much of the loss of strength that would ordinarily occur between ages 30 and 80. With training and subsequent maintenance, older adults who have already lost strength can regain some of it, even if they have never trained before.

Guidelines for Training

In addition to the five basic principles discussed above, it is important to keep in mind some guidelines for making training safer and more effective.

Breathing

During resistance training, time spent "holding the breath" should be minimized. Holding the breath—this is known as the "Valsalva maneuver"—causes dangerous fluctuations in blood pressure: a rapid increase in blood pressure is quickly followed by a rapid decrease. Holding the breath too long can actually lead to "weight lifter's blackout," which occurs because the heart is not able to get enough blood to the brain. A useful rule is to "exhale with effort." The Valsalva maneuver should be maintained just long enough to get a weight moving. Then, one should breathe out as the weight (or resistance) is lifted and breathe in as it is returned to the starting position.

Lifting Speed

In strength training, there is no universally accepted speed of movement. As a general rule, though, the lifting phase of a repetition should be faster than the lowering phase. For example, some trainers suggest that if it takes 2 seconds to lift a weight, the weight should be lowered back to the starting position in about 4 seconds. The most important point with regard to speed is that lifting speed should be controlled at all times: there should be no bouncing and no momentum. Bouncing a weight, in particular, does nothing to improve strength, and it can lead to serious injury.

Recovery Time

Recovery time is an important consideration in strength training. When muscle cells repeatedly contract against a load, they eventually become fatigued, and fatigued muscle cells cannot contract as fast or generate as much force as they could when they were rested. However, muscle fatigue is a temporary phenomenon: when a muscle is allowed to rest after the onset of fatigue, it can recover its ability to contract forcefully. The time needed for recovery depends on the duration and intensity of the exercise that caused the fatigue—the more intense and repetitious the exercise, the longer the recovery time. The concept of recovery time in strength training can apply to three different situations: (1) rest between sets of repetitions, (2) rest between different exercises, and (3) rest between workouts. Research has not established an ideal rest interval between sets or exercises, though in general an adequate recovery time is 3 to 5 minutes. A reasonable guideline is to allow enough recovery time so that you can resume the exercise with confidence, control, and good form.

Recovery time between workouts is another matter. Research has shown that a muscle group should be allowed at least 48 hours of rest before being trained again. Many people believe that experienced weight lifters and bodybuilders must train every day. This may be true in a sense; but what actually happens is that weight lifters and bodybuilders train different body parts on different days, to allow for adequate recovery of individual muscles and muscle groups. For example, a power lifter may train the legs on one day, the chest and triceps on the next day, and the back and biceps on the third day; then the cycle is begun again. As a result, there is a rest period of about 72 hours before any given workout is repeated.

Balanced Workouts

For the musculoskeletal system to work, muscle groups must oppose one another. When one muscle (agonist) causes a particular movement, the opposing group (antagonist) pulls the limb back to the starting position. In designing a strength training program, opposing muscle groups should be trained equally. It is important to avoid training only those muscles that are important to a particular sport or activity. Training opposing muscles helps prevent strength imbalances that can lead to injury.

Full Range of Motion

When performed correctly, strength training can improve flexibility. The key is to use good form and move the resistance through the full range of motion. As a muscle is contracted against resistance, it undergoes some internal stretching—like a rubber band. To get a feel for the dynamics of muscle stretching, tie a weight to one end of a rubber band, and then begin to lift the weight by holding the other end of the band: the band will stretch (lengthen) before resistance is overcome and the weight begins to rise. The heavier the weight, the greater the elastic stretch before it begins to rise.

There is a similar phenomenon when muscles contract against resistance. As a muscle begins to develop force against resistance, its elastic components (connective tissues surrounding the muscle and muscle proteins themselves) are stretched. The heavier the weight, the greater the initial stretch. This is one reason why certain athletes with great muscular strength also have great flexibility. Olympic weight lifters are one example; for some muscles, their flexibility is second only to that of gymnasts.

All too often, though, average people fail to move a resistance through the full range of motion, either because the resistance is too great or because they do not know how to perform the exercise properly. Training through the full range of motion not only ensures adequate stretching of the elastic components of the muscle but also increases strength throughout the range of movement.

Keeping Records

Keeping records of training resistances, sets, repetitions, and exercises is a good way to save time and provide an incentive. Often, people find it difficult to keep their own progress in focus. Written records document gains in strength and thus contribute to motivation.

Aids for Strength Training

Many magazines devoted to bodybuilding and weight lifting give the misleading impression that strength training requires belts, wraps, and straps. While such equipment may be useful for competitive

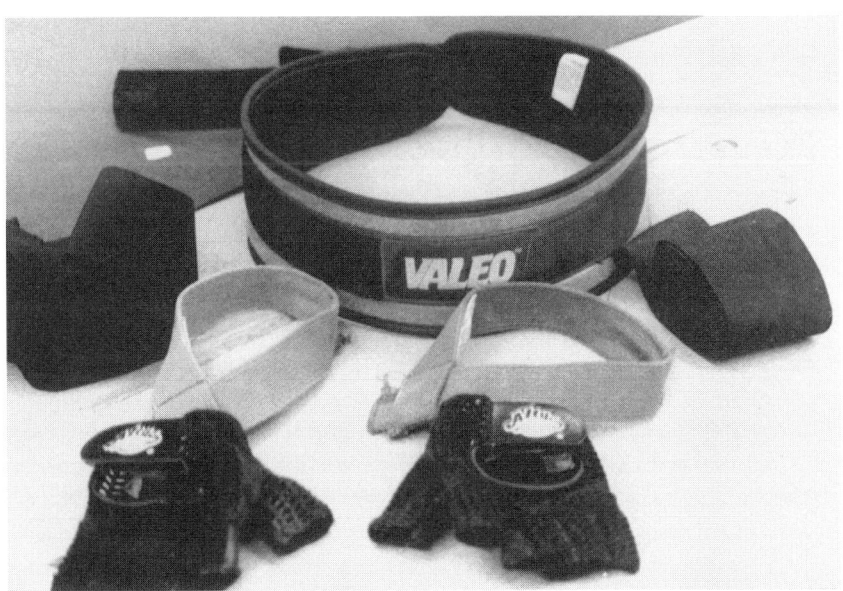

Figure 3. *Strength training aids are not prerequisites for a safe, successful program*

training, it is not necessary for general fitness (*see Figure 3*). In fact, training without belts, wraps, and straps can be more beneficial than training with them.

Knee and elbow wraps, for instance, lend support to the joint and remove some of the stresses that might otherwise be encountered by the connective tissue surrounding it (*see also KNEE*). As a result, the strength of the connective tissue does not develop to the same extent as the muscles. For most people, then, it is best not to wear wraps.

Straps are used to help the forearm muscles maintain a grip on bars, dumbbells, or weight machines. While they are certainly effective, they prevent the forearm muscles from getting stronger. Functionally, this is a problem: it does little good to increase the strength of the larger upper-extremity muscles if the strength of the forearm muscles—the grip—does not keep up with it. In other words, unless straps are worn all the time, the strength of the forearm muscles will be a limiting factor.

The weight-lifting belt is another piece of equipment that has become almost synonymous with strength training. Research has shown that weight-lifting belts can decrease stress on the lower back; they do this by assisting the muscles of the abdominal area. During lifting, the abdominal muscles (obliques and rectus abdominus) contract, increasing pressure within the abdominal cavity. This increased intra-abdominal pressure helps make the torso rigid and redistributes some of the load away from the spinal column. The abdominal muscles give the muscles of the extremities a rigid torso against which to contract, thus enabling the extremity muscles to generate even more force. The belt gives support to the abdominal muscles and keeps them from bulging out, so that the intra-abdominal pressure is not lost under a heavy load (*see Figure 4*). For example, if the abdominal muscles bulge out because they are not strong enough to maintain a squeeze, then the intra-abdominal pressure decreases and the torso loses some of its rigidity; this results in a drop-off of strength.

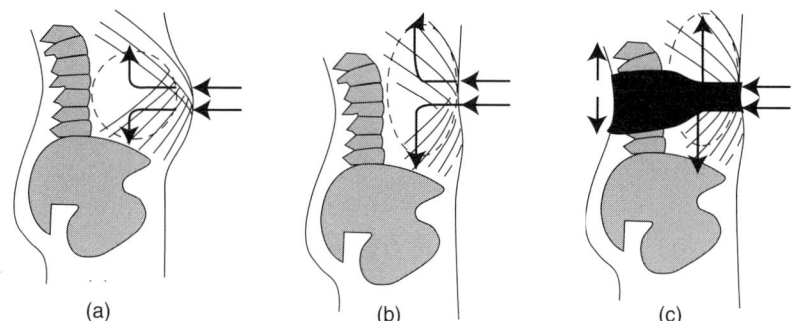

Figure 4. *Abdominal muscles, which are the main "unloaders" of the lower back during lifting, increase abdominal pressure upon contraction (a and b). The abdominal belt (c) assists the abdominal muscles; but it should be used only for lifting near-maximum weights, so that the abdominal muscles can keep up in strength with gains at the extremities.*

However, like most other training aids, weight belts can become a crutch. Because a belt reduces stress on the abdominal muscles, the strength of these muscles fails to "keep up" with gains made by the extremities. Therefore, it is a good idea to avoid becoming dependent on a weight belt. Instead, the abdominal muscles should be strengthened, and the belt should be used only for lifting near-maximal weights.

By contrast, weight-lifting gloves are highly recommended, particularly for lifting barbells and dumbbells. Gloves help maintain a good grip on the equipment and protect hands from the knurling on the handles, thus preventing calluses. Gloves are relatively inexpensive and can be bought at any store that carries sporting goods.

Types of Strengthening Exercises

There are two major categories of strengthening exercises: static and dynamic. In static exercises—more commonly known as isometric exercises—the muscles push or pull against an immovable object, as in pushing against a wall. Although the muscles are generating considerable force, there is no movement of the limbs or trunk. Dynamic exercises, by contrast, allow for movement; that is, when the muscles being worked develop force, the result is movement of the trunk, arms, or legs. Dynamic exercises are the exercises most people associate with strength training, such as working out on machines and lifting dumbbells.

Static Exercises: Isometrics

The advantage of static, or isometric, exercises is that they do not require special (and often expensive) equipment. A wall, a doorjamb, a heavy table—these can all be used to perform isometrics. Also, since no special equipment is needed, isometric exercises require little space and can be performed almost anywhere.

On the other hand, isometrics have several disadvantages. First, any gain in strength is specific to the body position used in training. Second, gains in isometric strength do not carry over to dynamic strength. Third, since most sports and most daily activities are dynamic in nature, relying solely on isometric strength training is a questionable practice. Fourth, isometric strength training is not suitable for everyone: it raises blood pressure, and this is a serious potential problem for anyone with, or at risk of, cardiovascular (heart and circulatory) disease. Fifth, the psychological factor can be a problem: daily isometric training can become very tedious, because isometrics do not provide feedback about resistance or about gains in strength.

Dynamic Exercises

Dynamic exercises, as mentioned earlier, involve movement. They include not only the exercises normally associated with strength training, but also some types that are less familiar.

Isotonic exercise. Isotonic exercise, also called dynamic constant-resistance exercise, is the type most often associated with strength training (*see Figure 5*). It involves lifting dumbbells and barbells which provide a fixed amount of resistance—hence the term *isotonic* (from the Greek *iso*, "same," and *tonos*, "tension"). This term, however, has

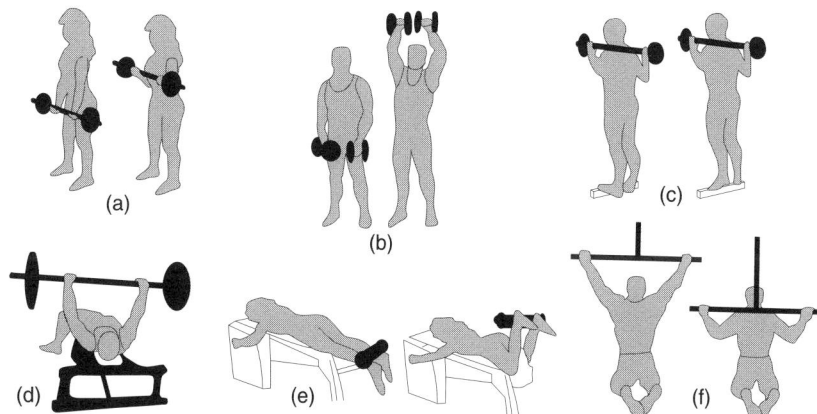

Figure 5. *There are hundreds of dynamic resistance exercises, so an appropriate combination should be chosen with the guidance of a strength training coach. A few examples of standard exercises are shown: (a) bicep curls, (b) lateral shoulder raise, (c) standing heel raise, (d) bench press, (e) hamstring curls, (f) latissimus pulldown. (For the half squat, or parallel squat, see the essay "Squats: Worthwhile or Too Dangerous?") Advantages: (1) Cost. Equipment is relatively inexpensive; (2) Size. Most free weight equipment (dumbbells, barbells, weight plates, etc.) do not take up much space; (3) Loading and lifting approximate daily activities. Disadvantages: (1) Safety. A lifting partner or spotter is usually necessary, particularly with exercises involving lifts from under the bar; (2) Setup time. Changing exercises involves unloading and loading weights; (3) Limitations. Weight lifted is limited by the weakest point in the range of motion.*

caused some confusion, particularly among muscle physiologists. It suggests, misleadingly, that the tension or forces being produced by the muscle do not change. In fact, as a joint is moved through its range of motion, the force produced by the muscle does change, because the positions of the bony levers change. For this reason, the term *dynamic constant-resistance exercise* is now widely used instead. In this more accurate term, *dynamic* indicates movement, and *constant resistance* indicates that the weight of the object being lifted does not change.

The major advantage of isotonic exercise is that sports and activities of daily living require isotonic movements. As the principle of specificity (*see above*) indicates, the more closely training mimics an actual sport or activity, the greater its potential for improving performance.

The major disadvantage is that the weight lifted is limited by the weakest point in the range of motion. In other words, a muscle is stressed most at the weakest point in the range of motion—the point where leverage is poorest—and is less stressed at the other points in the range. For example, in the bench press exercise the weakest point in the range of motion is usually the "middle": the point at which the barbell is 6 to 10 inches (15–25 cm) above the chest. The muscles are stressed maximally through this 6- to 10-inch range of motion, and only to a lesser extent at the beginning and end of the chest press. Ideally, however, a muscle should be stressed maximally throughout its range of motion, not just at its weakest point.

Variable-resistance exercise. Variable-resistance exercise is a popular type of dynamic exercise. This type of training requires machines, many of which are provided by health clubs. The exercise machines use lever systems or offset cams to change the resistance as a person moves through a range of motion while performing an exercise. Variable-resistance machines were designed to better accommodate the changes in force produced as a joint is moved through its range of motion. In other words, unlike dynamic constant-resistance exercise, variable-resistance exercise is designed to stress a muscle throughout its range of motion rather than just at the weakest point (*see Figure 6*).

Training using variable-resistance exercise machines is time-efficient: because each machine is designed to work specific muscle groups, setup time is mininized. A major disadvantage is that the machines tend to be prohibitively expensive.

Isokinetic exercise. The term *isokinetic* is from the Greek *iso* ("same") and *kinesis* ("motion"). Isokinetic exercise involves training on computerized equipment, which not only changes the resistance encountered but also controls the speed of the exercise movement (*see Figure 7*). It is not commonly used for strength training; its primary use is in clinical tests and for rehabilitation.

The advantage of isokinetic exercise over other forms of strength

Figure 6. *Variable-resistance exercise machines, common in health clubs, offer relatively easy, safe, and timesaving strength training. Advantages: (1) With the machines, a lifting partner or spotter is unnecessary. (2) Exercises require little skill or balance, since the weights merely move up and down on guide rods. (3) The machines allow specific muscle groups to be worked. (4) There is no need to load and unload barbell weights. (5) Variable resistance is designed to stress muscles more effectively through the range of motion. Disadvantages: (1) The machines are expensive. (2) The machines tend to be large and bulky. (3) Joint and limb movements are restricted to those allowed by the machine and thus do not mimic everyday or sports-related movements. (Photo: Comstock, Inc,)*

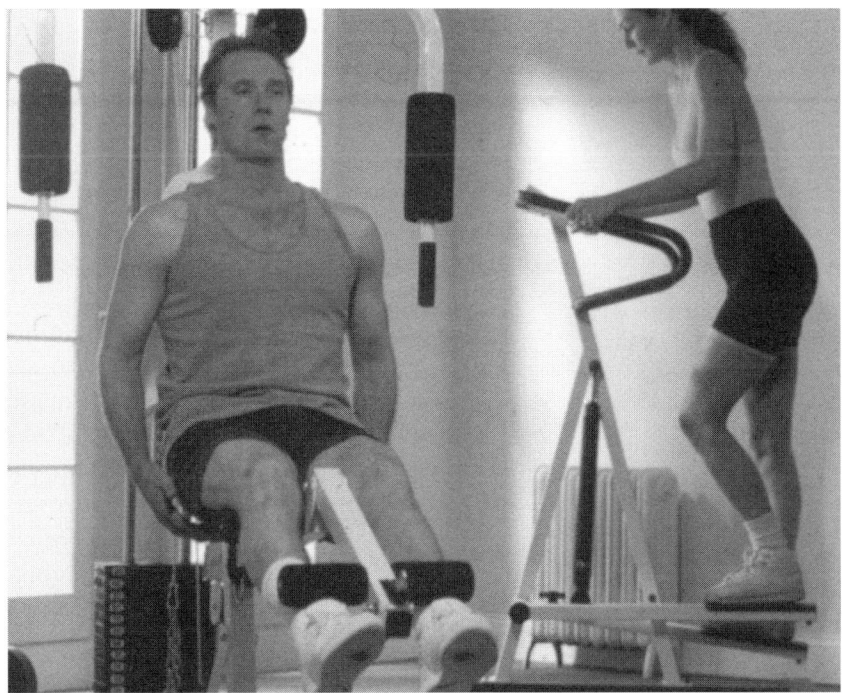

training is that the muscles are worked maximally throughout the range of motion. However, isokinetic machines are not a real option for most people: they are enormously expensive, and a technician is needed to run them.

Figure 7. *Isokinetic exercise. Advantages: (1) The machine provides resistance which precisely matches muscle force, thereby giving maximal resistance throughout the range of motion. (2) These machines can be set up to isolate particular muscle groups—this is very useful in rehabilitation and clinical strength testing. Disadvantages: (1) The machines are very expensive. (2) Setup time for different exercises is lengthy. (3) Technicians are usually required to run the machines. (4) Strength gains are limited to the speeds used when training.*

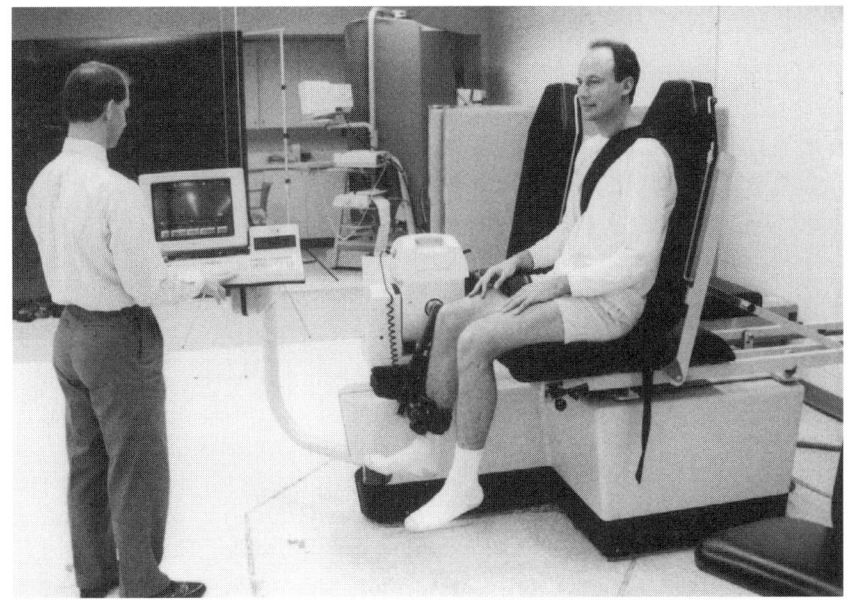

Physiological Adaptations

Obviously, muscle strength increases with strength training. But why? At a "macro" level, strength training stresses muscles beyond normal use, and the muscles change in order to meet this challenge. At the "micro" level, since the muscles must generate more force, they respond by making more contractile proteins—the proteins inside the muscle cells that are directly responsible for these cells' capacity to generate force. By producing more contractile proteins, each muscle cell becomes stronger, in turn strengthening the entire muscle. As more contractile proteins are made by the muscle cells, the cells themselves get bigger around, and eventually the entire muscle becomes larger. This enlargement of muscles from strength training is known as muscle hypertrophy. Extreme muscle hypertrophy is seen, of course, in professional bodybuilders and other strength athletes.

In addition to the enlargement of muscle cells, another factor contributing to muscle hypertrophy is hyperplasia—production of new muscle cells. Research involving animals has shown that weight lifting can cause the number of muscle cells to increase; and as the number of muscle cells increases, the muscles can become larger and stronger. However, the extent to which humans add new muscle cells is unclear. Thus although hyperplasia contributes to muscle hypertrophy, physiologists believe that the primary factor in hypertrophy is enlargement of existing muscle cells.

Physiology and Fitness

Strength training not only increases the size and strength of muscles but also contributes to other components of fitness: muscular endurance, muscular power, body composition, and flexibility, or full range of motion (*for range of motion, see earlier discussion*).

Absolute muscular endurance—the ability of a muscle or group of muscles to lift a given weight repeatedly—improves with strength training. For example, before beginning strength training, a person might be able to perform 8 biceps curls with 30 kilograms (66 lb.); after training, the same person may be able to do 20 biceps curls—more than twice as many repetitions—with the same weight.

Muscular power, like muscular endurance, is a vital factor in performance in sports. "Power" is not the same thing as mucular strength, although muscle strength is the basis of muscle power—and it is power, not strength, that ultimately affects performance. Power involves not only the muscle's ability to generate force, but also the rate at which force is generated; thus power is sometimes referred to as speed-strength. Shot putters are a good example of muscular power: to throw a 7.2-kilogram shot (16 lb.; this is the weight for men) 18 meters (60 ft.) or more, a shot putter must generate a tremendous amount of force in a very short time. Strength training improves power; and when strength training is combined with movement drills specific to a given sport, there is a dramatic improvement in power specific to that sport (*see also* MOTOR CONTROL).

Strength Training for Children: A Taboo?

Four common misconceptions about strength training for children are (1) that it is not effective, (2) that it impairs motor development, (3) that it damages muscle and bone, and (4) that it stunts growth. None of these notions is supported by research. A few studies do indicate that strength training before and during early puberty does not produce muscle hypertrophy, but such training is still a good way to prevent injuries.

A strength training program for children differs from a program for adults or adolescents in emphasis, intensity, and duration. Here are some guidelines:

- Strength training should be only a small component of a child's sports and fitness activities.

- Calisthenics are an effective way to begin building muscle strength and endurance.

- Resistance training technique should be developed under the supervision of an experienced coach.

- Warm-up exercises should be done before training and flexibility exercises after training.

- Children should avoid lifting heavy loads; a weight should be light enough for the child to lift 10 to 15 times.

- Absolutely no maximum lifts.

Weight Loss and Strength Training

A sedentary person on a weight-loss diet will experience a decrease in not only in fat but also in muscle mass. Strength training decreases this loss of muscle mass, ensuring a healthier ratio of muscle to fat. Strength training also helps a dieter maintain a higher energy level and metabolic rate, contributing to overall well-being and thus to further weight loss.

Strength training also improves body composition by increasing muscle mass and decreasing body fat (*see also* BODY COMPOSITION). The body must expend more energy (calories) to maintain muscle tissue than to maintain fat cells; therefore, when muscle mass is increased through strength training, the metabolic rate also increases. A higher rate of metabolism not only results in a loss of body fat but also helps in controlling and maintaining body weight once a desired weight is achieved (*see also* ENERGY AND METABOLISM). There is a second reason why strength training should be part of any weight-loss plan: dieting alone results in a decrease of muscle mass as well as fat. Resistance training decreases the loss of muscle mass during dieting, so that the ratio of muscle to fat is healthier. It is common knowledge that aerobic exercise (such as walking, running, or swimming) helps people lose weight; but the role of resistance exercise is not as well known. In addition to the effects just noted, strength training helps a dieter maintain a higher energy level and thus contributes not only to a higher rate of metabolism but to overall well-being.

Physiology and Prevention of Injuries

Muscle strength can decrease the risk of injury both directly and indirectly. One direct effect is on the muscles surrounding joints. The joints are crisscrossed by muscles and muscle tendons that enable us to move and also give the joints structural integrity. A joint surrounded by strong muscles and the tendons of strong muscles is less easily disrupted—and thus less vulnerable to injury—than a joint surrounded by weaker muscles.

A less direct effect of strength training has to do with the connective tissues associated with muscle. Connective tissue (as the term implies) connects, anchors, and supports body structures; it also forms the tendons connecting muscle and bone. Connective tissue

Squats: Worthwhile or Too Dangerous?

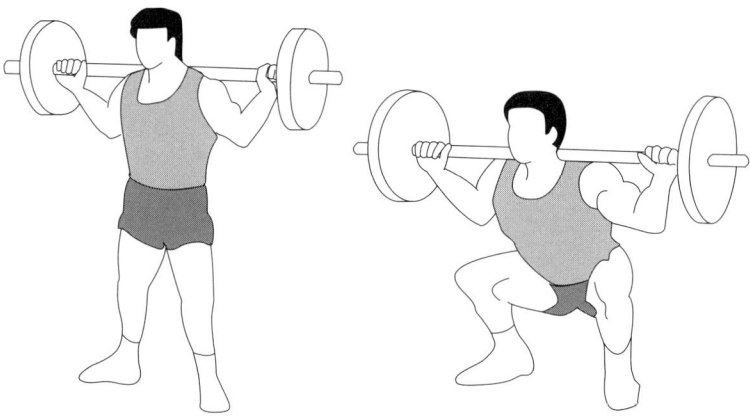

A properly executed half squat.

No muscle strengthening exercise has been more controversial than the knee bend, also known as the squat or full squat. The full squat involves going from a standing position to a squatting position in which the buttocks touch the heels, and then returning to the standing position.

The full squat was introduced as a strengthening exercise in the early 1920s by a German immigrant to the United States, Heinrich Steinborn. Steinborn's physique and his feats of leg strength drew tremendous attention, and soon articles on the benefits of squatting began appearing in weight training magazines such as *The Strong Man*, *Strength*, *Strength and Health*, and *The Iron Man*. By the late 1950s, the full squat was considered a mainstay of any serious strength training program.

In 1961 and 1962, however, Karl Klein published a series of studies in which he claimed that the full squat is injurious to the knee joint; he argued that the full squat causes the ligaments to become permanently stretched, making the knee joint loose and unstable, and suggested that only half squats should be used. A half squat stops at the point where the thighs are parallel to the floor; thus it is also called a parallel squat.

Klein set off a debate that was still going on in the 1990s. In the heat of the controversy, many people lost sight of the fact that Klein had not proposed eliminating squats as a strength exercise—he had simply recommended using half squats instead of full squats. Some people who were opposed to squats used Klein's argument to de-emphasize squats in general and perpetuated misconceptions about squats.

One misconception—still widely held—is that any type of squatting is bad for the knees. Research has suggested otherwise. One study compared laxity in the knee joints in leading power lifters, Olympic lifters, physical education students, and a control group of people who had never before performed squats. (In this study, the athletes did both full and half squats; the control group did only half squats.) These researchers found that the squat did not appear to cause instability. In fact, many of the elite athletes had "tighter" knees than the control group—the subjects who had never before performed squats at all. The conclusion is that squats do not appear to stretch the ligaments of the knee joint permanently and thus do not make the joint unstable.

The National Strength and Conditioning Association currently recommends the half squat. To date, there is no evidence that joint laxity results from performing half squats. Moreover, half squats performed with good technique effectively increase lower body strength, and the gains are comparable to those achieved with full squats. In fact, so many muscles are involved in performing a parallel squat that it has been called the "king of exercises." The parallel squat has become a key component of almost all strength training programs.

cells produce collagen, a fibrous protein that gives this tissue its tensile strength and helps it hold together the hundreds of thousands of cells that make up muscle. These connective tissues, like the muscle cells themselves, can become thicker and stronger when stimulated by strength training. Further, as muscle strength increases, so does the connective tissue. The resulting thicker, stronger connective tissue prevents muscles from tearing or ripping as training loads increase (*see also* REHABILITATION).

Strength training also contributes indirectly to the prevention of injury in another way—by increasing the strength of bones. All too often, bone is thought of as lifeless, because that is how it is presented in anatomy or physiology laboratories: a skeleton hangs in a closet, white, dry, and dead. It is important to realize that the bones of a living animal consist of living cells—just like any other bodily tissues. And like the cells of muscles and connective tissue, bone cells also respond to strength training. The increased loading during strength training stimulates certain bone cells, the osteocytes, to make denser, stronger bone. This is particularly important for anyone who has or is at risk of osteoporosis, a condition characterized by porous, brittle bones (*see also* SKELETAL SYSTEM).

In Conclusion

Finally, and arguably most importantly, strength training can improve the quality of life. Although research is inconclusive regarding the ability of strength training to lengthen life, this training certainly improves our lifelong options. Too often, older people must give up activities they once enjoyed because these activities have become too strenuous to be rewarding. By maintaining or building strength throughout life, we can continue to participate in activities we enjoy, and this in turn contributes mightily to our overall well-being.

Alan E. Mikesky

References

Baechle, T. (ed.) *Essentials of Strength Training and Conditioning*. Champaign, Illinois: Human Kinetics, 1994.

Flech, S., and W. Kraemer. *Designing Resistance Training Programs*. Champaign, Illinois: Human Kinetics, 1987.

Sale, D. "Strength Training in Children." In C. Gisolfi and D. Lamb (eds.), *Perspectives in Exercise Science and Sports Medicine*. Vol. 2, *Youth, Exercise, and Sports*. Indianapolis, Indiana: Benchmark, 1989.

Westcott, W. *Strength Fitness*. 4th ed. Dubuque, Iowa: Brown, 1995.

Swimming

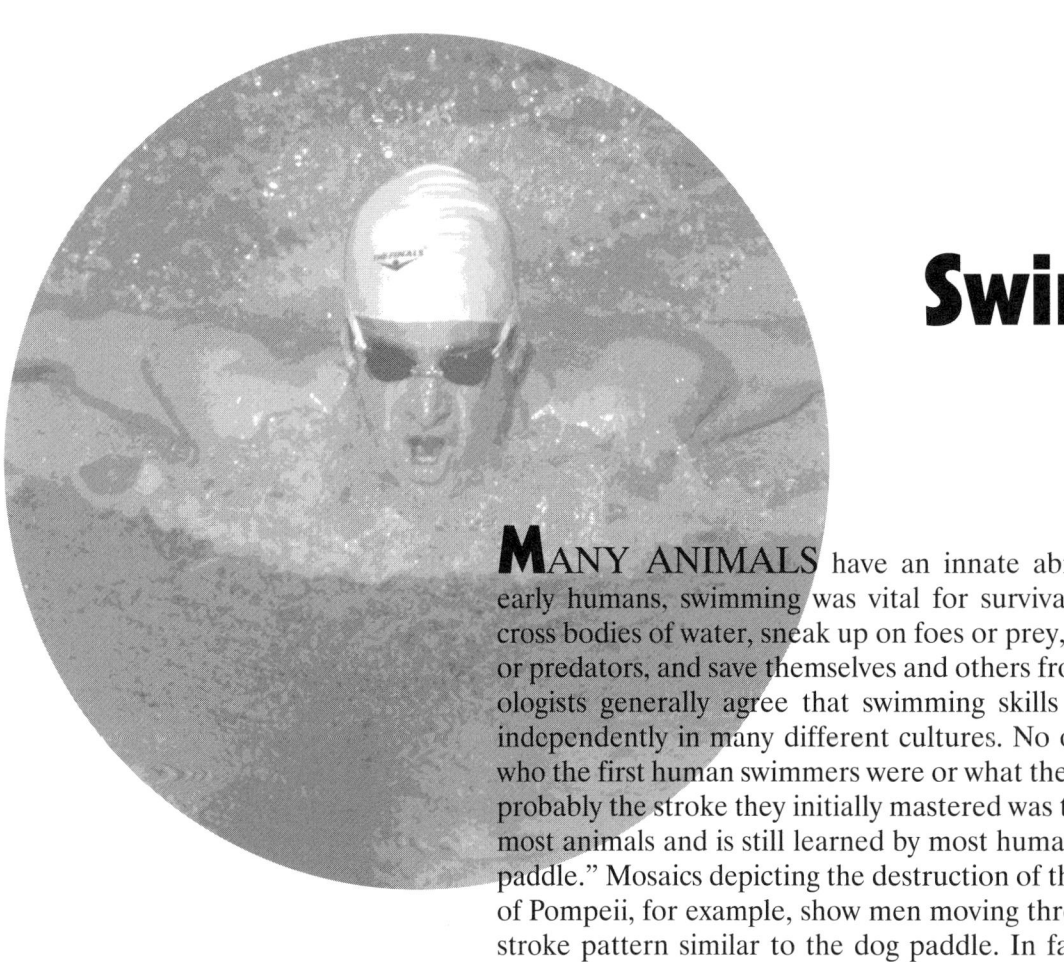

MANY ANIMALS have an innate ability to swim, but for early humans, swimming was vital for survival: it allowed them to cross bodies of water, sneak up on foes or prey, escape from enemies or predators, and save themselves and others from drowning. Archaeologists generally agree that swimming skills developed early and independently in many different cultures. No one knows, of course, who the first human swimmers were or what their first stroke was, but probably the stroke they initially mastered was the one that is used by most animals and is still learned by most human beginners: the "dog paddle." Mosaics depicting the destruction of the ancient Roman city of Pompeii, for example, show men moving through water by using a stroke pattern similar to the dog paddle. In fact, the Romans were great proponents of swimming. Julius Caesar prided himself on his ability to swim and often challenged others to follow. Legend has it that whenever a river obstructed the advance of Caesar's army, he himself was the first one in and the first one out at the other end, all the time urging his men on. Since these early days, swimming has always remained a major sport.

Science and Swimming Records

Over the past few decades, swimmers have shown an amazing ability to break records—even more so than runners. Olympic record times have declined at a faster rate for swimming than for any other clocked sport. It is interesting to compare world record times set by 100-meter (110-yd.) swimmers and 400-meter (440-yd.) sprinters (*see Figure 1*). From 1960 to 1996, male sprinters reduced their Olympic record times by 1.41 seconds, while male swimmers reduced their Olympic record times by 6.46 seconds.

One case in point is the gold medal performance by the Australian John Devitt in the 100-meter freestyle in 1960: 55.2 seconds. This is 6.46 seconds slower than the men's time achieved by Alexandre Popov (Russia) at the 1996 Summer Olympics in Atlanta—and slower than times for the women's 100-meter freestyle in 1988, 1992, and 1996. Nothing this dramatic has been seen in sprinting records. For instance, in 1996 the women's 400-meter time, 48.25 seconds (by Marie-Jose

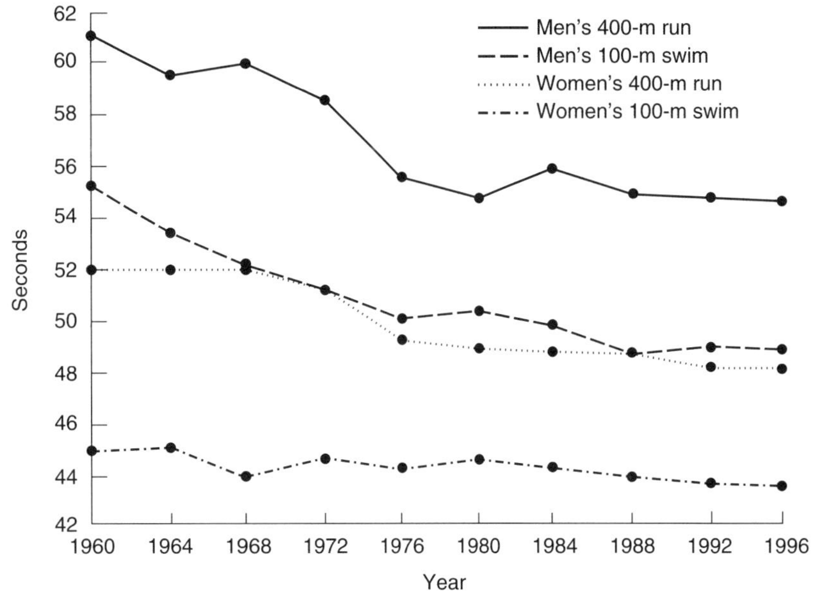

Figure 1. *The rate at which Olympic records have fallen over the last three decades is much greater for swimming than for running. Times for the men's 400-meter sprint dropped by 1.7 seconds between 1960 and 1992; times for the 100-meter swim dropped four times that much—by 6.6 seconds. One factor is a better understanding of the physics of fluids—how to maximize propulsion and minimize resistance.*

Perec, France), was still far behind the men's time achieved in 1960, 44.9 seconds (by Otis Davis, United States).

Another example is Mark Spitz, who won seven gold medals at the 1972 Munich Olympics. This was one of the greatest accomplishments of all time in any sport, and it brought him fame and a following that still endured 20 years later, when he tried for a comeback at the 1992 Olympics. The attempt was ill-fated: in preparation for the Olympic trials, Spitz opposed Matt Biondi, the 1988 Olympic gold medalist, in a 100-meter freestyle race and was soundly defeated. This came as no surprise to the experts, and not only because Spitz was by then 20 years older and had to face the enormous task of getting into top shape again. Another important factor was that there had been revolutionary advances in swimming technique over those

FREESTYLE WORLD RECORDS

Men:

50 m: 21.81—Tom Jager (United States), Nashville, March 1990
100 m: 48.21—Aleksandr Popov (Russia), Monte Carlo, 18 June 1994
200 m: 1:46.69—Giorgio Lamberti (Italy), Bonn, Germany, 15 August 1989
400 m: 3:43.80—Kieren Perkins (Australia), Rome, 9 September 1994
800 m: 7:46.00—Kieren Perkins (Australia), Victoria, Canada, 24 August 1994
1,500 m: 14:41.66—Kieren Perkins (Australia), Victoria, Canada, 24 August 1994

Women:

50 m: 24.51—Le Jingyi (China), Rome, 11 September 1994
100 m: 54.01—Le Jingyi (China), Rome, 5 September 1994
200 m: 1:56.78—Franziska van Almsick (Germany), Rome, 6 September 1994
400 m: 4:03.85—Janet Evans (United States), Seoul, 22 September 1988
800 m: 8:16.22—Janet Evans (United States), Tokyo, 20 August 1989
1,500 m: 15:52.10—Janet Evans (United States), Orlando, 26 March 1988

20 years, making it necessary for Spitz to incorporate the latest research in stroke mechanics.

These differences in records over the past 30 or 35 years cannot be attributed to steroids, diet, or improved physiological training; if these were the reasons, sprinters would have been breaking records at the same rate as swimmers. There must be something else—something unique to swimming.

Undoubtedly, a great deal of the credit must be given to sports science. The earlier haphazard technique of "slash and splash" has given way to modern smooth, serpentine stroke mechanics. In the past 30 years or so, sports scienctists have developed a far more accurate and complete understanding of the complexities of moving efficiently through water. This understanding has been transferred to swimmers and coaches in terms of better ways to use the hands, arms, and feet. In the 1990s, swimmers were continuing to make advances in moving through water quickly and efficiently—learning to model themselves on sleek, high-speed powerboats rather than on plodding paddleboats.

The Body in Water

Water—the enviornment in which a swimmer must execute propulsive movements—is a complex medium: the swimmer is suspended in a fluid with dynamic three-dimensional characteristics. Thus swimming is very different from land sports. In most sports, athletes propel themselves by pushing off a solid surface (e.g., shoe against floor), but swimmers must propel themselves by pushing against a fluid. Because a fluid such as water has no constant proportions, it is difficult to move through or around. Similarly, it is much more difficult to throw than a solid object; anyone who tries to throw water from cupped hands soon realizes that although some of the water may hit the target, a great deal will simply fall through the fingers.

Not only is forward propulsion initially more difficult through water than over land; once swimmers are moving, they encounter considerably more resistance to forward movement, because water is 832 times denser than air. To understand the difference between air and water resistance, consider the deceleration of a boat and an automobile, both moving at, say, 65 kilometers per hour (about 40 MPH) and then suddenly placed in neutral—the propeller is stopped or the engine is disengaged. The car, of course, will decelerate only gradually; but because of the water resistance acting on its hull, the boat will decelerate immediately. In other words, the deceleration forces acting on the boat are far greater than those acting on the car. It is for this reason that passengers standing in a boat must be prepared to react to differences in pressure: their feet are planted on the deck, which is subject to water resistance; but their bodies are subject only to air resistance and thus will decelerate much more slowly than the boat—so that the passengers lunge forward abruptly.

What swimmers try to accomplish is to maximize the propulsive force they can generate while simultaneously minimizing resistive forces. This is no easy task. One difficulty in swimming is that increasing propulsive force means more movement of the limbs, which, in turn, usually increases resistance. Theoretically, the only way to reduce resistance is to reduce propulsive force. Thus swimmers must find a delicate balance between maximizing propulsion and minimizing resistance.

Buoyancy and Flotation

If they are thrown into water, most untrained people will tend to sink. In fact, this tendency was the basis of a grim medieval practice: people accused of witchcraft were sometimes thrown into a body of water to determine their guilt or innocence, on the assumption that an innocent person would sink and drown—only a witch would be able to float. To understand how swimmers propel themselves, it is necessary to understand how water sometimes provides support (floating) and sometimes fails to provide support (sinking).

Floating depends on the effects of gravity, a force to which everything on earth is subject. In water, or any fluid, gravitational effects create a phenomenon called hydrostatic pressure: any given layer of fluid must hold up the layers of fluid above it (*see also* PADDLE SPORTS). In other words, every layer creates a force exactly counterbalancing the layers above it. The amount of pressure is determined by the force per area. When an object, such as a body, is placed in water, it will seek a point of equilibrium, determined by an upward force called buoyancy. The object—a swimmer, say—will sink to a point where the hydrostatic pressure from all directions is equal (*see Figure 2*).

The concept of buoyancy was first explained in the second century B.C.E., by the Greek mathematician and scientist Archimedes. He discovered that any object submerged in fluid is buoyed up by a force equal to the weight of the fluid it displaces. If the object's weight is greater than the buoyant force, it sinks. If the object's weight is less than the buoyant force, it floats. At the equilibrium point, the weight of the displaced water equals the weight of the object. For example, consider a beach ball—a highly buoyant object that floats when very little of it is submerged. If you try to submerge a beach ball any farther, it will typically pop up into the air, propelled by an increased buoyant force; the more the ball is submerged, the higher it will pop up. The term *specific gravity* refers to the weight of a body compared with the weight of an equal volume of water; that is, it quantifies the buoyancy of a body or object:

$$\text{Specific gravity} = \frac{\text{weight of body}}{\text{weight of equal volume of water}}$$

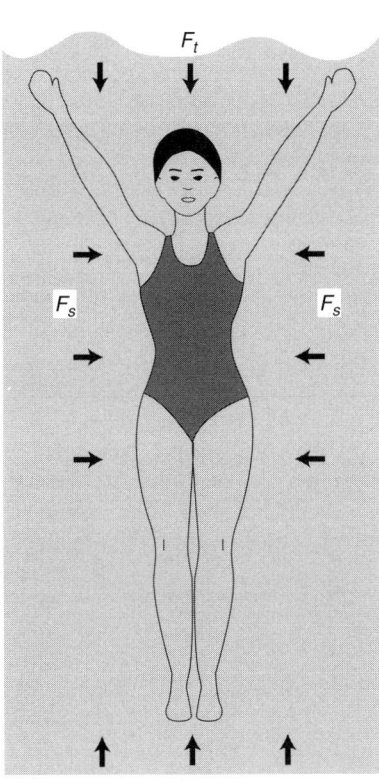

Figure 2. *Hydrostatic pressure on a swimmer = hydrostatic pressure × surface area. F_t = hydrostatic pressure on top; F_b = hydrostatic pressure on bottom; F_s = hydrostatic pressure on sides; buoyant force = $F_b - F_t$. (Adapted from Brancazio, 1984)*

Water Training and Water Therapy: A "Miracle" Environment?

To gain a "competitive edge"—even a small edge—athletes continue to experiment with different training methods. The tried and true rule for developing technique is "Practice, practice, practice"; but this often has its limitations. One limitation is simply that maneuvers may take place at such high speeds that it is difficult for the athlete to be aware of them: this is true, for example, when a gymnast or a pole vaulter is airborne. But there is a way for athletes to slow down their motions: they can practice in water.

Whereas the average density of air at sea level is 0.075 pound per cubic foot, the density of freshwater is 62.4 pounds per cubic foot. In other words, water is 832 times denser than air. By practicing in this much denser medium, athletes can slow down their movements to a point where they can form a full mental picture of exactly what is involved, step by step, from start to finish. To put it another way, a land-based activity is simulated closely, but at a greatly reduced speed. Movement in any direction is slowed down by the three-dimensional effects of water resistance.

Billy Olson, one of the top pole vaulters of the 1980s, and the first to clear 5.9 meters (19 ft. 4 in.) indoors, was an early proponent of underwater training. Wearing a mask and staying underwater for about 30 seconds, Olson tried to perfect his technique by making subtle adjustments that would correct bad habits.

Anyone who has ever attempted a pole vault will acknowledge that there is an element of fear to overcome (*see also* FIELD ATHLETICS: JUMPING). Fearing injury, vaulters tend to rush the action: they "hug" the pole, trying to pull up with the arms; thus they do not let the shoulders and head drop smoothly back so that the hips can be raised over the bar. Underwater training reduces fear and helps vaulters learn to slow their motions. Moreover, the added resistance in underwater training makes it easier for a vaulter to relax and perfect the motor skills necessary to catapult the hips over the head and shoulders to clear the bar.

Pole vaulting is a complex action, but water training is also appropriate for some very simple actions, such as running, because it improves overall balance and coordination (*see also* RUNNING AND HURDLING). For example, a runner thrusts downward simultaneously with the left arm and right leg in what is called "cross-crawl patterning." That is, because of an imbalance in strength between the two legs—and also because of injuries—stride mechanics differ between the right and left side of the body. The added resistance of water permits runners to develop a better overall awareness of running mechanics and a more balanced stride, and it can help eliminate jerkiness.

Although pool training began as a means of perfecting motor skills, it has been increasingly used for preventing injuries and for rehabilitation (*see also* REHABILITATION). The development of current and treadmill pools has certainly contributed to this trend. A treadmill can be set at, say, 11 to 12 kilometers per hour (7 MPH), and a current pool can also be adjusted to variable speeds. An athlete can achieve a uniform pace by "running forward" while actually staying in one place: any forward progress made in the propulsive stride is negated by "pushing" the runner back between strides (the runner rises from contact with the bottom between strides).

One kind of therapeutic pool uses a variable-speed reversible treadmill instead of a current. The floor of such a pool moves at speeds ranging from a crawl to 16 KPH (10 MPH), giving a

Human bodies vary widely in specific gravity, and this explains the wide variations in buoyancy among humans. How well a body floats is largely a function of individual bodily components (*see also* BODY COMPOSITION). Other things being equal, a person with a higher proportion of body fat has a lower specific gravity (less than 1) and thus floats more easily. Estimated specific gravity of various body parts is usually close to 1, but some components are higher and some lower: for example, the specific gravity of fat is 0.8, of muscle 1, and of bone 1.5 to 2.

The survival float is a good example of specific gravity in human terms. In this float, a person fills the lungs with air: this lowers the sensation of running on moist sand. Working out in this pool allows an athlete to begin rehabilitation much sooner after major surgery, particularly surgery for an injury to a weight-bearing joint like the knee (*see also KNEE*). In the immediate postoperative period, the knee joint is not yet capable of absorbing the impact forces entailed in running on land; but in water an athlete can engage in fairly rigorous workouts at a very early stage of rehabilitation.

The principle operating here is quite simple: because of hydrostatic pressure, only about 10 percent of the force of gravity that a land-based person experiences is exerted on a person standing shoulder-deep in water; in effect, the person in the water is 90 percent weightless. This means that impact forces against the bottom of a pool are greatly reduced.

Hydrostatic pressure acts as an extraordinary cushion for weight-bearing joints, limiting and preventing some of the drawbacks of traditional rehabilitation, such as joint stiffness, loss of circulation, muscle atrophy (shrinking), and difficulty exercising body parts surrounding an injured area. Moreover, hydrostatic pressure stimulates and accelerates the formation of stronger, more functional scar tissue.

Actually, water acts like a resistance weight machine—the harder you push, the greater the resistance you encounter (*see also STRENGTH TRAINING*). But water is superior to resistance weight machines in that water exerts a force against movement in three dimensions: up-and-down, back-and-forth, and side-to-side. As a result, the muscles get a much better—that is, a more balanced—workout because they work in synchronized pairs. When the quadriceps contracts, for example, the hamstring relaxes, and vice versa.

For any movement, a force must be applied to accelerate the body; and (obviously), the greater the force, the greater the acceleration. A contraction of the hamstring driving a runner's leg back must be stronger than the contraction of the quadriceps pulling the leg forward. Water workouts require a more equivalent use of both halves of each muscle pair—in this example, a nearly equal effort from the quadriceps and hamstring. The buoyancy of water diminishes the effect of gravity and thus reduces the work required of the hamstring, while simultaneously increasing the force necessary from the quadriceps.

As noted, water training permits earlier and more rigorous initial rehabilitation, which in turn allows an athlete to return to action sooner.

However, athletes should think twice before completely replacing land-based training with pool training. This is because pool training places less demand on the cardiovascular system.

For one thing, hydrostatic pressure assists cardiac performance by improving venous blood return. Therefore, the heart does not beat as fast for any given expenditure of energy. Second, increased body temperature is directly correlated with increased heart rate; therefore, because a submerged body stays cool, the heart rate is lower at the same pace of exercise during a water workout. Third, the buoyancy of water means that the muscles do not work as hard against the force of gravity with each stride. These three factors reduce oxygen uptake in a water workout by 10 to 15 percent compared with a dry-land treadmill workout, and by 5 to 10 percent compared with typical running.

Still, this cardiovascular effect is a minor drawback; the benefits of water rehabilitation far exceed its deficiencies. During the early stages of recovery from an injury or operation, water rehabilitation offers an effective way to maintain fitness and retain muscle tone. It is destined to grow as an excellent alternative to what is often the only other option: inactivity.

John Zumerchik and Steve R. Geiringer, M.D.

body's specific gravity by enlarging the chest cavity. If the arms and legs are allowed to relax, they will sink, their specific gravity being higher than that of the chest. To put this another way, inhaling deeply—filling the lungs and expanding the chest—increases the volume of the body so that it displaces more water; this decreases the body's specific gravity and thus increases the buoyant force keeping it afloat. However, people with heavier and denser bone mass and low body fat may not be able to float: they may sink no matter what they do.

Being a floater or a sinker has little or nothing to do with swimming speed. Powerful swimmers do not need good buoyancy to keep themselves from sinking: their propulsion generates more than

Long-Distance Swimmers

Swimmers who cross the English Channel and compete in other long-distances races tend to have a higher proportion of body fat. For these events, more body fat is an advantage because it increases buoyancy and helps reduce the dissipation of body heat into the surrounding water—this dissipation steals energy.

enough force for them to maintain horizontal hydrodynamics. However, buoyancy does become a factor in long-distance swimming: in fact, the longer a race, the more important buoyancy becomes (*see also* SKELETAL SYSTEM).

An interesting aspect of buoyancy is saltwater versus freshwater. Because it contains dissolved salt, saltwater—such as ocean water—has a higher density than freshwater. Buoyant forces are approximately 3 percent greater in the ocean than in, say, a freshwater lake. Therefore, swimmers in the ocean can propel themselves with a larger percentage of the body above the surface than swimmers in a freshwater lake. Having a greater percentage of the body above the surface of the water—that is, out of the very dense water and in the less dense air—is a major reason why most long-distance swimming records have been set in ocean water.

Drag: Resistance and Swimming Speed

Because water is so much denser than air, a swimmer must exert five to ten times as much energy as a runner to cover any given distance. As noted above, buoyancy has little to do with swimming speed; resistance, or drag, is much more important.

Humans—unlike, say, dolphins—are inefficient swimmers. Dolphins move through water with 80 to 90 percent efficiency; the best world-class swimmers achieve only about 10 percent efficiency. One reason for this is simply that the human body is not designed for swimming; it is not streamlined, and so humans must try to propel themselves by thrashing through the water. Dolphins, by contrast, are highly streamlined: they have a very tapered shape, with the thickest portion of the body well behind the midpoint of snout to tail; and this allows them to propel themselves effortlessly, without churning up large masses of water. Aquatic creatures in general, of course, attain much faster swimming speeds than humans (*see Table 1*); many of them swim much faster than the best humans sprinters can run on land.

The deficiencies of the human body are compounded by the nature of water—the resistance a swimmer encounters and creates. *Drag* is a term used to describe resistance forces that impede the movement of objects through water. Drag is always exerted in the opposite direction to the swimmer's movement. It is partly a function of the shape, size, and speed of the swimmer. Whatever the size and shape of the body, though, the major factors in resistance (and thus the major impediments to swimming speed) are the same: (1) water flow, incuding the formation of eddies (whirling water); (2) waves, specifically those created by the swimmers themselves; and (3) body surface friction. Although the human body is not naturally streamlined, there are many techniques human swimmers can use to reduce resistance significantly and propel themselves more efficiently.

TOP SPEEDS OF HUMAN AND AQUATIC ANIMALS

Species	MPH	KPH
Sailfish	68	110
Bluefish; tuna	43	70
Blue whale	40	64
Sperm whale	20	32
Humpback whale	9	14
Human	8	13

Table 1. (*Source: Guinness Book of Speed Records*)

Water Flow and Resistance

One factor affecting drag is the pattern of water flow—either laminar or turbulent—as it makes its way around the contours of a swimmer's body. The flow of water molecules tends to be laminar—a smooth unbroken pattern—until the molecules encounter an object that interrupts their movement. Such an interruption is called turbulence; it sets water into random motion.

Usually, the more laminar a flow of water, the less resistance a swimmer encounters; this is because laminar water flows in the same direction and at a uniform speed. However, swimmers themselves disrupt laminar water. When a laminar flow encounters a swimmer, or any other object, the molecules become turbulent: they begin to rebound randomly and wildly in every direction. These rebounding molecules begin a chain reaction: they reach out, crossing paths with other laminar molecules, which then also become turbulent. This effect continues to multiply: the newly turbulent molecules in turn spread out to disturb still more laminar molecules, creating an ever-widening path of turbulence.

This churned-up, turbulent water usually creates a high-pressure zone in front of the swimmer, but the water toward the rear of the swimmer remains in a lower-pressure laminar pattern. Thus a pressure differential develops between the water in front of and behind the swimmer, creating a drag that greatly impedes swimming speed. This drag will be proportional to the amount of turbulence: the greater the turbulence, the greater the pressure differential and the greater the drag.

High-pressure turbulent water at the front of a swimmer develops "gaps" or "holes." This creates low-pressure swirling water, called eddy currents, near the swimmer's legs. Thus, swimmers have two turbulence effects to be concerned about: they are "pushed back" by frontal resistance and "pulled back" by a pressure differential caused by eddy currents. Minimizing turbulence reduces the detrimental effects of eddy currents, because the water "gaps" are smaller, are fewer, and fill in more quickly.

Anyone with paddling experience understands why a canoe can be propelled much faster than a rowboat—a canoe encounters less resistance. This is because the canoe is tapered: given the same propulsive force, a tapered shape like a canoe entails much less drag than a squarer shape like a rowboat. The reason for this, in turn, is that water flows differently around tapered and square objects (*see Figure 3*). A tapered object and a square object will each change the direction of water molecules as they make their way around it, of course, but there is a great difference in the amount of turbulence created. A tapered (oval) object causes only a small amount of turbulence, since it affects the path of the molecules path only slightly. Eddy currents also are minimized by a tapered shape, because the narrower rear allows water to quickly fill in the "gaps" behind the object. By contrast, the rectangular object causes the water molecules to smatter randomly across its squared-off front, creating turbulence.

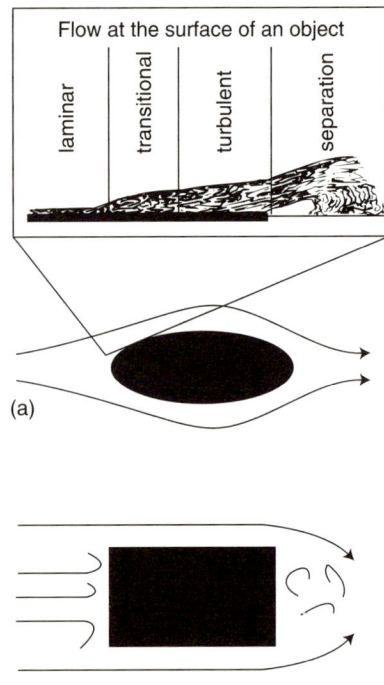

Figure 3. *The shape of an object affects the transition from laminar to turbulent flow as water moves around it. A tapered shape (a) creates less turbulence and thus less drag than a rectangular shape (b).*

The rear end, also squared off, creates additional drag. A significant low-pressure area develops behind a rectangular object because the water must fill in behind a significant area very quickly, and this creates eddy currents. (Eddy currents are very apparent in canoeing; *see PADDLE SPORTS*.) There is also a pressure differential between the front and rear of a square object that severely reduces speed.

Accordingly, swimming favors certain physiques. Barrel-chested men and big-breasted women are at a competitive disadvantage because their frontal profile is proportionately large. It is true that a heavily muscled, bulky physique was once typical in world-class swimming, but in the 1980s and 1990s tall, lean swimmers have become predominant. Apparently, tall, lean swimmers have a more optimal ratio of height to weight and height to volume. In other words, they have a more gradually tapered shape that allows water to flow more laminarly around it. This lets them maintain a more consistent pace between strokes.

Obviously, swimmers can do little to change their hereditary size or shape. Regardless of physique, however, there are several adjustments swimmers can make to minimize their frontal area, or profile, as they propel themselves through water. In fact, their foremost concern is to maintain a streamlined profile; this—not propulsive power—is primarily what separates world-class swimmers from everyone else. Even world-class swimmers cannot maintain a perfectly streamlined, tapered profile, because in order to generate propulsive force they continually need to change positions. But what they do better than the average swimmer is generate propulsive forces while maintaining a more horizontal profile from head to feet and minimizing side-to-side movement (*see Figure 4*). They are better able to balance the need to remain level with the need to apply propulsive force. On the other hand, trouble often begins when swimmers become obsessed with maintaining a good horizontal hydrodynamic profile. They may achieve the desired profile, but it comes at

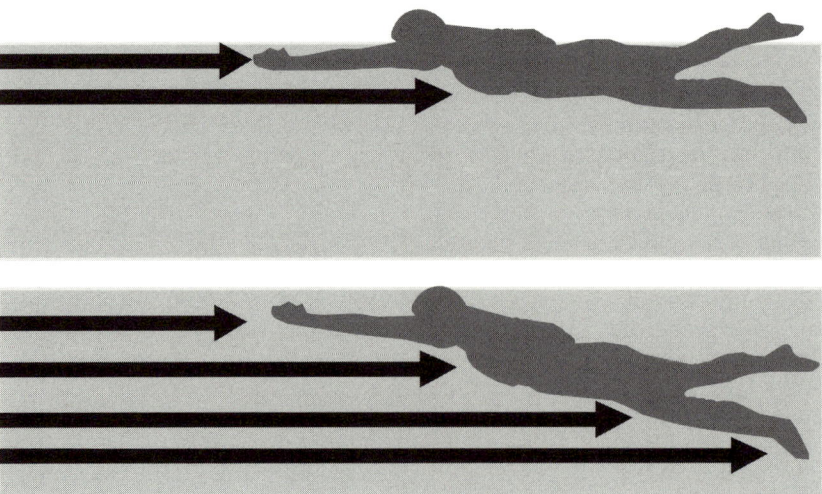

Figure 4. *The best swimmers can minimize drag and maximize thrust and lift. Here, the swimmer shown below takes up more space (has a less horizontal profile) and thus will encounter more drag than the swimmer shown above.*

the expense of reduced propulsion. The greatest contribution a coach can make is to help the swimmer increase propulsion without sacrificing hydrodynamic profile.

Waves and Resistance

The most underappreciated factor contributing to the remarkable improvement in record swimming times is reduced wave drag in pools. Advances in technology have made possible pools that are much better at keeping water still. First, Olympic pools are now deeper—all of them are at least 7.5 feet deep—and this significantly reduces wave rebound off the bottom. Second, at the walls, contoured gutters engulf waves to eliminate turbulence from waves rebounding off a wall. Third, there have also been advances in lane dividers. Dividers now have finned disks that further "damp out" waves. Until quite recently, wave turbulence off the wall made it disastrous for a swimmer to draw an outside lane; now, although the outside lane is still a disadvantage, it is no longer a catastrophe. All in all, better pool technology allows every swimmer in every lane to swim in minimal turbulence.

Swimmers have no control over waves created by other swimmers, but they can control their own waves. Swimmers create frontal waves with the head and trunk as they push water forward. This is particularly evident when a freestyle swimmer is slapping the arms against the surface during the stroke recovery phase—such a slapping motion can reduce speed by as much as 30 percent. Not only do the arms create turbulence by pushing forward, improper recovery of the hands in the backstroke and freestyle also creates a problem. When the hands enter the water, the palms should not slap the surface; rather, the hand should cut into the water like a knife, with the palm edgewise—perpendicular to the surface. These are the only causes of wave drag that swimmers can control, and so a great deal of effort is made to limit them.

Friction and Resistance

It is believed that friction between the water and a swimmer's skin pulls along water molecules. This frictional drag is probably the least important form of drag a swimmer must contend with. Still, considering that the margin of victory in some events is less than 0.01 second, reducing the drag caused by water molecules adhering to the body may provide a significant, if slight, advantage. The frictional drag of a body is affected by three variables: surface area, surface texture, and velocity. Of these, surface area is essentially uncontrollable, and velocity is an objective rather than a factor to be controlled. Thus swimmers concentrate on surface texture.

For the past three decades, swimmers have "shaved down"— shaved their bodies and sometimes their heads—before major competitions to reduce frictional drag; the idea is that clean-shaven skin will be more likely to repel water molecules than drag them along. In a study of blood lactate concentrations (a physiological measure of

Effects of Water Temperature

The viscosity (thickness) of water is in large part a function of its temperature: as temperature drops, viscosity increases rapidly. Theoretically, then, in terms of physics, a swimmer should be able to record faster times in water at 5 degrees C (41° F) than at 20 degrees C (68° F). However, the physiological deficits of swimming in colder water (greater heat loss, muscular inefficiency) may outweigh the benefits of increased viscosity and thus reduce speed (*see also PADDLE SPORTS*).

work) and stroke length before and after shaving, sizable differences were recorded. This study found that shaved swimmers increased their stroke length by 10 percent and completed their paced swims using less energy: their blood lactate values were 21 percent lower (Sharp and Costill, 1989). The researchers also found that shaved swimmers did not decelerate as quickly after pushing off and gliding away from the wall. These results were even greater than had been expected—and they are the reason why every world-class swimmer shaves down today.

Advances in swimsuit technology have also helped greatly in reducing frictional drag related to surface texture. Thinner, tighter, and much slicker swimsuits and caps have been designed to reduce drag by sealing the countours of the body as tightly as possible.

The next advance may come in the form of high-tech skin treatments. For example, just as swimmers shave down, sailors lightly sand the hull of a boat before a race: a hull sanded in this way repels water molecules. (It might seem more logical to wax the hull, but water molecules actually adhere to wax; *see also SAILING*.) Perhaps the day is not far off when swimmers will treat their skin in some way to produce the effect of light sanding.

Propulsion in Water

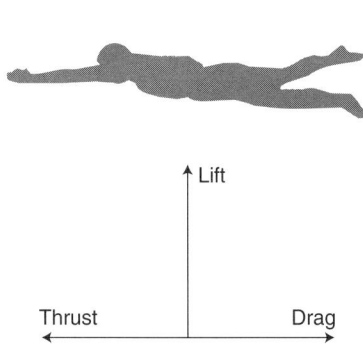

Figure 5. *In swimming, resistive forces (drag) and propulsive forces (thrust and lift) have different sources. Drag comes from profile friction, surface friction (hair and skin), and waves. Thrust is provided by the arms and legs. Lift is the body's angle of attack. The arms, and especially the hands, provide far more propulsive lift than the body. The angle of lift is always perpendicular to drag, though it changes continually during the serpentine stroke motion of the arms and hands.*

Humans cannot fly because without wings it is impossible to generate enough interaction (resistance) with air to create the necessary thrust or propulsion: there is no way to interact with a large enough volume of air at a fast enough pace. Water is different: because it is so much denser than air, humans can generate enough force in water—move a large volume of water at a fast pace—to propel themselves forward. However, the complexities of both human anatomy and the flow of water make it difficult to develop a definitive model of how swimmers actually propel themselves through water

Swimmers try to minimize the drag of the body through the water, but at the same time they try to maximize the drag created by the arms and hands—that is, they try to push back as much water as possible. In part, Newton's third law of motion explains how swimmers propel themselves through water: to every action there is always opposed an equal reaction. In the case of a swimmer, pushing water back (the "action") accelerates the body forward with a force of equal magnitude (the "reaction").

Lift

In theory, the swimmer's arms are pulled straight back to push water straight back. In reality, however, Newton's third law requires some qualification here, because swimmers do not only pull their arms straight back. During the stroke cycle, they change the angle of attack (tilt) of their hands and also use serpentine diagonal move-

Swimming 499

ments. Much like an airplane foil, the hand creates a lifting force during the diagonal stroking motion. An airfoil deflects oncoming air downward and thus adds a downward component of momentum (mass × velocity). Similarly, water is deflected from the leading edge to the trailing edge of the hand. This means that as the hand exerts, say, an outward force on the water, according to Newton's third law the water must exert some inward force on the hand. A good demonstration of lift is putting a hand out of the window of a speeding car: if the hand is tilted upward, the arm will rise as the rapidly oncoming flow of air caroms against the palm.

How much lift is created in swimming depends on the velocity of the hand relative to the water, the density of the water, the area of the hand, and—most important—the hand's angle of attack; cupping the hand creates lift, but not as much lift as changing the tilt of the hand relative to the flow of air. This lifting force, in combination with drag forces created as the hand pushes water back, results in forward propulsion (*see also* GLIDING AND HANG GLIDING).

In an airplane, as the airfoils create lift, power comes from the engine; in swimming, by contrast, both lift and propulsion come from the hands. Thus in order to create the proplusion and lift necessary to maximize forward speed, the hands' angle of attack needs to be very precise. However, because a complex lever action is involved, and because the surface of the human body is nonuniform, this task is very difficult to perform effectively.

Swimming and Propeller Propulsion

Swimming mechanics are difficult to master, primarily because the swimmer must get the arms and hands to act simultaneously like a canoe paddle and airplane foil. The action needed is most comparable to that of the propeller of a speedboat, although in terms of shape and size propeller blades and human arms and hands have very little in common. Unlike hands, propeller blades rotate about a fixed axis in a perfectly circular pattern; the propeller accelerates the boat by displacing water from the front to the back of each blade. A swimmer displaces water similarly—from the leading to the trailing edge of the hand (*see Figure 6*). However, because a three-dimensional S-shaped motion is used in all swimming strokes, the leading edge and the tilt angle of the hand vary as the arm is accelerated and decelerated through the stroke pattern. Each change in direction of the arm can be thought of as forming a "new blade" cycle. Because propulsive force can be increased by accelerating slow-moving water backward, swimmers use two or three "new blade" movements—acceleration pulses—per stroke cycle.

When a swimmer pulls a hand backward, the high-pressure zone in front of the palm accelerates water molecules straight back in the same direction as the pulling motion. To involve the greatest amount of slow-moving water throughout the stroke cycle, swimmers use a sweeping S-motion. By locating the slowest-moving water, each stroke creates more propulsion, and the length of the propulsive

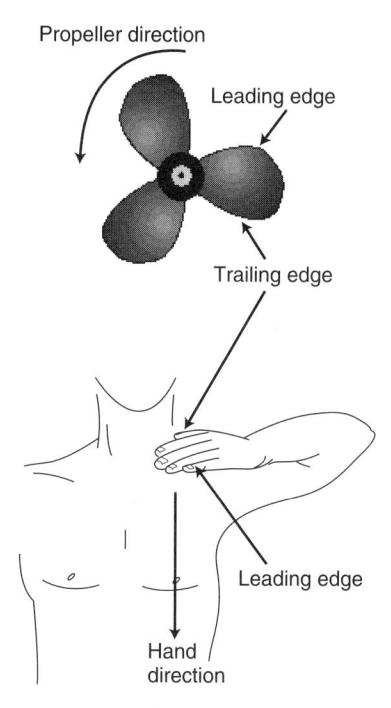

Figure 6. *The way a swimmer displaces water backward with a diagonal motion has many similarities to the way the propeller of a powerboat displaces water backward.*

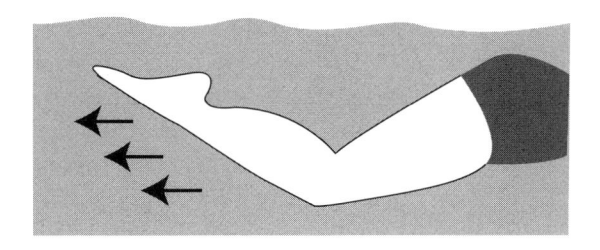

Figure 7. *There is considerable debate about how much kicking contributes to propulsion. The dolphin kick (above) in the butterfly stroke is probably the most propulsive. With legs together, knees bent, and toes pointed up, an effective hydrofoil is created. Considerable water is displaced back from the kick as the knees form a leading edge and the toes a trailing edge. Without an effective dolphin kick, swimmers would be unable to propel themselves upward and forward between stroke cycles. The dolphin kick creates a minimum of turbulence and continues to move out of the area of potential turbulence. The kick in the front crawl is another matter: estimates of its contribution to propulsion range from zero to 30 percent. The greater specific gravity of the legs, mainly from their high content of bone and muscle, requires a moderate flutter kick just to keep them horizontal—to compensate for the fact that they are less buoyant. However, excessive kicking robs the body of energy needed by the arms.*

force can be increased. The best swimmers are said to have a "feel" for the water, an uncanny ability to find the greatest amount of still water during a stroke cycle and thus to maximize the lift effect.

To visualize this phenomenon, consider swimming in a current, as in a river. It is difficult to swim upstream because the water is moving in the opposite direction; this is analogous to trying to run up an escalator that is moving down. In swimming upstream, the water is considered fast-moving because it is traveling in the same direction as the limbs are attempting to create propulsion. Much more propulsive force can be generated swimming downstream, because the water flow runs directly counter to the propulsive force. Once swimmers start moving forward, they are in effect swimming upstream because of their own speed relative to the water. Thus the higher a swimmer's speed, the harder it is to create resistance with the arms and hands, because the water is moving faster past the swimmer (*see also* PADDLE SPORTS).

Angle of Attack

Swimming requires continual shifts in the center of gravity to transfer the propulsive forces generated in the hand and arm (or the foot and leg) relative to the direction of travel. Stroke efficiency depends greatly on the angles of attack of the hands, the arms, and even the feet: to generate the most forward pressure with a given expenditure of energy, it is necessary to use the best angle of attack. Since the human body is not designed to rotate like a propeller, finding the appropriate angle of attack is an ongoing, dynamic process throughout the stroke cycle, from the moment the forward surface is broken until the arm breaks the surface near the thigh. The hand's angle of attack is the foremost concern, because the hands contribute most to propulsion and are most controllable. The hand creates much more propulsive force than the arm by virtue of its greater profile; also, the hand has greater rotational inertia (greater force is needed to set it in motion) because it is farther from the axis point (the shoulder joint). It is highly controllable because it can rotate nearly 180 degrees. (If the arm is extended palm-down, it can be rotated so that the palm is up.)

The flow of water around the hand depends on the position of the tilted hand—its leading edge and trailing edge. As the terms suggest, the *leading* edge is the first part of the hand to encounter the water flowing around it; the *trailing* edge is the last part of the hand to contact the flow of water. At various times during the underwater stroke cycle, these edges can vary—from the fingertips to the wrist, the thumb side, or the little-finger side.

Propulsive forces vary depending on the angle of attack: thus if the angle of attack is too great or too small, propulsion will be significantly affected. To determine the angle of attack, the hand's position must be considered in three dimensions. Suppose that the hands are moving at each of the following angles: 0, 40, 70, and 90 degrees (*see Figure 8*). At 0 degrees, lift is minimal. At 40 degrees, lift is increased

Lift as a Function of the Angle of Attack

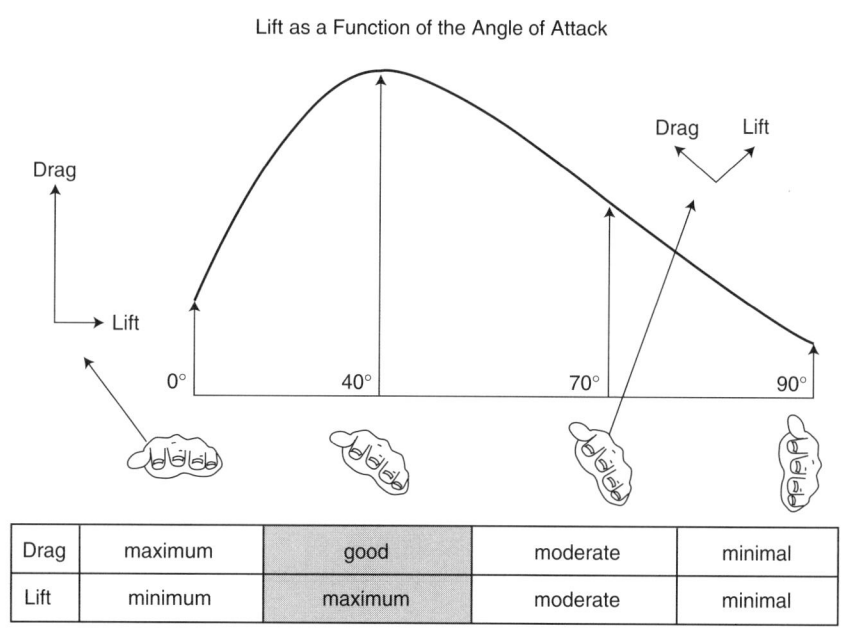

	0°	40°	70°	90°
Drag	maximum	good	moderate	minimal
Lift	minimum	maximum	moderate	minimal

Figure 8. *The angle of attack of the hand is important because it creates both propulsive drag and lift. As with an airplane foil, a 20- to 60-degree angle of attack creates a greater propulsive force than a flat-palm motion (0 degrees). Cupping of the palm should be kept to a minimum: tilting without cupping increases lift. Stroke power has also been found to increase when the fingers are slightly spread apart rather than kept together. This is because drag between the fingers—the effect of water passing between them—creates a larger cross-sectional area, so that the hand works more like the webbed appendage of a water animal like the seal. In other words, spread fingers present a larger cross-sectional area to create propulsion. (Adapted from Costill, 1992)*

considerably: water passes under the leading edge (thumb side) to the trailing edge (little-finger side) to create an optimal lifting force. This is the ideal angle of attack for the sweep under the swimmer's body. At 70 degrees, the angle of attack is too flat to create optimal lift. At 90 degrees, there is no leading or trailing edge: the hand acts more like a paddle than a propeller. As a result, a great deal of water bounces off the hand; also, significant eddy currents are created on the knuckle side, further slowing forward momentum.

To generate the greatest propulsion, then, swimmers should maintain a hand angle of attack somewhere between 20 and 60 degrees during the underwater stroke. Cecil Colwin, one of the foremost authorities on swimming, explains that the lifting force generated by the hand is directly proportional to its speed through water, so that a 40 percent increase in the speed of the hand—positioned as an effective foil—almost doubles the propulsive force (Colwin, 1992). However, a swimmer cannot always keep an ideal angle of attack throughout the wide range of movements of the hands and arms. A fixed airplane wing maintains an ideal angle of attack that produces the steady flow necessary to generate lift propulsion; but in swimming, there are constant changes in the hand's angle of attack. As a result, propulsion in swimming mainly occurs in what is called an unsteady flow.

An interesting point about angle of attack underwater is how to monitor it, since coaches cannot easily observe it. Actually, coaches monitor underwater mechanics by paying attention to the amount of air bubbles (turbulence) created—one of the few clues available to them. For a coach observing from above, excessive air bubbles usually indicate that a swimmer is not using the right limb positions and angle of attack. Air bubbles are to be expected around the hands and arms between the entry phase and the catch phase (where propulsion begins), but it is widely agreed that during and after the propulsive phase of the stroke cycle, the best swimmers are those who create the least air bubbles.

Arm Speed

When young children compete in swimming, there is tremendous variation in their arm speed: some flail away with abandon; others take a more controlled approach, trying to maximize the propulsive force delivered in each stroke; and who will win is unpredictable. But arm speed becomes more uniform as swimmers mature: they learn from their coaches and their own experience that they need to balance speed and power, and they develop a feel for optimum limb speed.

World-class swimmers all accelerate the arms and hands from the beginning to the end of the underwater stroke. In swimming, however—unlike most athletics on land—this acceleration is not slow and steady from start to finish; instead, swimmers use a pulse method. During the underwater arm stroke, arm velocity is increased and decreased with every major change of direction. The arm accelerates, then slows to change direction, and then accelerates again. Nevertheless, for all strokes, it is generally agreed that hand velocity reaches its peak near the end of the underwater movement.

It is highly likely that there is an optimal speed for the arm and hand at each stage of the underwater stroke, just as there is an optimal angle of attack. But these velocities have not yet been quantified by researchers—perhaps because of the complexity of the movements involved and because of physiological and mechanical variations among individual swimmers. Nevertheless, as noted above, swimmers develop a "feel" for an optimum hand velocity through midstroke, followed by a shift to maximum power for the final propulsive sweep.

Sweep Actions

The front crawl, butterfly, breaststroke, and backstroke seem to use very different sweep strokes, but their appearance is deceptive. This popular misconception arises because spectators usually see only what happens out of the water, not what is happening underwater. Although arm motions outside the water are indeed very different, the sweeps a swimmer uses underwater are remarkably similar from one stroke to another.

The propulsive arm movements of swimmers underwater can be broken down into four basic sweeps: outsweep, downsweep, insweep, and upsweep (*see Figure 9*). Water makes the mechanics of these sweeps much different from what might be expected. As noted above, in land sports—whether throwing or running—athletes try to accel-

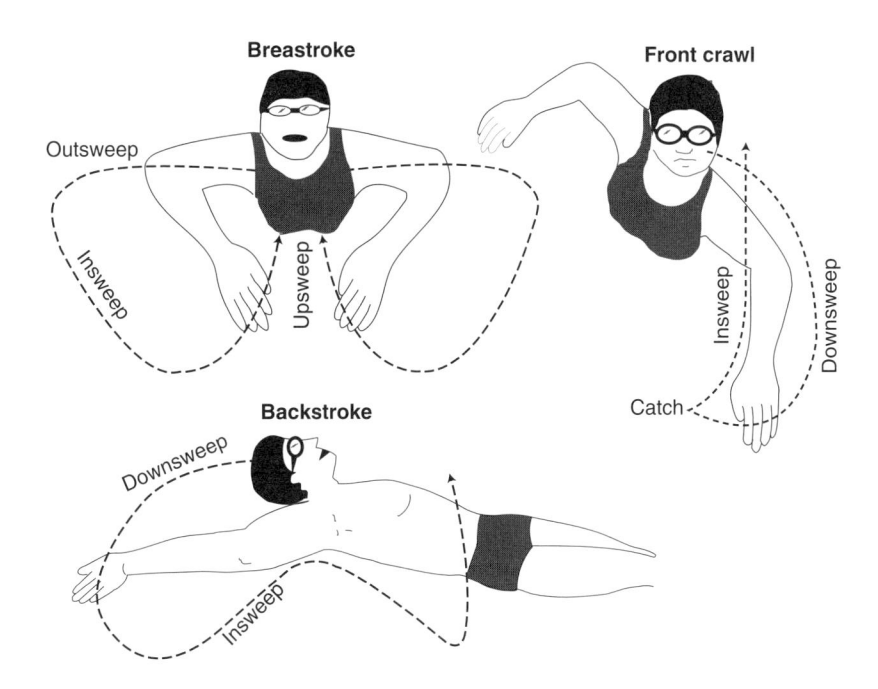

Figure 9. *Arm stroke patterns used in the front crawl, breaststroke, and backstroke consist of four basic sweeps.*

Hip Rotation in Freestyle

World-class swimmers train constantly to perfect the sweeping S-curve arm motion, but there is a growing consensus among coaches that in the freestyle improving hip rotation is just as important. According to the biomechanist Bob Pritchard, who worked with Amy Van Dyken (the 50-m sprint champion in the 1996 Olympics), developing a fluid early hip rotation is far more important in generating power than developing greater strength in the chest and arms.

erate steadily from start to finish. But swimmers need to accelerate and decelerate in pulses, and these four sweeps categorize the pulses they use.

Outsweep and Downsweep

For the butterfly and the breaststroke, the outsweep motion is the initial underwater movement. It starts with the swimmer's hands and arms entering the water in front of the body. Then, the arms are swept out beyond shoulder width in a flat curved path. Toward the end of the outsweep, the hands are rotated out and back in preparation for the first propulsive sweep to begin the "catch" and create useful forward lift through the outsweep and insweep.

The downsweep in the freestyle and backstroke is analogous to the outsweep in the butterfly and breaststroke. As it enters the water, the hand moves diagonally forward to prepare for the "catch." The hand naturally slides out diagonally during the downsweep because of the roll-over motion of the shoulder. It is important that this motion should remain natural and not exaggerated, for an exaggerated slide out will increase drag without increasing propulsion. Since the outsweep and downsweep form the first "pulse," hand movement should nearly stop at the "catch."

Insweep

The insweep is the first propulsive stroke that begins at the "catch." From the catch, the swimmer sweeps the arm and hand down, in, and then up to a point where they are directly under the midpoint of the body. The hand begins parallel to the wrist and flexes back at a moderate pace until it reaches a 90-degree angle at the end of the insweep.

Among world-class swimmers, there is tremendous variation in the length of the insweep. Some sweep their hands well beyond the midpoint of the body; others finish the insweep at the midpoint. Because these two styles seem equally effective, this variation is probably a matter of swimmers' individual biomechanical strengths and preferences. One factor may be the starting width of the swimmer's hands. Swimmers who start with the hand far outside shoulder width, and sweep over a greater area, feel that they achieving great "mileage" with the insweep and are ready to begin the outsweep earlier. Swimmers who begin with the hand inside shoulder width feel that they need to sweep across the body's midpoint in order to use the full potential of the insweep. Another factor is differences in propulsion: some swimmers generate more propulsive force in the insweep and less in the upsweep; some generate less force in the insweep and more in the upsweep. This is much more a matter of preference based on "feel" than of any biomechanical advantage.

Upsweep

The upsweep begins when the insweep is completed; it continues until the swimmer's hand reaches the thigh. There is an acceleration pulse in the transition between insweep and upsweep: hand speed slows during the transition and then accelerates rapidly through the remainder of the upsweep. Much of the success of the upsweep depends on the ability to keep the hands hyperextended (bent back) at the wrists. The more perpendicular the hand is to the water, the more propulsion can be achieved during the final portion of this movement. A well-flexed back hand allows a swimmer to continue to generate significant propulsion even though the forearm is well beyond a position to generate much velocity. Because this hand position feels unnatural, however, it is very difficult to teach.

Breaststroke: Velocity Fluctuations

The breaststroke has the dubious distinction of being the slowest of the competitive strokes. This is not due to any lack of force: it has been found that during the propulsive phase, more force is generated in the breaststroke than in any other stroke. The greater propulsion, however, is more than offset by the large deceleration force that occurs each time the breaststroke swimmer recovers the legs in preparation for the next kick.

The English physicist Malcolm Kent, after serving several years as a swimming instructor in the Royal Navy, conducted a study to measure instantaneous velocity and relate it to average velocity per stroke: he developed an analytic model of velocity through the stroke cycle by recording instantaneous velocity at different intervals. Kent believed that one "best" stroke cycle could be discovered—a cycle that would result in a higher average velocity per stroke. Determining a "best" stroke cycle would imply that it could be repeated; and if it could be repeated without introducing adverse effects, overall speed would increase.

Kent calculated velocity, acceleration, water resistance, and propulsive power throughout the breaststroke cycle (*see Figure 10*). According to the principle of conservation of linear momentum, the total linear momentum of an object remains the same unless an external force acts on the object. An accelerating force from the swimmer's strokes causes momentum to increase (peaks of curve), but there are continuous external retarding forces from the water, which is dense and viscous. The retarding force becomes very significant when a greater frontal area develops as the arms and legs complete stroke recovery, causing momentum to decrease further (troughs of curve). The greatest retarding force comes from the legs as they recover before the propulsive drive. According to Kent, the key to improved performance would be maintaining a more constant velocity—that is, minimizing fluctuations in velocity. Any changes that maintain horizontal momentum better within the cycle could save energy, and the energy saved would then be available for improving overall performance.

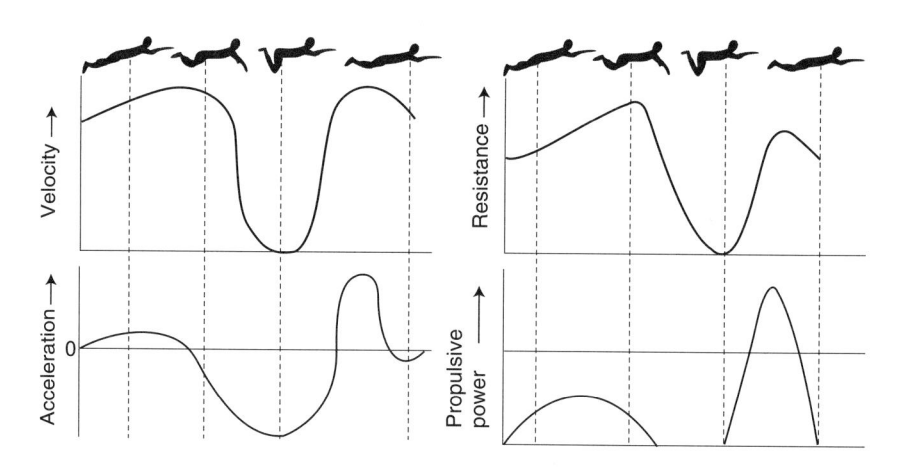

Figure 10. *Acceleration, velocity, resistance, and propulsive power change during the wave breaststroke cycle; shown here are Kent's calculations. Limiting the resistive forces as the legs recover before the propulsive drive means that velocity fluctuations will be limited. This is the major reason that few breaststrokers use the flat style.*

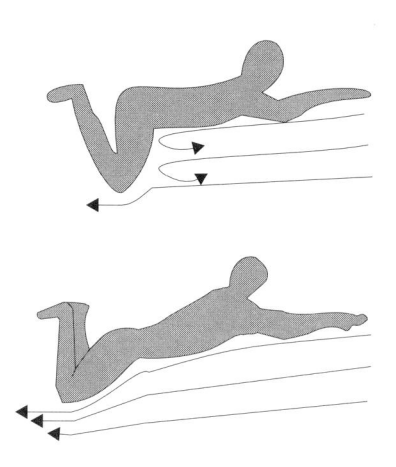

Figure 11. *Most breaststroke swimmers now use a wave style (below) rather than a flat style (above). One advantage of the wave style is that it involves less fluctuation of velocity because the legs create less resistive drag.*

In recent years, there has been debate among coaches over three different timing techniques: continuous, glide, and overlap. Much of this debate has involved the focus of Kent's study: reducing drag and minimizing fluctuations in velocity. In glide timing, there is a short interval between the completion of the kick and the beginning of the arm stroke, during which the swimmer glides along (hence the term). In continuous and overlap timing, the arm stroke begins before the kick is completed or just at the moment when the kick is completed.

Most coaches believe, and Kent would probably concur, that glide timing is least effective because of the lengthy deceleration time from the end of the kick to the beginning of the propulsive arm stroke. Most now use the overlap method. This timing is best at reducing the deceleration period between kick propulsion and arm propulsion: the arm stroke can begin early because the arms are swept out as the the legs finish the last portion of their insweep. The "catch" and the start of propulsion begin just as the propulsive phase of the kick ends. Although it is debatable whether drag is reduced, there certainly is a reduction in velocity fluctuations.

A recent change in the rules allows swimmers to drop the head underwater for portions of each stroke cycle. This has increased the use of what is referred to as the "wave" style for the breaststroke, rather than the traditional "flat" style (*see Figure 11*). Much of the controversy over these two styles centers on the question of which creates less "form" drag. Proponents of the flat style claim that it has less form drag; however, this profile forces the swimmer to push the legs down and forward against the water. There is an extended period when the legs are at a right angle to the surface of the water, creating a very large drag and thus entailing greater fluctuations in velocity (go-stop) between cycles. The wave style does involve more angular bodily motion, and it does present more frontal area; but the change in direction of the water (the necessary change in momentum of the water) is small compared with that in the "flat" style: although the frontal area may be smaller in the flat style, the change in momentum is probably larger.

Many world-class breaststrokers have adopted the wave style;

they believe it aids propulsion and reduces the deceleration force during leg recovery. As noted, in 1980 Kent used his model to predict that improvement in breaststroke times would come mostly from maintaining a more consistent velocity through the stroke cycle—a prediction that has proved to be very accurate.

Dive Starts

Significant advances have been made not only in reducing resistance and increasing stroke propulsion, but also in improving the dive. To maximize the speed and distance of their flight off the platform, swimmers (much like high jumpers and long jumpers) need to generate explosive leg force. They also need to enter the water in a way that will conserve as much momentum as possible and let them begin propelling themselves forward as quickly as possible. The principles of flight and water contact may seem quite elementary, but swimmers have been able to improve their times appreciably by incorporating a number of subtle techniques.

Pike versus Flat Dive

Almost all world-class swimmers use a pike dive; but before the pike dive emerged, in the 1960s, they used a flat dive. In the flat dive, the swimmer would extend straight out from the blocks and skim across the water at a very low trajectory, trying to contact the water like a skipping-stone. The pike dive quickly became more popular because of its distinct advantages. With a pike dive, the swimmer can leave the block at a higher trajectory and thus land farther out. Maximizing airborne time in this way is useful because less resistance is encountered in air than in water. On landing, there is an additional benefit: by bending at the waist, the swimmer enters the water at a steeper angle—that is, more "cleanly," encountering far less resistance and creating far less turbulence. As a result, the swimmer travels much faster in the glide phase before the first propulsive stroke. A flat diver creates a great deal more turbulence on entering the water because much more surface area is contacted (*see Figure 12*).

It is worth noting that swimmers should not allow the glide phase to last too long, but it is equally important not to start propulsion too soon. Propulsion should begin when the body decelerates to race velocity.

Grab and Track Starts

The grab start was introduced in the late 1960s. It allows a faster start because instead of using a circular backswing at the gun, the swimmer pulls up against the starting platform. A swimmer using the grab start may decelerate somewhat more quickly than a swimmer using the arm-swing style, but this is more than compensated for by increased acceleration off the platform: pulling up on the platform

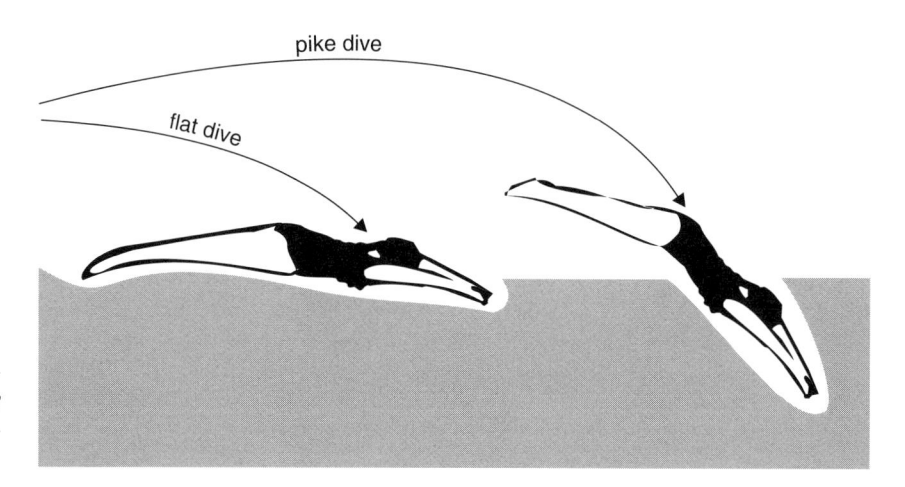

Figure 12. *The pike dive is superior to the flat dive because it creates far less splash—that is, less energy-stealing turbulent resistance.*

increases the amount and speed of the force the feet can generate off it. The swimmer can lean forward more—move the center of gravity farther forward—without losing balance.

The track grab start (*see Figure 13*) adds an innovation to the grab start. In the track start, instead of squaring both feet up to the end of the platform, the swimmer staggers the feet, just like a sprinter in the blocks. Although the superiority of the track start has not yet been conclusively established, it does offer at least two clear advantages. First, by pushing initially with the rear foot and then with the front foot, the swimmer can leave the blocks faster and with greater acceleration (quicker forward rather than upward acceleration). Second, the track start gets swimmers into the water sooner because they seem to leave the platform accelerating faster and at a slightly lower trajectory. Because more and more coaches had adopted the track start, in the 1990s it was becoming the prevalent technique among top swimmers.

John Zumerchik*

*The author thanks James Koehler and Eric Sprigings for providing useful suggestions and comments.

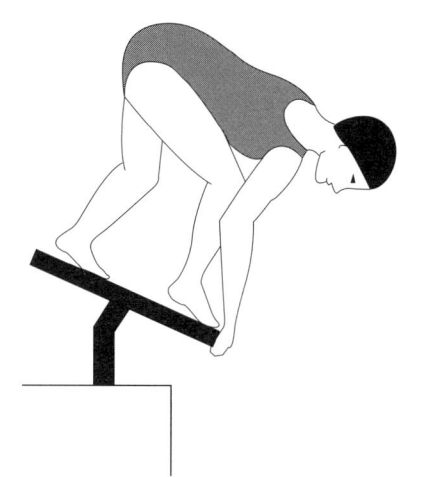

Figure 13. *In the track grab start, the swimmer pulls up hard on the underside of the block and drives off with the rear leg first.*

References

Brancazio, P. *Sport Science*. New York: Simon and Schuster, 1984.

Colwin, C. *Swimming Into the 21st Century*. Champaign, Illinois: Human Kinetics, 1992.

Costill, D., et al. *Swimming*. Boston: Blackwell Scientific Publications, 1992.

Hay, J. "The Status of Research on the Biomechanics of Swimming." In J. Hay (ed.), *Starting, Stroking, and Turning*. Iowa City: Biomechanics Laboratory, University of Iowa, 1986.

Huey, L., and P. Forster. *The Complete Waterpower Workout Book*. New York: Random House, 1993.

Jerome, J., "Propellers, Paddle Wheels, and Swimming Faster." In E. Schier and W. Allman (eds.), *Newton at the Bat: The Science in Sports*. New York: Scribner, 1987.

Kent, M. "The Physics of Swimming." *Physics Education* 15, no. 5 (1980): 275–279.

Kreighbaum, E., and K. Barthels. *Biomechanics*. Minneapolis, Minnesota: Burgess, 1985.

Larue, R. "Future Start." *Swimming Technique* 21 (1985): 30ff.

Locke, L. *The Name of the Game: How Sports Talk Got that Way*. Whitehall, Virginia: Betterway, 1992.

Schmidt-Nielson, K. "Locomotion: Energy Cost of Swimming, Flying, and Running." *Science* 177, no. 4045 (1972): 202–227.

Sharp, R., and D. Costill. "Influence of Body Hair Removal on Physiological Responses during Breaststroke Swimming." *Journal of Medical Science, Sports, and Exercise* 21, no. 5 (1989): 576–580.

Ungerechts, B., K. Wilke, and K. Reischle. *Swimming Science V*. Champaign, Illinois: Human Kinetics, 1988.

Tennis

THERE ARE MANY THEORIES about the origin of tennis. One links it to a game that was part of ancient Egyptian and Arabian fertility rites; another links it to games developed and played by the ancient Greeks and Romans.

The first game that closely resembled what we now call tennis was an indoor game played in medieval France, called court tennis. This began as a sport for royalty during the reign of Louis X (1314–1316) and was fervently supported by most of his successors. There was considerable betting on court tennis; in fact, the penchant for gambling, and the debts that mounted up because of it, caused widespread anxiety among the French royalty and aristocracy. Although modern tennis is very different from court tennis, it has retained an interesting legacy from the earlier version: scoring. A game in court tennis was worth 60 points, counted by fifteens—0, 15, 30, 40 (an abbreviation for 45), 60. The number 60 was chosen because it had special significance: it indicated completion or coming full circle, since there are 60 seconds in a minute and 60 minutes in an hour.

Throughout the seventeenth and eighteenth centuries, court tennis was played indoors on a flagstone floor. But around 1870, technology allowed the game to evolve: rubber balls were developed that would bounce on grass. The game was thus taken outside, ushering in the era of "lawn tennis." By 1880, lawn tennis was played virtually worldwide. Wimbledon, the ancestor of all tennis tournaments, began in 1877 for men and added a women's tournament soon thereafter, in 1884. In the twentieth century, other playing surfaces also came into use for lawn tennis, including clay, composition (grit), and various hard all-weather materials—a variety of legitimate playing surfaces unique among sports. Lawn tennis is still the official name, but the modern game is usually called simply tennis.

Lawn tennis was part of the first modern Olympics in 1896; and although it was (mysteriously) dropped after the games of 1924, it was restored for the Olympics of 1988. For most sports, nationalism is most prominent in the Olympics; for tennis, however, nationalistic feelings have been stirred more by the Davis Cup. During the years when tennis was divided into amateur and professional competition (until the late 1960s), the Davis Cup, which was for amateurs, drew as much attention as any of the other major tournaments (also amateur). One feature of the Davis Cup that makes it especially interesting, and unpredictable, is that the host country chooses the playing surface. Even if the host country is the underdog, it still has a competitive chance, since it can choose a surface that favors its best players. For example, Spain and Italy usually select clay; Australia usually selects grass. The playing characteristics of these two surfaces differ tremendously—clay is very slow and grass is very fast—and the surface chosen has actually been the deciding factor in some outcomes.

Around 1970, tennis competition became "open," and the game rapidly developed into a major professional sport, focusing much more on the achievements (and sometimes the antics) of individual players, a number of whom have become superstars. Several tennis stars—such as Chris Evert, Jimmy Connors, and John McEnroe—retired in the 1990s, and popular interest in the game waned somewhat. But prize money and endorsement contracts in tennis are enormous, and the best male and female professionals continue to rank among the highest earners in sports.

Although professional tennis may be at a crossroads, recreational tennis remains very popular. Tennis courts have become a fixture of city parks and school playgrounds around the country, and most people in the United States live within a few minutes of a tennis court. Tennis is accessible, simple, and moderately paced—a sport that can be enjoyed by young and old alike.

Tennis Rackets

Tennis was revolutionized in the late 1970s when Henry Head—the inventor of fiberglass skis—shifted his attention to designing tennis rackets and began to market the Prince, an aluminum racket with a large head that almost doubled the previous hitting surface. Henry Head had taken advantage of one aspect of the rules that no one else seemed to have noticed: only the length of the official racket was specified—not the size of the head.

The Prince was so successful that within a few years small-frame rackets, and many of their manufacturers, had disappeared. In the late 1970s, tennis officials, in an attempt to halt a progression toward larger and larger heads, imposed a maximum size. This change in the rules, however, had the effect of accelerating innovations in rackets, because it forced designers to focus on making improvements elsewhere. There are still no restrictions on the materials used for the frame or strings of a tennis racket, the number of strings, the shape of the racket, the thickness of the frame, or the distribution of weight; thus designers have enormous scope for experimentation.

In the 1990s, almost all tennis rackets sold had a midsize or an oversize head, and many were made of the latest space-age composites. Composite material for tennis rackets is a combination of polymers and graphite, and it achieves what until relatively recently would have been considered mutually incompatible goals: the strength of

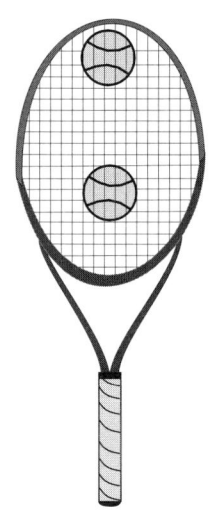

Figure 1. *The larger the coefficient of restitution, the greater the rebound height of a ball. For a ball dropped from the same height, an off-center contact (above) results in a smaller coefficient of restitution than an on-center contact (below). The farther off-center a shot is, the more energy is diverted to rotation of the racket.*

steel and the lightness of balsa wood. In other words, these composite materials are stiff (for control) and strong (for power), but at the same time are very light.

The Size of the Head

One reason why a racket with a larger head is superior to the earlier standard-size racket is obvious: a large head makes missing the ball less likely. But there is also an advanage that may be less obvious: the larger head is almost foolproof because any type of contact produces better results. To understand this effect, it is useful to consider the physics of the contact between racket and ball.

Contact can take one of two forms: on-center or off-center. To evaluate a collision—in this case, the impact of racket and ball—physicists measure the coefficient of restitution: the relative velocity of two elastic objects before and after direct impact. Coefficient of restitution can vary from 0 (no rebound) to 1 (perfect elasticity), and it differs markedly for an on-center versus an off-center hit (*see Figure 1*). Hitting the ball off-center, away from the long axis of the racket, twists the racket in the player's hand. With an on-center hit, the ball rebounds much farther, because energy is returned to the ball rather than being diverted toward rotation of the racket. In order to achieve consistent, accurate, powerful shots, on-center contact is of course the goal; but because of the velocity of the ball (which is often just a blur to the player), even the best professionals cannot always hit it on-center. There are two ways in which the larger head makes an off-center hit less detrimental.

First, a racket with a larger head has more rotational inertia (resistance to rotational change), which depends on the distribution of mass relative to the axis of rotation. In other words, such a racket is less likely to twist in the player's hand because it is more stable along its long axis.

Second, a racket with a larger head increases the high-power area—the area with a high coefficient of restitution. This is because the large-head racket is no longer than a standard racket (as noted above, overall length is specified in the rules); instead, the racket head is extended farther down the shaft. In other words, the shaft is shorter and the head longer, and this configuration means that the primary contact point (the center of the strings) and the balance point are farther up the handle toward the head. This effectively makes the racket stiffer, and the stiffer the racket, the less it flexes, so that—again—a greater proportion of energy is returned to the ball.

Another advantage of the larger head is, of course, an enlarged "sweet spot." The sweet spot is discussed later, after the following brief consideration of the frame.

The Racket Frame

Most players on the professional tour tinker with their rackets to improve playability. For one thing, they may try to increase rotational inertia by using perimeter weights, such as lead tape, to add mass along the frame. Perimeter weights increase both the rotational inertia of the racket and its linear momentum (mass × velocity).

In the 1970s and 1980s, for example, Jimmy Connors was using a heavy steel Wilson T-2000 with a standard head, which he customized by adding significant mass around the frame. Since linear momentum is the product of mass times velocity, it can be increased by increasing either of these, but Connors increased only the mass of his racket. Unlike the "big hitters," he did not try to increase its velocity. His technique was unusual in that he used a slow, deliberate swing, "driving" through the ball rather than relying on the speed of the racket. Many of Connors's opponents said that he hit the "heaviest" ball in the game. However, even Connors eventually acknowledged the value of the new rackets. He switched to a larger-head composite racket in the late 1980s, at a time when his career was resurging. (He would go on to give a series of exciting performances in the prestigious United States Open in the early 1990s.) One of the major reasons for this switch was that with his standard-head racket, his customized perimeter weighting increased rotational inertia only linearly; with a large-head racket, by contrast, rotational inertia increases as the square of the head width.

Balance of weight is a significant feature of a racket, and this differs radically between modern and earlier designs. In the 1960s and 1970s, the classic wooden racket weighed about 0.4 kilograms (15 oz.) and was neutrally balanced: that is, its center of gravity was the same as its geometric center. Modern rackets, on the other hand, weigh only around 0.28 kilograms (10 oz.) and are top-heavy—that is, "head-heavy."

Because of this reduction of weight in the handle and shaft, along with the use of lightweight composite materials, a racket that is 30 to 40 percent lighter can still impart as much momentum to the ball at any given velocity of swing. Slow-motion films of racket-ball collisions show that the old rackets flexed backward, with the ball leaving the strings well before the racket flexed forward again. The balance of weight in the modern frame, along with a design based on composite materials, makes it better "tuned" to ball-string contact: it flexes backward and forward in conjunction with the time of contact.

Racket designers continue to seek still better performance. A recent trend is toward wide-body rackets. Standard frames are 15 to 20 millimeters (0.6 to 0.7 in.) wide, whereas wide-body frames range from 25 to 35 millimeters (1 to 1.4 in.). The increased width—this increase is greatest near the top of the head—helps damp the frame where it is most flexible. This is important because the more a racket flexes, the more it vibrates; and since vibration wastes energy, less energy is imparted to the ball. A wide-frame racket also encounters less air resistance during the swing because, being wide but thin, it presents less frontal area in the direction of the swing.

What makes the wide-body racket possible is the use of composite materials, which allow added width without added weight. A wooden wide-body racket—if anyone wanted to make it—would be a loglike object that only a player with the strength of a lumberjack could handle (*see also EQUIPMENT MATERIALS*).

The Evolution of the Tennis Racket

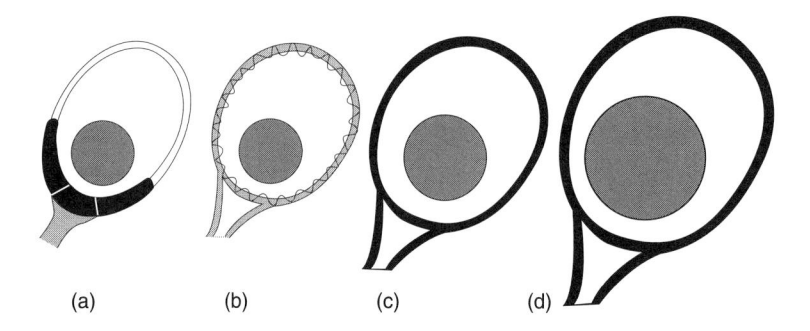

(a)   (b)   (c)   (d)

Wood: *(a)* This was the standard racket for nearly a century, from the game's origin until the late 1970s. With a head of about 75 square inches, the sweet spot is close to the throat of the racket.

Metal: *(b)* Stiffer steel and aluminum rackets appeared in the early 1970s, but they had no advantage over the wooden rackets they tried to replace: the size of the head and the sweet spot was unchanged. The racket shown, the Wilson T-2000, was Jimmy Connors's favorite.

Graphite: *(c)* Bigger, wider graphite frames—as large as 120 square inches—were introduced in the late 1970s. These rackets had a bigger sweet spot that was nearer the center of the strings.

Composite: *(d)* Today's "head-heavy" rackets now have most of their weight toward the head and away from the throat. This enlarges the sweet spot by bringing it farther up toward the top of the strings.

The Sweet Spot

Many people believe that modern rackets generate much more power than earlier rackets. This is not entirely true: in the 1970s, service speeds of 190 to 215 kilometers per hour (120–135 MPH) were recorded for players like Roscoe Tanner and John Newcombe—about the same range as the best servers were achieving in the 1990s. Still, the men's tour in the 1990s was indisputably characterized more by a "power game." Some of the increase in power could be attributed to stronger, better-conditioned players, but the major reason was the consistency of power made possible by the modern racket. Roscoe Tanner, for instance, might hit about 20 serves per match in the 190- to 215-KPH range; but the big servers of the 1990s—Pete Sampras, Goran Ivanisevic, Boris Becker—hit about 60 to 70.

The reason for this increased consistency is that the newer large-head rackets have a bigger "sweet spot," or effective rebound area. Given the same swing speed as was used with earlier rackets (such as wooden rackets), the player can generate as much or more power with equal or better accuracy.

In fact, some people argue that technology has gone too far—that men's tennis has become too much of a power game, and less of a serve-and-volley game requiring finesse. They point out that although there are more "big servers" than ever before, there have been fewer serve-dominated matches in the 1990s than in the 1960s. The larger sweet spot of modern rackets has negated much of the advantage of a big serve: a growing number of players can return it with stunning pace, consistency, and effectiveness.

An impressive example is Andre Agassi's Wimbledon championship in 1992. Few observers would have predicted it, because Wimbledon has always been dominated by big servers. It is a grass-court tournament; and on grass—a very fast surface—a baseline player like Agassi (that is, a player who rarely comes to the net) finds it difficult or impossible to neutralize a big serve. Nevertheless, Agassi defeated Boris Becker (a three-time Wimbledon champion) and Goran Ivanisevic (a booming server), to a large extent by counterattacking with a powerful, adept return of service. His service returns reached nearly the velocity of the serves themselves. In this, he was definitely helped by the enlarged sweet spot of his modern racket.

The term *sweet spot* means different things to different people. It can refer to the maximum-power spot (the point with the highest coefficient of restitution), the minimum-vibration spot (node), or the point of minimum initial shock (center of percussion). Most racket manufacturers seem to define it as an oval-shaped area encompassing a combination of these three spots (*see Figure 2*). The minimum-vibration point is at the edge of the sweet spot, the length midpoint of the racket face; hitting a ball away from the node—toward the top of the racket—means that contact occurs farther away from the racket's center of mass, increasing vibration.

Racket manufacturers adjust their designs in several ways to change the sweet spot: by altering flexibility, by adding weight to the top of the racket, by modifying the strings, and by changing the size and shape of the head. On the modern racket, which has a stiffer, heavier head, the sweet spot is much farther up the strings than it was on the more flexible, neutrally balanced racket of the early 1980s; and the trend among manufacturers is to continue to raise the sweet spot higher and higher. This gives big servers a twofold advantage: first, they can contact the ball at a higher point in the toss; second, the racket will be traveling faster at contact because the sweet spot is farther from the axis of rotation (the hand).

Interestingly, among professional players the transition to modern rackets has been slow, and this has to do at least partly with these changes in the sweet spot. The dynamics of the racket-ball collision change as the sweet spot moves higher and higher, requiring a major adjustment in motor memory, and touring professionals often cannot take the time needed to make that adjustment.

This problem with the sweet spot is a specific instance of a more general phenomenon: very few touring players "trade up" to new tennis equipment. Ivan Lendl, for instance, played with a small-headed

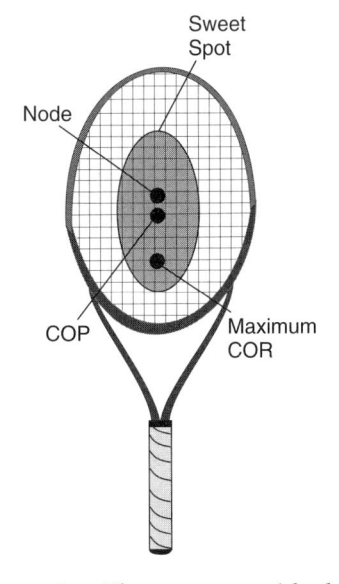

Figure 2. *The sweet spot (shaded area) can be defined as a combination of node, center of percussion (COP), and maximum coefficient of restitution (COR). In a wooden racket, COP was near the throat; in a modern racket, it is much closer to the center of the head.*

racket from the 1970s until he retired in 1994. It is true that for a veteran like Lendl, who used a great deal of wrist snap to create topspin, there would be less gain in overall power; but even Jimmy Connors, who used a flat power stroke, felt more comfortable keeping his outdated racket. (Although, as noted above, Connors did eventually use a large-head composite racket, he thought that changing to a widebody racket late in his career would impair his game.) Thus it is the junior players, the young players moving up the ranks, who benefit most from new technology, because they grow up with it.

The Strings

Historically, the reasons the tennis racket evolved with strings—instead of having a solid surface like a table tennis paddle—can only be a matter for speculation. Scientifically, however, the reason for having strings is quite clear: strings allow a low-velocity swing to launch a ball at a very high velocity. They are designed to return most of the energy they receive from the velocity of the ball. To put it graphically, strings act like a trampoline.

Tension of Strings

According to the principle of conservation of energy, energy is neither created nor destroyed; it merely changes from one form to another. The energy involved when racket meets ball must be transferred to the ball, the racket frame, the strings, the player's body, or some combination of these. Herbert Hatze, a biomechanicist at the University of Vienna, found that about 2 percent of this energy is dissipated (lost) in the hand; 2 to 4 percent of energy in the strings; a substantially higher proportion, 15 percent or more, in the ball; and 58 to 64 percent in the frame (see Table 1). Of these factors, energy lost in the ball is the most variable, because it increases exponentially with increased swing velocity on impact. By far the largest loss of energy is obviously the 58 to 64 percent dissipated in the postimpact recoil and internal vibration of the frame. All this leaves a surprisingly small proportion of the original kinetic (movement) energy for propelling the rebounding ball back over the net—only about 20 percent.

At the moment of contact, most of the impact energy is stored in the ball, the frame, and the strings. The ball returns about half its energy (when a ball is dropped from any given height, it bounces back halfway). The racket, however, returns much more of the impact energy, because of the deformation of the strings. Strings at lower tension—that is, loosely strung—show greater deformation, storing more energy and dispersing less, than strings at high tension (tightly strung). In other words, low-tension strings allow more kinetic energy to be returned to the ball. The difference in coefficient of restitution

ENERGY LOST DURING RACKET-BALL COLLISION

Hand	2%
String damping	2–4%
Ball damping	15+%
Racket (recoil and internal vibration)	58–64%
Energy available for ball propulsion	20%

Table 1. *(Source: Hatze, 1993)*

(rebound) between low-tension and high-tension strings can be demonstrated by lying a tightly strung and a loosely strung racket on the floor and dropping a ball onto each racket, and the floor, from the same height. The ball will bounce highest off the loosely strung racket; the bounce off the tightly strung racket will not be as high, though it will still be considerably higher than the bounce off the floor.

Loose strings, then, result in more power; in fact, when a racket is strung very tightly, it feels more like a table tennis paddle than a racket. Why, then, do most manufacturers recommend stringing their rackets between 25 and 29.5 kilograms (55 and 65 lb.) of pressure? Why not 20 kilograms (45 lb.), or even less? The reason is simply that power is not everything. Because every shot in tennis needs to be directed, a balance must be struck between power and control.

A loosely strung racket increases power because it prolongs the contact between ball and strings (dwell time)—but for this same reason it also impairs control. First, as has been noted, the strings produce a "trampoline" effect: the ball is harder to control because it accelerates off the strings more quickly. Second, the speed of the ball as it leaves the strings depends more on the pace of the opponent's shot than the direction of the player's own swing. The longer dwell time with a loosely strung racket means that the arm and hand experience less of the shock of contact, because the magnitude of the force is spread out more. Third, the ball does not flatten out as much as it would with tight strings. This means that the ball-string contact area is smaller; and the smaller the contact area, the less the control. Fourth, when dwell time is increased, the racket is more likely to twist or turn, sending the shot off course.

It is generally agreed that players should string their rackets at the upper end of the manufacturer's tension range for control, and at or below the lower end of the range for power. It should be noted, however, that looser strings do not necessarily decrease control; they may actually increase control if the swing is modified. Because looser strings send the ball off the strings at a higher speed, it is not necessary to swing as hard; a slower, more precise swing can be used to give more control over where the ball is going. But looser strings require a player to convert the opponent's shots more efficiently—that is, the power of the opponent's shot must be used to generate power for the return. And for players who "blast" at the ball or use a lot of spin, a tightly strung racket might be better.

An educated decision about tension must also take into account the flexibility of the racket. The earlier wooden rackets all played similarly with similar tension; different modern rackets, by contrast, may play differently at the same tension. For example, a stiff racket frame requires higher tension than a more flexible frame, to complement its design characteristics.

All in all, there seem to be no clear-cut answers to the question of tight versus loose strings. However, Jack Groppel, chairman of the United States Tennis Association's National Sport Science Committee, has found that the coefficient of restitution is greater for moderately and loosely strung rackets during on-center contact and is far superior when the impact is off-center (Groppel, 1987).

Tension and grip. Tension is not the only factor in rebound velocity; another factor affecting rebound is the firmness of the player's grip. Hatze (1993) found that with an on-center hit, a tight grip increased the coefficient of restitution slightly for both loosely and tightly strung rackets. The real advantage of a tight grip, however, occurs when contact is off-center. In an off-center contact, racket vibration increases significantly, but a tight grip enables the hand, arm, and body to damp this vibration. This increases velocity after impact because more energy is transferred to the ball and less is absorbed by racket vibration.

Tension and time. With continual use, a spring will eventually spring back more slowly. Similarly, the strings of a tennis racket eventually lose tension. If a tennis racket is initially strung at, say, 29.5 kilograms (65 lb.), in a year the tension may drop to 27.2 kilograms (60 lb.). Racket strings lose tension whether or not they are used—whether the racket is played with every day or sits in the closet—but of course more tension is lost with use. At a microscopic level, this loss occurs because the original tension exerts a stretching force on the strings that gradually breaks the molecular bonds (Brody, 1987). Thus the strings can no longer assume their original shape and are said to be permanently strained. Old strings are less elastic—they stretch without springing back—and therefore are less effective. This is why serious players regularly restring their rackets (*see also ARCHERY and EQUIPMENT MATERIALS*).

Thickness of Strings

Tennis racket strings have been made from literally hundreds of different natural materials (such as catgut) and synthetic materials (such as nylon). Manufacturers of various string materials naturally make claims about superior playability, but there is actually little evidence to suggest that any one material is better than another. For example, Groppel (1987) found that in oversize and midsize rackets the string material did not result in any clear advantage; in particular, gut (which is more expensive) was not superior to nylon. Thus many experts believe that recreational players, at least, would be wiser to concern themselves less with materials and more with the thickness—the gauge—of strings.

Strings come in three thicknesses: 15-, 16-, and 17-gauge. The thickest is 15-gauge string, which is 12 percent thicker than 16-gauge; in turn, 16-gauge is 11 percent thicker than 17-gauge. How strings of different thicknesses play is not directly related to thickness; rather, it is related to the area of cross-section: to how much string area overlaps. If string thickness is increased by 11 percent, the area of cross-section increases approximately twice as much, about 22 percent. This area of cross-section determines strength, durability, stretch, and elasticity—how quickly the strings rebound (Brody, 1987). Thicker strings are of course stronger and more durable, but they stretch less and are less elastic; thinner strings stretch more and are more elastic.

Elasticity is the most important factor in playability: it is the elasticity of strings that determines "feel," the player's sense of control over the shot. For an on-center shot, the longer the ball remains on the strings, the greater the accuracy and the greater the likelihood of imparting the desired spin to the ball.

Selecting the thickness of strings therefore comes down to choosing between durability and playability: thick strings are more durable, but thin strings are more playable. A player who is unlikely to break strings, or who does not mind breaking them regularly and often, is better off with thin gauge. However, "blasters" and players who use exaggerated spin are better off with medium or large gauge.

Tennis Shots

This section will consider various aspects of tennis shots, beginning with spin—an important part of the game, and of the related sports science.

Principles of Spin

The most obvious advantage of the large racket head, as noted earlier, is a decrease in mishits—off-center impacts where the ball hits the strings and then the frame. This is true of both flat shots and shots with spin, but the effect is more important with spin.

In a flat shot—a shot without spin—the racket is moving along the horizontal plane, close to the ball's line of flight. Because the racket is swung on the same horizontal plane as the ball, the ball strikes and leaves the strings in the same spot. Thus, even if the racket's line on the ball is inaccurate, string contact is still likely to be somewhere near the center.

By contrast, in a spin shot—topspin (forward spin), underspin (backspin), or slice (exaggerated underspin or sidespin)—the ball strikes the racket at one spot on the strings, spins across them, and leaves from another spot. Spin requires the racket head to move not only in a horizontal plane but also in a vertical plane, either up or down. Precise timing is required so that the racket head will meet the ball at the proper height; even a slight miscalculation can cause a mishit, sending the ball off in an unwanted direction, with a flight path like that of a knuckleball. (If such a shot does somehow land in-court, however, it will bounce unpredictably and will thus be extremely difficult to return.)

Applying spin reduces the margin for error in making contact with the strings, and also makes it more likely that the ball will carom off the frame, though a larger (wider) racket head gives a greater margin of error at contact and reduces the probability that the ball will contact

Will High-Tech Rackets Put an End to Tennis Elbow?

When a tennis player returns a ball traveling at 150 kilometers per hour (92 MPH), the force of the impact is comparable to that experienced by a weight lifter trying to jerk-lift 75 kilograms (170 lb.). When this is multiplied by the number of strokes in a match, there is obviously a substantial amount of repetitive stress. In addition, whether the ball is hit off-center or on-center, the racket vibrates; and whatever vibrational energy is not absorbed by the racket is, of course, absorbed by the hand, arm, and elbow. Tennis elbow, a form of overuse tendinitis, results from the inability of the muscles, tendons, and joints in the arm to effectively absorb vibrational energy from the tennis racket (see also SHOULDER, ELBOW, AND WRIST).

Tennis elbow is not caused by the racket, although a racket can compound the problem. Many studies have shown that tennis elbow is most prevalent among novice players whose technique is poor. In particular, it is the weekend hacker's backhand technique that causes most cases of tennis elbow: the shoulder is raised, the forearm is slightly flexed, and the tip of the elbow is pointed toward the net.

A hacker is also more likely than a good player to hit off-center, and the physicist Howard Brody has found that the oscillation, or vibration, caused by a ball hit at the sweet spot is different from the vibration caused by an off-center hit: the off-center hit creates much more high-frequency vibration (see the figure). This higher-frequency vibration causes much greater stress on the joints of the hand and arm.

Another major factor in tennis elbow is frequency of play. Forty-five percent of recreational players who play daily develop symptoms of tennis elbow, compared with 7 percent of those who play only two or three times a month (Adrian, 1989). Obviously, the more often poorer players play tennis, the more they use poor form, and the more off-center hits they make.

Even among very good players, there is considerable potential for tennis elbow. During a serve by a male professional, racket velocity can reach 500 to 560 kilometers per hour (300–350 MPH). On impact, the kinetic energy of the swing is absorbed in the elastic deformation of ball and racket, and the speed of the racket head is abruptly reduced to 240 KPH (150 MPH)—or less, if a hit is off-center. This is a massive deceleration for the body to absorb.

The new composite rackets greatly reduce the vibrational energy that the muscles and joints must "damp," or "dampen"; thus in theory, cases of tennis elbow should decline as these rackets replace older rackets, and as even newer designs are developed. There are several reasons why the new rackets reduce vibration.

First, the larger-head composite rackets have a larger sweet spot: this means fewer off-center hits.

Second, "dwell time"—contact time of strings and ball—is increased. This means that vibrations are less intense because they are spread out over a longer period.

Third, the newer rackets allow looser stringing. Looser strings do not require as hard a swing; and when the swing is less hard, the chance of making contact in the sweet spot increases greatly.

Fourth, with the new rackets, the risk of tennis elbow can be reduced by installing a small vibration "damper" in the strings near the throat of the racket. (Such a device does indeed damp string vibrations, although it does nothing to damp frame vibrations.)

According to the manufacturers, there is also a fifth way in which these rackets reduce vibration: by improvements in grips and the grip-racket

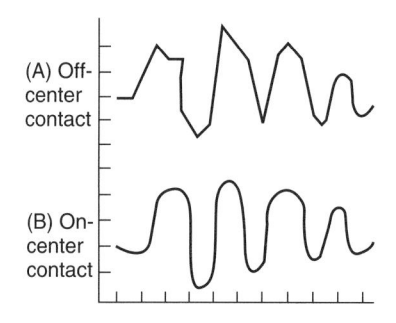

(a) An off-center contact (near the tip of the racket) creates higher-frequency (less smooth) vibrations than (b) an on-center contact. These higher-frequency vibrations send a painful "chattering" vibration up the arm. (Source: Adapted from Brody, 1987)

the frame as it leaves the racket. How far the ball slides across the racket depends on the swing and the dwell time of the ball on the strings. Players who use a lot of spin usually string their rackets more tightly to reduce dwell time. This decreases the distance the ball moves across the strings and consequently increases their margin for error.

Developing a variety of spin shots is an important part of a well-interface. However, this claim has been questioned by scientists, who point out that the hand (mostly because of its location)—not any materials built into the frame—damps most vibration (Brody, 1995). Some players help the hand damp vibrations by using a spongy grip overlay. Such overlays are actually designed primarily to absorb sweat (which can cause the hand to slip), but they also damp some vibrational energy.

Few studies have been conducted to determine the prevalence of tennis elbow among players using the new rackets, but there does seem to be a decline in incidence. In the early 1980s, it was estimated that 20 to 30 percent of professionals had tennis elbow, but by 1990 the estimate had dropped to only about 10 to 20 percent (Sobel, Pettrone, and Nirschl, 1990). This significant decline can certainly be attributed in large part to improvements in rackets. For all tennis players, the incidence of tennis elbow has also declined, though not as much as among professionals.

As noted above, the incidence of tennis elbow will probably continue to decline as more and more damping technology is incorporated into tennis rackets. For example, in a racket called the Kinetic (maufactured by ProKennex) the German aircraft engineer Roland Sommer adapted technology used to reduce flutter on aircraft wings and rudders (*see the figure*).

Around the head of the Kinetic are 100 hollow plastic chambers arranged in two-by-two grids, each chamber holding 100 free-flowing microbearings made from powdered metal oxides. The plastic weighs about 2 grams (0.07 oz.) and the microbearings weigh about 8 grams (0.28 oz.) total. The free-flowing bearings will always shift in the opposite direction of racket acceleration. Thus as the player moves the racket forward, the microbearings gather at the back of the chamber. On impact with the ball, as the strings deform and the racket flexes backward and vibrates, the microbearings shift forward.

The Kinetic operates on the same principle that makes drivers of tractor-trailer tankers avoid traveling with much less than a full load. A tanker carrying, say, only half a load is very difficult to stop because of the inertia of the liquid, which surges forward when the driver hits the brakes. In the Kinetic, this effect is an advantage: the bearings continue forward as the racket flexes backward, and their inertia imparts more energy to the ball, expands the racket's sweet spot, and damps vibrations—particularly for off-center shots. A study at the Massachusetts of Technology found that the Kinetic reduced shock by 20 percent, reduced vibration by 43 percent, and expanded the sweet spot by 12 to 15 percent (Sandomir, 1995).

Despite racket technology, tennis elbow is likely to remain fairly prevalent among recreational players who do not hit the ball on the sweet spot and may sometimes even hit it off the frame. There is not much to be done to rehabilitate the elbow, except rest. One of the few available options is manipulating and stretching exercises to increase the flexibility of the muscles and tendons around the elbow. These exercises will not cure tennis elbow, but they do reduce the pain associated with it (*see also SHOULDER, ELBOW, AND WRIST; and REHABILITIATION*).

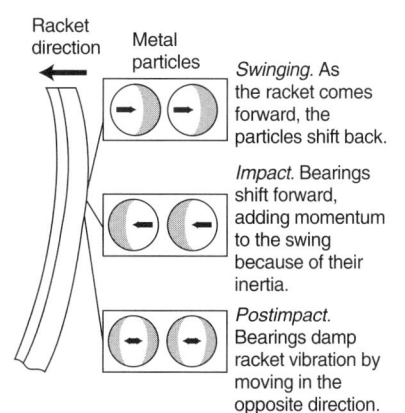

The ProKennex kinetic racket. (Adapted from Sandomir, 1995)

SELECTING A RACKET TO PREVENT TENNIS ELBOW

1. Midsize rather than oversize (for less off-center shot torque).

2. Graphite or fiberglass composite (aluminum is worst).

3. Well-balanced, medium-weight frame (not unbalanced or lightweight).

4. String tension at lower end of manufacturer's recommended range.

5. Large sweet spot.

6. Grip overlay and string-damping technology.

John Zumerchik

rounded game: well-executed kick serves, chip approaches, and topspin lobs are all very useful excessive-spin shots. In fact, however, every shot is affected to some degree by spin. Even when a ball is hit with no spin (flat), its contact with the court surface will create forward spin—that is, topspin—because at the moment of contact the bottom of the ball is slowed down by friction.

"Spaghetti" Rackets

The oddest spins tennis has seen so far were those produced by the spagehtti racket. The ingenious designer, a German, took a standard-size racket, fitted it with double strings, and wove plastic tubes and other objects around the strings. "Spaghetti" rackets were not only bizarre to look at but generated some bizarre bounces: for instance, a topspin lob that landed near the baseline might easily bounce extremely high—far over the opponent's reach—and off into the stands. American officials hurriedly added a new provision to the liberal rule allowing rackets "of any material, weight, size, or shape"; they specified that attachments to the racket must not alter the flight of the ball and that the strings must be evenly spaced.

Topspin

When a player deliberately hits a shot with topspin, it will slow down less on contact than a ball hit flat. This effect is so pronounced that the ball looks as though it were jumping forward—picking up speed. To repeat, this is an illusion: what really happens is simply that the ball does not slow down as much. However, a topspin shot does actually bounce higher than a flat or underspin shot. Howard Brody studied spin and height of bounce and found that at the same rate of spin (32 revolutions/sec.) a topspin shot bounced (on average) 24 percent higher than an underspin shot (Brody, 1987). This is because a ball hit with topspin curves in flight, giving the ball greater vertical velocity, which in turn results in a higher bounce.

For spectators, the topspin lob is one of the most exciting shots in tennis. It is typically used when an opponent has made a good approach (aggressive shot) and closes in on the net. To return such a shot, it is usually necessary to stretch to reach the ball—a weak position. Instead of directing a shot toward the net, then, where the opponent would probably be able to put it away easily, it is often more effective to flick a topspin lob over the opponent's head. Once a topspin lob clears an opponent's head, pursuing it is usually futile, because on landing it will bounce away at a high speed.

Using topspin, particularly for a lob, has three major advantages: (1) There is greater margin for error; (2) The trajectory of the shot makes it more difficult for an opponent to reach; (3) After bouncing, the ball carries away at a fast speed.

To determine the effectiveness of topspin, Brody (1987) calculated the speed needed to make an underspin shot, a flat shot, and a topspin shot land at the same point, if they are hit from the same point at the same angle (*see Figure 3*). Brody calculated that to land in-court, a backspin shot from the baseline could not be hit at a velocity greater than 125 KPH (78 MPH), but a topspin shot could be hit at about 160 KPH (100 MPH) and still land inside the baseline. For a waist-high 107-KPH (67-MPH) shot from the baseline, a topspin shot had almost four times more margin for error than a backspin shot. To put this another way, Brody found that the ball hit with topspin came back to earth fastest. It follows that the harder a player wants to hit a ball, the more important it is to apply topspin.

By applying tremendous topspin, big hitters—like Pete Sampras and Andre Agassi in the mid-1990s—can hit the ball with nearly their own maximum physical force. Topspin is also recommended for recreational players. It is admittedly a difficult skill to master, but heavy topspin is not necessary to improve one's game—even slight topspin will significantly increase the margin for error.

Touch Shots

In the 1990s, traditionalists often complained that most tennis players no longer used touch shots, such as drop shots and soft, sharply angled volleys. They felt that men's tennis had turned into a shooting match.

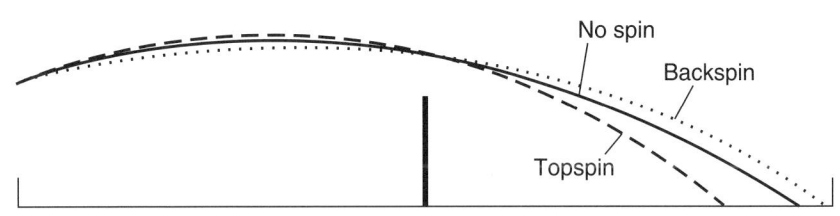

Figure 3. *Brody calculated the effect of topspin (16 revolutions/sec.), underspin (16 revolutions/sec.), and no spin on the flight of a tennis ball. (Source: Brody, 1987)*

Here, each ball is hit waist high, and at the same speed (107 KPH, 67 MPH). For the same net clearance, the topspin shot bounces shortest and gives the greatest margin for error—that is, the best chance to keep the ball in the court. The backspin shot bounces the deepest in the court and thus has the least margin for error (the least chance to keep the ball in the court).

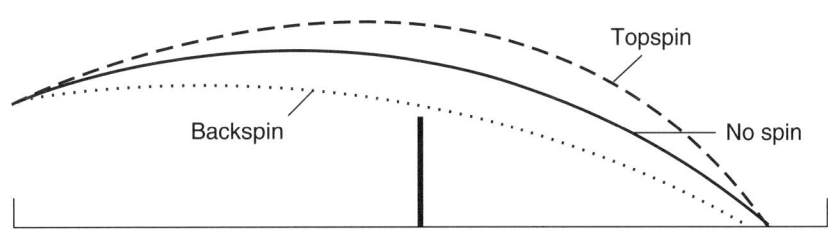

Here, each ball leaves the racket at the same speed but lands at the same spot in the backcourt. There is a considerable difference in the margin of error for net clearance. The topspin shot clears the net by the most and gives the greatest margin for error; the backspin shot clears the net by the least and gives the smallest margin for error.

Keeping Tennis Balls Cool

Fact 1: On a cold day, a tennis ball becomes noticeably slower: a cold ambient temperature lowers the air pressure inside the ball, reducing its rebound velocity.

Fact 2: A new ball has the greatest coefficient of restitution (rebound velocity) when the can is first opened; through play, it gradually loses some pressure, and this causes its coefficient of restitution to fall. These two facts explain why during a tennis tournament, the balls are kept in a cooler, or at least out of the sun, until they are used. The balls will play more consistently throughout nine games (the standard interval on the professional tour) if kept in a cooler beforehand. As the balls lose pressure through play, this is offset somewhat by the fact that they are warming up.

John McEnroe, in the 1980s, is often cited as the last champion with a full range of touch shots. Not coincidentally, McEnroe was also the last great champion to use a wooden racket. In a touch shot, the player makes contact with a ball traveling at high velocity and returns it at a very low velocity; this is done by damping—absorbing—most of the energy from the initial velocity, and damping requires a coordinated effort by the racket and the body's muscles and joints. Because wooden rackets have much greater flex and are heavier than composite rackets, the ball remains on the strings longer; hence, it is much easier to return a ball with a soft touch. A wooden racket, having a much smaller sweet spot, also increases the probability of a mishit—and some of the worst off-center hits turn out to be effective drop shots. An off-center hit reduces the coefficient of restitution by increasing the recoil impulse of the racket or the twisting of the frame, or both. It is possible, then, that the touch shots favored by earlier players were a reflection of the kind of rackets they were using.

Baseline Shots and the Margin of Error

Commentators announcing televised tennis matches often explain a missed shot by saying that the player "tried to hit too good a shot." What they mean is that the player did not allow enough margin for error. It is clear from statistics why players need to leave themselves a margin for error: about 66 percent of all points are determined by someone's mistake, and in about 75 percent of these the ball fails to clear the net (Hensley, 1979)

One way to leave a margin for error, as already discussed, is to use topspin. The other factors in making a shot are the height of the ball at contact, the position at contact, and the velocity at which the ball is struck.

Regardless of the velocity of a shot, for ground strokes made at waist height or lower, the margin for error increases the farther back the player is in the court. In other words, the farther back the player is standing, the safer these shots become. One reason for this is that even the best players cannot precisely control the vertical angle at which the ball comes off the racket: it will always vary at least a few degrees from what is intended. Some balls will take a trajectory higher than intended; some will take a trajectory lower than intended. At a given speed, then, because of the variability of this rebound angle, the safer ground strokes are those taken farther back behind the baseline (endline).

Two other reasons for playing farther behind the baseline are that this gives the player more time to prepare for the opponent's approaching shot, and it gives air resistance more time to slow down the approaching shot.

Note, however, that stepping back farther from the baseline to create a margin for error is appropriate only for ground strokes taken at a relatively low contact point. Obviously, an overhead smash (to mention one counterexample) is much more likely to go in if it is made near the net than if it is made from the baseline.

Accuracy: Controlling Shots

Some people have the mistaken idea that the direction a ball will take is determined by the direction in which the player is facing—that is, by the player's stance. In fact, what determines where the ball goes is the angle of the racket face and the direction of racket velocity at contact. A shot will be "off course" (going too far left or too far right) when a player misjudges the speed of the incoming ball and therefore swings too early or too late.

A swing in tennis can be described as an arc of a circle; somewhere along this arc, the racket makes contact with the ball. An early swing will "pull" the ball; a late swing will drive the ball off course in the other direction. Even average players usually have little problem timing contact in a rally (an exchange of shots) where the pace is controlled; but as soon as the opponent puts pressure on them—by hitting harder or by hitting shots that must be run down—the probability of mistiming increases dramatically. The same is true when players swing harder to try to increase the pace of their own shots. Accuracy and control can be improved by increasing the swing radius: lengthening the swing reduces errors in timing.

The swing radius is greatest at the shoulder, smaller at the elbow, and shortest at the wrist (*see Figure 4*). Because of this, coaches advise generating most of the power at the shoulder. Almost all professionals use a bent-elbow forehand, which would seem to shorten the radius of the swing. But because they straighten the elbow as the racket comes forward to hit the ball, it actually lengthens the arc of the swing. Many professionals also use considerable wrist action. For recreational players, however, imitating the professionals' wrist snap can be disastrous because wrist action requires extraordinary timing: the small swing radius allows very little margin of error. Professionals can use wrist action safely because they practice enough to develop consistent timing, but recreational players can rarely achieve this. For most players, then, a firm wrist minimizes timing errors.

Keeping the wrist firm and enlarging the swing radius—lengthening the arc—will greatly reduce the chance of horizontal angular errors. To further increase swing radius, players should begin their swing with the elbow somewhat bent and let it straighten as they follow through. Keeping the elbow slightly bent gives the added advantage of being able to adjust the swing, and knowing what direction the ball will take makes it possible to hit with more power.

Serving

Tennis is unique in that the server gets two chances to put the serve in. This leads many players to reason as follows: "I might as well go for broke and blast my first serve. If it's in, I'll probably win the point outright; if not, I'll 'dink' the second serve in and play the point." This does make sense at some level, but it is by no means a universal principle on which to base a service strategy. Following are some factors to be taken into account.

One factor is the player's height. The taller the player—more precisely, the higher the contact point—the greater the probability of getting the serve in: that is, the higher the ball is hit, the greater the margin of error. Moreover, as the speed at which the ball is hit increases, the more important height becomes. Consider, for example, three velocities for a flat serve hit down the middle of the court: 107, 144, and 179 KPH (67, 90, and 112 MPH). Brody (1987) calculated that a flat serve hit at 179 KPH from a height of 2 meters (80 in.) has no chance of going in; at 136 KPH (85 MPH) a serve from that height still has only a slight chance of going in. However, if the ball is hit at 136 KPH from a height of 2.6 meters (105 in.), the chance that it will go in is increased by 400 percent. For many players, height of contact—hitting the ball at 2.6 meters, say, rather than 2 meters—can be controlled by adjusting the swing. By reaching overhead for the ball instead of hitting the ball close to the head or out to the side, many players can significantly improve their serving percentages.

Another factor is spin: applying a little topspin can greatly increase the probability that a serve will go in. In fact, the effect of topspin is so great that a short player who hits the ball with topspin from a height of 2 meters is more likely to get the serve in than a taller player hitting a flat serve from a height of 2.6 meters. A topspin serve crosses the net with more clearance and bounces shorter than a serve with no spin.

Still another factor is where the server stands. For most players

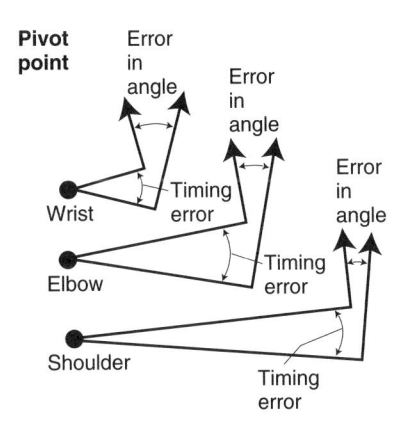

Figure 4. *The larger the radius of a swing, the smaller the angle of error; therefore any given error in timing—either an early or a late swing—results in a less dramatic error. Wrist, elbow, and shoulder are the three major pivot points or axes of rotation. Most instructors warn against using too much wrist action, because the wrist has the most potential for a timing miscue—a large angle of error.*

Shuttlecock: The Fastest and Slowest Projectile in Sports

An unusual Indian game called *poona* was brought to England around 1860 by men returning from service in the colonial army. With a few changes, the game—renamed badminton—quickly became popular and spread to other English-speaking countries, including the United States, Canada, and Australia. Today, badminton is immensely popular in Europe and in some parts of Asia, particularly southeast Asia, where it is a fiercely competitive sport.

The badminton racket resembles a tennis racket, although it is much lighter in weight. Unlike the other racket sports, however, badminton is played not with a ball but with a unique object called a "shuttlecock," "shuttle," "bird," or "birdie." The shuttlecock consists of a half-round cork head 2.5 to 2.6 centimeters (1 to 1 1/18 in.) in diameter, with 14 to 16 feathers embedded in its flat surface. The feathers rise like a crown, forming a circle 6.25 centimeters (2 1/2 in.) in diameter at the top. A shuttlecock weighs only 5.12 grams (0.011 lb.). All this gives it unique aerodynamic properties that make the game of badminton far different from other racket sports.

Another feature that sets badminton apart from, say, tennis and table tennis, is that the shuttle must remain airborne during play—much like a volleyball. Players do not have the option of playing the shuttle off a bounce: when the "birdie" lands, the point ends. This makes the game extremely fast-paced. Also—again as in volleyball—points can be earned only on serve. In a game involving equal players, the scoreboard often remains unchanged during endless "side-outs."

Paradoxically, the badminton shuttle has the distinction of being the fastest as well as the slowest projectile in sports. To understand this, it is useful to consider the concept of terminal velocity—perhaps the most important quantity used in studying the aerodynamic properties of projectiles. The terminal velocity of an object is its limiting speed in a free fall under gravity; this velocity can be calculated or experimentally determined for projectiles of all kinds, from rockets and satellites to cannonballs to sports projectiles. Whatever its initial speed, a falling object will, given enough time, eventually attain its terminal velocity. Specifically, if the object is moving at less or more than its terminal velocity, it will speed up or slow down to this limiting speed.

Terminal velocity depends on air resistance, which is a function of the mass and the cross-sectional area of an object. Because of its unique construction, a shuttlecock has a small mass but a large effective cross-sectional area (measured at the top of the feathers); thus it encounters the greatest air resistance for its mass, and this means that it decelerates rapidly during flight. Consequently, the terminal velocity of the shuttle is only 24.3 KPH (15.2 MPH). This makes the shuttle the slowest free-falling object of all sports projectiles—for example, it is more than 20 times slower than the heavier, denser shot (*see table*).

In an overhead smash by a world-class badminton player, the shuttle is "fired" off the racket strings at a scorching velocity—often exceeding 320 KPH (200 MPH), or 90 meters (297 ft.) per second. This is—to take one example—almost twice as fast as a tennis player can hit a ball. But air resistance quickly applies the brakes, slowing the shuttle down dramatically in a fraction of a second. This near-instantaneous change in the velocity of a shuttlecock, from very fast to very slow, seems almost incredible to many observers.

In addition to the peculiarites of the shuttlecock, the badminton racket

Projectile	Weight (lb.)	Diameter (in.)	Drag factor (ft.$^{-1}$ estimated)	Terminal speed (MPH)
16-pound shot	16.0	4.72	0.00014	325
Baseball	0.32	2.90	0.0016	95
Golf ball	0.1	1.68	0.0018	90
Tennis ball	0.13	2.56	0.0030	70
Squash ball	0.07	1.77	0.0048	55
Volleyball	0.59	8.43	0.012	35
Ping-Pong ball	0.006	1.47	0.037	20
Shuttlecock	0.011	2.50	0.064	15

who do not hit the ball extremely hard—less than 144 KPH (90 MPH)—a position closer to the alleys should, theoretically, improve serving percentages. The reason is that air resistance will slow the ball down more and thus cause it to fall sooner after clearing the net. However, serving right on the baseline—trying to get as close to the service court as possible—is an advantage only for powerful servers,

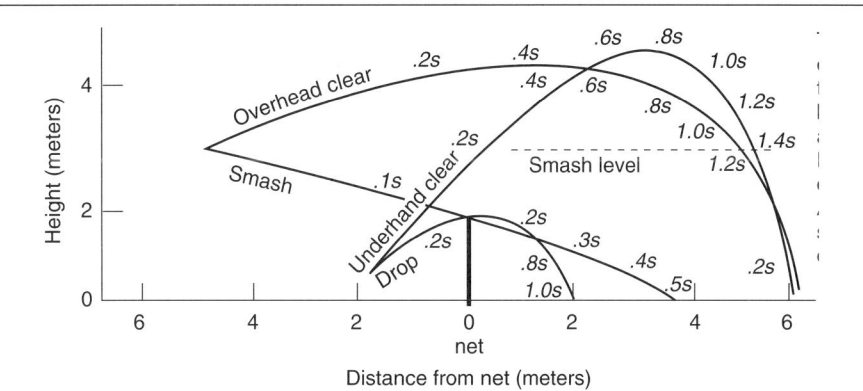

Typical velocities and trajectories for the smash, drop shot, underhand, and overhand clear. The two deep clear shots are excellent for defense because of their less-than-parabolic trajectories and their airborne time (1.1 to 1.4 seconds). Keeping the shuttle between 5 and 6 meters deep during clears is optimal and usually not difficult. Any clear shot that stays airborne for over 1 second gives ample time to assume a good defensive position.

is also of interest: its extreme lightness is what makes the blazing shuttle speeds possible. The rotation speed of a badminton racket is three times that of a tennis racket (Adrian and Cooper, 1989), and the technique used to accelerate it is similar to snapping a whip.

The body movement starts from the trunk and proceeds through the arm and the wrist to the racket strings, where contact with the birdie occurs. Timing, coordination, flexibility, and agility—more than sheer strength—are of paramount importance in achieving a fluid swing that can generate the very high racket speeds.

Watching the unique flight path of the shuttle once it leaves the racket is a pleasure. Because the shuttle encounters so much air resistance, its path deviates significantly from the near-parabolic path of the more familiar ball projectile with low air drag. A shuttle lofted high into the air will descend almost vertically, reaching a very slow velocity—almost a crawl—near its terminal speed. To gauge the flight path of the shuttle so that they can position themselves appropriately, players must rely on their understanding of and feel for the effects of air drag.

The trajectories of the basic strokes in badminton can be graphed (see the figure). The overhand and underhand "clear" shots are defensive strokes lobbed deep into the opponent's backcourt. They are an integral part of the game and are used often because they give a player more time to get into position and more time to react to the opponent's next stroke, since it will be coming from farther away. Also, a backcourt smash by the opponent rarely becomes a kill, thanks to the shuttle's aerobraking. During a point, several "clearing" or "recovery" shots can be made safely, keeping an opponent deep in the backcourt without jeopardizing the point by giving the opponent an opportunity to attack. By contrast, the defensive lob in tennis is a low-percentage shot, almost a desperation shot: unless it is executed with perfect timing and trajectory, it is usually smashed back by the opponent for an easy winner.

In badminton, a well-executed defensive clear lets the player switch quickly from defense to offense; this gives the game an added dimension and makes a match between two evenly matched opponents spectacular to watch. The paradoxical "fast-slow" nature of the shuttle also contributes to the fascination of the game. Players must make split-second decisions when reaching for smashes but must also exercise judicious patience when waiting for a floating "bird" to fall. Badminton involves tracking and contacting a shuttle that is moving at ever-changing velocities, and thus it demands the utmost in visual acuity, dexterity, and foot and hand speed.

Unlike most sports, badminton favors light, agile players—players who can move forward, backward, and sideways with great efficiency. According to one of Newton's laws, the heavier a body, the more force is needed to change its direction. It is not surprising, then, that the vast majority of top badminton players are lean.

Arjun Tan

and even for them it is at best a slight advantage. Brody calculated that for a 179-KPH (112-MPH) serve, if the player crowds up to the baseline instead of remaining 2.5 centimeters (1 in.) back, the chance of getting the serve in will be improved by just 1 more time per 100 tries. (In comparison, using topspin might result in an improvement of 2 or 3 times per 100 tries.)

Surface Effects

The "grand slam" in tennis consists of Wimbledon and the French, United States, and Australian opens. Very few players, even the greatest champions, have been able to win the grand slam, because these tournaments are played on different surfaces: the French Open is played on clay; Wimbledon is on grass; the Australian and United States Opens (although they were originally on grass) are now on composition. In tennis, the outcome of a match is highly dependent on the court surface; rarely, for instance, will a player be able to win on both the slow red clay at the French Open and the lightning-fast grass at Wimbledon.

How the tennis ball loses speed at the bounce is a combination of its angle at landing and the coefficient of friction (*see also* BOWLING). On a low-friction surface, like grass, the ball loses only a small amount of its forward speed. On a high-friction surface, like clay, the ball loses much more of its forward speed—as much as 40 percent. For lobs, there is actually very little difference between a slow and a fast surface with regard to the speed of the ball after the bounce, because the ball has landed at a high angle. But for low-trajectory shots, the contact time between ball and surface is shorter; consequently, on a high-friction surface the ball is less likely to roll after the bounce. Another effect of surface friction is the angle of rebound. Rebound is greater on a higher-friction (slow) court, like clay, than on a low-friction (fast) court, like grass. On a fast surface, a slice or an underspin shot seems to slide or skip, especially if the court is dusty (*see Figure 5*).

Playing on fast and slow courts is probably the single most difficult adjustment a touring professional must make. In fact, some players cannot adjust to different surfaces; they remain clay-court or grass-court specialists throughout their careers. Clay-court specialists are usually steady baseline players; they prefer a slow surface because a point tends to last longer (the players can run down more balls), and powerful serves and ground strokes are less effective. Grass-court specialist are usually big servers and volleyers who feel more comfortable on a court where it is easier to hit a ball out of an opponent's reach; they want to win each point quickly by overpowering the opponent.

Many recreational players find clay courts particularly enjoyable. Although recreational players (in the United States, at least) seldom encounter grass, there are other fast recreational surfaces, including concrete and asphalt-base courts. Clay offers two distinct advantages over these surfaces. First, clay is a softer surface and is thus less painful to the joints. Second, as a softer—and more porous—surface, clay slows the ball more, allowing the player more time to get to it.

However, clay also changes the dynamics of the ball-string collision. As a match proceeds, the balls get heavier and heavier because they collect more and more clay particles. The weather is a significant factor in this effect: humidity will make the ball even heavier. The

Figure 5. *Whatever the spin of the ball on contact with the surface, the force of friction creates a rotating force in the direction the ball was hit. The way the ball bounces is affected by four factors: (1) its velocity, (2) its angle of approach to the court, (3) its spin, and (4) the court surface. These four factors are all interrelated, making it difficult to generalize about the angle of reflection (R) on the basis of angle of incidence (I).*

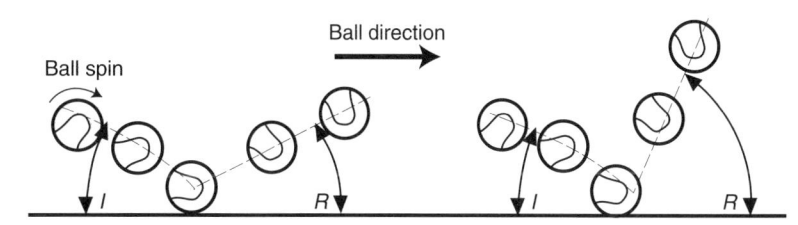

Left: In theory, a topspin ball should dip downward and bounce off at a smaller angle than it approached. *Right:* But in practice, excessive spin or a high-friction court (like clay) can send the ball upward at a much steeper angle than it came down.

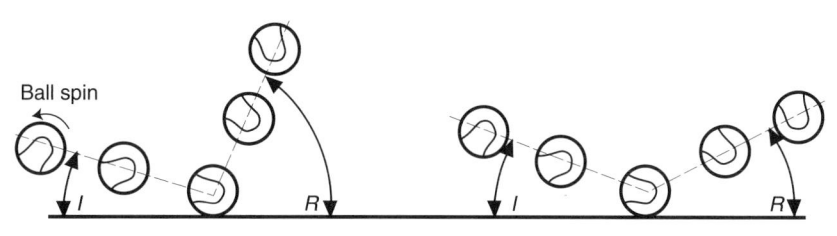

Left: In theory, an underspin ball should "grip" the court and cause a steeper upward bounce than the angle at which it came down. *Right:* But in practice, a high velocity and a low angle of approach can cause the ball to bounce upward at a very low angle, especially on a fast asphalt surface.

heavier the ball, the longer the ball-string dwell time; and increased dwell time increases the coefficient of restitution. This tendency of the ball to become heavier means that the player must make some adjustment. A player who ordinarily has a racket strung at, say, 27.2 kilograms (60 lb.) for use on a hard court might consider increasing the tension to 28.5 to 29.5 kilograms (63 to 65 lb.) for a clay court.

Biomechanics

Recreational players often spend considerable time and money taking tennis lessons to improve the mechanics of the swing; this is a good idea, but unfortunately many of them want to imitate a favorite professional—which is not always a good idea. For example, as noted earlier, a professional like Andre Agassi can use tremendous wrist snap for ground strokes; but the wrist snap requires such a high degree of precision, acquired through extensive practice, that it is not within the scope of a beginner or even an intermediate player. Recreational players should develop their own strokes, strokes that adhere to basic physical principles.

Biomechanics of the Serve

For many recreational tennis players, the serve is the most neglected—and least practiced—stroke. This is illogical, because the serve is very important. It is meant to put the ball into play, and it can significantly shape the play of a point. Moreover, a good serve can be the only stroke in a point—an outright winner—and a double fault (failure to put in both the first and the second service) is of course an outright loser. Professionals, obviously, focus intensely on the serve. On the men's tour, the majority of players consistently serve over 175 KPH (110 MPH), and some serve well over 190 KPH (120 MPH). Such speeds are particularly impressive because the velocity of a serve must be generated entirely by the swing of the racket; the toss-up adds no horizontal momentum.

The key to a good serve is developing a fluid swing. A good service looks effortless: it is a smooth coordination of body segments in a sequence that produces optimal racket position, trajectory, and velocity at impact. The upper limbs must be coordinated with the lower limbs, and acceleration must take place smoothly through the lower limbs and trunk, the hips and shoulder, and finally the racket arm to produce maximum velocity at impact. As in other sports involving a swing, the impact occurs after the racket has reached its maximum velocity.

The serving motion in tennis is often compared to the pitching motion in baseball, and it is sometimes argued that in order to serve well, a player must be able to throw well. However, although the same muscles are used to execute a serve and a pitch, both the range of motions and the sequence and timing of muscle activity vary tremendously. One major difference is that in a serve there is a pause beween bursts of muscle activity. This pause occurs after the knees bend and the server rocks back on the rear foot, and for almost all world-class players it is a vital part of the rhythm of a serve. It gives the center of gravity a chance to move forward as the knees and back extend (straighten) and the shoulder rotates.

This coordinated kinetic chain culminates with a powerful wrist snap that greatly accelerates the racket. The wrist snap is another difference between serving and pitching: a strong wrist snap is more important for servers than pitchers because the racket, in effect, is an extended lever. Tennis players often fail to develop a strong wrist snap, but this snap is critical to the velocity of the racket. The angular velocity of the wrist has been measured at 1,087 degrees (slightly more than 3 revolutions) per second just before impact (Jack et al., 1979), and since racket velocity at this point is 2,200 degrees per second, the velocity of the wrist is a large part of the total. (Wrist velocity quickly drops to 600 degrees per second at 0.1 second into the follow-through.)

At ball contact, the center of gravity varies, depending on the serve: for world-class players, it is about 25 centimeters (10 in.) forward of the front toe in a flat serve, and 41.5 centimeters (16.6 in.) forward in a slice or kick serve (Smith, 1979). Hyperextending the back accounts for most of this difference (*see also* FIELD ATHLETICS: JUMPING).

A slice or kick serve—typically used for the second serve—requires a more exaggerated back bend than the flat first service because the racket is used to "peel" the ball rather than pass straight through it. The swipe across the back of the ball (which is analogous to peeling an apple) results in a longer dwell time than occurs with a flat serve.

Holding the center of gravity back over the rear foot also brings the body's center of gravity farther into the court, and at a lower plane, which makes it possible to close in on the net rapidly. For instance, the Swedish superstar Stefan Edberg, perhaps the best player of the early 1990s, "crowded" the service line, and used a very exaggerated hyperextended back motion for his slice and kick serves; his center of gravity was already far out over the court by the time the ball left the strings. It was widely acknowledged that no one closed in on the net faster after serving than Edberg.

Circular versus Straight Forehand

Before the modern era of tennis, almost all tennis players used a straight-back motion for the forehand. In the mid-1960s, however—around the beginning of the modern era—players began experimenting with a sweeping circular-motion forehand. For example, John Newcombe, a legendary Australian of that time, had an exaggerated motion that he affectionately called a "buggy whip."

In the 1990s, almost all professionals were using a circular motion similar to Newcombe's. The circular forehand stroke maintains the momentum of the racket, making it easier to increase velocity as the racket moves through the backswing. In comparison, a straight-back forehand requires a stop-and-start motion in which the player must overcome inertia (the racket's tendency to remain in motion) when bringing the racket to a stop, and then overcome inertia again when starting the racket forward (because now the racket has a tendency to remain at rest).

A circular motion, therefore, does allow a player to generate more power. But it should be noted that without accuracy, this additional power really does not matter—a fact that is well known to tournament players.

One-Handed versus Two-Handed Backhand

The backhand is more difficult to master than the forehand because it is a less natural motion. The forehand has many similarities to a throwing motion and relies on the inner-arm muscles, which are very often used; the backhand relies on the outer-arm muscles, which are not used that often (*see also* SHOULDER, ELBOW, AND WRIST). The backhand also differs from the forehand because it requires a combination of forward body motion, rotation of the trunk at the hip joint, and rotation of the arm and racket from the shoulder.

It is often debated which is better, a one-handed or a two-handed backhand. (The two-handed backhand was introduced in the 1950s and was popularized in the early 1970s by Jimmy Connors and Chris Evert.) The two-handed backhand does have a significant disadvantage: it reduces the length of the lever; particularly, it reduces the distance a player can stretch for wide returns. However, that seems to be its only disadvantage. Studies have shown that the one-handed backhand does not offer any advantage except when the player is forced to stretch for a ball—although it should be noted that with regard to the relative accuracy of the one-hand and the two-hand stroke, studies done so far have been inconclusive.

Theoretically, a one-handed backhand should be able to generate more racket velocity, because the swing encompasses a larger arc. In practice, though, most people find it easier to generate velocity with a two-hand stroke, because two hands can produce greater momentum than one. The two-hand stroke is simpler and more compact: the hips and the trunk and upper limbs act as a single unit. In effect, the smaller swing arc of the two-hand stroke reduces the moment of inertia, allowing greater angular velocity. But the primary reason for the prominence of the two-hand backhand is that the one-hand stroke is harder for young players—it requires more strength, particularly wrist strength, to counteract torque (rotation about an axis) created by off-center hits. Evidently, the younger players are when they take up the game, the more likely they will be to use the two-hand stroke

Even for beginners, the difference between the two-handed and one-handed backhand is insignificant. All in all, neither stroke seems to be inherently superior. Given the differences among individuals in anatomy, physiology, and motor control, most coaches believe that the choice can be simply a matter of personal preference.

John Zumerchik

References

Adrian, M., and J. Cooper. *Biomechanics of Human Movement*. Indianapolis, Indiana: Benchmark, 1989.

Ariel, G., et al. "Biomechanical Analysis of Ballistic versus Tracking Movements in Tennis Skills." In J. Groppel (ed.), *Proceedings of the National Symposium of Racket Sports*. Champaign: University of Illinois, 1979.

Brody, H. "How Would a Physicist Design a Tennis Racket?" *Physics Today* 48, no. 3 (March 1995): 26–31.

Brody, H. *Tennis Science for Tennis Players*. Philadephia: University of Pennsylvania Press, 1987.

Elliot, B., and R. Kilderry. *The Art and Science of Tennis*. Philadelphia: Saunders, 1983.

Flink, S., "The Mechanics of a Power Serve." *Popular Mechanics* (September 1993).

Groppel, J, "Effects of Different String Tension Patterns and Racket Motion on Tennis Racket-Ball Impact." *International Journal of Sports Biomechanics* 3, no. 2 (1987): 142–158.

Groppel, J. *Tennis for Advanced Players and Those Who Would Like to Be*. Champaign, Illinois: Human Kinetics, 1984.

Hatze, H. "The Relationship between the Coefficient of Restitution and Energy Losses in Tennis Rackets." *Journal of Applied Biomechanics* 9, no. 2 (1993): 124–129.

Hensley, L. "Analysis of Stroking Errors Committed in Championship Tennis Competition." In J. Groppel (ed.), *Proceedings of the National Symposium of Racket Sports*. Champaign: University of Illinois, 1979.

Jack, M., et al. "Selected Aspects of the Overarm Stroke in Tennis, Badminton, Racketball, and Squash. " In J. Terauds (ed.), *Science of Racket Sports*. Del Mar, California: Academic, 1979.

Liu, Y. "Mechanical Analysis of Racket and Ball during Impact." *Journal of Medicince and Science in Sports and Exercise* 15, no. 5 (1983): 388–392.

Sandomir, R. "It's New, Costly, and High-Tech. Is It Better? Perhaps." *New York Times,* 19 February 1995, sec. 3, p. 9.

Smith, S. "Comparison of Selected Factors Associated with Flat and Slice Serves of Male Varsity Tennis Players." In J. Gropel (ed.), *Proceedings of the National Symposium of Racket Sports*. Champaign: University of Illinois, 1979.

Sobel, J., F. Pettrone, and R. Nirschl. "Prevention and Rehabilitation of Racket Sports Injuries." In J. Nicholas and J. Hershman (eds.), *The Upper Extremity in Sports Medicine*. St. Louis: Mosby, 1990.

Tan, A. "Shuttlecock Trajectories in Badminton." *Mathematical Spectrum* 19 (1986–1987): 33ff.

Terauds, J. (ed). *Science in Racquet Sports*. Del Mar, California: Academic, 1979.

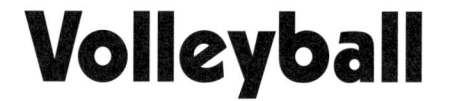

Volleyball

VOLLEYBALL WAS DEVELOPED around 1895, a few years after basketball. The inventor of volleyball, William Morgan (like James Naismith, who invented basketball), was looking for a new indoor sport for a YMCA gymnasium—in this case, in Holyoke, Massachusetts. Morgan invented volleyball as an alternative to calisthenics (which can become monotonous), indoor track events (which are difficult to stage), and gymnastics (which have a slow learning curve). The story is that he strung a tennis net across the gymnasium at a height of 7 feet (just over 2 m), divided a group of athletes into two teams, gave them a basketball bladder, and instructed them to use their hands to bat it back and forth over the net. The name *volleyball* was chosen because the ball is "volleyed" back and forth: that is, it remains in the air (the derivation is from the French *vol*, "flight"). At first, the rules of volleyball were quite simple: when one team knocked the ball out of bounds, or failed to get the ball over the net, or allowed the ball to drop to the ground, the other team won the point.

Volleyball caught on very quickly, flourishing in the midwest and along the Pacific coast. For some reason, Fort Wayne, Indiana—with a population of only 114,000—became a center of volleyball. By the mid-1930s, it had 200 organized teams and more than 8,000 players. During the Depression, volleyball was one of the most popular recreational sports. For one thing, it was portable: not only was it an excellent indoor sport, but a game could be put together quickly at a beach or park when the weather was warm enough. Also (as noted above), the rules were simple, and little equipment was needed.

In the 1950s and 1960s—as basketball, football, bowling, and golf became more prominent—the popularity of volleyball waned in the United States. But interest continued to grow overseas. During and after both world wars, Americans stationed abroad had helped to spread volleyball; in fact, this is in large part the reason that more than 30 countries now have teams in international competition.

Japan was one country that fell in love with the game. A Japanese women's team, Nichibo, dominated international volleyball for most of the 1960s and had one of the longest winning streaks in all sports: 150 matches. Nichibo also won the gold medal at the 1964 Olympics in Japan—the first Olympics to include both men's and women's volleyball.

In addition to the continuing interest abroad, in recent years television coverage of beach volleyball and Olympic competition has led to a resurgence of interest in volleyball in the United States. Along with Brazil, Cuba, and China—to name just a few examples—the United States now has excellent volleyball teams.

William Morgan would be surprised by the volleyball of the 1990s. The game is no longer a leisurely patting of a basketball bladder back and forth across a net but has evolved dramatically, showcasing powerful athletes with impressive skills who sprint, jump, and dive to keep the ball in play. Perhaps more than any other sport, "power" volleyball requires excellent teamwork. In basketball, a great player can dominate a game both offensively and defensively, ripping down a defensive rebound, speed-dribbling up the court, and scoring at the offensive end. Power volleyball is different. It is highly preferable—in fact, almost necessary—for two or three players to touch the ball every time it comes over the net: the ball moves from passer (digger) to setter to spiker. Blockers force opposing spikers to redirect the ball toward the digger, who is positioned to pass the ball to the setter; and the setter checks the opponent's defense and tries to select a spiker with the best chance of achieving a "kill."

Aerodynamics and the "Floater"

In volleyball (as in a number of other sports), the serve puts the ball into play and largely determines the offensive and defensive characteristics of the point. A team with effective servers dramatically improves its chance of winning; by producing serves that veer unpredictably, a team can run up long strings of service points, often turning the tide of a match. All experienced volleyball players are familiar with the "floater" serve, which has a pronounced, unpredictable flutter if the velocity is high enough; but exactly what causes this remains somewhat mysterious. Several explanations have been offered.

First, the popular explanation is that the inflation point of the volleyball puts the flutter into the floater serve. It is reasoned that because the ball is so light, the inflation point creates a mass imbalance—a center of gravity or mass that is actually off-center—and that this produces the characertistic movement of the serve. This explanation, though plausible, is mistaken, at least for tournaments, because the official volleyball has a counterweight opposite the inflation point.

A second and more plausible explanation has to do with air resistance. Resistance in the direction opposite to a given motion (drag) depends on the viscosity and velocity of the medium (in this case, air) through which an object (in this case, a volleyball) travels, and on the texture of the object's surface. When air passes by one side of a ball, the air pressure at the surface remains unchanged at the forward panel, drops to a minimum over the windward panel, and rises by an equal amount over the leeward panel. A simple way to visualize this pressure differential is to tape the strings of two helium balloons to a table, positioning the balloons about 0.3 meter (1 ft.) apart and at the same height; then blow a stream of air straight between them. Instead of moving apart—as many people would predict—the balloons will move toward each other. This effect is described by Bernoulli's principle: whenever streamlines of airflow come together or increase in velocity, there is a corresponding drop-off in air pressure. In this demonstration, the constant air pressure on the outside of the balloons and the reduced pressure between them combine to push them together.

This example explains the effect of laminar (smooth) drag on the surface of the volleyball, but it does not explain another drag factor—pressure drag. Pressure drag occurs once boundary-layer separation takes place, that is, the change of airflow from laminar to turbulent. The surface flow begins at the leading edge of the ball as minimum-drag laminar flow but then makes a transition (a boundary-layer separation) to turbulent flow with a large drag. Pressure drag does not occur until boundary-layer separation occurs, and this depends on reaching a critical velocity. That velocity is highly dependent on the size of a ball; the smaller the ball, the higher the velocity needed for boundary-layer separation. For example, a baseball experiences boundary-layer separation at a much higher velocity than a volleyball. With regard to boundary-layer separation, scientists use a dimensional parameter called the Reynolds number; for boundary-layer separation to exist, this number must be within the range of 100,000 to 300,000 (*see Table 1*). Even when it is moving at a much lower velocity, the larger size of a volleyball gives it a much higher Reynolds number than a baseball or a golf ball. Note that the flutter effect occurs only when the ball is struck at a moderate pace; a jump serve (*see below*) struck at 27 meters per second (60 MPH) is actually traveling too fast to flutter (the Reynolds number is 358,000).

Surface drag and pressure drag can adequately explain, say, the knuckleball in baseball, and it is instructive to consider the knuckleball—a careening pitch—as an example of these two factors. In a knuckleball, it is the seam of the baseball that creates the boundary-layer separation responsible for the careening effect. The slowly rotat-

REYNOLDS NUMBERS

Ball	Diameter (m)	Velocity (m/sec.)	Reynolds number
Golf ball	0.043	67	190,000
Baseball	0.071	45	212,000
Volleyball	0.20	27	358,000 (jump serve)

Table 1. *The "Reynolds number" must be between 100,000 and 300,000 to create boundary-layer separation, which causes a ball to move erratically. This happens at a much lower velocity with a volleyball than with a baseball or golf ball. Boundary-layer separation has been offered as one possible explanation for the flutter in a floater serve.*

ing ball jumps, or "breaks," because the seam disturbs the air flowing around it. When the ball rotates so that the seam protrudes from the bottom, the ball drops. In the region of laminar flow at the top of the ball, the airflow from leading to trailing edge is slowed by surface friction; however, there is not enough friction for the laminar flow to become turbulent—the airsteam does not break away (there is no boundary separation) before it reaches the trailing edge. Simultaneously, however, the seam along the bottom of the ball does create boundary-layer separation (a turbulent airflow). The turbulent airflow along the bottom of the ball is not slowed as much by surface friction as the laminar airflow along the top. This is important because, according to Bernoulli's principle, the pressure of an airflow is reduced as its speed increases. Airflow along the bottom of the ball hugs the surface farther to the rear before it separates. This airflow actually has a small upward component of velocity; as a result, the trailing wake also has an upward component of velocity relative to the ball. According Newton's third law, if a collision of ball and air drives the air upward, the ball must be driven downward. The same effect applies for other random positions of the seams: the ball breaks in the direction the seam is positioned (*for further comparison, see Figure 1*).

However, this kind of analysis—based on drag—may not entirely explain the erratic movement of a floater serve in volleyball; additional factors may be involved. In other words, the aerodynamics affecting a volleyball are more complex than those of a baseball, and this is because of the nature of the volleyball. A baseball is small, solid, and dense, with rather large convex seams; the volleyball is larger, hollow, and relatively light, with small concave seams.

A third explanation has to do with shape and deformation: it is sometimes suggested that the floater serve wobbles and breaks primarily because the ball takes on an out-of-round shape when struck. A volleyball has such a thin shell that it deforms when struck by the server: its side panels expand outward, greatly increasing its frontal surface area. In flight, the ball then oscillates back and forth from round to out-of-round: that is, it goes from being spherical to being ovate (egg-shaped), with a large frontal surface area. As the ball's countour changes, the airflow pattern around the ball also shifts back and forth—and this causes the ball to flutter.

This theory has two serious flaws. First, the dimensional change in shape is rather small. Second, and more important, most of the deformation oscillations dissipate by the time the ball clears the net, and this is the point at which, according to many players, the ball breaks most. It seems unlikely, then, that the out-of-round distortion is responsible for much, if any, of the flutter.

A fourth analysis of the floater serve focuses on the postion of the inflation panel. This is another plausible explanation: that is, the position of the inflation panel probably contributes more to the flutter than the out-of-round shape. In fact, volleyball coaches tell servers to strike the ball on any panel other than the inflation panel. The goal is to serve so that the ball will behave unpredictably, break-

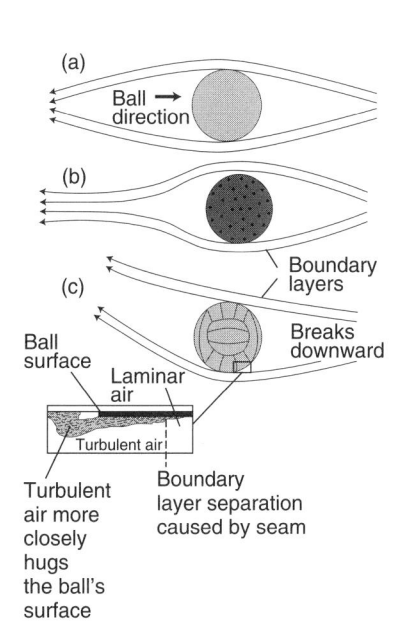

Figure 1. *Airflow differs around (a) a spinless, smooth ball, (b) a spinless, dimpled golf ball, and (c) a concave-seamed volleyball. Laminar airflow rushes past the smooth ball. Around the uniformly dimpled golf ball, airflow becomes turbulent and hugs the surface more. The wake over and under the ball narrows. When the seam of a spinless volleyball protrudes along the bottom, the airflow around the bottom hugs the surface while the airflow along the top rushes past the ball. The ball is in effect pushing the air upward, so, according to Newton's third law, the air must be pushing the ball downward.*

ing up, down, left, or right. To achieve this, the server repositions the inflation panel. With the inflation panel forward, toward the opponents' side of the court, the serve veers unpredictably left or right. The same is true in the vertical plane: with the inflation panel facing upward, the ball breaks upward; with the inflation panel pointing downward, the ball breaks downward. This probably occurs because of the slight difference in the surface texture near the inflation point, and because the inflation panel may have a slightly different curvature from the other panels when the ball is struck. Both of these factors, theoretically, could increase the probability of erratic airflow by increasing the probability of a transition from laminar to turbulent surface flow along the inflation panel. The seams of the inflation panel may indeed protrude farther than the seams of the other panels, thereby creating an effect analogous to a knuckleball.

Some coaches believe that an out-of-round shape is responsible for the ball's erratic flight and thus tell the players to maximize deformation. If, as the foregoing discussion suggests, the probability of an erratic flight path is not affected by an out-of-round shape but is affected by the position of the inflation panel, should a server still "bash" the ball in an attempt to maximize deformation? The answer may be yes if a hard hit does create a difference in contour between the inflation panel and the other panels. Nonetheless, it is hard to prove the merits of bashing. When a ball is bashed, it travels at a higher velocity relative to the air; thus, in the case of bashing, it is questionable whether an increase in breaking action is attributable to deformation rather than simply to increased velocity.

There do not seem to have been any studies measuring the oscillating frequencies of a struck volleyball, or tracking the breaking actions of a permanently deformed volleyball in flight. Such studies might reveal the relative contributions of the out-of-round shape and the inflation panel to the floater. For now, however, it is probably reasonable to conclude that a knuckleball effect is the major reason for the volleyball's breaking, and that the position of the inflation panel is a factor contributing to the knuckleball effect.

A note on deformation. Maximizing the deformation of the volleyball may prove to be useful in producing a floater serve, but this is not necessarily a simple task, for at least four reasons.

First, it is important for contact to occur at the center of the ball: an off-center contact not only decreases deformation but also impairs the server's accuracy.

Second, in order to maximize deformation, the server—like a punter in football who rotates the laces away before contact—needs to strike the ball at a point other than the inflation panel (*see also* FOOTBALL).

Third, bashing a ball to maximize deformation can easily send it sailing out of control. Thus, a good server maximizes deformation at impact by accelerating the hand as quickly as possible and then pulling back, retarding arm velocity in the follow-through. This maximizes the force imparted but limits the time this force is applied. To accomplish this, the service action should not rely on a large transfer of momentum from shoulder rotation and lower-body follow-through; rather, the serve should be a strong, snapping, "elbow-on-up" action. The striking motion is just the opposite of a karate strike (*see KARATE*). Karate experts try to hit through a target, somewhere between 30 and 37.5 centimeters (12 to 15 in.) past the contact point, by generating punching and kicking force with a kinetic chain involving many body segments. A server in volleyball, by contrast, should maximize acceleration at contact but limit the follow-through, by using only an elbow-through-wrist action.

Fourth, the striking force used also depends on position, but the best position from which to serve is a subject of considerable debate. Should the server toe the endline or stand well behind it? In this regard, players' preferences vary tremendously. To improve the chance that a serve will land in, many players stand far behind the endline—sometimes even a full court length, at the extreme end of the floor. In some respects, this is a good strategy: a server who stands farther back can strike the ball harder to create more deformation. However, the advantage of a harder strike may be offset by the fact that standing back gives the opposing passers more time to react to the serve. Thus the serving position is a choice between creating more deformation (to produce more breaking) and limiting the opponents' reaction time.

The Jump Serve: Endline "Spiking"

The jump serve—a "spike from the endline"—is relatively new in power volleyball. It was first used by several of the men's teams in the Olympics of 1976, in Montreal, and had become commonplace among both men and women by the Olympics of 1984.

The rationale for the jump serve is quite simple. By jumping up and into the court, the server strikes the ball at a higher point. This allows the ball to be hit downward into the opponents' court, and so the server can strike the ball harder, from a point closer to the target, leaving the opposing passers less time to react. However, a jump serve is difficult to master, and tremendous athleticism is needed to execute it consistently; thus it is usually seen only at the elite level.

Jump servers want to get as high and as close to the net as possible. But since jumping out over the court is legal only if the jump is initiated from behind the endline, it is important not to make an error in timing; therefore, most players limit the run-up to two or three steps. The ball is hit with topspin, like a spike, so that it will drop during flight. To apply topspin, the wrist snaps at contact, the hand wraps around the ball, and contact is made slightly above center, to produce a slow rotation. Topspin is vital. Without some topspin, most serves would land beyond the endline (*see also TENNIS*).

Plyometric Training: Can Jumping Ability Be Improved?

Volleyball players, like many other athletes, want explosive jumping ability. Unfortunately, not everyone has it.

The reason for good or poor jumping ability may have to do with genetics. There is some evidence that the position of the leg muscles on the bones determines—or at least affects—jumping ability. Usually, a person has a better vertical jump if the gastrocnemius and soleus muscles of the calf are located closer to the knee joint (that is, are higher up the leg). This is true for the same reason that it is easier to turn a nut with a 36-inch pipe wrench than a 12-inch wrench: higher calf muscles give the ankle joint more torque—rotational force about a pivot point—than lower calf muscles. A high ratio of the perimeter of the thigh to the weight of the body (lower) also seems to affect jumping ability (Adrian and Cooper, 1989). In addition, good jumpers have proportionately more explosive fast-twitch muscle fibers.

Another factor is motor control (*see MOTOR CONTROL*). Lengthening the calf muscle just before a contraction results in a stronger contraction. As the muscle spindles stretch, the ability to stimulate other receptors, and to increase the number of other motor units involved greatly influences the amount of muscle power delivered.

For the most part, genetics and motor control are givens. However, whatever an individual physique, a good jump training program can greatly improve the recruitment of muscle fibers and develop strong jumping skills.

Jump training relies heavily on plyometrics: the science of training fast-twitch muscles to use more fibers in each contraction so that they work synchronously and more effectively. It was once mistakenly believed that the explosive power generated by fast-twitch muscle fibers was determined largely by genetics. In fact, plyometric training helps coordinate the action of fast-twitch muscle fibers to generate more overall explosive power and improve jumping.

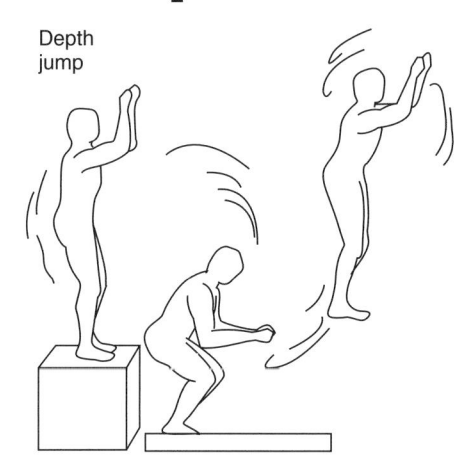

Plyometric training is different from strength training, which is focused primarily on generating a sustained force for an extended time by multiple repetitions, sets, and slow-velocity barbell work (*see also STRENGTH TRAINING*). Plyometric training involves fewer repetitions and less weight than strength training; it concentrates, instead, on improving the speed with which a person can move, or the speed at which the person can move weights.

Plyometrics maximizes the stretch reflex: an eccentric (lengthening) contraction, in which the muscle is fully stretched, precedes the concentric (shortening) contraction. The theory behind this technique is that the greater the stretch put on a muscle from its resting length, immediately before a concentric contraction, the greater the load the muscle will be able to lift or overcome. To maximize the stretch reflex, plyometric training concentrates on hops, bounds, and depth jumps. Drop training drills, which are probably the most popular among volleyball and basketball coaches, entail drop or rebound jumps. These drills involve jumping from a height of 0.3 to 1.1 meters (1 to 3.5 ft.), and then imediately jumping off the landing surface, preferably a mat (*see figure*). It is believed that depth jump drills optimize the stretching-shortening cycle to increase the elastic potential of leg muscles during extension.

In addition to the stretch reflex, quickness is an important component of jumping: a quick jump is needed to deliver a quick spike. However, quickness is often underrated; many coaches are preoccupied with improving vertical jumps and therefore tend to neglect quick-leaping drills. It is important to be aware of the importance of quick leaping in sports like volleyball and basketball, which require a fast reaction to an overhead ball—and plyometric training is an excellent way to improve quickness.

However, the relative merit of any one type of plyometric exercise over another is still a subject of debate. Thus, athletes should use a variety of plyometric drills (*see also MOTOR CONTROL and FIELD ATHLETICS: JUMPING*).

The Spike

A power volleyball team must have a powerful spiker: a "big gun" or "hammer" who can "kill"—that is, win the point—with great regularity. Great spikers have a sense of place, an awareness of opponents' positions that enables them to hit over, through, and around blockers. When they catch a blocker off-guard, they can drill the ball nearly straight down at a speed of over 160 KPH (100 MPH). A player with an acute awareness of the opponents' defensive positions will usually achieve a high percentage of "kills," despite having to hammer the ball through double- and triple-team blocks.

A powerful spike is extremely effective, and, like the jump serve, is not an easy skill to master. The ball usually comes from a position between 1 and 3 o'clock, but the distance from which it is coming and the trajectory it follows will vary, and the spiker must time and chart the approach and elevation to intercept it.

A high contact point is the spiker's foremost concern, because this widens the range of options for the attack. The chance of making a kill increases dramatically if the ball is contacted at its maximum height. Velocity is also important: an opposing passer is much better able to to run down a spike tipped at, say, 112 KPH (70 MPH) than a spike tipped at 160 KPH (100 MPH). However, because a number of factors are involved, spike velocity varies greatly among players.

In one sense, at least, the spike is much like a pitch in baseball or a serve in tennis (*see also BASEBALL and TENNIS*): the muscles function optimally when exerted in a definite sequence and with proper timing so that each muscle makes a maximum contribution to the velocity of the arm. Although the motion needs to be fluid, with no delay in the application of muscular force, for illustrative purposes it can be broken down into five phases: (1) approach, (2) takeoff, (3) acceleration and contact, (4) decleration and follow-through, and (5) landing.

Phase 1: Approach

For a typical high set, to generate kinetic energy the player uses an approach of 2.5 to 3.6 meters (8 to 12 ft.): a one-, three-, or five-stride run-up. The jumping motion then adds more kinetic energy; as a result, vertical momentum at takeoff is greater than it would be if the player had been just standing. The farther back the run-up starts, the greater the height reached. One study examined jump-and-reach scores recorded for elite spikers with jumps from a standing position and jumps following one-, three-, and five-stride run-ups (Enoka, 1971). The mean jump heights for the three run-up distances were 57.5, 63.2, and 63.7 centimeters (23 in., 25.3 in., and 25.5 in.) respectively—all significantly higher than the standing- jump height, 56 centimeters (22.4 in.). If time is not a factor, then, for maximum height a spiker should use a three- or five-stride run-up.

If a five-step approach (about 3.6 m) gives more height than a three-step approach, why not use, say, ten steps? There is one major reason spikers seldom use a longer run-up: timing. More height will do little good if the jump and the spiking motion are mistimed. In addition, the increase in height attainable by using more than 3.6 meters is only incremental and thus cannot compensate for the sacrifice in timing.

Phase 2: Takeoff

In a high set, the spiker takes off using both feet, and as with any jump, a forceful extension at the hips, knees, and ankles is needed. However, there is an erroneous popular notion that only the legs are responsible for height. The fact is that although the legs are obviously important, the head, trunk, and arms are almost equally important. When a vigorous arm swing is used to create additional force for takeoff velocity, height can be increased by as much as 15 percent: for a vertical jump of 50 centimeters (20 in.), for instance, that would be an increase of 7.5 centimeters (3 in.). (This effect is comparable to the increased jumping distance achieved in ancient Greece by the use of handheld weights; *see FIELD ATHLETICS: JUMPING*.) An increase of this magnitude can be achieved only by an excellent player—one who can bring the arms down as the lower body flexes and then bring the arms up and back as the lower body extends at the knees and hips. Average jumpers tend to extend earlier at the knees and hips and thus are less likely to get the full advantage of a forceful arm swing. Other factors limiting height include the quickness of the set, the angle of trajectory taken, and the length of the hurdle step.

For quick sets—commonly referred to as front or back one-sets—a one-foot takeoff is typical. A quick jump, rather than a high jump, is important for one-sets, especially if the spiker is tall. Quick one-step jumps permit spikers to pivot and position themselves more quickly to finish off these fast play patterns. In an elite volleyball match, the threat of a quick set and kill is vital, if only as a decoy.

Body positioning in spiking is a unique and underappreciated skill. A tennis player, or a batter in baseball, takes a stance perpendicular to the direction of the oncoming ball. In volleyball, however, a good spiker uses an approach at a 45-degree angle (*see Figure 2*). The spiker's hitting arm is positioned farther away from the ball than it would be with a more squared-off stance, and it is hidden so as not to reveal the intended hitting direction. The spiker must rotate smoothly through the large range of motion necessary to generate a high hitting velocity. For a strong side hit (*again, see Figure 2*), the spiker can rotate either partially to hit the ball cross-court or fully to hit it down the line. Fluid rotation with high arm velocity allows the best spikers to disguise their intent much longer than less skilled spikers can.

Phase 3: Acceleration and Contact

Before contact, the spiker counterrotates away from the ball and coils up like a spring: forearm flexed, upper arm rotated outward, and

Figure 2. *The two major spikes are (a) high outside and (b) quick low set to a middle hitter. Tennis players and batters in baseball take a perpendicular striking stance, but a spiker approaches at a 45-degree angle. This imparts more rotational momentum to the ball and also hides the hitting arm, concealing intent. To give the ball maximum angular momentum, the spiker must counterrotate (coil up). A deliberate motion is used for a high outside spike; a quick set depends on the element of surprise, so the spiker uses a quicker leap, along with a more compact arm motion and less body rotation.*

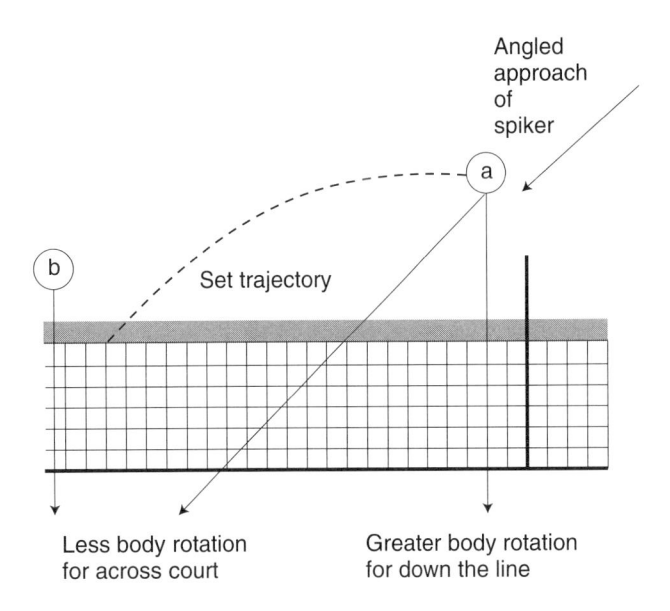

hand hyperextended. This increases the distance over which velocity can be generated. To further increase that distance, the trunk is hyperextended, the hips and shoulders are rotated, and the striking arm is cocked back behind the ear. The ability to hyperextend and rotate effectively is the major reason for the spike velocity generated by elite players.

As the body starts forward, the left arm and shoulder drop quickly and the right arm accelerates toward the ball, with the elbow leading. The drop of the left arm and shoulder raises the potential contact point. The trunk pikes, flexing from hyperextension to a forward curl; this greatly increases the body's horizontal momentum. The velocity of the spike is determined by the sequential timing of these movements more than by anything else.

Wrist action is important not so much to increase velocity as to impart topspin. Topspin is generated by a wrist snap at a contct point slightly above center, after which the hand wraps around the ball. Because the ball is hit with tremendous velocity—often exceeding 160 KPH (100 MPH) in international play—the proper wrist action to create topspin is vital. It significantly increases the chance that the ball will drop and remain in the court. The velocity and accuracy of spikes differ from player to player, and from time to time for the same player, depending not only on timing and mechanics but also on fatigue. One study found that fatigue greatly affects the efficiency of a spike (Sardinha and Zebas, 1986). Many players jump 300 to 400 times during a match, and this makes strength training imperative (*see also* STRENGTH TRAINING).

Phase 4: Deceleration and Follow-Through

For spikers in volleyball, as for pitchers in baseball, the deceleration stage is responsible for most injuries to the swinging arm; but spiking involves other risk factors in addition to those present in pitching (*see BASEBALL* and *SHOULDER, ELBOW, AND WRIST*). To avoid injury, an athlete should maintain good mechanics; but often a spiker must pull up jerkily to avoid hitting the net, or must make last-minute adjustments (also jerky) to the swing to compensate for misplaced sets.

Because deceleration forces can be twice as great as acceleration forces, deceleration should start shortly after contact. At contact, the body is so loaded up with energy that the possibility of injury is high, unless there is a smooth deceleration as the swinging motion comes to a stop. In particular, average (as opposed to elite) players commonly fail to fully rotate the hip and shoulder forward; this limits the body's ability to absorb the energy created by the swinging arm. Overuse injuries occur when the swinging arm comes around while the body stays behind.

Phase 5: Landing

When possible, a landing should be made with both feet, to increase the area over which the landing force is distributed. This lessens the chance of tendinitis in the knee joints. Playing on more forgiving surfaces and selecting the right shoes (*see the essay "Selecting Shoes"*) will also help prevent injury.

Passing

The volleyball pass is perhaps the most impressive "touch" shot in any sport. The receiving player must redirect a spike that may be moving at 160 KPH (100 MPH) and must control the pace and height so that a teammate can set the ball for an offensive return.

To appreciate the passing shot, it is helpful to compare volleyball with a sport like tennis. In tennis, the ball is moving faster but the contact area available for hitting it—the racket face, which in modern rackets has a large sweet spot—is significantly greater; also, the longer dwell time (contact between ball and strings) enhances control (*see TENNIS*). In volleyball, a passer does not have either of these advantages, because the ball is hit with the flat inside of the lower forearm. About all the passer can do to increase control is turn the thumbs out as far as comfortable to increase the surface area of the arm. The greater the surface area used to pass a ball, the less the force per square inch on the ball, and this improves the chance of executing a controlled pass.

Furthermore, in tennis a well-centered hit will give a fairly uniform coefficient of restitution, that is, a relatively constant rebound (*see also BASEBALL*); but in volleyball, when the ball hits the passer's forearm the coefficient of restitution varies, depending on muscle tension. In other words, the tenser the muscles and tendons in the arms, the greater the rebound.

To better understand the dynamics of passing, consider the rebound of a volleyball off the passer's forearms versus a rebound off

Selecting Shoes: Thick or Thin Soles?

Movements in volleyball include—among many others—jumping, lunging, twisting, and stretching, along with split-second stops and explosive starts. In volleyball, as in many other sports, the appropriate shoes can improve performance and prevent injury; but until relatively recently the selection of footwear was so limited that athletes rarely thought about it. Throughout the 1950s and 1960s, in fact, almost everyone wore the same shoes for volleyball, basketball, tennis, and running: Chuck Taylor Converse All-Stars. Today, there is a wide selection of footwear, often designed for specific sports, and athletes have much to consider in choosing a shoe.

Because we ask so much of our feet, it is important to select shoes that meet their biomechanical needs. Shoes serve four critical functions: (1) they absorb shock (that is, cushion landing forces); (2) they provide "spring" to return more energy for running and jumping; (3) the outer sole provides friction for lateral movement; (4) the uppers support and protect the foot and ankle.

Shoes for a given court sport—such as basketball, racketball, or tennis—are often similar in design, with only cosmetic differences. This is not true of volleyball, however. Footwear for volleyball ranges from very thin-soled shoes with little cushioning to basketball-type shoes with a great deal of cushioning. As recently as the 1980s, almost all volleyball shoes had thin soles. Volleyball requires a great deal of lateral—that is, side-to-side—movement (more even than basketball), and it was believed that thin-soled shoes accommodated quicker lateral movement and also reduced the risk of ankle sprains. In the 1990s, thicker soles with more cushioning became popular because many players wanted shoes that felt springier and would absorb landing impacts better.

Before deciding on a volleyball shoe, it is useful to understand the forces involved in a jump landing. One study found that the impact force ranged from 1,000 to 2,000 newtons (225 to 450 lb.) under the forefoot and up to 6,495 newtons (1,460 lb.) under the heel (Stacoff, 1986). The elastic limit of cartilage—approximately 5,000 newtons (1,125 lb.)—was exceeded in more than 10 percent of the jumps recorded. For an athlete weighing, say, 72.5 kilograms (160 lb.), an impact force of 6,495 newtons is enormous—approximately nine times body weight. This fact highlights the importance of biomechanical studies designed to improve playing (landing) surfaces, athletes' landing technique, and the springiness and absorbancy of shoes.

Studies have found that thicker-soled volleyball shoes can reduce landing impact forces on the body by 30 percent more than thin-soled shoes. Thick-soled shoes are usually recommended for athletes suffering from jumper's knee (tendinitis; *see also* KNEE). However, if a player has weak ankles, thicker-soled shoes are not recommended, because thicker soles involve greater torque (rotational force about an axis) and thus exacerbate sprains. For this reason, and because explosive lateral stops and starts put a lateral stress of three or four times body weight on various parts of the foot, specialists recommend that weak-ankled players wear thin-soled shoes, strengthen the peroneal muscles around the ankle, and consider wearing high-topped shoes, ankle braces, and tape to increase ankle stability.

For the unfortunate few who have both jumper's knee and weak ankles, it is difficult to know what kind of shoe to recommend: neither thick nor thin soles will work miracles. Actually, only rest and conditioning will bring relief. Obviously, forgoing rest and then jumping 200 to 300 times during a 3-hour practice session or match will aggravate any existing injury (*see also* EQUIPMENT MATERIALS and ANKLE, FOOT, AND LOWER LEG).

IMPACT ON THE FOOT

Mode	Force (newtons)	Force (pounds)
Running	2,263	495
Jumping	6,495	1,460
Stop and go	2,915	655

a floor (Adrian, 1989). A volleyball dropped onto a wooden floor from a height of 7 meters (23 ft.) will rebound almost 2 meters (6.6 ft.). From the same height, the rebound off a maximally tensed tendinous surface—in this case, the forearms—will be only 1 meter (3.3 ft.). This means that the arms deaden or damp much more of the ball's energy than the floor does. Damping can be even greater—as much as 80 percent greater—if the forearms remain relaxed. Thus, accurate and consistent passing requires players to maintain consistent tension in the passing "platform," the tendinous surface of the forearms.

There is evidence that among elite players, contact time between ball and forearm is longer, and this would seem to indicate that elite players maintain less tension in the tendinous surface of the forearm (Ridgway, 1987). A longer contact time increases the player's ability to absorb the ball's force and pass the ball. An exaggerated pullback at the shoulders and a forward thrust of the hips will help the forearms absorb the ball's energy. Although these additional mechanics generally play a minor role, they can become critical when a ball arrives at nearly 160 KPH (100 MPH).

Variations in muscle tension explain, in part, why many passers "choke" under pressure—why a passer who can ordinarily place the ball right on target will suddenly send it sailing long and far off course. These players are tensing up without realizing it. Tennis is often cited as a sport infamous for "choking" situations, but with regard to handling pressure, the demands of tennis pale in comparison with volleyball. Tennis players who tense up can still perform effectively because they are contacting the ball with a racket, which is one step removed from the tense body—the inconsistent hitting surface formed by living tendinous tissue. In volleyball, whatever tension builds up in the player's body is delivered directly to the ball.

Before passing, a volleyball player needs to have kinesthetic awareness of tension in the arms (motor-control feedback). Passers should try to remain consistent. Some coaches advise players to shake their arms between points to relax the muscles and tendons. Releasing excessive tension, especially before pressure points, allows them to pass the ball from a more consistent platform.

Setting: What Is a Legal Set?

In basketball, the point guard calls the plays and runs the offense; in volleyball, the focal point of the offense is the setter. A setter needs to be accurate, deceptive, and capable of changing the pace of a game by varying the height and speed of sets to the spikers. This is not easy, and it is made even more difficult because setters are usually performing under pressure. Setters must also deal with unpredictability: "float" serves, for example, and errant passes caused by 160-KPH (100-MPH) spikes. In addition, setters must often perform acrobatic sets on the run and from a variety of squatting positions (*see also ACROBATICS*). In fast-paced play, setters usually do not have time to position themselves to use their legs as well as their arms. Thus for the most part the set is an arm-dominated skill.

A set starts with an absorption phase, and this is followed by a projection phase. How a setter handles the absorption phase makes an illegal set—a violation—a very subjective decision for the net judge. According to the rules of the United States Volleyball Association, "the ball may touch any number of parts of the body, provided that touches are simultaneous, and that the ball is not held, but rebounds properly. The ball must be hit and rebound cleanly. When a ball rests momentarily between the hands or arms of a player, it is considered to be held. Scooping, lifting, pushing, or carrying the ball shall be considered as holding." This sounds reasonable in theory, but in reality enforcement is difficult because the ball is being received in one direction and launched in another. Although the set occurs in less than 1/10 second, the ball must come to rest—even if for only 1/1,000 second—after the absorption phase and before the propulsion phase. In other words, the ball is always held momentarily. Is the time dividing legal from illegal sets absolute: a specific maximum during which the ball may rest on the setter's fingertips? Or is the time relative, depending on the setter or the type of set? The rules give officials little guidance.

One study measured "set time"—time from contact of ball and fingertips to release of the ball—and found a wide range of times, varying with the technique used. Average times were 0.054 second for a low set, 0.072 second for a high outside set, and 0.086 second for a high back set (Ridgway, 1986). This means that the high back set is held significantly longer (60 percent longer) than the low set. The contact time in the back set is longer because the back is hyperextended and the ball is launched overhead with one thumb and not all four fingers (typically, just the index and middle fingers are used). The longer contact time in the back set explains why it is notoriously "whistled" as a violation of the rule against momentary holding.

The apparent arbitrariness of judgments of violations often incenses coaches and fans. Although officials may not admit it, calling illegal sets is often a matter of preference with regard to style. Many net judges will rule a set illegal not because the ball was actually held too long but because the setter seemed to be in an awkward or otherwise poor position. Conversely, if officials like a setter's style—particularly, if the energy of the oncoming pass is smoothly converted to the set—they are more apt to allow a questionable set. To repeat, then, distinguishing between legal and illegal sets is often subjective. Many observers believe that volleyball officials are just as likely to overlook questionable sets as referees in the National Basketball Association (NBA) are to overlook traveling and carrying (palming).

John Zumerchik and David Lind

References

Adrian, M., and J. Cooper. *Biomechanics of Human Movement*. Dubuque, Iowa: Benchmark, 1989.

Enoka, R. "The Effect of Different Lengths of Run-Up on the Height Which a Spiker in Volleyball Can Reach." *New Zealand Journal of Health, Physical Education, and Recreation* IV (November 1971).

Ridgway, M., and N. Hamilton. "The Kinematics of Forearm Passing in Low Skilled and High Skilled Volleyball Players." In J. Terauds et al. (eds.), *Biomechanics of Sports V*. Del Mar, California: Academic, 1987.

Ridgway, M., and J. Wilkerson. "A Kinetic Analysis of the Front Set and Back Set in

Volleyball." In J. Terauds et al. (eds.), *Biomechanics of Sports III, IV.* Del Mar, California: Academic, 1986.

Sardinha, L., and C. Zebas. "The Effect of Perceived Fatigue on Volleyball Spike Skill Performance." In J. Terauds et al. (eds.), *Biomechanics of Sports III, IV.* Del Mar, California: Academic, 1986.

Stacoff, A., et al. "Foot-Movement, Load, and Injury in Volleyball." In J. Terauds et al. (eds.), *Biomechanics in Sports III, IV.* Del Mar, California: Academic, 1986.

Volleyball: Official Rules and Interpretations. Washington, D.C.: American Alliance for Health, Physical Education, Recreation and Dance, 1979.

Wilkerson, J., "Vertical Jump Utilized in the Volleyball Spike." In D. Winter et al. (eds.), *Biomechanics IX-B.* Champaign, Illinois: Human Kinetics, 1985.

Weight Lifting

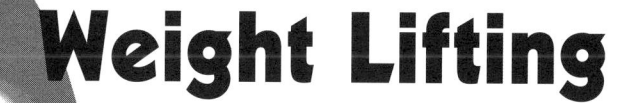

WEIGHT LIFTING goes back to ancient Greece and Rome. Though it was never an event in the ancient Olympics, one Greek athlete, Milon of Croton, may have been the first to employ the approach to weight training now known as progressive increased resistance, or progessive loading. Legend has it that he acquired a newborn calf and lifted it over his shoulders every day; as the calf grew, Milon's strength increased, until eventually he was able to lift the full-grown bull. This may just be a story, but it is based on an actual principle of weight lifting: the only way to make muscles grow stronger and stronger is to make them work harder and harder by moving more and more weight. Continually lifting a calf that is gaining a pound or so a day would be a perfectly valid way to do this; in fact, although computers and specialized high-tech equipment have replaced calves, Milon's basic approach still remains the cornerstone of weight lifting and weight training (*see also* STRENGTH TRAINING).

In recent decades, weight lifting has become more popular mainly because of weight training, which has proved beneficial for almost every conceivable sport. Almost all world-class athletes participate in some sort of weight training program, and many colleges and universities, and even high schools, have a strength training coach on their staff. Athletes must have strength as well as speed and stamina, and coaches began to realize in the 1960s that the best way to achieve this combination is through weight training. As a result, most top athletes in all sports have a new appreciation for the sport of weight lifting—for those who lift weights as an end, not just as a means to an end.

In developing weight training programs for specific sports, to improve the strength and endurance of muscles and joints, coaches naturally borrowed principles and techniques developed successfully over the years by world-class weight lifters. Today "explosive" throwing sports (e.g., shot put and discus), and jumping sports (e.g., volleyball, basketball, and high jump) use their own versions of weight training programs based on the tried and true methods of weight lifters. This is the best training for getting the large-muscle groups moving at ever higher speeds.

Although muscular strength and endurance can be improved, weight lifting is also highly dependent on inherited abilities. Not everyone has the potential to be a world-class weight lifter. It takes a combination of inheritance, determination, and years of training to produce the necessary progressive gains in strength.

Principles of Weight Lifting

Anyone who has seen a solid steel barbell bent by the weights hanging from its ends can understand the almost superhuman effort involved in weight lifting. Weight lifters train for competition by repeatedly stressing their muscles. The muscles respond by producing more actin and myosin—proteins found in muscle fiber. As the muscles become thicker, more blood vessels form to serve them, and this in turn allows the muscles to become even larger and stronger, capable of lifting ever greater weights (*see also* SKELETAL MUSCLE).

Work and Energy

At the beginning of a lift, the lifter faces two adversaries: inertia and gravity. *Inertia* refers to the tendency of an object to resist any change in its state of motion. A massive object at rest is difficult to get moving; a massive object in motion is hard to stop. The more mass an object has, the larger the effect of intertia. Obviously, it is harder to shove a battleship away from a dock than a canoe; and a battleship colliding with a dock at a speed of, say, 10 knots will demolish it, while a canoe will not even make a dent. *Gravity* is perhaps a more familiar term to most people. This is the weight of a massive object: the force exerted by the earth pulling the object toward its center.

In weight lifting, the lifter must first exert an upward force sufficient to overcome the downward force of gravity—that is, the pull of the earth, or the weight of the object. Then, to accelerate the weight upward—to get it moving—the lifter must exert more force, to overcome the effect of inertia. Once the weight starts moving, however, inertia will tend to keep it moving, so at this point inertia becomes an advantage: the lifter can use it to get past the phases of the lift where the human body is less capable of exerting upward force.

To move a barbell, a weight lifter exerts force on it, moving it in the direction of the force. Lifting anything against the force of gravity requires *work*, in a special, physical sense of the word. For a constant force, the amount of work a weight lifter does on a barbell is the product of force times the distance the barbell travels while the force is acting (force × distance). Thus two repetitions involve twice as much work as one, and lifting the barbell only waist-high involves half as much work as lifting it overhead. To put this another way, as the barbell ascends, the weight lifter is doing work by exerting force through a distance.

In this sense of *work*, a weight lifter holding a barbell motionless overhead is doing no work at all on it. The muscles might be stretching and contracting—"working" in a physiological sense—but the lifter is not doing work in a physical sense, because the distance the barbell moves is zero. This point is worth repeating: weight lifters may expend considerable energy extending their arms or "locking out" their knees, but if the barbell does not move, no work is being performed on it.

Another point to be noted is that although work equals force times distance, "force" is not consistent in weight lifting: the amount and direction of the force exerted change while the barbell is being lifted.

The more work a weight lifter does on a barbell, the greater the speed of ascent and the greater the height that can be reached. In this regard, another crucial concept is *energy*—the capacity to do work. Energy cannot be created or destroyed, but it can be transferred; in weight lifting, it is transferred from the lifter to the barbell. To transfer energy to a barbell, the weight lifter must use energy.

The work done on the barbell gives it both potential energy, which is proportional to the height it is raised; and kinetic energy, which is proportional to the square of its speed. Thus as the speed of the upward ascent slowly diminishes, its kinetic energy diminishes but its potential energy increases. At full extension, its kinetic energy is zero and its potential energy is maximized.

Not all the energy expended by a weight lifter results in useful work: some dissipates as heat, and some is expended within the lifter's own body. If timing is off or technique is poor, some of the energy used to lift the barbell is "wasted." Energy spent regaining balance or lifting with the bar too far from the body is considered wasted because the barbell will not travel as high as it would if an equal amount of energy were expended with perfect execution. To limit the amount of energy expended within the body, weight lifters devote considerable time to improving their mechanics.

Strength versus Power

At the beginning of a lift, the lifter tries to get the barbell moving upward as fast as possible—that is, with as much kinetic energy as possible. To lift the maximum weight, the lifter needs to impart the maximum velocity to the mass being lifted; thus it is necessary to apply maximum force for as long as possible. This is analogous to a cannon, which has a long barrel in order to prolong the time that the force of the exploding gunpowder acts on the cannonball. The longer the force acts, the greater the increase in kinetic energy. But not all guns are cannons: some have a short barrel and use more explosive force. Similarly, weight lifters do not always act like a cannon: they can use a "cannon" strategy in which relatively less explosive force is applied over a longer time; or they can use a strategy that involves generating a very explosive force over a short time (like a short-barreled gun).

This dichotomy between the short-barrel and the cannon strategy divides weight lifting into two entirely different categories: Olympic and power. Olympic and power weight lifting are sports which make vastly different demands on athletes, and lifters follow very different training regimens depending on which category they fall into.

Olympic lifting is like a short-barrel gun. The two Olympic lifts—the snatch and clean-and-jerk—depend on high power applied over a shorter time. In both, the lifter must raise the weight to an overhead position with elbows "locked out." The difference between the two lifts is in the motion. Whereas the snatch requires one continuous motion from floor to overhead, the clean-and-jerk allows two: the lifter first brings the weight to the chest and then raises the bar overhead. Olympic weight lifters are much like sprinters and shot putters, though they look very different from either. All these athletes have a high proportion of explosive fast-twitch muscles (*see also* RUNNING AND HURDLING). Perhaps surprisingly, many Olympic weight lifters can move as fast as sprinters, if only for the first few steps.

Oddly enough, although Olympic lifting depends on high power, it is the *other* category that is actually called power lifting. This second category—the cannon strategy—relies on steady strength applied over a longer time. It includes three lifts: dead, squat, and bench press. In the dead lift, the lifter raises the weight from the ground to a point at midthigh; the back remains straight and the knees remain locked. In the squat, the barbell stays on the lifter's shoulders while the lifter squats down and then straightens up again. In the bench press, lying on the back, the lifter brings the weight down to the chest and extends and locks out the arms. Unlike Olympic weight lifters, power lifters do not need a high proportion of fast-twitch muscles. For some reason, power lifting is considered less glamorous than Olympic lifting, a sort of stepchild.

To understand the concept of strength versus power, and Olympic versus power lifting, it is useful to understand something about how muscular power is defined and calculated. Muscle power is a rate of energy expenditure, and it depends on the amount of energy available and the time taken to expend it. It is impossible to measure muscle power internally—that is, the rate at which muscles are actually producing and transferring mechanical energy—so the only real clues are external: the amount of weight lifted, for example, and the time involved.

As noted earlier, there is a difference between *work* in the physiological sense and in the physical sense, and there is also a difference between the physiological and physical meanings of *power*. Physiologists associate power with mechancial force—how much force is being produced—but physicists define power as the rate at which work is done or energy is transformed:

$$\text{Power} = \text{work/time}$$

Physically, the relationship between power and force is:

$$\text{Power} = \text{force} \times \text{velocity}$$

According to the physicists' definition, a lifter who raises a heavy weight quickly generates a lot of power; a lifter who raises the same

What Is Power?

Physiologists associate power with mechanical force: how much force is being produced. Physicists, on the other hand, define power as the rate at which work is done or energy is transformed. According to physicists, the term *power lifting* is something of a misnomer because power lifters raise tremendous weights a short distance at lower speeds. Olympic lifters must generate far more power because they explosively raise barbells more quickly, over a greater distance: from the ground to directly overhead in a split second.

weight or possibly even a heavier weight more slowly is generating less power. Thus, as we have noted, the term *power lifting* is something of a misnomer for a sport in which power, in this sense, is actually less.

In the physicists' sense, then—to repeat—it is Olympic weight lifters who depend more heavily on power, while power lifters are much more dependent on strength (sustained force). Therefore, Olympic lifters rely on instantaneous muscle recruitment: getting as many muscle fibers contracting as simultaneously as possible; this is not necessarily the case for power lifters. Olympic lifters raise the barbell explosively; power lifters take a much more deliberate approach. In terms of time, an Olympic snatch lifter will take 227 kilograms (500 lb.) from floor to overhead (about 2 m, or 7 ft.) in about 0.6 to 0.9 second (this represents 8.4 to 5.6 horsepower). A power lifter will take about 2 seconds to lift 454.5 kilograms (1,000 lb., or half a ton) 0.6 to 0.9 meter (2 to 3 ft.). Olympic lifters move the barbell faster, over a greater distance. Because of this, there is a substantial difference in output of power, as we have just defined it.

To make this clearer, keep in mind the difference between power and work. Lifting, say, a 200-kilogram (440-lb.) barbell 2 meters (6.6 ft.) involves the same amount of work whether it takes 2 seconds or 2 hours. However, the power input is much different with these two times. To raise the barbell in 2 seconds requires 1,960 watts of power, that is, 2.63 horsepower; to raise it in 2 hours requires only 0.52 watt, or 0.0007 horsepower. (Note: The watt, abbreviated W, and the kilowatt are units of power; the kilowatt-hour is a unit of energy.) Olympic lifters, as we have seen, generate much more power than power lifters (*see Figure 1*).

We can now return to the idea of strength versus power. The ability of the muscles to generate power is limited by the ability of the body to deliver oxygen to them. As the example above indicates, a human being can generate several horsepower over a period of less than 1 second. However, the ability to sustain this high level of power drops off quickly; in fact, only well-trained athletes can maintain a power level of over 1 horsepower for more than a few seconds. Practitioners use the term *strength* to refer to the ability of muscles to exert maximal force at a specified or determined velocity; they use the term *power* to refer to explosive force.

Olympic lifters need to lift weights farther; since this requires more work, they try to generate explosive power from the start so that the inertia of the barbell will help them through the segments of the lift in which leverage is poor. Power lifting depends far less on inertia. Olympic lifters tend to do poorly at power lifting, and one reason may be that they experience difficulty producing a sustained force at a very low velocity. They depend on their upper motor centers to generate muscle contractions, and their rapid movements make it unnecessary for them to develop kinesthetic feedback (motor-control memory) regarding how much force to generate. Power lifters, by contrast, depend heavily on kinesthetic feedback and train to develop

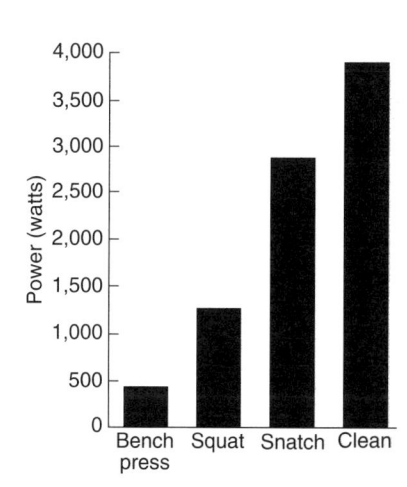

Figure 1. *Paradoxically, Olympic weight lifters depend much more on high power than power lifters do. John Garhammer, a biomechanicist and an expert on weight lifting, developed a model giving maximal values for power that are very close to actual measurements. His measurements for world-class athletes in the clean-and-jerk ranged from 31 to 37 W/kg in the clean-pull and 45 to 60 W/kg in the jerk-thrust. He believes that both ranges are very close to the theoretical human maximum. (Data from Garhammer, 1989)*

it—to sense how much force they are generating (*see also* BASKETBALL and MOTOR CONTROL).

The "Sticking Point"

Strength or power determines the extent of force applied, but leverage is what determines the effectiveness of an application of force. Force generated by the human body depends greatly on the bodily lever system—the mechanical system for performing work. Thus the concept of leverage is important for understanding any of the factors involved in physical skills: position, sequence, direction, timing, and speed.

The human lever system consists of the bones and joints. Each joint is the fulcrum (pivot point) of a particular lever that comes into action when force is applied by the muscles. Movement occurs because the muscles contract (pull) their respective bones. In physics, there are three classes of levers; the type that is most common in the human body is the third-class lever (*see Figure 2*). In a third-class lever, the pivot point (such as a joint) is at one end, the source of force is in the middle, and the resistance is at the other end. For example, when a weight is lifted with the arm, the force is exerted between the elbow and hand by the biceps muscle.

An effective lever does one of two things: (1) it increases the amount of work per given force, or (2) it causes work to be done at a faster rate than the application of the force. The first effect is achieved when the fulcrum is located closer to where the force is applied than to where it is executed: the amount of force increases to produce greater output at the other end. A crowbar is an example of this first effect. In the human body, however, the first effect is rare; the body is built not for strength but for speed. For example, the biceps is attached to the radius (a bone in the lower arm), very close to the fulcrum, and a weight in the hand is far from the fulcrum: that

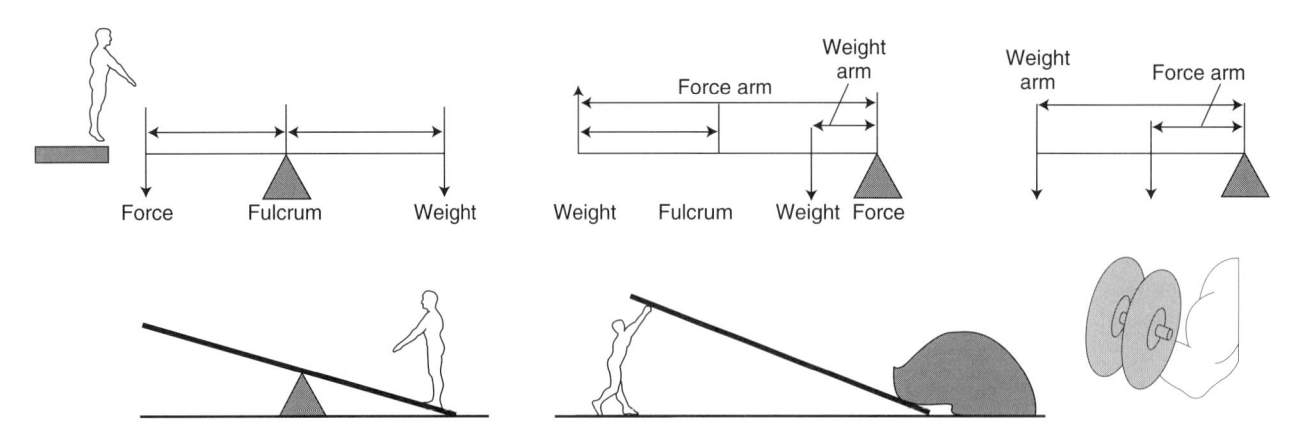

Figure 2. *There are three types of levers (left to right): a first-class lever is the kind seen at circuses; a second-class lever is the kind used to move a rock; a third-class lever is the kind used to curl a weight. The third-class lever is most important in human motion; such a lever favors speed and range of motion at the expense of force. Thus the human body performs fast movements with light objects well (e.g., throwing a baseball) but is less efficient at heavy work (shot putting or lifting a heavy barbell).*

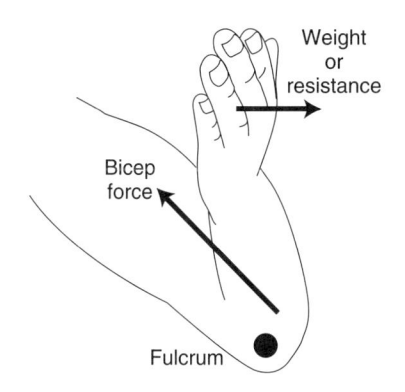

Figure 3. *The biceps is attached close to the elbow joint (the fulcrum); this means that the hand can move very fast, but with less force.*

is, the fulcrum is closer to where the force is executed than to where it is applied (*see Figure 3*). Therefore, it is the second effect that operates here: this lever allows a force at the elbow to make the hand move considerably faster, though with less force. To quantify this, when the hand lifts, say, a 1-pound (0.45-kg) weight, the biceps works at a disadvantage of about 7 to 1: lifting 1 pound requires a force of 7 pounds (3.1 kg; Ariel, 1985).

Whether the requirement is speed or strength, the efficiency of a lever is a function of the particular task. At some positions, a lever is very efficient, at others less so. A less efficient position is what weight lifters call a "sticking point." This is a point of resistance—a critical joint configuration that pushes the muscle to its limit—and it almost always occurs somewhere in the midrange toward full arm extension, where there is significant bending at the joint. Once a lifter gets past a "sticking point," resistance diminishes greatly, and the weight can be lifted much more easily.

When the elbow is straight, the axial arm load is transferred to the body without muscular action through the joints. A relatively small muscular force at the elbow holds or straightens the arm. Very little torque about the joint is necessary. On the other hand, when the arm is bent sharply, 90 degrees or more, the muscles must exert enormous forces to provide enough torque at the joint to keep it from collapsing. This is the reason that the anterior cruciate ligament in the knee gets torn in many sports (such as skiing), and why strength training is so important: it raises the collapse threshold (*see also KNEE*).

Whatever a weight lifter's ability, at certain positions of the barbell in relation to the body the muscles are not as effective. Anyone who has worked under the hood of a car knows that it is not only important to get the wrench onto the right nut but also, and equally, important to have the wrench in the right position to exert the greatest torque on the nut—the most rotational force about an axis. The same is true of a crowbar, which may be ineffective at one angle but, with only a slight adjustment, very effective at a different angle.

A sticking point occurs during the short period when the lifter's upward force on the barbell falls below the gravitational downward force on the barbell. It is necessary to produce vertical momentum so that the inertia of the barbell overcomes the segments of the lift where there is a natural slowing of the barbell. To get past a sticking point, then, weight lifters try to generate maximum barbell velocity. In fact, unless the lifter develops enough barbell momentum, it is impossible to overcome a sticking point. To repeat: it is necessary to develop the highest possible bar velocity before the sticking point. In this way, linear momentum (vertically) maintains enough velocity so that the barbell's inertia will help "drive" the barbell through the sticking point.

A common characteristic of any lift with a sticking point is that more than one joint is involved. The bench press, for instance, involves the shoulder and elbow; the squat involves the hip and knee. All these joints operate at a wide range of angles. The muscles working these

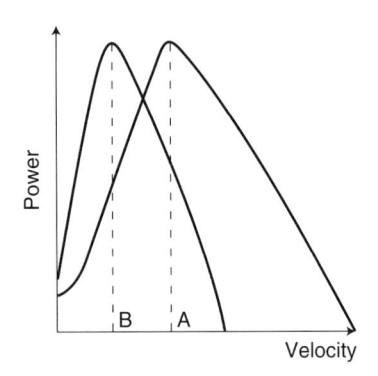

Figure 4. *Two people pushing a car out of the mud will work more successfully if they push in concert. The same is true of individual muscles. The curves here show theoretical potential power (maximum velocity of contraction) of two muscles, A and B. The dashed lines indicate the velocity where peak power output occurs. Peak power of A occurs at twice the velocity of B; moreover, the range in velocities through which muscle A can produce power will be twice that of B. Although there is a link between muscle mass and potential power, the peak power potential of individual muscles cannot be considered cumulatively unless the muscles function similarly in terms of fiber lengths and biochemical processes. This phenomenon contributes to the "sticking point." (Adapted from Edgerton, 1986)*

joints can generate tremendous torque at some angles but are far less efficient at other angles. Sticking points, then, are areas where the combined power from the angles of muscles and joints is not in the peak power range for either joint. Once the sticking point has been passed, both joints reach a more optimum power range, so that barbell velocity naturally increases. This is analogous to two people who are trying to rock a car stuck in mud: they will find it far more effective to coordinate their efforts than to push independently (*see Figure 4*).

For the squat, the biomechanist John Garhammer reported that knee torque was greatest at the bottom and declined gradually during extension, while hip torque was near maximum at the sticking point (Garhammer, 1988). Hypothetically, this means that at the sticking point the knee joint may be operating at 50 percent of its peak power and the hip joint at 20 percent of peak power. After the sticking point has been passed, the barbell quickly accelerates as the hip increases to, say, 60 percent of peak power, and the knee increases to 80 percent.

The "transitional zones"—the areas of poor leverage—that cause a sticking point are difficult to measure accurately. One of the major problems in measuring is that the actions of muscles and joints at a sticking point are not uniform. Factors influencing the location and magnitude of a sticking point include musculoskeletal leverage, body build, different levels of strength in individual muscles, flexibility, and stamina. Thus if two athletes with different physiques attempt the squat, their different weight lines and joint angles may result in entirely different sticking.

The "Bounce Effect": Muscle Meets Material

The squat and the clean-and-jerk are two lifts in which the concept of *elastic energy* becomes important. In both events, the weight lifter uses a "bounce effect" to generate elastic energy for the thrust up. This bounce effect is not applicable in the bench press because the bar must come to a stop; nor is it applicable in the snatch and dead lift, because one continuous motion must be used.

Springs, bungee cords, bowstrings, hockey sticks, barbells, and even muscles all store elastic energy, but magnitude and dynamics differ dramatically among them. The elastic energy of any material is determined by mass and stiffness. A material with greater mass responds more slowly, because greater mass usually means greater inertia; but the stiffer a material, the more quickly it returns energy. Elastic energy is complicated, though, because the stiffer the material, the less energy can be stored. That is, given the same force, a stiffer material flexes less and stores less energy than a flexible material of the same mass. Bungee jumping is the most graphic example of "weak" elastic energy. A heavily weighted barbell is at the other extreme: this is "strong" elastic energy, having the same properties as a very stiff spring.

Energy cannot be created or destroyed; it can only be transferred. Thus it must either remain with the lifter or be imparted to the barbell. In the jerk-lift, kinetic energy is developed by raising the bar slightly so that it falls to the chest from the force of gravity; this allows the elastic energy of the barbell to assist the muscles in "powering" the bar overhead. As it flexes at its node (center point) against the chest, the barbell begins to oscillate (move back and forth). The weighted elasticity of the bar acts like a very stiff spring—such as a leaf spring in a car—and considerably more barbell elastic energy helps raise the weight (resulting in greater gravitational potential energy). The elastic energy of a car spring, which can cause an occupant's head to hit the roof if the car goes into a pothole, is analogous to the elastic energy of a barbell.

In the clean-and-jerk, the bounce effect is very beneficial because the joints are in a locked position, and this is a better position to sustain the jolt from the force of gravity as the barbell strikes and leaves the chest. The elastic energy given to the bar increases the application time of the force for the same total work; thus, the instantaneous force demanded of the muscles is reduced when the joints are in a position less favorable for generating the large forces needed to make the barbell overcome gravity.

In the squat, the bounce effect occurs while the athlete is in a crouched position (joints unlocked); thus more is required from the lifter in order to absorb the weight, and it is more difficult to time the thrust upward. However, the bounce effect still plays a crucial role in the squat, because muscle itself is a very elastic fiber. Research has shown that muscles actually brake the body as well as "propel" it. Part of the energy in braking during the downward phase is stored in the elastic elements while the contracting muscle stretches. This stored energy is then used to "propel" the barbell during the upward phase as the muscles are called on to do work. The elastic nature of muscle allows more power than would be produced solely by contraction, because part of the stored energy is released. (It also explains why athletes can jump higher in a vertical drop jump than a standing vertical jump.)

A telling study by biomechanicists at Indiana University proved this by finding a larger force at the knee during the squat when it was performed fast than when it was performed slowly (Andrews, 1980). Not only does slower motion create less force, but the elasticity of the body falls out of sync with the elasticity of the barbell. This situation is very similar to the timing of a golf swing and the flexibility of the shaft of a golf club. The bounce effect used by weight lifters is an enlightening example of how human (muscle) elasticity works in conjunction with mechanical (barbell) elasticity.

Olympic Weight Lifting

Olympic and world weight lifting championships are decided by two types of lifts: the snatch and the clean-and-jerk (often called simply the jerk). The weight lifted during the jerk is almost entirely determined by the lifter's ability to generate power, while the snatch requires more of a balance between power and technique. Usually an overall winner will outlift the opponents in both the snatch and the jerk, but this is not always the case. If only power mattered, the lifter who could generate the greatest power would of course dominate in both; but in the snatch an athlete with superior technique can and frequently does outlift an athlete with superior power. Much as in boxing, where most of the attention centers on the heavyweight division, in Olympic weight lifting attention centers on the superheavyweight division. Athletes in this division, who weigh 300 pounds (136 kg) and more, are competing not only for official championships but also for the informal title "strongest man on earth."

The most impressive superheavyweight lifter thus far has undoubtedly been Vasily Alexeyev (*see Figure 5*) of the former Soviet Union, who dominated the division throughout the 1970s, was undefeated for 9 years—from 1970 through 1978—and set 82 world records. (The Soviet government is said to have offered him a bounty every time he broke a world record.) John Goodbody, an English expert, wrote that no other athlete in any sport could match Alexeyev's achievements.

In a sport where very little time is actually spent lifting and a great deal of time is spent waiting and mentally preparing in back rooms, the sight of the massive Alexeyev striding around (he weighed 350 lb., or about 160 kg) could be intimidating. Alexeyev's strategy was also intimidating. Each lifter is granted three opportunities in the snatch and three in the jerk, and customarily the competitors match each other lift for lift. But Alexeyev would sit back in the wings until all the other competitors had made their final attempts and only then would take his own first attempt. He assumed, confidently, that he himself was his only real competition. Usually, his first attempt would be for the victory, and in the remaining two lifts he would compete against his own world records. In his prime, he broke a record almost every time he went to a meet. He was the first man ever to break the 500-pound (227-kg) barrier for the jerk, and he came close to being the first to pass the 600-pound (272-kg) barrier. His record 255-kilogram (562-lb.) jerk lift in the 1976 Olympics in Montreal stood until 1996 (when Andrey Chermerkin set a new record of 573 lb. at the

WEIGHT LIFTING RECORDS

Men over 108 kilograms

Snatch: 205 kilograms (452 lb.)—Aleksandr Kurlovich (Belarus), Instanbul, Turkey, 27 November 1994

Jerk: 260 kilograms (573 lb.)—Andrey Chemerkin (Russia), Atlanta, 30 July 1996

Women over 83 kilograms

Snatch: 105.5 kilograms (232.5 lb.)—Li Yajuan (China), Hiroshima, Japan, 5 October 1994

Jerk: 155 kilograms (341.5 lb.)—Li Yajuan (China), Melbourne, Australia, 20 November 1993

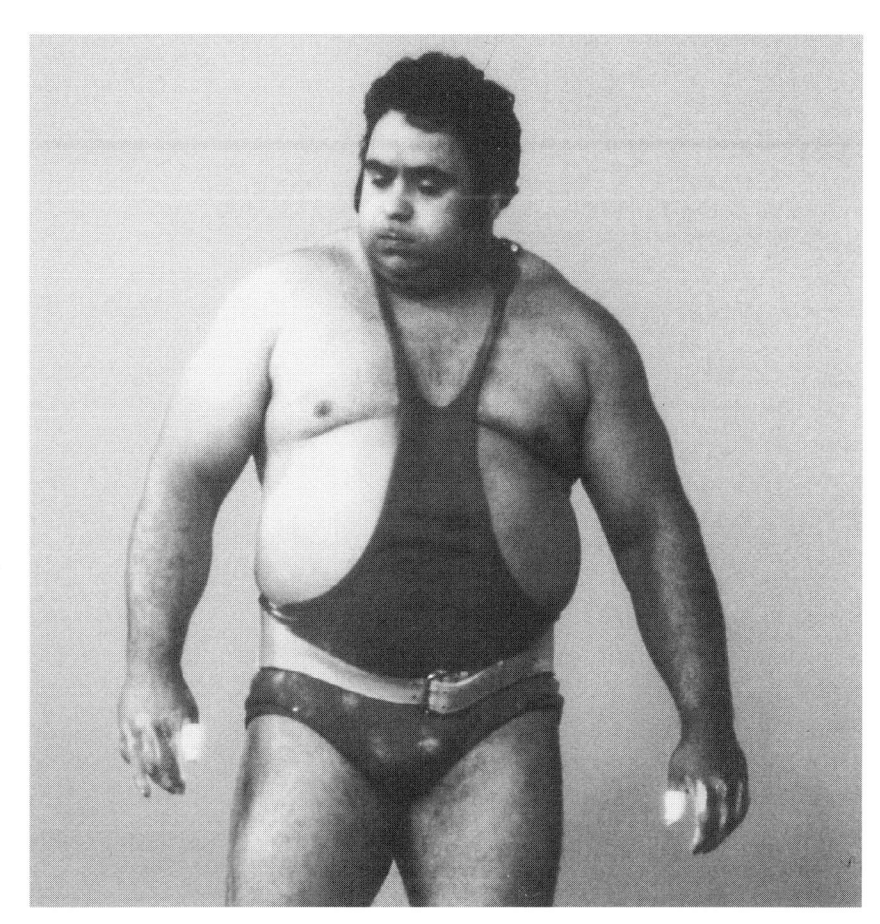

Figure 5. *Vasily Alexeyev was "the strongest man on earth" for most of the 1970s, although his physique was atypical: massive on top and with comparatively spindly legs. In weight lifting, the athletes' peak years are the early thirties—much later than in other sports. It is noteworthy that Alexeyev was in his prime from ages 30 to 35, a time which coincided with his peak skeletal mass. (Photo courtesy of Allsport Photography, Inc.)*

Olympics in Atlanta). During Alexeyev's years as champion, there was no debate about who was the strongest man on earth.

However, in terms of physique Alexeyev cannot be considered a typical weight lifter. When he began competing internationally in 1970, he weighed about 300 pounds, but by the time of the 1980 Olympics he weighed more than 360. This was a consequence of his diet, which would have dismayed any sports nutritionist of the 1990s. He loved to feast; and at the 1972 Olympics in Munich, he was once seen breakfasting on a huge steak and 26 eggs. This type of diet not only filled out his large frame but gave him an ever-expanding belly. It is true that because his frame was so large, he carried his excess weight well, and it is also true that all superheavyweights are enormous; but Alexeyev contrasted sharply—especially later in his career—with the well-proportioned muscularity of his opponents. Eventually, he became even more saggy on top, with a belly that kept increasing and legs that looked disproportionately thin.

Alexeyev's body can only have been detrimental to his performance. Early in his career, he overcame its disadvantages through sheer ability, but finally it proved too much of a handicap. In 1980, at the Olympics in Moscow, Alexeyev—then age 38—tried to make a comeback, after having been injured in the world championship of 1978, but he was eliminated early. He failed three times to snatch 180 kilograms (397 lb.), a weight he had handled easily a few years before. All this is easy to explain biomechanically: to put it simply, Alexeyev's girth—his protruding belly—got in his way. It moved his center of gravity (point of mass concentration) farther forward, so that it was no longer directly under his center of support, making it more difficult for him to maintain his balance. As a result, he had great problems in the snatch. He could still achieve the explosive power necessary to raise the bar quickly, yet he had a problem once the bar came to shoulder height. To counter the change in the position of the weight when it reaches shoulder height, lifters must alter their center of gravity from a position where the weight is below the body to a position where the weight is above the body. Alexeyev's belly created difficulty during this transition. (He did not have this difficulty in the clean-and-jerk, though, because that lift occurs in two stages, and the break between the two occurs at the shoulders.)

It is interesting to speculate—considering Alexeyev's obvious genetic gifts—whether he might have dominated weight lifting even longer if he had followed a better diet and controlled his girth.

Snatch

For spectators, of all the ways weights can be lifted, the most athletic method is surely the snatch. The snatch requires strength, speed, coordination, timing, and balance. This is perhaps the one event in which technique is just as important as power: as noted earlier, in the snatch a very powerful lifter with mediocre technique will usually lose out to a slightly less powerful lifter with good technique. This is because good technique allows a lifter to make use of the maximum available explosive power. World-record lifts are considerably lower in the snatch than the clean-and-jerk, because the weight must be lifted overhead in a single motion rather than two motions.

An ongoing debate about the snatch is whether the double knee bend or the split leg method is better (*see Figure 6*). The knee bend relies on knee extension to accelerate the barbell during the later portion of the lift (middle to top), whereas the split leg method depends on the thrusting ability at the hip joint. The deep knee bend is more popular among elite lifters. It is believed that this is so because the powerful knee extensor used during the later portion of the lift occurs during the strongest range of motion for the knee. It is also believed that a certain amount of elastic energy comes into play during the double knee bend.

Clean-and-Jerk

The clean-and-jerk is the final lift in a competition, and it is a telling test of maximal muscle power. In the 1990s, world-record weights in this event were about double the body weight of the lifter. Because the clean-and-jerk is actually two lifts and involves a much heavier weight, it requires considerably more muscle stamina than the snatch.

Lifters begin by positioning their feet under the bar to place their center of gravity as close to that of the weight as possible. The arms

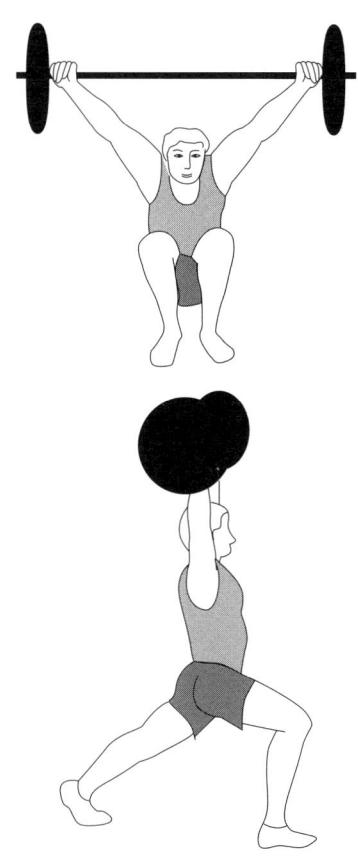

Figure 6. *The two techniques used in the snatch are the double knee bend and the split leg method. The double knee bend is preferred by most world-class lifters.*

are perpendicular to the bar so that they act more efficiently, like cables, pulling the barbell straight upward. This is possible because extension of the knees and hips is mainly responsible for overcoming inertia to get the barbell moving upward. Midway through the clean, the shoulders elevate and the elbows flex to bring the barbell to rest across the chest. Although the jerk seems to take place with the arms extending straight upward, the barbell is actually launched upward only about halfway to full extension by a slight knee flex, followed by an explosive extension. Once the barbell starts upward, lifters have a brief "window of opportunity" to shift their center of gravity by slipping under the barbell with a quick leg split: one leg moving forward and the other backward.

Films of weight lifters in action reveal that they raise themselves off the ground during this split: in essence, a lifter drives the body plus the barbell into the air—although with a quarter-ton weight overhead, it does not take long for gravity to bring lifter and barbell back to earth. This technique allows the arms to "lock out" at a lower height, so that the thicker, more powerful muscles in the lower body can finish the lift with an explosive knee extension to a "locked out" position. Most of the power generated during both phases of the clean-and-jerk comes from the very effective muscles that control knee extension. Although the popular stereotype of a powerful athlete has a massive, chiseled upper body, it is the power generated in the lower body that really counts. A top-heavy body builder, for instance, would have little or no chance of becoming a top Olympic lifter.

Power Lifting

As mentioned above, power lifting is something of a stepchild or poor relation, without the fame or glamour of Olympic weight lifting. Still, it remains widely admired because so many athletes use the three power lifts—bench, squat, and dead—as part of their in-season and off-season training.

One of the most interesting power lifters of all time was Lamar

POWER LIFTING RECORDS

Men over 125 kilograms

Squat: 447.5 kilograms (989 lb.)—Shane Hamman (United States), 1994
Bench press: 310 kilograms (685 lb.)—Antony Clark (United States), 1994
Dead lift: 406 kilograms (897 lb.)—Lars Noren (Sweden), 1988

Women over 90 kilograms

Squat: 277.5 kilograms (613 lb.)—Juanita Trujillo (United States), 1993
Bench press: 157.5 kilograms (348 lb.)—Ulrike Herchenhein (Germany), 1994
Dead lift: 240 kilograms (530 lb.)—Ulrike Herchenhein (Germany), 1994

Gant of the United States. Gant was endowed with incredible natural strength. In 1971, at the age of 14—on his first visit to a gymnasium, and never having lifted before—he set a bench press record in the 123-pound class for the city of Flint, Michigan. Gant immediately fell in love with weight lifting, and he could not get enough of it, often training so hard that his hands would bleed. His training soon paid off: in 1975, at age 18, Gant became the youngest man ever to win the world power lifting championship. Over the next 16 years, he won a record 15 world titles. Many people considered Gant the strongest man in the world, pound for pound, an assessment that is hard to dispute. In 1985, when Gant, weighing 132 pounds (60 kg), lifted 661 pounds (just over 300 kg), he became the first man to dead-lift more than five times his own weight.

Gant was hypermuscular, even for an athlete. His body fat was only 2 percent of his body weight; by comparison, most collegiate athletes average 10 to 15 percent, and even most bodybuilders cannot get down to 2 percent. Moreover, Gant did not resort to the near zero-carbohydrate diet that bodybuilders use to approach 2 percent. Nor did he use steroids. (With regard to steroids, he offered to take polygraph tests, because he wanted everyone to know that all his records were clean.)

Although Gant set world records in the bench and the squat, it was the dead lift in which he was truly exceptional. Biomechanically, the dead lift is the simplest of all lifts, but it is nevertheless amazing to watch the herculean effort involved: the athlete must lift a barbell so heavily weighted that it actually bends. Gant's dead lifts looked superhuman; his arms seemed to stretch. This was an illusion, of course—his arms did not really lengthen—but what did happen was that his back in effect became shorter.

The reason for this phenomenon was that Gant had a spinal condition called scoliosis, in which there is a lateral curvature of the spine (*see Figure 7; see also SPINE*). Scoliosis affects 5 percent of the general population. Onset usually occurs at puberty, when there are

Figure 7. *Lamar Gant's scoliosis, a curvature of the spine, gave him a significant advantage over his opponents in the dead lift. A normal spine "shortens" as the disks compress each other, but a scoliotic spine "shortens" much more because the spine curves more. An athlete with a normal spine finishes the lift at midthigh; Gant was able to finish his lift with the barbell just above the knee.*

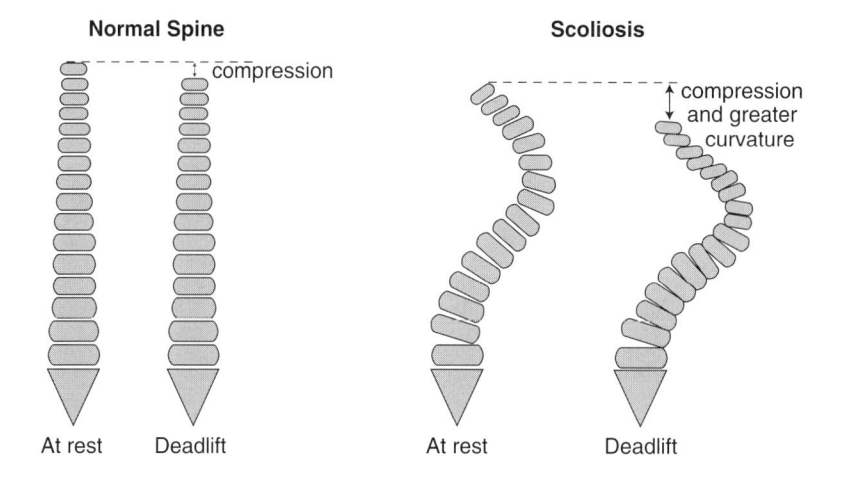

hormonal changes; after a rapid initial curvature, the condition continues to worsen by about 1 degree a year. As a general rule, a brace is prescribed for a curvature of 20 to 40 degrees; surgery is performed when the curvature is greater than 40 degrees. Gant's curvature was between 74 and 80 degrees, and once when he was X-rayed while lifting 425 pounds (193 kg), the curvature reached 90 degrees. In fact, it has been estimated that in his world-record dead lifts, his curvature was as much as 100 degrees. To spectators, as the weights Gant lifted became heavier, his trunk appeared smaller: his collarbone seemed to drop almost to his waist. (Gant's scoliosis was so advanced that he probably was 4 to 6 inches shorter than he would have been with a straight spine.)

Most people who have scoliosis are weaker than average. However, Gant started weight training at adolescence, at the onset of the condition, and—as has been noted—kept training harder and harder. The hypermuscularity he developed then acted as a natural brace.

Because of his scoliosis, Gant's trunk was shortened in relation to his height. This meant that he had a shorter shoulder-to-hip lever to work, which altered his "sticking point." In the dead lift, there are ordinarily two major sticking points: one is at the bottom, because of insufficient strength in the leg, hip, and back; the second is at around knee level, when the body weight shifts from toes to heels. At knee level, where most lifters experience a "sticking point," Gant was strongest, and it was at this point that he began the "lockout" (final extension) of his knees and trunk. Gant's own sticking point was much lower, at around midshin. Thus he finished his lift with the bar just above the knee—an advantage over his competitors, who finished about midthigh.

The hip and the knee are the two joints experiencing torque during the dead lift. Because Gant's scoliosis allowed his spine to bend more than normal—the greater the load, the more the curvature—the torque at the hips and the torque at the knees were reduced and evened out. Therefore, the load was distributed more evenly throughout all segments of the lift. In addition, Gant's arms were longer than normal, and this meant that he did not have to lift the bar as far or as high. Taking all this into account, Gant's dead lift would be the equivalent of a dead lift in which an athlete with arms of average length started with the weight not on the ground but on a block 3 to 6 inches (7.5–15 cm) high. This partially explains why as recently as 1996, Gant still held the world record for the 56-kilogram class: 289.6 kilograms (640 lb.), a record he had set in 1982. In 1996 he also still held the record for the 60-kilogram class: 310 kilograms (685 lb.), which he had set in 1988.

However, it would be a mistake to attribute Gant's success entirely to his scoliosis and his long arms. Although these factors did give him a definite advantage in the dead lift, they were irrelevant in the squat and disadvantageous in the bench press—and Gant excelled at all three events.

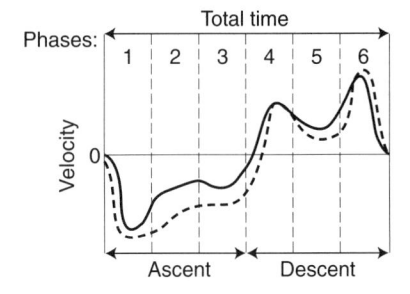

Figure 8. *In the squat, barbell velocity varies for elite lifters (solid line) and skilled lifters (dotted line). But less skilled lifters have shown much greater fluctuations in velocity. (Adapted from Garhammer, 1989)*

Squats

In one regard, the squat—sometimes called the deep knee bend—has been controversial over the years: is it beneficial in a strength training program? The answer usually given is yes, but with an important caveat: proper technique. It is believed that a full squat may stretch the medial and lateral ligaments of the knee joint, decreasing stability. Although there is virtually no evidence to support this belief, most professionals in the 1990s were recommending the half squat, in which the thighs are parallel to the floor. This is the depth used by world-class power lifters, and it is also considered the right depth for strength training (*see* STRENGTH TRAINING).

In the squat, one of the most important factors is the velocity of the barbell. Barbell velocity during the six phases of the squat differs significantly between elite and less skilled lifters (*see Figure 8*). More proficient lifters descend at a slower rate. This means that they approach the bottom in a more controlled manner, so that they can coordinate their stopping muscle force during the descent to begin the ascent in conjunction with the elastic nature of the barbell. They maintain a more vertical torso position during the entire lift to limit the load on the lower back, and they maintain a higher vertical bar velocity through the sticking point (phase 5).

Early during the descent, there is a shift in balance toward the heels. Later in the descent, and early in the ascent, weight shifts to the toes. This creates a slight rocking motion—from downward and slightly backward to forward and slightly upward. This very slight, very slow shift in the center of gravity should not sacrifice stability, however; without stability and timing, the muscles cannot be evenly loaded. Once the bottom is reached, the ascent should begin immediately so that stored elastic energy can be recovered to aid it. Stored elastic energy is critical early, from midway through the ascent until the point where superior leverage takes over.

Actions of the hip and knee are of primary and equal importance. Knee torque peaks at the lowest position of the squat (the point of greatest knee flex). To counter this, a slow descent is recommended, because the greater the speed of descent, the greater the peak knee forces. It has been argued that at the lowest position, recovery of elastic energy through interactions of the muscle fibers is an important factor in generating power for the ascent (Cavagna, 1977). As with a spring, muscle contractions and stretching during the descent and at bottom, followed immediately by rapid muscle contractions, greatly assist in the ascent (*see Figure 9*).

Bench Press

For athletes in rigorous strength training programs, and even for neophytes, the bench press is the most popular and best-known power lift. In the bench press (unlike the squat), elastic muscle energy does not play a significant role, because the bar must come to a complete stop before the lifter can proceed upward. Therefore, world-class lifters lower the barbell at a much slower rate and gener-

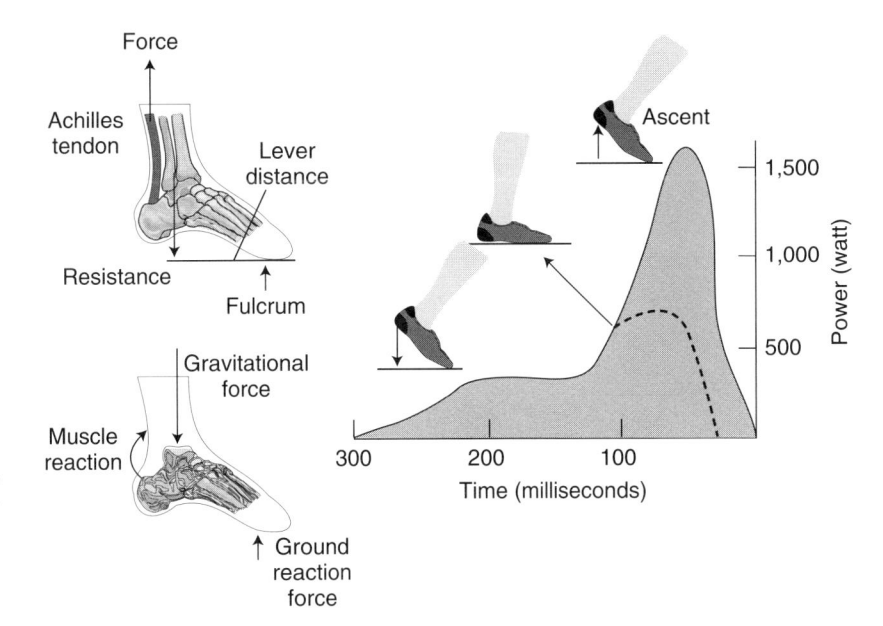

Figure 9. *Shown here is the elastic potential of muscles and tendons at the ankle joint during the squat: solid line = elastic potential; dashed line = no elastic potential. A power lifter who attempts a squat flat-footed cannot take full advantage of the elasticity of muscles at the ankle. (Adapted from Huijing, 1992)*

Bench Press Technique

One of the major differences in technique between world-class and novice weight lifters is the barbell's path during descent and ascent. Expert lifters bring the barbell up and down in a more vertical path.

ate a more consistent level of force. The more slowly the barbell descends, the less energy the lifter needs to expend to overcome inertia. Inertia is an advantage in lifting upward, so the barbell should be raised quickly. In descending, however, inertia works against the lifter, who therefore tries to lower the barbell slowly.

One factor that distinguishes world-class bench pressers is the path the barbell follows during the lift. Expert lifters shorten the lever from the shoulder—a superior technique in which the path of the barbell is closer to the shoulder joints on the way down and is more vertical (and thus more efficient) during the ascent. Studies have found that the spacing of the hand grip, the angle of arm and forearm, and the angle of arm and torso are also significant in the bench press.

John Zumerchik*

*The author owes special thanks to Don C. Hopkins for his assistance in putting together the section "Principles of Weight Lifting."

References

Andrews, J., et al., "The Concept of Joint Shear." In *Proceedings of the Biomechics Symposium, Indiana University, October 1980*. Indianapolis: Indiana State Board of Health, 1980.

Ariel, G. "Principles of Biomechanics." In C. Lietz (ed.), *The Scientific Basis of Sports Medicine*. Toronto: Decker, 1989.

Cavagna, G. "Storage and Utilization of Elastic Energy in Skeletal Muscle." In R. Hutton (ed.), *Exercise and Sport Science Reviews*, vol. 5, 1977, 89.

Chang, D. E., et al. "Limited Joint Mobility in Power Lifters." *American Journal of Sports Medicine* 16 (1988): 280–284.

Danoff, J. "Power Produced by Maximal Velocity Elbow Flexion." *Journal of Biomechics* 11, nos. 10–12 (1978): 481–486.

Edgerton, V. "Morpholological Basis of Skeletal Muscle Power Output." In N. Jones et al. (eds), *Human Muscle Power*. Champaign, Illinois: Human Kinetics, 1986.

Garhammer, J. "Biomechanical Profiles of Olympic Weight Lifters." *International Journal of Sport Biomechanics* 1, no. 2 (1985): 122–130.

Garhammer, J. "Power Output as a Function of Load Variation in Olympic and Power Lifting." *Journal of Biomechics* 13 (1980): 198ff.

Garhammer, J. "Power Production in Olympic Weight Lifters." *Journal of Medicine and Science in Sports and Exercise* 13, no. 3 (1981): 198–204.

Garhammer, J. "Weight Lifting." In C. Vaughan (ed.), *Biomechanics of Sports*. Orlando, Florida: CRC, 1989.

Huijing, P., "Elastic Potential in Muscle." In *Strength and Power in Sports*. Boston, Massachusetts: Blackwell Scientific, 1992.

Kulig, K., et al. "Human Strength Curves." In R. Terjung (ed.), *Exercise and Sports Science Reviews*, vol. 12. Lexington, Massachusetts: Collamore, 1984.

Madsen, N., and T. McLaughlin. "Kinematic Factors Influencing Performance and Injury Risk in the Bench Press Exercise." *Journal of Medicine and Science in Sports and Exercise* 16, no. 4 (1984): 376–381.

McLaughlin, T., et al. "Bench Press Techniques of Elite Heavyweight Power Lifters." *Journal of the National Strength Conditioning Association* 6 (1984): 44.

Menz, P. "The Physics of Bungee Jumping." *Physics Teacher* 31, no. 11 (1993): 483–487.

Niles, R. "Forward Is Faster." *Bicycling* (November 1992): 162–163.

Perrine, J. "The Biophysics of Maximal Muscle Power Outputs." In N. Jones et al. (eds.), *Human Muscle Power*. Champaign, Illinois: Human Kinetics, 1986.

Whittle, M., et al. "Computerized Analysis of Knee Moments during Weight Lifting." In G. de Groot (ed.), *Biomechanics XI-B*. Amsterdam, Netherlands: Free Press, 1988.

Wrestling

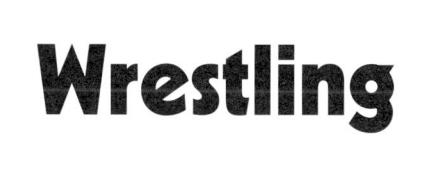

WRESTLING IS AN ANCIENT SPORT, but it certainly originated long before it became a sport. For prehistoric peoples, wrestling, like running and jumping, was probably a skill essential for survival. It is impossible to say exactly when it evolved into a sport. Most people associate the sport of wrestling with ancient Greece and Rome. However, it dates back much farther. Excavations in Mesopotamia, near Baghdad, uncovered a bronze Sumerian statuette of two wrestlers grasping each other's hips; this figurine is at least 5,000 years old. Still, the association of wrestling with Greece and Rome is accurate in that it was prominent in both cultures and was one of the main features of their festivals. The ancient Greeks may have revered the discus thrower as the greatest of all athletes, but the wrestler was a close second. One of the Greek wrestling champions was Milon of Croton, who for many years defeated all comers. Ancient wrestling matches seem to have had an element of superstition and mysticism: if wrestlers showed weakness, anger, or fear, that was considered an ill omen.

For centuries, wrestling took many different forms, with many countries developing their own unique styles. At one time, these forms included the glima style in Iceland, the schweitzer schwingen style in Switzerland, and the particularly savage cumberland style in Ireland. Most versions were rough and tumble—the approach could be summed up as "no holds barred" or "any means necessary." Wrestlers would grapple, bite, gouge, clinch, strangle, punch, and kick.

Throughout much of western history, though, the Greco-Roman style of wrestling remained most prominent, and today it is still popular in Europe. Worldwide, however, freestyle has become far more popular. Actually, Greco-Roman style and freestyle are quite similar, except for the fact that the Greco-Roman style does not allow any holds below the waist.

Concurrent with the development of wrestling in the west, the Japanese began to create their own form, called sumo wresting. The first records of sumo date back to 23 B.C.E., when, according to legend, the emperor Suinin asked a potter named Sukune—now immortalized as the father of sumo—to take on a bully and braggart named Kehaya. After a prolonged fight, Sukune finally delivered some debilitating kicks to Kehaya's stomach and solar plexus, mortally wounding him.

Japanese sumo is one of the few national styles to remain very popular today. It also spawned two other popular styles—ju-jitsu and judo—though these are employed more for self-defense than competition.

Wrestling was relatively late in coming to the Americas, and it was not until the mid-nineteenth century, about the time of the Civil War, that the United States took a fancy to freestyle wrestling; Americans liked the catch-as-catch-can grappling style that allowed them to grip wherever and whenever possible. Today, freestyle wrestling is the version practiced in American colleges and high schools. Intercollegiate wrestling is not as prominent, of course, as intercollegiate football or basketball, but there are a few areas where it is hugely popular. One example is Iowa, which has become a center of amateur wrestling. The annual wrestling competition between the University of Iowa and Iowa State is a notable rivalry.

Throughout the history of wrestling, there have always been some people who consider it not only the oldest but the only worthwhile sport. One reason may be that it is a very natural sport, and an exciting way for athletes to exhibit their prowess as fighters. Also, although wrestling may look rather simple, its appearance is deceptive: every wrestling style depends on subtle and complex techniques, based on sound physical principles. That is why a neophyte—no matter how strong or how naturally talented—can be quickly disposed of by a seasoned veteran, and a perfect technique can more than make up for minor disadvantages in quickness and strength. In addition, wrestling requires no equipment, and it is an exhilarating way to contribute to health and to build muscular strength and endurance.

The Basics of Wrestling

Wrestling comes under the category of combative sports. Its objective is quite simple: to pin the opponent's shoulders to the mat for 2 seconds, or to outscore the opponent. When a pin—also called a fall—does not occur, the referee awards the match to the wrestler who has scored more points. Wrestlers are often referred to as grapplers because they are continually grasping each other in a long series of moves and countermoves.

Torque and Center of Gravity

Wrestling involves high impacts and pivot-point forces. For a wrestler, the main task is to maintain balance while compromising the opponent's balance. To take advantage of the small "windows of opportunity" that present themselves during a match, a wrestler must act and react quickly in both the offensive and the defensive mode. Although the timing and the execution of moves are critical, neither can be effective without a practical understanding of two important principles: torque and center of gravity.

In wrestling, center of gravity (COG) is the geometric center of a wrestler's mass distribution; for most people it is located between the spine and the navel. COG can be thought of as the point where gravity acts on the body as a whole to produce an observed motion—although one must keep in mind that the weight of the body is not concentrated at any one point but is distributed over its entirety. Torque is a twisting or rotational force. Just as linear force sets an object in linear motion, torque causes an object to rotate. Torque depends on the magnitude of a force and its distance from COG or the axis of rotation. The effects of torque are demonstrated in loosening a stubborn nut when changing a tire: a long-handled wrench makes the job easier. That is because the farther away from the rotation point torque is applied, the less torque—the less force—is necessary (*see also* FIELD ATHLETICS: THROWING).

Balance and Motion

From the first whistle, wrestlers engage in continual maneuvers involving force versus counterforce. They use very slight pushes and pulls to probe for the opponent's COG and changes in balance. According to Newton's third law of motion, whenever one body exerts a force on another body, it in return receives a force equal in magnitude and opposite in direction. Thus when a wrestler exerts a large force against an opponent, the opponent must be prepared to counter that force. In anticipation, a well-prepared wrestler drops one foot back to brace for a contact, or repositions the body to counter an expected force—for example, by leaning forward and crouching. Even when a wrestler is caught off-guard by a maneuver, there must still be a counterforce. If the counterforce isn't created by the wrestler receiving a force, it will be created when that wrestler is slammed down onto the mat.

Wrestlers often use a stance that places their COG slightly forward over their front foot, leaning toward the coming opposing force. Although they try to maintain this position as best they can, it is not always possible. By delivering a slight push, the offensive wrestler moves the opponent into a more upright position, which offers an opportunity to execute a takedown before the opponent can resume a forward-leaning position.

A good defensive position is assumed by flexing at the knees to lower the body's COG (*see Figure 1*). Wrestlers' stability is proportional to their base of support. A wrestler who stands with feet together can easily be thrown off balance. Thus, wrestlers use a wide staggered stance with their knees bent and their feet anywhere from 24 to 36 inches (60 to 90 cm) apart. This enlarges the base of support, making it much easier to keep from being knocked off balance. A secondary benefit of a wide staggered stance is that it lowers the COG. Bending at the knees and crouching will lower the COG more, for an even stabler base of support. Although this is a very simple principle, applying it takes considerable training because many moves tend naturally to raise a wrestler's COG.

Usually, the feet need to be about hip-width apart to provide the

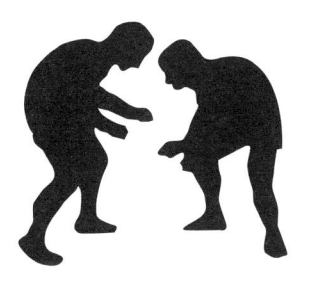

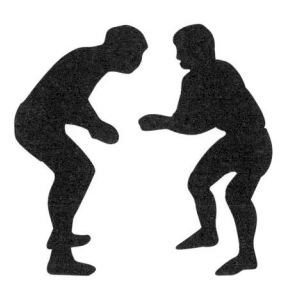

Figure 1. *For good balance and rapid movement backward and forward, wrestlers use a staggered stance with knees bent (top). For good balance and rapid movement left and right, they use a parallel stance (bottom).*

wrestler with stability laterally as well as backward and forward. In attacking, wrestlers all use short, quick, low-to-the-ground steps to keep the COG as low as possible. Such steps provide stability and maintain balance during the explosive locomotion of the attack.

The same principles apply when a wrestler assumes the "down" position (kneeling with hands flat on mat). The postion is very stable when the hands are placed out wider than the shoulders, and the knees are out wider than the hips.

Sometimes wrestlers attempt to keep the COG on the rear leg rather than the forward leg. During an offsenive move, this allows the wrestler to stop a forward thrust up to some midway point without losing control. If a wrestler launches a takedown move with the body weight over the front foot, there is no turning back after committing to the move. A rear-foot start allows time to reconsider the move during the moment when the wrestler rocks over the front foot. This is not true of a front-foot lead. Almost as soon as the front foot begins moving, the wrestler's weight moves forward and outside the base of support. However, there is sometimes a good reason for a front-foot lean: maintaining weight over the front foot allows the rear leg and foot to generate rotational velocity to swing around behind the opponent.

Many of the moves in wrestling center on manipulation and control of the opponent's head, since controlling the head position helps control the movement of the body as well. The principle operating here is that a wrestler who applies force above the opponent's COG can more easily develop rotation, because the distance from head to COG is much less than the distance from feet to COG. For another example of this principle, consider two small, light people—two children, say—who want to move a portable volleyball net post: they will soon figure out that it is much easier to push the heavily weighted circular base than to try to spin it by rotating the end of the pole.

Successful wrestlers are usually offensive wrestlers—those who continually drive forward. For one thing, the human body is not designed to move backward as easily or effectively as it moves forward. Also, any backward motion places a wrestler at a tremendous disadvantage in terms of momentum, which is equal to mass × velocity. Although this concept is very important for all wrestlers, it is particularly important for lighter wrestlers, that is, for wrestlers with less mass. An effective takedown attempt requires a combination of momentum, balance, leverage, and good timing. (*For a fuller explanation of momentum, see "Sumo Wrestling," below.*)

It is important to note that offensive wrestling includes not only movement forward, but also movement left and right. Continually moving to the right or left opens up new angles of attack, as both wrestlers shift their balance while circling. The strategy in circling to the left and right is to seek an opening for unleashing explosive force in the forward direction—accelerating mass toward the opponent to execute a takedown.

Leverage

No matter how great the natural strength of a wrestler may be, it is inconsequential without an understanding of leverage. In fact, wrestling is in large part a matter of leverage.

Leverage in throws. In a throw, the opponent is taken from a standing position to a prone position. Executing a throw requires a working knowledge of certain basic principles of physics: force, stability, torque, and rotational motion. Two other necessities are fluidity and timing, although these are not as easily described in terms of basic physics.

Stability of the thrower and instability of the opponent are of paramount importance. It is impossible to execute a throw without overcoming the opponent's stability. To a great extent, the success of a throw depends on anticipating a movement by the opponent that will create momentary instability, and then making a well-timed response. Unless the thrower quickly takes advantage of the opponent's momentarily unstable position, the opponent will be able to return to a well-balanced position and thus will be able to exert firm resistance to the throw. (In this scenario, neither wrestler will be thrown.)

Almost all throws rely on principles of rotational motion. To initiate rotational motion, torque is necessary. Applying torque involves two equal and opposite forces acting on an opponent's body. In wrestling (and in judo), one common form of torque occurs when the thrower applies pressure against the opponent's axis of rotation, usually the COG (for example, the waist), and then generates a throwing force at a point distant from the axis of rotation (for example, the shoulder). To calculate the torque involved, two forces must be multiplied: the force bringing about the rotation, and the lever arm between the pivot point (axis of rotation) and the force. Physicists refer to this type of lever as a first-class lever: the force and the weight are at opposite ends, with the fulcrum or pivot point somewhere between them (*see Figure 2; see also* WEIGHT LIFTING.)

One of the most common throws in wrestling (and judo) is the hip throw (*see Figure 3*). This is worth examining in some detail. First, the thrower must step forward toward the opponent, and specifically toward the opponent's COG, closing the distance between the thrower's hip and the opponent's COG to create a pivot point so that the force generated creates rotational motion about the hip. Next comes the pull. It is best for the pull to be to the right or left, because this shortens the distance that the opponent's COG must be displaced. In comparison, a pull straight toward the thrower keeps the opponent's COG more directly over the base of support, making it easier for the opponent to recover from the instability and to counter the thrower's rotation.

One key to wrestling (and, again, to judo) can be seen here: a chief aim is to dupe the opponent into assuming an unstable position. A wrestler who is in an unstable position, even for a brief moment,

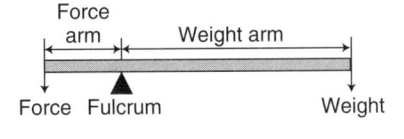

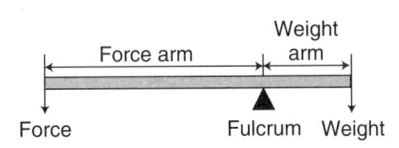

Figure 2. *Wrestling in large part is a matter of leverage. When a force is applied near the fulcrum (above), it requires much more torque than when the force arm is much longer than the weight arm (below).*

Figure 3. *(a) In an improper hip throw, the center of gravity (X) and pivot point (dot) do not match up. The lever arm of the opponent's weight works against the throw. (b) It takes an instability due to the weight of the opponent to execute the throw. (c) When the center of gravity and pivot point match up, the hip throw is much easier to execute. (Adapted from Walker, 1980)*

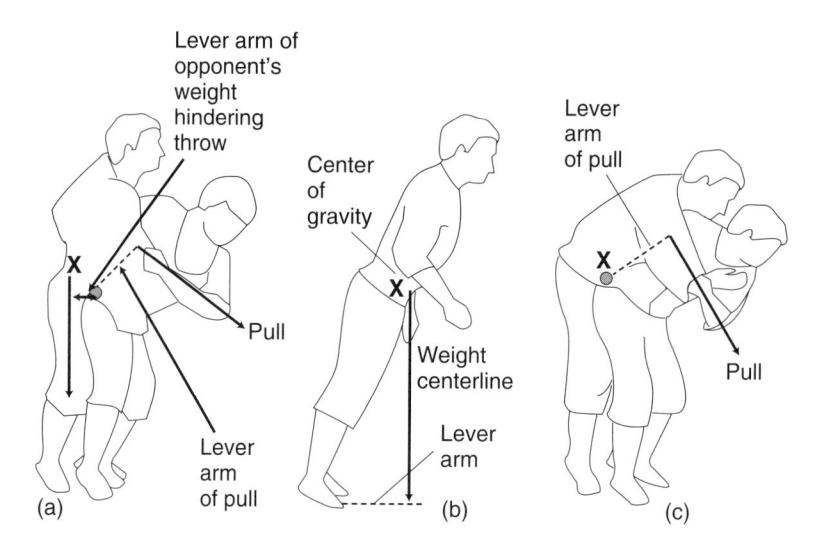

can usually be brought crashing to the mat before there is a chance to regain stability, if a skilled opponent applies torque.

In executing throws, wrestlers sometimes first push at—"straight-arm"—the opponent. This move forces the opponent's COG slightly away from the base of support; it also lengthens the thrower's force arm lever as the opponent is pulled back. Thus, more torque can be created by bringing the opponent back across the COG and executing a throw in the opposite direction.

A combination of good timing and proper positioning is critical. More often than not, when attempted throws are unsuccessful it is because throwers miscalculate the opponent's position or err in their own timing. With regard to timing, the margin of error is very slender—probably tenths of a second. Because wrestlers continually adjust their COG, any window of opportunity for executing a throw usually closes quickly.

To return to the hip throw: The pull brings the opponent's COG forward of the navel, that is, to a point outside the body. This is the point where the thrower's hip should be, the pivot around which the opponent can be rotated. There are actually two torques involved in the hip throw: one from the opponent's own weight and unstable position, the other from the pull the thrower exerts on the opponent. It is important to note that without shifting an opponent's weight and creating an unstable position (the first torque), the thrower could never generate sufficient pulling torque to finish off the throw.

Being short is an advantage in executing the hip throw, for two reasons. First, a short thrower has a lower COG and can thus more easily slide the hip under a taller opponent, and pull the opponent downward in a more smoothly curved rotational motion (more "over" than "up and over"). Second, a shorter person has a greater potential for generating pulling torque because of the longer lever arm as measured from the taller opponent's COG to the pulling torque exerted at the thrower's shoulder.

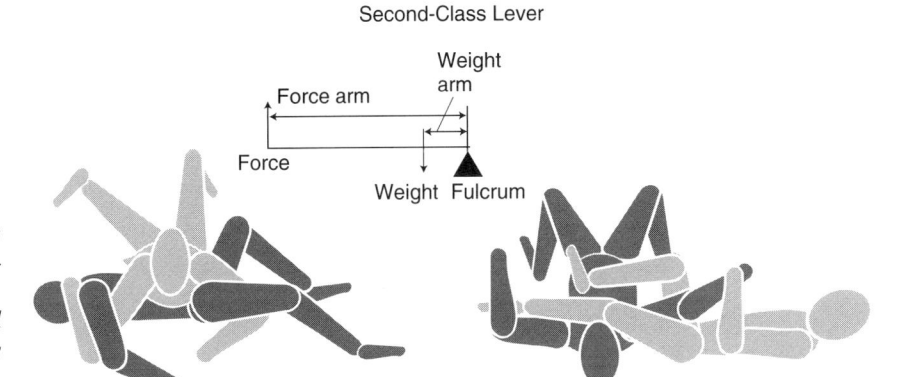

Figure 4. *Second-class levers are effective at maintaining a position—controlling an opponent's position. Left: Second-class lever being used in a pinning movement. Right: Cross armlock in judo.*

Leverage in the half nelson. Leverage is not only vital in throws but is also important for other moves, such as trying to turn an opponent from a face-down position. Wrestlers try to turn an opponent with a technique called a half nelson. In a typical half nelson, the wrestler places the right arm under the opponent's right arm with the forearm resting against the opponent's neck. Because wrestlers often cannot supply enough leverage to turn an opponent in this position, they move their forearm down from the neck to the shoulder. This increases the turning action that can be generated, because a shorter force arm can move faster than a longer one. However, repositioning the forearm is not always the best option, because the shorter force, although faster, is not as great. The better choice in many cases is a longer force arm: it is slower but stronger (there is more torque).

The half nelson, like the hip throw, involves a first-class lever.

Leverage in the press pin. A different kind of leverage applies in a body "press pin" combination. Here the wrestler creates a second-class lever using a long force arm hold (*see Figure 4*). The wrestler's body is anchored by the arms over the opponent's COG. With body and arms spread out in such a highly leveraged way, it is very difficult for the opponent to get up from the mat from a position flat on the back.

Sumo Wrestling

Wrestling is not widely popular in the United States, but in Japan the situation is very different: sumo wrestling is a national passion. It is so popular that the top sumo wrestlers are celebrities on a par with American rock stars and baseball superstars. In fact, sumo wrestling is more than a sport; it is part of a profound cultural tradition.

As a sport, sumo wrestling is very simple: it takes place in a sand ring 15 feet (4.5 m) in diameter, and the wrestler tries to push, twist, and throw his opponent either down or out of the ring. But sumo is also a spectacle. The wrestlers, who wear nothing more than the traditional mawashi belt, are enormous men, and they accelerate explo-

Wrestlers and the Hazards of Extreme Weight Loss and Gain

Weight loss in wrestling. Most high school and college wrestlers still abide by an old maxim: try to compete in the lowest weight class possible. The implication is that if you compete in a class below your normal or natural weight, you will be bigger and stronger relative to your opponents. Also, in wrestling (unlike most other sports), the existence of weight classes means that unless team members stay within their weight limit, the team's chance to win is jeopardized, because second-string wrestlers will have to substitute for them. During the wrestling season, therefore, some wrestlers are 10, 20, or even 30 pounds lighter than their normal weight. This is known as "making weight" or "weight cutting," and it has become almost a ritual.

The self-inflicted ordeal of making weight takes a terrible physical and psychological toll on a wrestler. Some wrestlers starve themselves; some use laxatives; some induce vomiting; some sit in a sauna for long periods of time. Whatever method is chosen, the result is the same: denying the body the food and water it requires.

Often, on the day before a match, wrestlers still need to lose 5 to 20 percent of their preseason weight. Because about 70 percent of body weight is water, wrestlers "sweat off" weight by wrestling vigorously, by running several miles in a rubber sweatsuit, or even by taking diuretics and laxatives. (A diuretic is a drug that causes the kidneys to exrete more water from the body; a laxative is a drug that causes the bowel to empty more rapidly.) Not only water but also fat, protein, and glycogen are lost in this process. The wrestler arrives at the weigh-in dehydrated and exhausted but makes the weight.

When wrestlers make their weight by dehydrating themselves, the quantity of blood in their veins is below normal, adversely affecting the heart: cardiac output is lower, stroke volume is smaller, and heart rate is higher. Another consequence of dehydration and decreased blood volume is a decrease in the filtration of wastes from blood by the kidneys. Also, there is a loss of electrolytes, and this can impair nearly every cellular process, including nerve transmission and heart function. Dehydration, by reducing fluid available for producing sweat, can make it more difficult for the body to keep cool while working. It is also suspected that reduced fluid may upset the chemical balance within the cells, making it more difficult for the body to utilize energy. In all, starvation and fluid deprivation wreak havoc on the body's internal regulators.

Many coaches believe that dehydration is a temporary phenomenon and that wrestlers can replenish the body's water supply, undoing any potential damage, in the time between weigh-in and match—an interval of 1 hour for high school matches and 3 hours for collegiate matches. But studies incorporating blood tests, urine samples, and biopsies (tissue extraction) have found that a wrestler is still dehydrated 1 hour after drinking large quantities of water. This lag occurs because it takes time for the body to replenish its water supply (see NUTRITION).

Besides dehydration, many wrestlers also engage in starvation dieting a few days to a week before competing. Dieting deprives the body of sugar, its main source of energy. In this situation, the body begins breaking down its supply of glycogen (the body's ready energy supply, used by exercising muscles) to form glucose (sugar), which is vital for brain function (see ENERGY AND METABOLISM). Most wrestlers are already very lean (they have no excess body fat), and so the body must begin to convert protein into glucose to maintain nervous system function. Wrestlers may lose up to several ounces of protein a day, much of it stolen from muscle tissue.

With this internal chaos, the wrestler steps onto the mat—where the muscles will be asked to perform at peak capacity. Not surprisingly, the muscles cannot respond at anywhere near their full potential: their energy supply has been depleted. No one doubts that a starving wrestler runs out of energy. Starved wrestlers are deprived of glycogen, the primary source of anaerobic power (the kind used by the explosive fast-twitch muscles), and they are therefore unable to summon the quick bursts of speed and power that are the basis of wrestling. At first, these wrestlers may show no appreciable loss in anaerobic power, but as a match wears on they simply run out of gas. The body is being asked to run at full speed, but there is no fuel in the tank to make that possible.

Nor is this the only liability caused by starvation dieting: a protein-calorie deficiency, along with other specific nutrient deficiencies, has been shown to decrease the ability of the immune system to resist viral and bacterial infections.

Furthermore, besides the obvious outward signs of rapid, extreme weight loss—gauntness, weakness, and fatigue—there can be adverse effects on the body's hormonal functioning. The endocrine system includes all the hormone-secreting glands: pancreas, testes, ovaries, hypothalamus, kidneys, pituitary, thyroid, parathyroid, adrenal, intestinal, thymus, heart, and pineal. These glands are responsible for a multitude of chemical regulation and coordination functions.

Endocrinologists at Ohio State University have found that extremely low body fat—anything less than 5 percent—has the potential to impair the endocrine system (Strauss, 1993). In particular, wrestlers can experience a significant drop in serum (blood) levels of several hormones: testosterone, estradiol, prolactin, thyroxine, and luteinizing hormone. The mechanism that causes these endocrine changes in some wrestlers remains unclear, though it is widely believed that the drastic alteration of the internal environment somehow triggers a reduction in hormone secretion. Once body weight and the percentage of body fat return to normal, the endocrine system begins to function properly again. Whether or not this short-term "shock" to the endocrine system has any long-term effects on health is still uncertain.

Another serious implication of this kind of weight loss has to do with its effects on the immature body. The majority of wrestlers compete at the high school level, at ages 13 to 18, when they are still growing. Poor nutrition in these formative years is detrimental to health in both the short and the long term. Of course, at this age—as at any other—weight loss is sometimes necessary, but if so, it should be done gradually through reasonable exercise and sensible dieting.

Various steps could be taken to address the problem of dangerous weight loss in wrestling. For one thing, wrestling coaches should plan more realistically. Despite their best intentions, coaches often find themselves in a difficult situation: the two best wrestlers on a team naturally carry about the same weight. In this case, these two wrestlers are competing against each other for one weight-class position on the team, so only one of them will be able to wrestle at the natural weight; still, the coach should probably resist the temptation to have the other one drop down, rather than move up, a weight class.

Regulations could also help. In Wisconsin, for example, high school wrestlers are required to maintain a minimum 7 percent body fat and are allowed a maximum weight loss of only 3 pounds a week: this helps ensure that they will have enough energy to train and compete. If such safeguards were established nationwide, coaches would no longer be able to gain any advantage from risking their wrestlers' health, and thousands of young wrestlers would be protected.

Sumo wrestlers and weight gain. At the other extreme from wrestlers obsessed with losing weight are sumo wrestlers—who are obsessed with gaining weight. From the moment they step into their first practice ring, sumo wrestlers realize that a deficit in mass will be difficult to overcome. The only way to stop a freight train is to become a freight train yourself.

In order to gain as much weight as possible, then, sumo wrestlers eat enormous amounts. In fact, gorging is part of the lifestyle and lore of sumo: thirty-six trays of noodles at one sitting, fifteen platefuls of cutlets, twenty-four pounds of sweet potatoes—to mention just a few legendary instances. One traditional sumo dish, eaten in tremendous quantities twice a day (at lunch and dinner), is *chankonabe*, a stew of fish, stalks of greens, and rice.

But it is not simply the amount eaten that is significant here; another factor is the pattern of gorging itself. In experiments with rats, those fed one large meal gained 25 percent more weight than those fed the same amount of food in six small meals. A few studies with human subjects have also found this difference between "gorgers" and "nibblers." When a large amount of food is consumed quickly—this is the definition of gorging—the fuel-regulating hormone, insulin, is released more quickly and is then sustained longer in the bloodstream. For sumo wrestlers, large meals ensure that their insulin levels remain elevated longer after they eat. Insulin allows cells to absorb energy-packed nutrients from the blood; it helps the muscles replenish their store of glycogen and also helps fat cells take up and store fatty molecules (*see also ENERGY AND METABOLISM*). Gorging thus increases the likelihood that the body will have a large excess of fuel and, therefore, that a considerable portion of the fuel will be converted to fat.

Another factor in weight gain among sumo wrestlers is the timing of their meals, specifically in relation to the times when they sleep or nap. Sumo wrestlers traditionally do not eat breakfast, because (to put it bluntly) they don't want to vomit during their belly-slamming morning practice. Thus by the time they have lunch, after the morning practice, they have gone 12 to 16 hours without eating. Moreover, the 6 hours of morning exercise preceding this meal consist of bumping, grinding, and sweating. Exercise normally increases metabolic rate, but for sumo wrestlers it has the opposite effect: their morning exercise on an empty stomach signals the body that more calories are being spent than consumed, and so their metabolic rate drops. After a huge lunch, they nap; and after a huge dinner at night, they go to bed.

This schedule of fasting, exercising, eating, and sleeping is highly conducive to weight gain. Eating a large meal before a long nap or before a night's sleep ensures that most of the ingested nutrients will turn to fat. On top of that, in the morning these sumo wrestlers train on an empty stomach, which "tricks" the body into operating

(continued)

Wrestlers and the Hazards of Extreme Weight Loss and Gain (continued)

at a slower metabolic rate. And sumo wrestling itself involves expending energy in short, intense bursts that do not burn body fat. Burning fat requires moderate energy-expending (aerobic) workouts of 20 minutes or more, but such workouts are not part of a sumo wrestler's daily practice sessions.

As noted, all this is ideal for gaining weight, but it is dangerous for long-term health. Actually, there are no studies of the long term health of sumo wrestlers or former sumo wrestlers; but there has been an informative study, by the National Institutes of Health, of a similar group: retired professional football players (*see also* FOOTBALL). This study found that life expectancy for linemen—who are the largest players—was lower than that for men who had played other positions. The overriding reason for a shorter life was apparently heart disease. This does not indicate that larger people necessarily die earlier. Rather, it seems that once players stop competing at a high level, they stop or greatly decrease their physical activity but continue to eat, and even to gorge, at their former rate. Eventually, their tremendous muscle mass declines, and in its place they develop a large increase in body fat. Inactivity and a high level of body fat, taken together—not size—are what lead to heart disease (*see also* AGING AND PERFORMANCE, ENERGY AND METABOLISM, and NUTRITION).

HEALTHY WEIGHT CONTROL

Sumo wrestlers are experts at putting on weight, but most athletes want to maintain their weight or lose weight. A healthy program of weight control should abide by a few simple principles:

- *Weight loss should occur over an extended period, and only the loss of excess fat—not water or lean tissue—is desirable.*
- *Drink plenty of water. Water is a nutrient, and a deficiency of water—more quickly than a deficiency of any other nutrient—can lead to premature fatigue and possible illness.*
- *Eat small meals, and do not exercise on an empty stomach. This practice will maintain fuel in your tank—that is, keep a more even energy supply available—so that your body will not have to lower its metabolic rate to compensate for a lack of fuel.*
- *Avoid skipping breakfast; on the contrary, concentrate most of your eating early in the day. Meals eaten early in the day have a better chance of being burned rather than being stored as body fat. Napping soon after a large meal is a sure way to gain weight.*
- *Limit your intake of fat. Fat is a highly concentrated source of energy that, pound for pound, provides far more calories than carbohydrates or proteins.*
- *Get most of your calories from complex carbohydrates like corn, potatoes, rice, pasta, cereal, and bread—rather than from sugars. Complex carbohydrates are broken down more slowly and are less readily stored as body fat.*
- *Do not limit activities to those involving brief intense bursts of energy (like sprinting and weight lifting). Sustained exercise—of either low or high intensity—burns calories.*

John Zumerchik

sively toward each other like freight trains, with a bellowing "Ahhhhhg!" When they collide belly to belly, a loud splatting noise resoundes through the arena. On contact, sumo wrestlers lock up, each securing a firm grip on the opponent's belt. An interesting feature of sumo is that it begins with a prolonged war of nerves called *niramiai*, in which the combatants size each other up. During *niramiai*, wrestlers must maintain their concentration and try to read the opponent's intent—will his first move be to the right or the left? Many sumo wrestlers and experts in sumo believe that a wrestler can break an opponent simply by staring him down at this point.

Wrestlers who reach the pinnacle of sumo are called *yokozuna*, and they are the kings of the sport—the top of a hierarchy of 800 wrestlers. There are very few *yokozuna*, so when they compete they are a huge box-office draw; scalpers ask for, and often get, as much as $4,000 for a ringside seat. *Yokozuna* cannot be demoted, but a *yokozuna* often retires in his mid-thirties, when he starts to lose more than he wins.

In the early 1990s, one of the most popular figures in sumo was Konishiki (*see Figure 5*), a wrestler of Samoan descent who was born in Hawaii. Konishiki was a living testament to the advantages of greater mass: he was 6 feet 1 inch tall (1.8 m) and weighed 580 pounds (263 kg). He was one of perhaps a dozen sumo wrestlers (including Kotogaume and Kushimaumi) weighing over 400 pounds (180 kg), but he weighed 175 pounds more than most elite sumo wrestlers, and 300 pounds more than the average sumo wrestler. Konishiki's body was almost cubical: he was almost as wide and thick as he was tall. If genetic engineers set out to create a perfect sumo wrestler, they probably could not do much better than Konishiki. Many observers believed that Konishiki often won bouts in *niramiai*, without having to take a step; his opponents felt that he grew larger and larger the longer they looked at him.

Actually, some sumo traditionalists have been concerned that giants like Konishiki will change the sport: that its character as an ancient and almost mystical art form will become less important, and that victory will depend more on mass than on skill. This concern seems warranted, although other observers tend to disagree, arguing that quickness and timing are just as important as mass.

The Sumo Association officially recognizes 70 moves. These 70 moves fall into four categories: throws, trips, bending, and twisting. Almost all moves use *yotsu-zumo* and *tsukioshi-zumo*. *Yotsu-zumo* entails the use of the mawashi belt to lift and throw an opponent out of the ring; *tsukioshi-zumo* entails pushing and thrusting to drive an

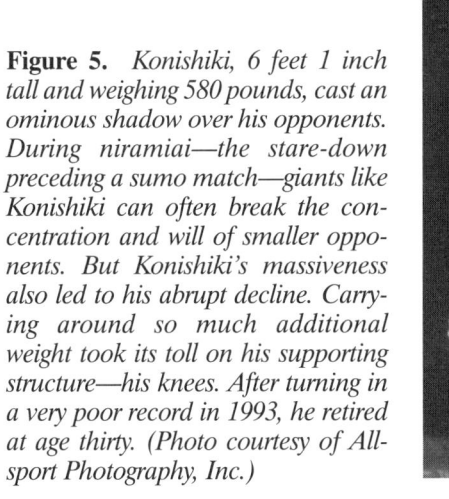

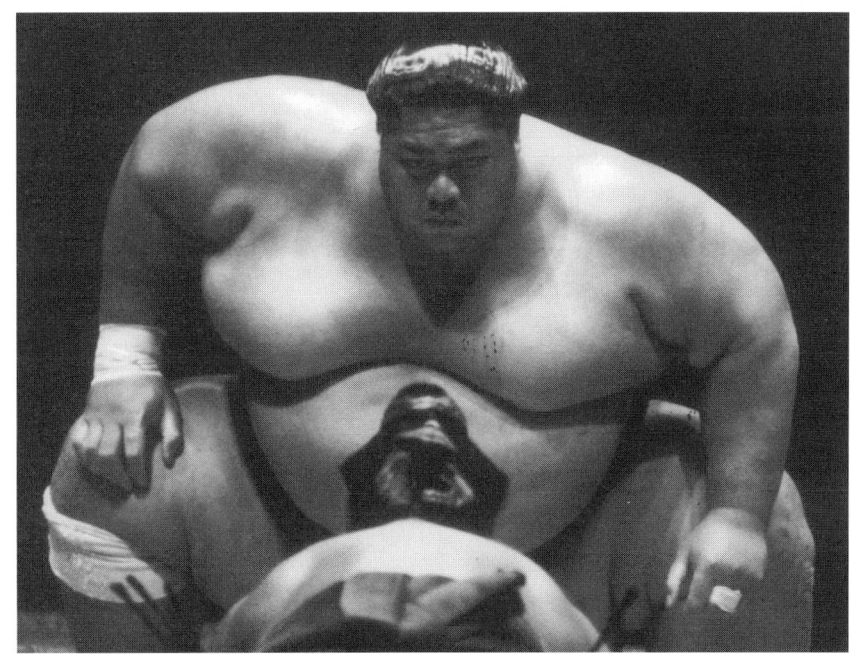

Figure 5. *Konishiki, 6 feet 1 inch tall and weighing 580 pounds, cast an ominous shadow over his opponents. During niramiai—the stare-down preceding a sumo match—giants like Konishiki can often break the concentration and will of smaller opponents. But Konishiki's massiveness also led to his abrupt decline. Carrying around so much additional weight took its toll on his supporting structure—his knees. After turning in a very poor record in 1993, he retired at age thirty. (Photo courtesy of Allsport Photography, Inc.)*

opponent out of the ring. Wrestlers who rely solely *tsukioshi* (pushing) maneuvers must strike fast because they will soon be at a disadvantage: the longer a match lasts, the more important *yotsu-zumo* becomes.

Collisions in Sumo

Any one of the 70 moves a sumo wrestler decides to use involves controling the initial collision. Probably the most pertinent formula of physics applicable to collisions in sumo is

$$\text{linear momentum} = \text{mass} \times \text{velocity}$$

Mass is a measure of inertia—the tendency of an object at rest to stay at rest, and the tendency of a body in motion to maintain motion. Velocity is the rate of motion. The momentum of an object—moving or stationary—can be changed only by applying force to the object. An accelerating force from a push or pull causes momentum to increase. A decelerating force—from a collision or friction—causes momentum to decrease. When there is no net force, momentum remains constant.

The key to sumo is maintaining momentum, which means controlling the collision with the opponent through a combination of strength, speed, and balance. Sumo wrestlers maintain a low COG, accelerate as quickly as possible, and on contact use balance and strength to move the opponent out of the ring. However, although these wrestlers attempt to keep their COG low, they must be careful not to touch the floor. When any part of the body other than the foot touches the floor, even momentarily, the match ends and the wrestler who touched the floor loses. A sumo match rarely lasts more than a few seconds, because one wrestler usually gains a small advantage on contact and then uses that advantage to drive the opponent down or out of the ring.

To decelerate an opponent, the countering force applied must be enough to bring the opponent's momentum to zero. Naturally, the more momentum the opponent has, the more force is needed to stop him. The time interval also must be considered. A small force acting over an extended period is as effective as a large force acting for a shorter period. In other words, the longer a force acts, the more change in momentum it will produce. When two sumo wrestlers surge toward each other, each of them experiences a tremendous decelerating force. In the simplest sense, the one who is better able to continue driving forward—to maintain his own linear momentum—is likely to come out victorious.

According to the law of conservation of momentum, when two wrestlers collide the increase in the momentum of one must be equal to the decrease in the momentum of the other. Assume that two sumo wrestlers have the same COG, the same strength, and the same ability to maintain balance, but that one weighs 380 pounds (173 kg) and the other is Konishiki, weighing 580 pounds (263 kg). In a collision in which both are moving at a velocity of 10 feet (3 m) per second, Konishiki's momentum will be 52.6 percent greater than that of his lighter opponent. The net effect is for his opponent to come to a stop and then go backward at a velocity of 2.08 feet per second. Greater speed contributes to greater momentum, though. In this example, if the 380-pound wrestler increases his velocity to 16 feet (just under 5 m) per second, his momentum will be more than Konishiki's (190 versus 181.25 momentum units), and he will drive the heavier Konishiki backward. However, this second scenario is only hypothetical with regard to sumo. In football, collisions often do take place in which there is a tremendous difference in velocity between the colliding players; but in sumo, the small size of the ring makes it unlikely that either wrestler can move at high speed.

Technique in Sumo

In the example above, it is assumed that the collision is head-on, and that the collision point coincides with COG for each player. Of course, this is not always the case. In collisions in sumo, the importance of linear momentum is somewhat diminished because a collision is rarely direct or centered. In fact, if collisions were direct and centered, the wrestler with the greater mass would win almost every time.

Almost all wrestlers use two moves in which mass is less important: *oshidashi* and *tsukioshi*. These are the open-palm slapping moves usually seen at the beginning of a match. In these moves, the intent is not to knock the opponent down or out of the ring but simply to knock him slightly off-balance. Knocking the opponent off-balance in this way gives a wrestler a great advantage: while the opponent is briefly unbalanced, he himself can quickly lock up in a balanced position.

The concept of center of gravity (COG) is therefore very important in sumo technique. Not only does a comparatively lower COG assist in moving an opponent backward, but it also gives a wrestler a distinct advantage in leverage. By grabbing an opponent's mawashi belt while driving his own legs forward and arching his own back, a wrestler can further raise the opponent's COG. This will increase the propulsive force he himself can generate from the ground and lower the propulsive force his opponent can generate from the ground. Maintaining good ground contact, with feet driving forward, means that the deliverable force is equal to the sum of the wrestler's momentum, plus the force being generated from the ground through the legs.

Sumo wrestlers are, in effect, human bulldozers. They scoop up their load, raise it, carry it, and then dump it.

John Zumerchik

References

Benjamin, David. *The Joy of Sumo: A Fan's Perspective*. Rutland, Vermont: Tuttle, 1991.

Chiba, K., et al. "Cefatium Disposition in Markedly Obese Athlete Patients, Japanesse Sumo Wrestlers." *Journal of Antimicrobial Agents Chemotherapy* 33, no. 8 (1989): 1188–1192.

Lidz, Franz. "Meat Bomb." *Sports Illustrated* 76, no. 68 (18 May 1992), 68–82.

Northrip, J., et al. *Introduction to Biomechanical Analysis of Sport* (2nd ed.). Dubuque, Iowa: Brown, 1979.

Piscopo, J., and J. Baley. *Kinesiology: The Science of Movement*. New York: Wiley, 1981.

Sackett, Joel. "Sumo Wrestling." *Health Magazine* (March–April 1993).

Sandoz, P. *Sumo Showdown: The Hawaiian Challenge*. Rutland, Vermont: Tuttle, 1992.

Sharnoff, Lora. *Grand Sumo: The Living Sport and Tradition*. New York: Weatherhill, 1989.

Strauss, R., et al. "Decreased Testosterone and Libido with Severe Weight Loss." *Physician and Sports Medicine* 21, no. 12 (1993): 64–71.

Walker, J. "In Judo and Aikido Application of the Physics of Forces Makes the Weak Equal to the Strong." *Scientific American* 243, no. 1 (July 1980): 150–156.

Webster, S., et al. "Physiological Effects of a Weight Loss Regimen Practiced by College Wrestlers." *Journal of Medicine and Science in Sports and Exercise* 22, no. 2 (April 1990): 229–234.

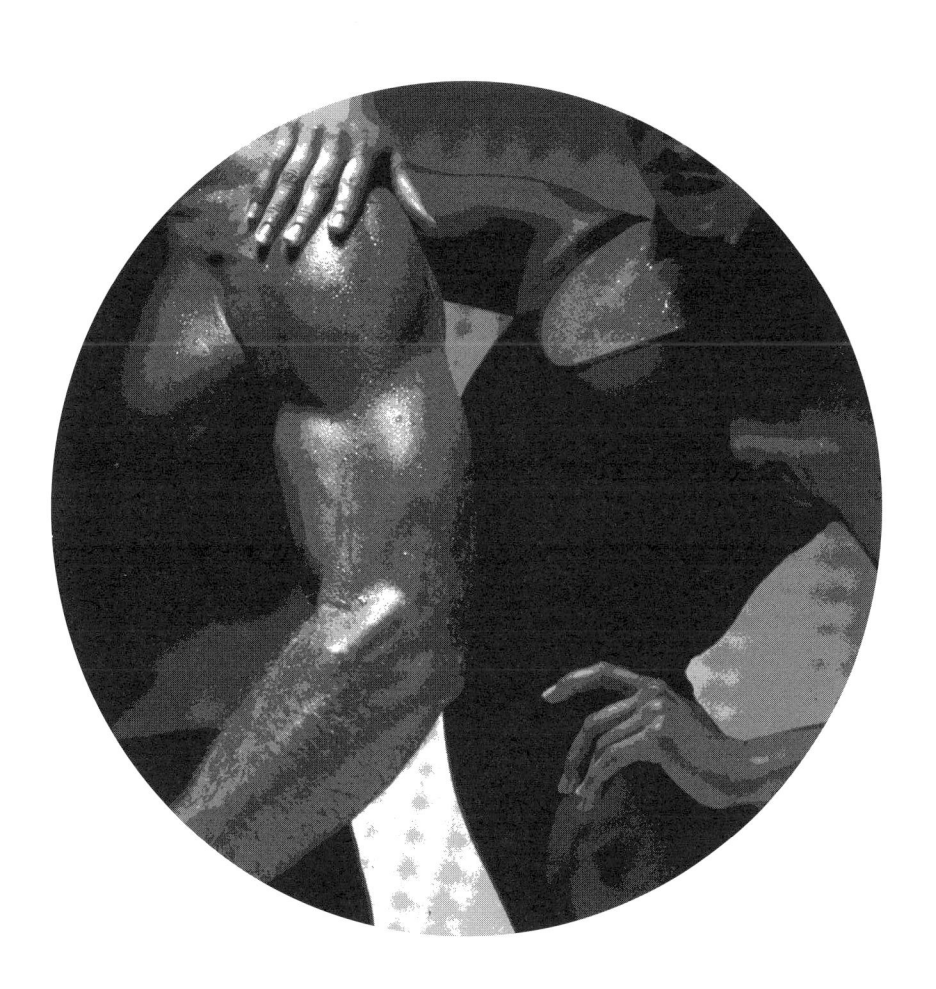

Part Two

The Body

Aging and Performance

ALL HUMAN SOCIETIES recognize a number of life stages. In the United States, people may be identified as children, teenagers, young adults, middle-aged, or elderly. Each category influences perceptions about what physical activities are appropriate for people of that "age." As recently as the 1960s, many people believed that the elderly should curtail their activity because exercise could be hazardous to their health. Sports, particularly competitive sports, were the domain of the young. Despite widespread scientific evidence of the benefits of regular physical activity, even in the 1990s many people continue to believe that the final years of life should be sedentary. The elderly often live in retirement communities, somewhat separate from the rest of society, and this tends to create a sedentary lifestyle.

Aging is one of the great mysteries of life. No two people age in exactly the same way or at the same pace. Aging and the condition of the elderly also vary from society to society; an extended life span without a high quality of life is certainly not the same as an extended life span with health and physical mobility. The United States, Japan, and Europe are considered "aging societies." By the year 2030, more than 20 percent of the population in the United States will be 65 or older. The percentage of people over 65 in the United States nearly tripled from 1900 to 1980 (4.1 percent to 11 percent), and the number of people over 65 in the United States is expected to nearly triple again by the year 2030 (Institute of Medicine, 1990). The elderly (ages 60 to 75), old (ages 76 to 90), and very old (more than 90 years old) make up one of the fastest-growing minority groups in the country.

The number of people age 85 and older is expected to swell to 18 million by the year 2050, by which time the average life expectancy in the United States is expected to rise to more than 82 years ("Geographic High Life Expectancy," 1993). Some policy makers are concerned by this dramatic increase in life expectancy because of the potential burden on the health care system. Some assume that the elderly are less productive and incur more disabilities, injuries, and diseases than the rest of the population. While these generalizations may be accurate statistically, research shows that the time-related changes in the body do not necessarily mean disability or dysfunction. Lean body tissue and bone density tend to decline, and other age-related changes seem to increase the incidence of cardiovascular disease, but it now seems clear that the pace of aging varies with heredity, environment, and the level of physical activity.

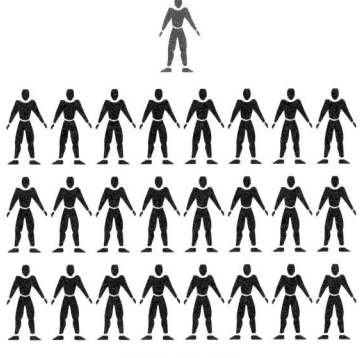

1905: 1 in 25

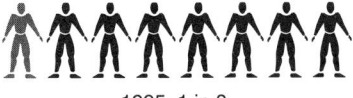

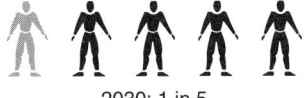

1995: 1 in 8

2030: 1 in 5

Figure 1. *Past, present, and projected demographic changes in the U.S. population over the age of 65. The dramatic increase in the number of people age 65 and higher is primarily attributable to better health care, which has increased the average life expectancy (Farrell, 1995).*

583

Biological Theories of Aging

Physiologists define aging as a process that involves a loss of capacity to withstand physical or environmental stress, which leads to functional impairment and eventually death (Spirduso, 1995). Most people associate aging with its outward signs: graying hair, wrinkles, and decreased mobility. But the process of aging also has internal and psychological impacts.

Two important events occur with aging. First, there are structural and physiological changes to the body, which are usually considered irreversible. Second, the biological changes frequently trigger psychological, emotional, and social changes that require adaptation. A loss in reserve energy capacity, or an inability to adapt to environmental stresses, is a good indication that aging has begun in body cells or in body systems. In the last stages of aging, the body fails to maintain itself through repair and replacement. It deteriorates and eventually fails to function.

The exact process of aging is a topic of extensive scientific research. Scientists have studied many aspects of aging, such as cellular deterioration and increased vulnerability to illness, disease, accidents, musculoskeletal pain, and discomfort. However, no single theory explains the aging process or the reasons that one person lives longer than another. Most theories about aging are based in large part on the following assumptions: Cells can divide only a fixed number of times; cell death is a genetically "preprogrammed" event; an accumulation of toxins can damage and eventually kill cells; and an accumulation of mutations can lead to cell death. Many theories propose that aging involves two or more of these general processes, or that the processes trigger one another.

Age-Related Changes and Exercise

This section describes the changes that occur in the various systems of the body during the aging process and investigates the effects that exercise may have on these age-related changes. Many of the elderly are paying a high price (poor health and premature mortality) because they were not physically active as their bodies aged. Exercise can help slow the decline in muscle strength and flexibility and may even improve the functional status of many organ systems.

Integumentary System

The body's exterior, known as the integumentary system, visibly changes with aging. Exterior wound healing slows due to changes in blood vessels that impede circulation to the skin. The skin starts to develop "age spots" and loses its elasticity, producing wrinkles. While these changes are not life-threatening, they are very obvious markers of aging.

Hair is often a highly visible marker of change. It changes in both qualitative (thinning and greying) and quantitative (balding) ways. As the level of pigment in the hair and cellular material production decline, it turns gray. This decline in pigment levels and cellular production also affects related glands and the nails.

The breakdown of collagen and elastin fibers over time causes another marker of aging, the thinning of skin. Skin becomes more susceptible to sun damage, bruises more easily, and may develop pressure sores. Decreased tolerance to cold is also common; this is due to thinning of the insulating layer of fat below the skin and a decrease in blood flow to internal body tissues.

Collectively, these changes often result in an altered body image that may negatively affect sexuality and self-esteem. Regular exercise may help in maintaining a positive self-image and attitude because it generates feelings of endurance, strength, and vitality.

Sensory System

Although it is not a threat to vision, *arcus senilis* may occur as the eye ages. This condition is characterized by an infiltration of lipids (insoluble molecules made of carbon and hydrogen) into the cornea around the outside of the iris (*see Figure 2*). Numerous other changes may occur as well. The lacrimal canal (tear ducts) may clog, the lens may become less elastic, the eye's ability to change the shape of the lens (affecting accommodation) may suffer, and its ability to focus may become impaired (presbyopia; *see also VISION*).

For several reasons, hearing also declines with age. Age-related deafness appears to result from hypersensitivity to loud noise. A loss in the ability to distinguish pitch, particularly sounds of high frequency, is also very common. A decline in the number of hair cells and nerves of the ear is a primary factor responsible for this decline.

Hearing loss may also be caused by a thickening and subsequent loss of elasticity of the eardrum, or tympanic membrane, and the growth of spongy bone in the inner ear, a condition known as otosclerosis. Excess wax in the external auditory meatus, or middle ear fluid, atherosclerosis, and chronic infection are other common causes contributing to a decline in auditory ability.

Skeletal System

While other symptoms of aging may vary, the loss of calcium from bones is almost universal. If the loss in bone mass is severe, bones become porous, more fragile, and brittle. Osteoporosis results when bone mass is sufficiently reduced to cause, for example, compression fractures of the vertebrae, back pain, and decreased stature.

The decrease in bone mass makes the body more prone to fractures of the hip, involving the neck of the femur (*see also PELVIS, HIP, AND THIGH*), or at the wrist, in which the distal ends of the radius and ulna are broken (Colle's fracture). There also may be associated postural or alignment problems including humpback or flexed posture (kyphosis) and swayback (lordosis).

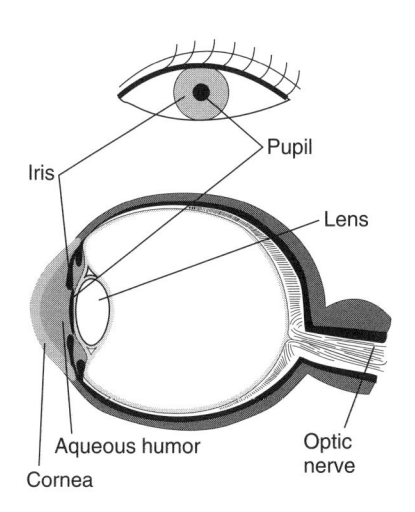

Figure 2. *Numerous age-related physiological changes occur to the eye that affect vision.*

Osteoporosis is a multifaceted disease in which the rate of bone resorption is greater than bone formation. The skeletal instability caused by porous bone increases the likelihood of significant pain, disability, and restricted mobility. Treatment of osteoporosis may require surgery, hospitalization, or placement in a nursing home.

Regular weight-bearing exercise plays a major role in retarding the loss of bone mass. When bone is stressed, bone-forming cells are activated to increase bone mineralization. This retention and development of bone, specifically in the spine and lower limbs, helps maintain the structure and integrity of the musculoskeletal system.

Changes of this type not only help prevent the age-related increase in bone fractures but also improve mobility. For example, a limited musculoskeletal range of motion may complicate an existing heart condition because tight joints require increased effort to move about, increasing the heart rate. An increase in heart rate requires an increase in oxygen to the heart. Given existing coronary artery disease, if oxygen does not increase, the heart becomes ischemic and chest pain (angina pectoris) ensues.

When joint flexibility is increased, the heart may not have to work as hard and therefore does not need a significant increase in oxygen. As a result, the reduction in the intensity and frequency of anxiety-provoking chest pain decreases the likelihood of a heart attack and susceptibility to an irregular heart rhythm.

Nervous System

It is believed that a loss of myelin (nerve cover and insulator) from some nerves is responsible for the slight decrease in the speed of nerve conduction in the peripheral nervous system as the body ages. In addition to this decline in speed, the number of motor neurons declines. Both factors adversely affect performance because they contribute to a decrease in reaction time.

Overall health is also a factor. Muscle atrophy and a decline in muscle strength adversely affect balance, which in turn requires changes in posture. Posture changes can increase pressure or friction against nerves that result in peripheral nerve pain (*see Figure 3*). Sciatica, for example, is a condition in which severe pain runs along the back of the lower leg. The sciatic nerve is compressed as nerve routes pass between the individual vertebrae. Age-related bone loss, which affects posture, may create problems with the spinal cord or spinal nerves. Displaced vertebral disks, vertebral fractures, and peripheral nerve pain are among the many structural changes with aging that can cause chronic pain and disability (*see also* SPINE).

The brain, the command and control center of the nervous system, experiences certain selective atrophy with aging. Although frequently difficult to locate and explain, some of the most common changes include neuron losses in the cerebral cortex, causing a decrease in brain weight; increase in the size of the two hemispheres and their ventricles (cavities); and extracellular deposits of amyloid polypeptides, various cell organelles, and degenerating nerves in the

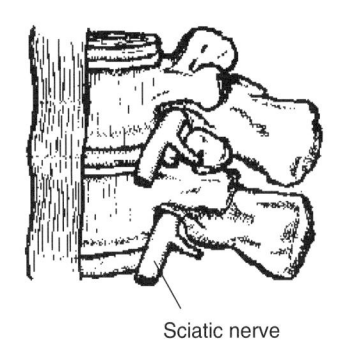

Figure 3. *Posture changes can increase pressure or friction against nerves. This may cause peripheral nerve pain, such as sciatica—a shooting pain that runs along the back of the lower limbs.*

cerebral gray matter, which may be associated with senility (also called senile dementia, or organic brain syndrome). Other frequent problems resulting from these changes are mental confusion and short-term impairment of memory, judgment, and the ability to learn.

Changes that occur in the central and peripheral nervous system might not be the result of aging alone. For example, regular physical activity may reverse the decline in the speed of nerve conduction that accompanies aging, so it is possible that disturbance of the nervous system is a function of inactivity rather than age. Many researchers believe that regular physical activity delays the age-related changes in the nervous system, particularly reaction time. While the exact mechanisms are not yet entirely understood, it seems that regular exercise provides the structure and function of the central nervous system with sensory input that overcomes a type of sensory deprivation associated with the aging process.

Similarly, exercise helps alleviate age-related changes in sleep patterns, and appears to reduce anxiety and promote a sense of well-being. Regular exercise may also play a role in the rate of deterioration of sense organ function. Aging and inactivity are associated with an increase in the auditory threshold, decrease in taste sensitivity, lessened intellectual capacity, and behavioral alterations, particularly depression. Regular exercise may delay these changes because they appear to be a function of disuse of the body as well as aging. The magnitude of the impact exercise has on these processes is unknown, but researchers suspect these changes may be offset significantly by exercise performed on a daily basis.

Muscular System

Age-related changes in the speed and ease of mobility are caused mainly by muscular and postural changes. Because of aging and inactivity, the number and diameter of muscle fibers decrease, and the muscles atrophy. They are replaced with fat and collagen, a protein found in connective tissue. Atrophy and poor posture result in muscle weakness and decreased blood circulation in specific areas of the body.

The neck region is one particularly susceptible area, as the age-related forward tilt of the head frequently causes pain and discomfort. The forward position of the head and neck creates instability of the head on the cervical vertebrae of the upper spine. The offset misalignment created by bone and muscle changes in the upper spine region causes the trapezius muscle at the back of the neck either to stay in a constant state of tension or to contract eccentrically; that is, the muscle contracts while it is lengthening. Both conditions may cause pain and discomfort in the neck region.

Moreover, the thoracic region between the neck and abdomen may tend to curve with age, causing a hunched appearance of the shoulders. To compensate for the movement of the body's center of gravity forward and away from the body, a broader gait and flexed-knee position are usually necessary to increase stability. As range of movement and physical activities decline, so does muscle strength, particularly in the lower limbs.

There also may be adverse postural adaptations in muscles under the trapezius muscle. Two such muscles include the levator scapulae and rhomboideus, which may atrophy. The first arises from the cervical vertebrae, while the latter arises primarily from the thoracic vertebrae, in the middle spine. Both muscles connect to the medial border of the scapula, or shoulder blade, to stabilize it during shoulder movements. When stressed, these muscles adjust by relaxing too much, thus causing a chronic lateral displacement, or protraction, of the scapula. This leads to a loss in effectiveness of the upper limbs, with increased atrophy and loss of strength.

Structural changes in skeletal muscles over time are similar to those observed with denervation. Hence, even though the muscles are connected to functional nerves, the effects of aging on muscle fiber structure result in significant changes in their function. This functional denervation with aging is characterized by a decrease in both the number of fibers and their capacity to generate energy for muscle contraction. The result is a reduction in the amount and activity of enzymes for glycolysis and oxidative metabolism in fast-twitch fibers—those producing rapid, repeated contraction.

Fast-twitch fibers are structurally and metabolically designed to supply energy for muscle contraction via the glycolytic pathway rather than the oxidative pathway (*see also* ENERGY AND METABOLISM). This tendency to selectively alter fast-twitch fibers, which are responsible for producing maximal, instant force, may be responsible for some of the decrease in strength in the aging body.

The decrease in the energetics of muscle contraction may be partly explained by the decrease in adenosine triphosphate (ATP) within individual muscle cells. The decrease in energy currency is apparently due to the decline in energy transfer, sources, and mechanisms. Phosphocreatine (PC) and glycogen are also decreased, which ultimately leads to a reduction in the recovery or synthesis of ATP. Since ATP is used directly for muscle contraction, a decrease in the recovery of ATP results in less transfer of chemical energy into tension, or contraction, energy. Muscles then fail to contract with the integrity they once had.

Inactivity is the main cause of age-related decline in muscle strength and the cross-sectional area of muscles, or muscle mass. A sedentary lifestyle has been linked to significant muscle fiber atrophy and the loss of associated motor neurons. Conversely, exercise has been linked to the ability to maintain significant muscle mass and strength. One study estimated an average loss of about 30 percent of muscle strength and 40 percent of muscle size between the second and seventh decades of life (Rogers and Evans, 1993).

An active lifestyle can provide an indirect health benefit: self-sufficiency. By maintaining overall body strength and efficiency, the elderly may be able to avoid increased dependence on family and friends. Moreover, the risk of falling declines with improved muscle strength and its related benefits to the musculoskeletal system and to postural stability—steady gait and balance, and strong muscles and bones help to lessen the impact of injuries from falls, such as hip fractures. Many studies have shown that the adverse changes in the soft connective tissues of the muscles, tendons, and joint capsules are slowed through participation in regular exercise. Maintaining strength and range of motion makes the simplest activities, such as standing up from a chair, less troublesome because the lower back muscles are not as restricted. Other lower-body and limb muscles, such as gluteals, hamstrings, and posterior leg muscles, also function better with regular exercise. Enhanced self-esteem and confidence may result from increased self-sufficiency, which may in turn encourage further involvement in physical activity.

Strength training is one way to increase the body's capacity to engage in aerobic activities over time, even without necessarily improving the cardiorespiratory system. In one study, researchers trained 12 healthy older men (age 60–72 yrs) for 12 weeks using standard strength conditioning procedures for developing the lower limb extensors and flexors. The study found that resistance training produced a variety of local adaptations in the exercised muscles. Biopsies of the vastus lateralis muscle showed a 28 percent increase in mean fiber area, no change in the distribution of fast-twitch muscle fiber, a 15 percent increase in capillaries per fiber (yielding better blood flow), and a 38 percent increase in citrate synthase activity (an indication of metabolic activity). The respiratory system benefited as well. Maximum oxygen consumption by leg cycle ergometry increased by 6 percent, though there was no effect of training on the heart (Frontera et al., 1990).

Respiratory System

Aging causes a loss of pulmonary function and increases the work of breathing. These changes also increase the volume that remains in the lungs at the end of a maximum expiration, known as the residual volume. This change may be due to a decrease in the elasticity of the lung tissue. Other changes include a loss of functioning alveoli, the air sacs in the lungs, and the related network of capillaries; both decrease the surface area for alveolar-capillary gas exchange of carbon dioxide for oxygen. As this process of exchange is affected, respiratory efficiency falls.

The decline in elastic recoil of the lungs and a stiffer rib cage result in a less rapid expansion of the chest when the ribs are raised, via the external intercostal muscles, and the diaphragm is lowered. As a consequence of the decrease in elastic recoil, the reduction in chest wall pliancy, and the increase in residual volume, the volume of air inspired, called vital capacity, is decreased (Christiansen and Grzybowski, 1993). The drop in vital capacity results in a compensatory increase in the number of breaths to ensure an adequate respiratory volume during physical activity.

Other factors in aging that may affect lung efficiency include a

Can a Sprinter Over the Age of 35 Still Compete?

Growing evidence seems to indicate that sprinters can sustain their careers much longer than was previously thought. Linford Christie was 32 years old when he won the 1992 Olympic gold medal in the 100-meter sprint. He won several events in 1995 and was considered the favorite in the Olympics of 1996. The major disadvantage facing older sprinters is the 30 to 40 percent longer recovery time needed between workouts. Younger athletes can train longer, harder, and more often, and they are less likely to sustain serious injuries. Also, they recover much faster when injured.

decrease in the strength of the respiratory muscles that enlarge the thoracic wall and thus expand respiratory volume, and an increase in resistance during exhalation. Obesity, chronic poor posture, calcification of bronchial and costal cartilage, and vertebral osteoporosis may all increase resistance during exhalation. Ultimately, the body is unable to sustain the necessary level of ventilation to support the heart and vascular network in the uptake and delivery of oxygen to the active tissues.

Regular exercise benefits the aging respiratory system in many ways. It helps keep pulmonary ventilation from decreasing during maximal exercise and hastens recovery following exercise. The energy cost of respiration for a given physical activity increases with age unless chest-wall movement and elastic load can be reduced from regular training.

Part of the increased lung efficiency that occurs with regular exercise comes from a larger tidal volume, the volume of air breathed in per breath. Because ventilation is the product of respiratory rate and tidal volume, an increase in tidal volume allows for a decrease in breathing rate. In other words, when the capacity of the lungs is larger, the rate of breathing can be lower.

The ability to maintain the gaseous concentration at the alveolar-capillary membrane, known as alveolar ventilation, increases the ventilatory efficiency both at rest and during exercise. Alveolar ventilation is the actual amount of air in the alveoli from which oxygen diffuses to the pulmonary blood to associate with hemoglobin, which is then transported to all body tissues. Effective alveolar ventilation means that the lungs are able to increase tidal volume with only a small increase in breathing rate.

While the benefits of regular exercise on lung function are numerous, the most significant result is increased efficiency of the lungs. Increasing lung efficiency and tidal volume through physical activity and exercise allows for a much more active lifestyle without undue respiratory stress (*see also* RESPIRATION).

Circulatory System

As the circulatory system ages, arteries throughout the body become less elastic, more rigid, and less flexible. Their diameter may decrease as well, which increases resistance to blood flow. This is often especially apparent in the extremities, causing the sensation of perpetually cold hands and feet. Many people mistakenly attribute this to low blood pressure, but it is an arterial problem.

Although systolic blood pressure, the highest pressure in the arteries at any time, increases with aging, diastolic pressure, the lowest arterial pressure, either decreases or remains unchanged. The increase in systolic pressure corresponds to an increase in ventricular systole, or contraction, which pushes the blood through the arteries. This results in an increase in the heart's need for oxygen, since systolic blood pressure is directly related to the work of the heart.

With aging, the heart undergoes cellular and interstitial changes that decrease its structural integrity. Collagen cross-linking, interstitial fibrosis, and deposits of amyloid, a starchlike protein, decrease both the elasticity and motion of the cardiac muscle. Lipofuscin, fatlike substances cross-linked with proteins, accumulate in the muscle cells and appear to compromise cardiac function by displacing subcellular organelles and interfering with intracellular transport. Other structural changes may include a reduction in the size of the left ventricle; a small amount of valvular fibrosis and calcification; and changes within the sinoatrial and the atrioventricular nodes (the small masses of muscle tissue embedded in the heart that work to stimulate the heartbeat) and associated conduction system, which increase the effort required of the heart during physical work and the susceptibility to atrial tachycardia, or rapid heartbeat (see Figure 4).

Owing to the morphological and electrophysiological alterations of the aging conduction system of the heart, maximum heart rate is decreased. This leads to a decrease in the cardiac output—the maximum volume of blood pumped from the ventricles per minute. Cardiac output equals heart rate × stroke volume (the volume of blood pumped per beat from each ventricle). Even with no change in maximum stroke volume with aging—which is usually not the case—cardiac output decreases. Decreased heart rate automatically decreases cardiac output and thus decreases the volume of oxygen transported to the tissues for oxidation of fuel (McArdle et al., 1991). The age-related decrease in maximum stroke volume is primarily due to the increase in peripheral vascular resistance, which also elevates blood pressure at rest and during exercise.

Oxygen consumption is the ability of the body to take in oxygen, transport it, and use it to make high-energy phosphate compounds for muscle contraction and other cellular purposes. A sedentary lifestyle leads to decreased oxygen consumption during maximum work in the elderly, in part because of the related loss of lean muscle tissue, which uses oxygen for oxidation of fuel. Since they have a reduced capacity to fuel muscle contraction, vigorous physical work becomes more difficult for the elderly.

However, despite the aging process, regular exercise training

Figure 4. *The aging heart is susceptible to collagen cross-linking, interstitial fibrosis, and deposits of amyloid (a starchlike protein), all of which decrease elasticity and motion of the cardiac muscle. Other structural changes may include: (1) a reduction in the size of the left ventricle; (2) a small amount of valvular fibrosis and calcification; and (3) changes within the sinoatrial (SA) node and the atrioventricular (AV) node and the associated conduction system.*

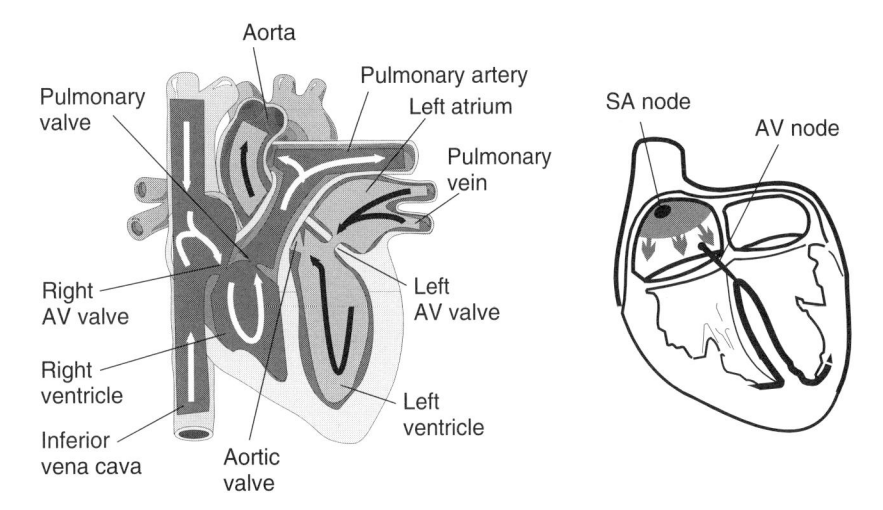

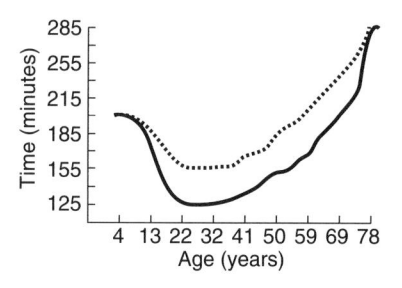

Figure 5. *Peak aerobic performance tends to occur from age 22 to 30. Although age-related cardiovascular decline sets in during the early thirties, among elite endurance athletes it is a very gradual decline. (Adapted from McArdle, 1986)*

Myth—"Cardiovascular disease is inevitable." *Reality*—In addition to hereditary factors, cardiovascular disease is affected by lifestyle. Poor diet, cigarette smoking, and lack of regular exercise may increase the risk of heart disease. Regardless of age, exercise can improve the rate of delivery of oxygen from the heart to the muscles.

results in a significant improvement in aerobic capacity. This outcome is achieved primarily by improving the rate of oxygen delivery from the heart to the active muscles and the improved extraction of oxygen by these tissues, which is known as the arteriovenous oxygen difference.

Other significant changes occur that can set the stage for either an increase in oxygen consumption during maximum exercise or a more economical usage of available energy during submaximal exercise. Since maximum heart rate in later life is generally fixed, an increase in cardiac output at maximal work levels is due primarily to the increase in maximum stroke volume. Regular exercise can improve myocardial contractility, though the volume of blood returning to the heart may stay the same. However, exercise training generally increases this volume, thus increasing cardiac filling. With more blood entering the heart and increased contractility, the volume of blood leaving the ventricles is increased (Mann et al., 1986). This appears to be related to the effect of exercise training on total blood volume (which is increased as plasma volume increases), and to the increased compliance of the ventricles.

In addition to the increase in aerobic power at maximal work, exercise training decreases myocardial oxygen consumption—the heart's need for oxygen—during submaximal exercise. This is achieved primarily by the reduction in heart rate: decreased heart rate results in decreased myocardial oxygen demand. The shift in autonomic balance favoring the parasympathetic (cholineric) division at the sinoatrial node may be more important for improved heart functioning than the adaptations that exercise generates in the peripherally active muscles.

A decrease in submaximal exercise heart rate is a positive physiologic adaptation to exercise training, because of its effect on the rate-pressure product. When this product (heart rate × systolic blood pressure) is decreased because one or both variables are decreased, the work of the heart is decreased. This finding is based on the fact that a high correlation exists between rate-pressure product and myocardial oxygen consumption. When the product is elevated, the heart will need more oxygen. If after training, the same exercise effort can be carried out with a reduction in heart rate, then the product is decreased. This means that the heart requires less oxygen than it originally needed to do the same amount of work; the body can exercise more economically and with less direct stress on the heart.

Exercise training also benefits the elderly by decreasing total peripheral vascular resistance, or afterload, which allows for an easier and more dramatic rise in cardiac output during increased physical work. The change in peripheral resistance is directly related to regular exercise, which increases the number of capillaries to the active muscles. Training also results in an increased tendency to vasodilate (open wider) the arterioles to the active muscles during exercise.

With the increase in capillaries and blood flow in the periphery, the increase in the diffusion gradient for oxygen (when cellular metabolism is increased), and the increase in the number of mitochondria and in mitochondrial enzyme activity, oxygen extraction is increased. The end result is that more energy is produced aerobically,

BENEFITS OF EXERCISE

Skeletal

Bone density (mass) increases
Risk of fractures decreases
Body alignment and posture improved

Neuromuscular

Central nervous system processing time improves
Nerve conduction velocity increases
Reaction and movement time improves
Neuromuscular function increases
Maximal voluntary strength increases
Fast-twitch muscle fiber function increases
Fast-twitch motor discharge increases
Rate of protein synthesis for muscle development increases
Muscle mass increases

Metabolic

Muscle concentration of ATP/PC increases
Muscle glycogen increases
Oxidative phosphorylation activity increases
Number of mitochondria increases
Mitochondrial enzyme activity increases

Respiratory

Vital capacity increases
Forced expired ventilation in one second increases
Lung and chest wall elasticity improves
Pulmonary ventilation improves
Tidal volume increases
Strength and endurance of respiratory muscles increases

Cardiovascular

Stroke volume increases
Oxygen consumption and cardiac output during maximal exercise increases
Oxygen economy during submaximal exercise increases
AV oxygen difference during maximal exercise increases
Blood volume increases
Hemoglobin increases

Psychological

Symptoms of anxiety, depression and insomnia improve
Cerebral function improves
Self-esteem improves
Sense of well-being improves

Table 1.

via oxidative phosphorylation, than anaerobically, via glycolysis. The body is thus able to exercise at a higher aerobic capacity or to sustain longer exercise periods at a comfortable percentage of maximum oxygen consumption. The improvement in cardiovascular fitness is clearly worth the effort, given that exercise slows the age-related decline in functional capacity and, quite possibly, increases active life expectancy (*see also* ENERGY AND METABOLISM, HEART AND CIRCULATORY SYTEM, *and* RESPIRATION).

Psychological Effects of Exercise

The psychological impact of aging may include changes in self-image, self-esteem, and general feelings of well-being. However, these factors can be improved by an active lifestyle. Exercise can decrease depression, anxiety, and other indicators of emotional instability. In one study, researchers examined the effect of 13 weeks of aerobic exercise training on the self-esteem of 50 adults age 60 to 79 (Moore et al., 1994). Results revealed significant improvements in fitness and self-esteem for the participants who exercised compared with the control subjects, who did not exercise.

Another study examined the benefits of regular exercise in 67 men and 87 women and found that those who consistently reported regular exercise also reported a significantly lower association between everyday problems and depression than those who did not exercise (Roth et al., 1994). The study therefore suggests that exercise may moderate the emotional impact of daily stress.

Long-term exercise training has also been shown to be associated with improvement in morale, as reported by the subjects of a 1993 study (Hill et al., 1993). Therefore, it is reasonable to conclude that exercise training may lower the risk of psychological distress.

Does Disuse Accelerate Aging?

The degree to which the biological process of aging can be stopped or slowed, and the extent to which the signs of aging may actually be caused by the environment, remain unclear. When coupled, inactivity and aging seem to accelerate the effects of aging. That is, aging is both a chronological process and a physiological process. While the former cannot be stopped, the latter can be slowed. The changes that characterize aging may be offset to some degree by keeping the mind-body complex active.

Not all the changes associated with aging can be slowed or lessened through exercise. Some changes, which involve the replacement of worn-out cells, may be affected by exercise. Other changes, such as impairment of the central nervous system, which involve the breakdown of cells that are not replaced, cannot be altered significantly.

The rate at which aging causes significant changes in functional capacity is influenced by a mixture of genetic and environmental factors. The relative importance of physical activity is difficult to gauge, although it is now generally accepted that lifestyle changes, such as increasing exercise, quitting smoking, and reducing stress, are related

EFFECTS OF AGING

Body Part	What Occurs	Repercussions
Skin	Loss of resiliency. Impeded circulation.	Increased bruising, pressure sores, and wrinkles. Intolerance to cold.
Bones	Decreased bone mass and strength.	Increased probability of fractures from falls and stress fractures from overuse.
Joints and cartilage	Cartilage becomes drier and more brittle and tends to wear away. Joints become stiffer as the body loses some of its ability to lubricate them.	Cartilage loses its capacity to cushion spaces between the bones, particularly the knees. Range of motion declines and there is an increased likelihood of arthritic pain in the ankle, knee, hip, and elbow.
Ligaments and tendons	Decreased elasticity and range of motion (flexibility).	Injuries are more common. It is not possible to run as fast, jump as high, or throw as hard or as far.
Muscles	Decreased number and size of fibers. Decreased enzyme activity. Reduced fast-twitch-fiber activity.	Loss of muscle strength and endurance. Loss of muscle efficiency and increased instability. More pain, quicker fatigue, and less energy. Loss of ballistic strength (explosiveness).
Nerves	Loss of myelin. Decrease in activity of motor neurons. Altered muscle function. Selective atrophy of the cerebral cortex.	Slower nerve conduction. Decreased reaction time and ability to balance. Increased probability of pressure (friction) against nerves, resulting in pain. Increased mental confusion; decreased ability to learn.
Eyes	Decreased lens elasticity and reduced ability to change the shape of the lens.	Accommodation is affected and the ability to focus is reduced (presbyopia).
Ears	Increased sensitivity to loud noise. Thickening and loss of elasticity of tympanic membrane.	Age-related deafness (presbycusis). Hearing loss (otosclerosis).
Arteries	Decreased elasticity and inability to increase size, reducing blood flow.	Increase in systolic blood pressure, which in turn increases the work of the heart.
Heart	Increased collagen cross-linking, interstitial fibrosis, and amyloid deposits. Decreased ventricular size. Changes in the sinoatrial and atrialventricular nodes and conduction system.	Decreased elasticity of the heart and associated function. Decreased stroke volume leading to a decrease in maximum cardiac output. Increased susceptibility to atrial tachycardia as heart rate decreases, which decreases the maximum volume of oxygen that can be transported to the muscles.
Lungs	Atrophy of the alveolar-septal membrane, increased size of alveoli and ducts, and decrease in size of lungs. Decreased strength of respiratory muscles.	Decreased gas exchange. Decreased elastic recoil of lungs and chest wall, which decreases lung efficiency.

Table 2.

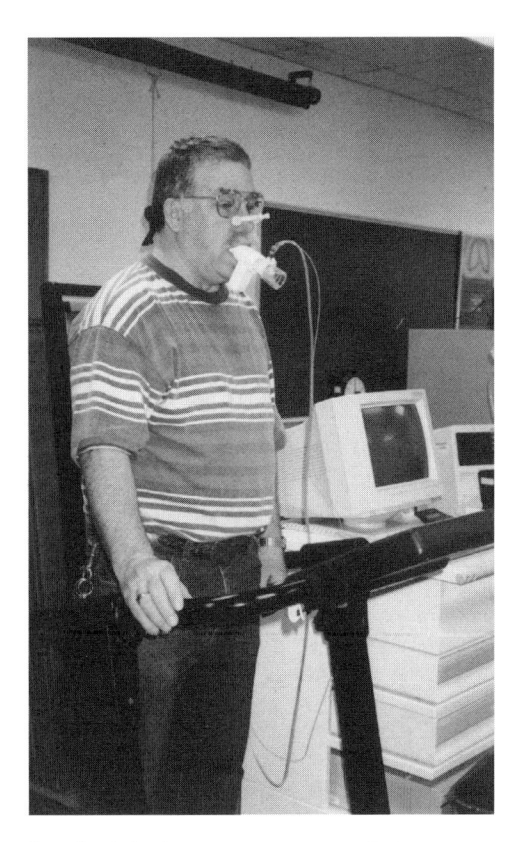

Figure 6. *Exercise physiologists test oxygen uptake to measure changes in aerobic capacity.*

to an increased life expectancy. Because inactivity appears to accelerate the aging process, the progressive loss of tissues of muscles, nerves, and various vital organs may be delayed, regardless of chronological age, by participation in a regular exercise program. The proverbial wisdom "use it or lose it" is especially pertinent for the elderly.

As explained elsewhere in this article, the level of physical activity may affect illnesses, such as coronary artery disease, high blood pressure, osteoporosis, and depression; as well as aspects of the body's general functioning, including muscle strength, endurance, flexibility, and aerobic exercise capacity. Many researchers have found a connection between regular physical activity and the rate of deterioration of organ systems. Through aerobic and resistance training, cardiorespiratory function and musculoskeletal integrity can be preserved and even improved over time.

However, many studies have found that the elderly often do not exercise regularly. According to one study, two-thirds of the elderly are either irregularly active or completely sedentary (Rooney, 1993). The 1985 National Health Interview Survey of 27,000 persons age 65 or older found that only 7.5 percent participated in regular physical activity (Caspersen et al., 1986). A sedentary lifestyle, in conjunction with poor health habits, may contribute to the deterioration commonly associated with aging. By constrast, the benefits of regular exercise include improved self-esteem, higher ratio of lean muscle tissue to fat and bone mineral mass, a stronger cardiovascular system, improved reaction time and balance, stronger muscles and tendons, and possibly improvements in memory, judgment, control of urination, absorption and metabolization of drugs, and gastrointestinal function.

It is important to note that the optimal level of activity is not necessarily the highest. Regular exercise can be achieved through a simple, nonstrenuous activity. Walking briskly for 30 minutes four times a week is not strenuous, but it will improve the cardiorespiratory system. Lifting weights 10 to 15 minutes a day twice a week will develop strength and maintain the physical appearance of the body. Exercise need not be difficult or strenuous to enhance the transport and extraction of oxygen and provide the proper stress to increase the integrity of the muscles.

It's Never Too Late

In *Richard II,* Shakespeare wrote, "I wasted time and now doth time waste me." Yet the inevitability of aging need not be as dire as Shakespeare makes it. A properly designed exercise program may slow the decline of physical abilities in older people relative to those who do not exercise. However, the relative benefits of exercise for different people vary with the extent of the damage from prolonged inactivity, initial fitness, motivation, and age. Anatomical and physiological differences also affect the level of benefits. Orthopedic problems can impose limitations on activity, and weak muscles and impaired joints may create unstable gait and posture, thus making it difficult to engage in certain activities. The response to training also has a genetic component.

However, initial differences in body capacity and ability can be compensated through training. Age-related impairments may result in a slower rate of improvement, but with persistence and regular activity, both muscle size and functional mobility may improve. Any level of activity may improve the condition of the body as it ages. Walking can maintain cardiac output and maximum oxygen consumption. Jogging at the right intensity, duration, and frequency will decrease exercise heart rate and improve exercise capacity, which also brings secondary health benefits, such as a reduction in serum cholesterol and an increase in high density lipoprotein (HDL) cholesterol. A strength-building program will improve muscle strength as well as endurance, range of motion, coordination, and balance (Rooney, 1993).

Older Adults Who Become Athletes

Active older adults who engage in regular physical activity may differ from athletes who are elderly, and both may differ from the aging population that is neither active nor athletic. The cardiorespiratory system declines more slowly for the active older adult than for

Does Exercise Help Prevent Cancer?

Many people believe that physical activity decreases the incidence of cancer and decreases mortality from cancer. However, there is little evidence that exercise enhances the body's natural immunity. It is true that many biochemical and physiological changes occur with exercise, but whether regular exercise prevents cancer or certain cancers is not known.

Numerous studies have reported on the incidence of cancer and the degree to which being physically active or inactive may be a causal factor. But there is a problem with causality. So many factors have been identified as causing cancer that it is difficult to identify physical activity as a clear cause.

Cancer is a complex array of diseases, perhaps more than a hundred. It is unlikely that exercise alone, however regularly practiced, could actually prevent cancer. What researchers may find instead is that when regular exercise is coupled with other factors, cancer may be retarded or put into remission.

Consider, for example, the relationship between colon cancer and physical activity. Data from a relatively recent study showed that men who were physically active had a reduced relative risk for colon cancer compared with subjects who were physically less active (Wu et al., 1987). There are similar hypotheses about the links between exercise and the incidence of breast cancer and cancers of the reproductive system (Albanes et al., 1989).

These studies do not necessarily imply, however, that cancer in general or one specific cancer will develop from lack of regular exercise. No data exist that support such hypotheses. Much of the published data are either conflicting or inconclusive. Further studies and clinical trials may help scientists reach more substantive conclusions. Even then, most research tends to assess more than one risk factor at a time, rather than isolating the level of physical activity.

The plausibility of links between physical activity, cancer, and natural immunity will probably depend on scientific analysis at the molecular level, rather than the more descriptive, epidemiological approach. Until such research is carried out, it may be difficult to make the case that regular participation in exercise will stop or put into remission the growth of cancer.

Athletic Training Later in Life

The trainability of 70- and 80-year-olds is not significantly different from that of younger people. While certain processes, such as oxygen uptake, decline in efficiency with age, others, such as heart output (blood volume and heart volume), can improve with training.

the sedentary adult. The lack of a systematic stimulus—physical activity—to maintain the oxygen transport and uptake components is the obvious reason for the decline.

Regular participation in exercise, at any age, improves the body's ability to take in oxygen, transport it, and use it to develop energy. The capacity of the body to conduct these processes in older active adults is equivalent to the maximum oxygen consumption of younger sedentary adults (Nieman, 1995). Older adults may achieve muscle mass and endurance comparable to that of younger athletes, but their cardiovascular capacity tends to remain lower than that of younger adult athletes. Few, if any, distance runners can effectively compete at a world-class level once they reach their mid-thirties.

Aging Athletes

Although age and inactivity contribute to a decline in physical ability, exercise training improves overall health to the point that participation in athletics can be safe. Regular exercise training helps offset the decline in physical structures and functions that are considered part of the aging process. Thus, regular participation in sporting activities may, indirectly, also improve the quality of life over time.

Some Remarkable Achievements of the Elderly (Adapted from Stones and Kozma, 1985)

At the age of 44, Bertil Jarloker ran the longest non-stop run ever recorded (568 km).

At the age of 64, Walter Polnisch completed the longest recorded ocean swim (208 km).

At the age of 65, Derek Turnbull ran 6 kilometers in 16:39.

At the age of 66, Luciano Acquarone ran a 2:38:00 marathon (a pace of 6 minutes per mile).

At the age of 70, Hilda Johnstone competed in equestrian dressage at the 1972 Olympics.

At the age of 70, Warren Utes set an age-group world record of 38:24 for the 10-kilometer race.

At the age of 83, Johnny Kelly finished the Boston Marathon in 5:42:54.

Between the ages of 70 and 87, Mavis Lindgren completed 65 marathons.

At the age of 91, Hulda Crooks climbed Mt. Fuji (3,776 meters).

At the age of 98, Dimitrion Yordanidis completed a marathon in 7:30:00.

One study found no decline in maximum oxygen consumption in 60-year-old athletes who had trained for the preceding 10 years. Comparable athletes whose training decreased over the same 10-year period demonstrated a 12.5 percent decrease in maximum oxygen consumption (Pollock et al., 1987). Another study found that aerobic training could improve the body's ability to withstand physiological changes in aerobic power (Pollock, 1973). The magnitude of the changes may reach 26 to 30 percent increases in maximal oxygen consumption after 6 to 12 months of training (Hagberg et al., 1989; Kohrt et al., 1991). Aging does not necessarily mean a loss in significant ability to compete in strenuous sports, nor does it shut the door on physical abilities, strength, or stamina. The list "Some Remarkable Achievements of the Elderly" illustrates the resiliency of the body.

Perceptions of the limits of the body over time have changed significantly. It was once considered impossible for men at the age of 80 to run 6 miles in little over 40 minutes. Many of these changes in perception have been sparked by achievements in competition, but it is not necessary to compete to achieve positive psycho-physiological results. Noncompetitive participation in regular exercise produces the same results, although probably not at the same intensity of development.

Do Athletes Live Longer?

It seems logical to conclude that participation in regular physical activity increases life expectancy. Some research seems to support this point, although the question is far from being resolved (Pekka-

Exercise and Longevity

Exercise may improve the quality of life, but the debate continues about whether it will lengthen the life span. Even though exercise improves the functioning of many bodily organs, there are only a few diseases that exercise helps prevent. In other words, exercise helps many of the body's organs to function better, but it cannot be credited with the ability to stop the onset of cancers and most other diseases.

nen et al., 1987). To begin with, being physically able to exercise does not mean that a person is necessarily healthy, and it is quite possible to be mentally and otherwise healthy without regular participation in strenuous activities.

In general, though, most middle-aged adults who exercise regularly will be healthier in later years. However, this debate is still quite contentious because of hereditary. A person endowed with few risk factors may experience only a small boost in life expectancy. However, for a person with numerous inherited risk factors, like coronary artery disease and high blood pressure, exercise can dramatically improve life expectancy.

Regular physical activity can decrease a number of important risk factors for coronary artery disease. It is reasonable to conclude that by decreasing the risk of cardiovascular disease (which might lead to death), life expectancy will be increased. In one study, when the alumni from a major university engaged in a loss of 2,000 to 3,500 calories per week in physical exercise, they experienced a 32 percent decrease in "all-cause" death rates (Paffenbarger et al., 1993). The authors of this study concluded that life expectancy was increased by 2 years when walking, stair climbing, and playing sports were part of the subjects' lifestyle. Likewise, data from the Aerobics Research Institute in Dallas seem to indicate that regular exercise lengthens life expectancy by about 2 years (Blair et al., 1989).

Which Sports Promote Longevity?

There is some evidence supporting the idea that only certain sports improve longevity (Sarna et al., 1993). In a cross-sectional Finnish study, researchers compared 2,613 world-class male athletes who competed during 1920–1965. The subjects participated in endurance sports (long-distance running and cross-country skiing), team sports requiring aerobic training (soccer, ice hockey, and basketball), and power sports (boxing, wrestling, and weight lifting). The reference cohort of 1,712 men was selected from the Finnish Defense Forces conscription register, and was matched according to age and area of residence. All referents were classified as healthy at the time of their induction into military service. The study made several conclusions: endurance athletes lived nearly 6 years longer than nonathletes, team athletes lived significantly longer than referents, and power athletes did not have increased longevity.

Regular physical activity probably contributes to longevity in many ways, primarily by preventing premature cardiovascular death. However, participation in athletics may also lead to positive behavioral changes, such as quitting smoking, eating a healthier diet, and having a better understanding of health-related matters in general.

The understanding of how regular exercise or a particular sport may affect later health status, incidence of chronic diseases, and longevity is not complete. Once the exact causes of the aging process are identified—particularly the microlevel effects of exercise on cells—more of the underlying reasons for variations in aging may be uncovered.

Tommy Boone and Michael Foley

References

Albanes, D., et al. "Physical Activity and Risk of Cancer in the NHANES I Population." *American Journal of Public Health* 79 (1989): 744–750.

Blair, S., et al. "Physical Fitness and All-Cause Mortality: A Prospective Study of Healthy Men and Women." *Journal of the American Medical Association* 262 (1989): 2395–2401.

Caspersen, C., et al. "Status of the 1990 Physical Fitness and Exercise Objectives: Evidence from NHIS-1985." *Public Health Report* 101 (1986): 587–592.

Christiansen, J., and J. Grzybowski. *Biology of Aging*. St. Louis, Missouri: Mosby, 1993.

Frontera, W., et al. "Strength Training and Determinants of VO_2max in Older Men." *Journal of Applied Physiology* 68 (1990): 329–333.

"Geographic High Life Expectancy." *Statistics Bulletin* 74 (1993): 28–35.

Hagberg, J., et al. "Effect of Exercise Training on 60–69-Year-Old Persons with Essential Hypertension." *American Journal of Cardiology* 64 (1989): 348–353.

Hill, R., et al. "The Impact of Long-Term Exercise Training on Psychological Function in Older Adults." *Journal of Gerontology* 48 (1993): 12–17.

Institute of Medicine, Division of Health Promotion and Disease Prevention. *The Second Fifty Years: Promoting Health and Preventing Disability*. Washington, D. C.: National Academy 1990.

Kohrt, W., et al. "Effects of Gender, Age, and Fitness Level on Response of VO_2max to Training in 60–71 Year-Olds." *Journal of Applied Physiology* 71 (1991): 2004–2011.

Mann, D., et al. "Effects of Age on Ventricular Performance During Graded Supine Exercise." *American Heart Journal* 111 (1986): 108–115.

McArdle, W. D., et al. *Exercise Physiology: Energy, Nutrition, and Human Performance*. Philadelphia: Lea and Febiger, 1991.

Moore, K., et al. "The Effect of Participation in an Aerobic Exercise Program on the Self-Esteem of Older Adults." Abstract presented at the 47th Annual Scientific Meeting of the Gerontological Society of America, Atlanta, Georgia, 1994.

Nieman, D. C. *Fitness and Sports Medicine: A Health-Related Approach*. Palo Alto, California: Bull, 1995.

Paffenbarger, R., et al. "The Association of Changes in Physical Activity Level and Other Lifestyle Characteristics with Mortality Among Men." *New England Journal of Medicine* 328 (1993): 538–545.

Pekkanen, J., et al. "Reduction of Premature Mortality by High Physical Activity: A 20-Year Follow-Up of Middle-Aged Finnish Men." *Lancet* 1 (1987): 1473–1477.

Pollock, M. "The Quantification of Endurance Training Programs." *Exercise Sports Science Review* 1 (1973): 155–188.

Pollock, M., et al. "Effect of Age and Training on Aerobic Capacity and Body Composition of Master Athletes." *Journal of Applied Physiology* 62 (1987): 625–631.

Rogers, M., and W. Evans. "Changes in Skeletal Muscle with Aging: Effects of Exercise Training." *Exercise Sports Science Review* 21 (1993): 65–102.

Rooney, E. "Exercise for Older Patients: Why It's Worth Your Effort." *Geriatrics* 48 (1993): 68–77.

Roth, D. L., et al. "Stress-Resistance Effects of Physical Exercise in 55–75-Year-Old

Adults." Abstract Presented at the 47th Annual Scientific Meeting of the Gerontological Society of America, Atlanta, Georgia, 1994.

Sarna, S., et al. "Increased Life Expectancy of World Class Male Athletes." *Medicine and Science in Sports and Exercise* 25 (1993): 237–244.

Spirduso, W. "Physical Dimensions of Aging." Champaign, Illinois: Human Kinetics, 1995.

Stones, M., and A. Kozma. *Aging and Human Performance*. New York: Wiley, 1985.

Wu, A., et al. "Alcohol, Physical Activity, and Other Risk Factors for Colorectal Cancer: A Prospective Study." *British Journal of Cancer* 55 (1987): 687–694.

Ankle, Foot, and Lower Leg

THE ANATOMY OF THE LOWER LEG, ankle, and foot is one of the most complex of the musculoskeletal system. As human ancestors evolved from quadrupeds to bipeds, so too did the lower extremity evolve. Early hominids had a foot structure that included an opposable digit like the thumb. But as the foot began to function almost exclusively as a means to get around, and less as a means for grasping objects, the foot adapted to the environment through the evolutionary process of natural selection, through which factors in the environment favor certain individuals over others to produce the next generation. In this case, individuals with a big toe parallel to the other toes could walk better and were favored over those with a big toe more perpendicular to the other toes.

The human foot and ankle are exercised with every step, so even for the most sedentary individuals, it is nearly impossible to neglect them completely. Walking to the bathroom, walking to the refrigerator, and stepping up a flight of stairs all exercise the ankle joint. The ankle joint—a complex system of bones, tendons, ligaments, and muscles—must support the body's weight as it is bent and straightened over a million times each year.

All this activity can come at some cost: injuries. However, though ankle and foot injuries are among those most commonly reported by athletes, it pays everyone to stay active and exercise, for the rewards of exercise far outweigh the risk of injury. To help avoid severe or permanent injury to the foot and ankle, fitness is of paramount importance. Once an ankle is badly sprained, the ligaments are never the same. Scar tissue forms in the damaged ligaments, which makes them less flexible and more vulnerable to future sprains. Even when a large amount of scar tissue does not form, injured ligaments may take up to 5 months to totally heal.

Functional Anatomy

The biomechanics of the ankle and foot allow both tremendous flexibility and impressive strength. However, since the foot and ankle come in direct contact with the playing surface, they suffer from a disproportionate number of injuries. Athletes at greatest risk are those

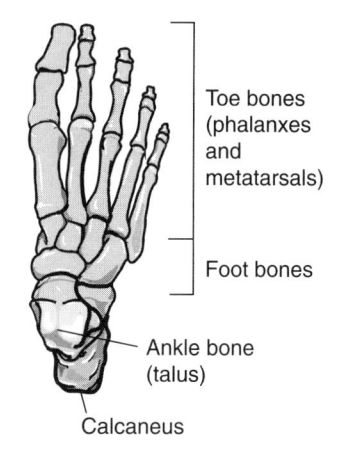

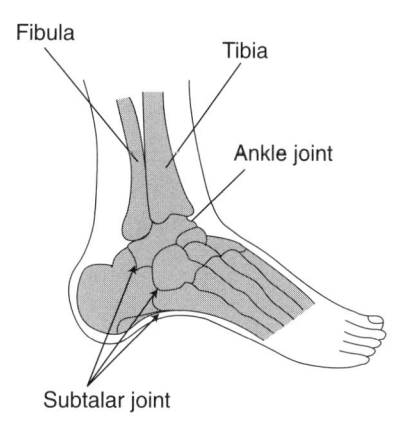

Figure 1. *The foot and ankle bones and joints.*

who participate in sports like tennis, football, basketball, volleyball, and skiing. All these sports require high-impact foot plants and quick changes of direction that stretch the physical limits of the foot and ankle.

Bones and Joints

The foot and ankle region is composed of an integrated group of 29 bones and 26 joints, each with a specific function (*see Figure 1*). The shape of each of the 29 bones suits the task or function it must fulfill. Similarly, each of the 26 joints has a specific purpose. Some, like the ankle joint, move a great deal; others, like the intercuneiform joints (located above the arch of the foot), move very little, if at all.

Since the ankle provides the foot's mobility, it is involved in many aspects of human locomotion, including walking, running, and jumping. The three bones that come together at the ankle are the tibia, the fibula, and the talus; and tightly packed into an area the size of a tennis ball, numerous tendons, ligaments, and muscles surround and support the joint. As they work to move the body forward over the foot, which is fixed on the floor, the curved dome of the talus rotates forward and backward under the tibia and fibula.

The ankle joint is well constrained by the ligamentary structures and bony architecture. Thus, when one plants one's foot and starts to fall, the leg often twists because the foot cannot. If the foot is hopelessly stationary (for example, when a football cleat is embedded in turf), the twisting continues until the foot becomes unplanted—in this case, when the cleat slips outward from the turf or when "something gives." All too often it is the ligaments of the ankle that must give. If the twisting continues, the bones of the leg—often just the fibula—

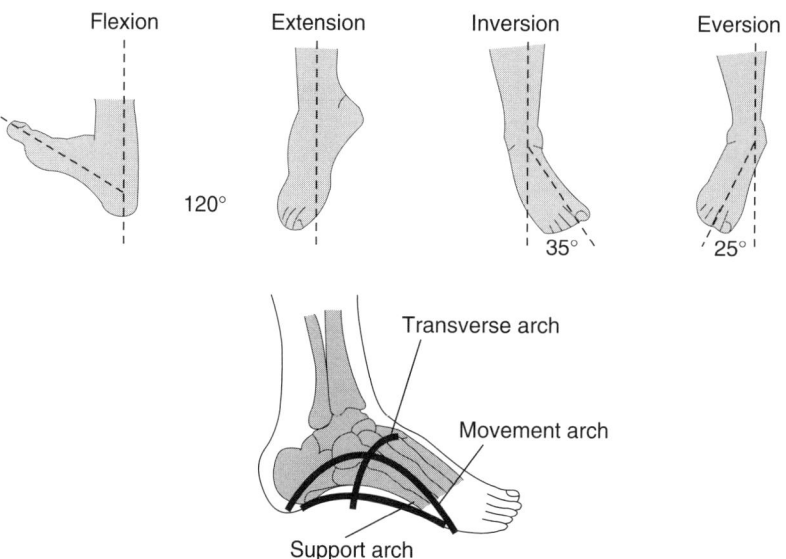

Figure 2. *The range of motion of the foot. Above: The ankle joint allows significant bending (flexion) and extension (straightening), about 120 degrees. The subtalar joint, the lower ankle joint, allows a moderate amount of inversion (pronation) and eversion (supination). Below: Shown here are the three arches (three dimensions). One of the major objectives of shoe design is to limit the stress on all three of these arches while maximizing support.*

may crack, or fracture, as the leg continues to rotate around the fixed talus bone. There are many types of ankle fractures. Some involve just the fibula, others just the tibia, and others involve both. Because there is such a wide range of potential fractures, it is important that each injury is individually assessed, treated, and rehabilitated.

The subtalar joint, located below the ankle joint and connecting the talus bone to the calcaneus bone, allows side-to-side movements of the heel (*see Figures 1 and 2*). This joint, which is often referred to as the "lower ankle joint," becomes very important when traversing uneven terrain. Its main function is to maintain balance, to shift back and forth so that a person's center of gravity lies as directly over the supporting foot as possible, regardless of the surface irregularities underfoot. The subtalar joint, although limited in its range of motion, provides a balanced platform of support for the ankle. Design research for running shoes is, for the most part, focused on ways to prevent this very important joint from turning excessively inward (pronation) or outward (supination; *see also EQUIPMENT MATERIALS*).

The joints of the midfoot provide stability and allow the foot's side-to-side movement. Such side-to-side action is critical for motions like striking a soccer ball with the arch of the foot. Without the action of the midfoot joints, far less force could be exerted on the ball, and it would be extremely difficult to kick it at a higher trajectory.

Near the toes, at the forefoot, are the critical metatarsophalangeal joints. They enable the toes to extend upward so that at push-off (running or walking), one bears the majority of one's weight on the ball of the foot, which is ideally designed for support just prior to push-off.

Muscles

A sophisticated group of muscles complements the bones, ligaments, and tendons of the foot and ankle (*see Figure 3*). While the calf muscles (the gastrocnemius, and the even stronger soleus) help to push off and jump, other muscles play less dramatic roles; the flexor digitorum brevis muscle, for example, supports the arch of the foot.

Muscles work in pairs; that is, as one muscle (the agonist) contracts, another muscle (the antagonist) must relax. For example, as the gastrocnemius contracts during foot push-off to run or jump, the tibialis anterior relaxes. Then as the tibialis anterior contracts to bend the foot for the next push-off, the gastrocnemius must relax. The ability of muscles like these to fire (to turn off and turn on) is one of many factors determining the top speed of a sprinter and, perhaps more important, the ability to stay at top speed without experiencing muscle fatigue. Two groups of muscles around the ankle serve a special stabilizing function during running: the anterior compartment muscles and the posterior calf muscles actually contract simultaneously at foot impact to absorb the very large impact force at the ankle. The muscles are, in effect, bracing for the impact that is sure to follow (*see also SKELETAL MUSCLE*). The anterior muscles then

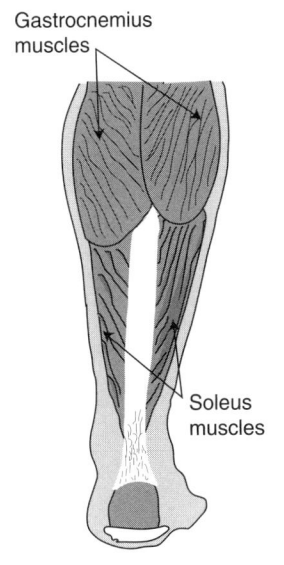

Figure 3. *The gastrocnemius and soleus are the powerful lower leg muscles that extend the foot at the ankle joint. These two muscles play an important role in determining how high athletes can jump and how fast they can run.*

very quickly relax so that the posterior calf muscles can contract to straighten the ankle for push-off.

Muscles are almost always at work to maintain the natural balance for normal standing, walking, and running. An injury to any one of the lower extremity muscles that results in pain or weakness may cause abnormal stresses and strains on the other muscles, impairing function, balance, and performance. For example, even a slight tear of the gastrocnemius muscle can affect a runner's performance. This injury would force a change in running mechanics, forcing an unnatural adaption to an unbalanced, labored running form. Such injury-related changes in running mechanics may require a greater energy expenditure at any given running speed. Running mechanics may not be normal again until the injury heals.

Ligaments

Figure 4 shows the ligaments, the sturdy tissues that hold the ankle joint together. Lateral support is mainly provided by the anterior talofibular ligament, which connects the end of the fibula to the talus, and the calcaneofibular ligament, which connects the back part of the fibula to the heel bone. The anterior talofibular restrains the talus from sliding forward, the calcaneofibular restrains the talus from twisting inward (inversion), and the posterior talofibular prevents the talus from sliding backward. Some additional lateral support is provided by the tough joint covering, or capsule, of the ankle joint. One or more of these ligaments usually gets stretched and torn when inversion ankle sprains occur. Of all ankle injuries, about 85 percent are of the inversion variety, in which the foot twists inward and the ankle turns outward toward the ground.

On the other side of the ankle is the deltoid ligament, which prevents the ankle from eversion, in which the foot turns out and the ankle turns in. The stout deltoid ligament—the strongest ligament in the foot—connects the medial malleolus (the distal end of the tibia) to the talus. If it is stretched or torn, its strength returns only after a lengthy period of healing. When the deltoid ligament is injured, it may take months to return to a pain-free, stable state.

Eversion stress may cause damage at the subtalar joint, the capsule and ligaments connecting the talus to the calcaneus. Prolonged stiffness and pain, especially when walking or running on uneven surfaces, may result.

The degree of ligament damage is described and graded on the basis of the amount of injury. Grade I injuries involve just a stretch of the involved ligament; grade II injuries involve a partial tear of the ligament, but some fibers remain intact; grade III injuries, the most extreme, involve a complete tear of the ligament. Surprisingly, only a few of even grade III ankle ligament injuries fail to heal. In these rare instances, recurrent instability or "giving out" episodes may require surgical reconstruction. Most ankle ligament injuries require rest, ice, compression, and elevation, followed by rehabilitation and muscle strengthening.

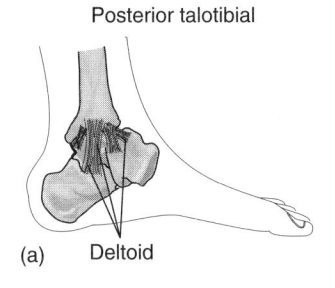

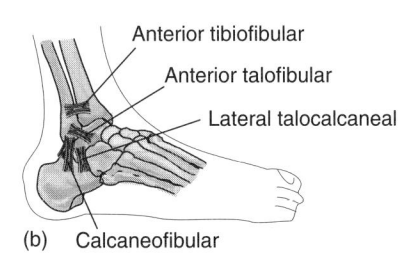

Figure 4. (a) The outside ligaments and (b) the inside ligaments surrounding and supporting the ankle joint.

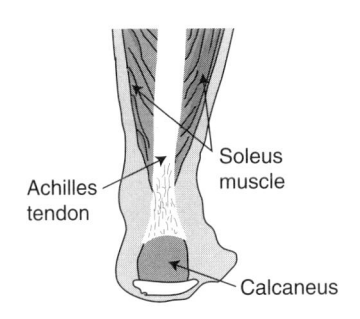

Figure 5. *The Achilles tendon connects the calf muscles (gastrocnemius and soleus) to the calcaneus.*

Tendons

Although the tendons located in the foot and ankle are some of the strongest in the body, forceful movements can result in serious, disabling injuries. Tears of these structures, which connect muscle to bone, range from minor stretching injuries to a severe rupture, or complete division, of the tendon.

Achilles tendon. A common overuse injury to the foot and ankle is damage to the Achilles tendon. This tendon connects the two powerful muscles of the calf—the gastrocnemius and soleus—to the calcaneus (*see Figure 5*). The function of this muscle and tendon complex is to plantar-flex the ankle (to point the foot down).

When the mechanical limits of the tendon are exceeded by forced dorsiflexion of the ankle (forcible upward bending) or a powerful contraction of the calf muscles, the result is a torn tendon. Complete tears of the Achilles tendon often follow a pattern. They frequently occur among court sport players who must constantly start and stop. At the moment of impact, the tear feels and sounds like a "pop," and the sensation of the tendon tearing often feels like a blow to the heel. Interestingly, despite losing the function of perhaps the strongest tendon in the body, a person can usually still weakly push off from the balls of the feet because of several secondary muscles that complement the Achilles tendon's function (tibialis posterior, flexor hallucis longus, flexor digitorum longus, peroneus longus and brevis).

Posterior tibial tendon. The tibialis posterior musculotendinous unit begins deep in the upper part of the leg, just below the knee. The muscle portion extends downward, ending just above the ankle. From this point on, the tendon extends behind the medial malleolus and follows the arch of the foot, finally ending up in the navicular bone and on the undersurface of the midfoot region. The function of this tendon is to help support the medial arch of the foot and to keep the foot from drifting laterally (to the outside). Eversion ankle injuries may put excessive force on this tendon, creating a tear. In young athletic individuals the tear is seldom complete, but rather more like "pulled taffy."

Injuries to the tibialis posterior frequently go undiagnosed and, if untreated, may lead to long-term pain and deformity. Severe ligament swelling often hides the injury inside an ankle sprain. If the tendon is torn, the pain persists well beyond the normal recovery period for a sprained ankle. It may be unrelenting, eventually leading to diagnosis and often requiring surgical treatment.

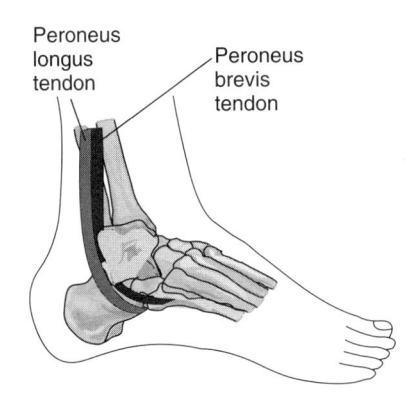

Figure 6. *The peroneus brevis and peroneus longus tendons lie on the lateral side of the foot and ankle. Along with the lateral ligaments, these two tendons are often overstretched and injured from an inversion ankle sprain.*

Peroneus longus and brevis. Located laterally about the ankle are the two peroneal tendons, both on the same side of the ankle (*see Figure 6*). The peroneus longus traverses to the opposite (medial) side of the foot and inserts at the base of the first metatarsal. The peroneus brevis inserts laterally at the base of the fifth metatarsal. Because both these tendons evert the foot, they are frequently injured by inversion ankle injuries, when they often experience a high tensile, or stretching, force. While most peroneal tendon tears go unnoticed because healing happens spontaneously, some may require surgical correction.

Overuse Injuries

Shin Splints: A Medical Mystery

No one knows for sure exactly what they are—just that they are an overuse injury that causes pain in the lower two-thirds of the shin area during running. Although this injury can occur suddenly, it usually develops gradually without any signs of swelling or bruising in the area feeling pain. Shin splints always go away with rest, but for many avid runners, rest is not an easy prescription to accept. Some recommendations for preventing shin splints include more stretching and warming up prior to and following running, proper shoes, running on grass rather than concrete, and improving running form.

The musculoskeletal system is composed of various subunits (bone, tendon, ligament, and other connective tissue), all of which are living cellular tissue. As such, these tissues are in a constant state of change. They become thicker or thinner, larger or smaller, depending on use or disuse. These changes in the various components of the muscular system usually represent either adaptive changes or age-related changes. The thickening of the outer covering of the leg bone of a long-distance runner is an example of an adaptive change; the thinning of the same bones, which may lead to hip fracture, is an example of an age-related change.

The normal process of musculoskeletal system adaptation, particularly for the foot, requires time. Therefore, regardless of the sport or activity, most training protocols recommend a gradual increase in repetitive activity. With enough time, appropriate healthy adaptive changes will occur and pretraining goals will be achieved.

Doctors often use the term *injury threshold*. Above a given threshold injury is likely; but a threshold is highly variable and depends on the activity and the individual involved. An overuse, threshold-exceeding injury may be something as simple as tendinitis, joint irritation (synovitis), and other forms of inflammation, or it might be more severe, such as a stress fracture of a bone.

Running and Injury

Biomechanical abnormalities of little if any significance during walking can take on great significance during running due to the much greater impact forces. Therefore, as an increasing number of people employ their feet to improve their bodies, their ankles and feet bear the brunt of their exercise and their desire for fitness.

Because of the repetitive nature of running, and the obsession some people have with the sport, overuse injuries are very prevalent among runners. Although the mechanics of walking and running are not that different, the impact forces are. Whereas during walking the impact force rarely exceeds 120 percent of body weight, during running the feet hit the ground 800 to 2,000 times per mile at a force of two to four times body weight. This extremely repetitive impact force is absorbed primarily at the ankle joint, and secondarily at the joints in the knee, hip, and lower back. Localized forces may reach 13 times body weight at the ankle and up to 10 times body weight at the Achilles tendon.

The force at the foot is much less because the 29 bones of the foot make it extremely flexible. It is designed to absorb impact forces and

Common Ankle, Foot, and Lower Leg Injuries

Injuries to the ankle and foot are extremely common. Of all the time lost from work and sports, foot and ankle injuries account for up to 25 percent of the total. Some injuries are specific to certain sports, like ankle sprains in court sports involving quick foot plants for changes of direction; other injuries, like Achilles tendinitis or strain, occur with relatively equal frequency in many sports.

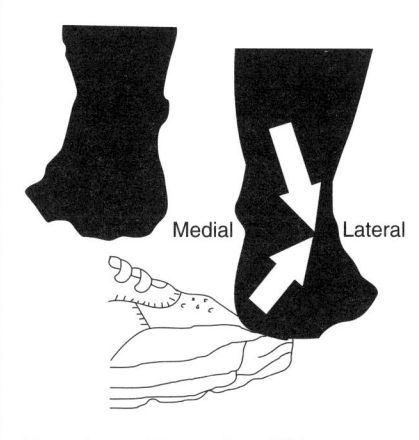

Inversion ankle sprain. This common injury is a stretching or tearing of the ligaments on the outside of the ankle. It typically occurs when the foot lands on its outside edge (fifth metatarsal), as shown here when a player steps on another athlete's foot. The ankle then twists inward as the athlete's full weight comes down on the foot.

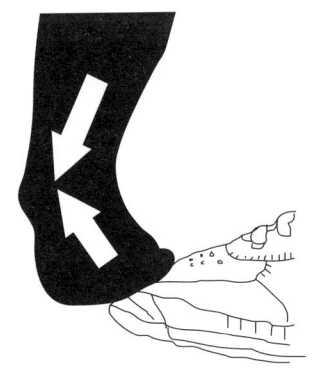

Eversion ankle sprain. This is a stretching or tearing of the ligaments on the inside of the ankle. It typically occurs when the foot turns sharply outward under the ankle and is sometimes more serious than the inversion sprain.

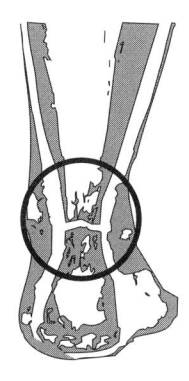

Achilles tendon rupture. When there is a tear in the Achilles tendon, a palpable defect or gap can be detected. Depending on individual circumstances, these injuries may be treated with or without an operation, although many orthopedic surgeons prefer operative repair, particularly for young healthy individuals. Rerupture rates for athletes treated with casting may be as high as 20 percent, compared with 2 percent for those undergoing operative repair. This injury often requires a prolonged recovery, commonly a year or more, before the tendon regains the level of strength it had prior to the injury.

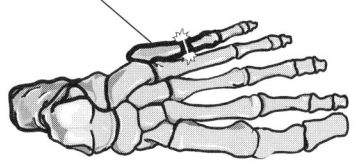

Toe fractures. A prevalent injury in contact sports, toe fractures usually occur from stubbing the toe or from someone stepping on the foot. The toe usually swells, turns black and blue, and causes considerable pain. Treatment is usually to tape the injured toe to an adjoining toe, with the adjacent toe acting as a splint. A fifth metatarsal fracture, usually from a blow, is far more serious. Many of these injuries require a cast, and may even require

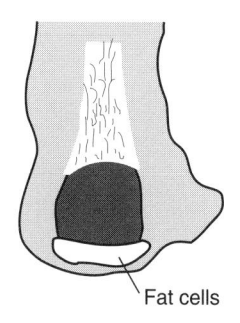

Heel injuries. The fat cells contained in the chambers formed by the fibrosepta in the heel pad act as one of the body's best shock absorbers. As fat under the heel is "pushed out" and away, heel spurs can develop. In rare instances the spur can contribute to heel pain. More commonly, pain results from inflammation of the thick plantar fascia. Repetitive microtrauma, excessive foot pronation, and worn shoeware all can result in plantar fasciitis.

conform to even the roughest surfaces. But as the foot reaches the toe-off position, it once again becomes a rigid lever trying to maximize leverage for the push-off. At this point, overpronation is a significant concern because the foot extends the period of pronation (the flexible foot period), and takes away from the period of supination (supination is necessary for the foot to become a rigid lever during push-off).

A smooth running style requires a coordinated action of a multitude of joints and muscles. One of the most important and underappreciated joint actions in running is the pronation and supination of the foot. At foot strike, as the lower leg internally rotates, the calcaneus everts or pronates. Ideally, running should entail some pronation, for pronation is one of the body's main mechanisms for absorbing shock, but athletes whose feet do not properly pronate—usually those with high arches—complain more often of sore feet than those with normal or low arches.

Interestingly, studies have found that running barefoot usually results in increased pronation. Without any shoe cushioning, most of this increase is attributed to biomechanical changes as the musculoskeletal system attempts to make up for the greater impact forces. On the other hand, runners experiencing excessive pronation with their shoes on tend to have a more neutral motion without them (Chan, 1994). Both these results point to the importance of selecting the right shoe, one that allows the foot to pronate properly without overpronating. The ideal shoe allows the calcaneus (the heel), which strikes the ground at about a 4-degree angle of inversion, to pronate to approximately 12 degrees. These figures will vary slightly, depending on the individual (*see Figure 7*).

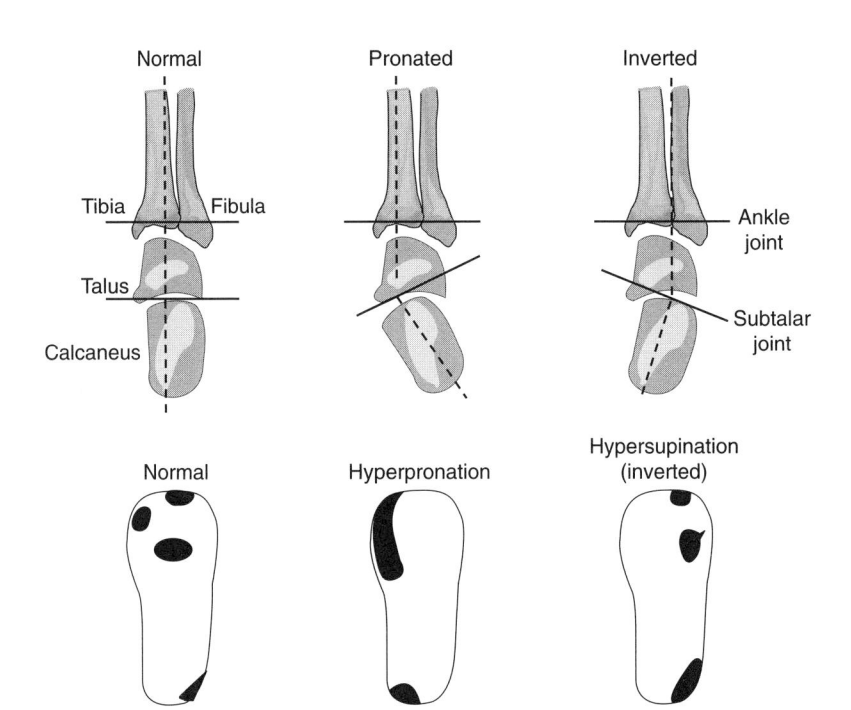

Figure 7. *Above: The right foot as viewed from behind. Although a certain amount of inversion and pronation is desirable while running, excessive pronation or inversion not only hurts performance but also can lead to injury. Below: Patterns of wear in shoes are a good indicator of a potential problems.*

If a runner experiences pain, she should try to determine the primary problem. For example, if the left ankle is slightly sprained, this can lead to a tibia stress fracture in the right leg. Attention is then placed on treating the "secondary problem" of the stress fracture, but the primary problem, or "trigger"—the sprained ankle—needs to be addressed. Considering the hundreds of thousands of foot impacts an average runner experiences each week, it makes sense to evaluate one's running mechanics to prevent overuse problems.

Prevention

Although ankle and foot injuries are very common, a number of preventive measures exist that can lower the risk of injury. These measures are especially important for athletes who have already experienced ankle ligament damage. Because scar tissue forms in their damaged ligaments, not only is it difficult to regain preinjury levels of flexibility and strength, but the chances of reinjury are also greater.

Stretching

After the ankle ligaments have been injured, usually the range of motion (ROM) is significantly restricted. Therefore, as soon as acute pain diminishes, during the several days following an injury, the emphasis of treatment should be shifted toward regaining ROM. Many simple exercises exist for improving ROM. To take the foot and ankle through a wide range of motion, one simple but effective exercise is to lift the foot into the air and "write" the alphabet with the tips of the toes. Unless proper attention is given to this phase of rehabilitation, residual stiffness can be a long-term complication after ankle sprains.

However, stretching is not just for rehabilitation after ankle injuries. Improving the ankle's ROM is a very effective way to prevent ankle injuries, even for those who have never experienced one. Improving the ankle's ROM enhances the "bending-before-breaking" threshold of the tendons surrounding the ankle. Figure 8 shows two of the most effective stretching exercises for improving the ankle's ROM: the straight-leg stretch and the bent-knee stretch.

Many young runners develop pain along the base of their heels. The Achilles tendon attaches to a tuberosity at the back of the calcaneus and is vulnerable to overuse injury. Stretching exercises are recommended for the calf muscles and the Achilles tendon, which often do not keep pace with an adolescent's rapidly growing skeleton. Frequent stretching, ice, and a heel lift are helpful in treating this condition.

Besides these linear stretches, athletes should engage in plenty of rotational stretching. For example, if rotation is limited at the hip or back, naturally more torque (rotation about an axis) occurs at the knee, lower leg, and ankle.

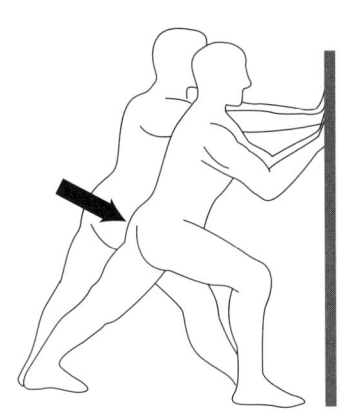

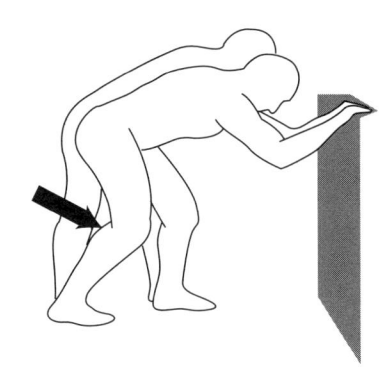

Figure 8. *Two effective stretching exercises for improving the ankle's range of motion: the straight-leg stretch followed by the bent-knee stretch.*

Strengthening

Crucial to prevention of ankle sprains is the strengthening of the supporting muscles. Strengthening begins as ROM nears normal. Isometric exercises are a good way to start rehabilitation without overloading the ankle. One effective exercise is to wrap an old bicycle tube, surgical tubing, or a rubber cord around the feet. Pull the forefeet apart by pushing against the tubing. Next, working one foot at a time, pull against the cord by raising and lowering the toes.

Proprioceptive exercises orchestrate the movement of the ankle with surrounding muscles to properly control the ankle at any given position. They can be used once the ankle has developed sufficient strength through isometric training. Proprioceptive training entails rapidly alternating movements in a controlled fashion. It is a crucial phase of rehabilitation as well as a much neglected strength-training exercise for athletes with normal ankles. Heel raises and hopping exercises are among the proprioceptive exercises used for the ankle.

Although heel raises are effective strength-training exercises for building muscle strength around the ankle, one should be careful not to lift excessive weight, for the gastrocnemius muscle of the calf may tear. This injury occurs when the power generated by the muscle exceeds the failure threshold of the muscle. Failure, or the tear, typically occurs at the junction of the tendon to the muscle, about one-third of the way up the leg from the ankle. It can be quite painful and can require several months to fully recover.

Improving Skills

Improving motor control and coordination through practice—kinesthetic awareness and feedback—not only improves performance, but can also pay a significant dividend in terms of preventing injury. Athletes with musculoskeletal dysfunction, usually after injury, become accustomed to the dysfunction when achieving certain positions and movements. Any effort made to improve skill or technique usually gives positive results because fewer muscles and less energy are used for any given movement, and this tends to raise the fatigue threshold. This is noteworthy because fatigue is a factor in poor running form (*see also* RUNNING AND HURDLING).

After an ankle sprain, a runner needs to be aware of ankle action and the different mechanics of the two ankles. The runner may need to relearn how to run and learn how to restore the injured ankle's performance, and condition the uninjured ankle.

Equipment

Advances in material science and a better understanding of the biomechanics of sports have resulted in shoes and other devices that have dramatically lessened the risk of injury and, in the case of injury, speeded recovery (*see also* EQUIPMENT MATERIALS).

Shoes. Athletes must make sure that their athletic shoes were designed for the sport in which they participate. When shoes wear out or "break down," they should be replaced. High-impact sports like running and basketball require maximum support and cushioning. Shoes also should fit in both length and width. Many women have feet wider than the typical B or C width of women's athletic shoes. Usually these women are better off wearing the wider athletic shoes designed for men.

For extra support following an ankle sprain, many doctors recommend high-top sneakers for sports like basketball, volleyball, and tennis. Whether or not high-tops lower the risk of injury or reinjury is still a subject of debate in the medical community, but most athletes believe they do, so at the least high-tops may provide more confidence when planting and changing directions.

Orthotics. Although there are literally thousands of different shoes, with hundreds of different features, some people still cannot find a shoe that addresses the particular needs of their feet. For those in this relatively small group, orthotic devices may be needed to provide ankle and subtalar support.

Whether or not to prescribe orthotics is a difficult decision for practitioners of sports medicine. If there is an anatomical abnormality that cannot be addressed by special athletic footwear, an orthotic device definitely makes sense. Yet it is rarely the sole answer and is usually part of a comprehensive prevention or rehabilitation program.

Taping and braces. Until the ankle has fully healed (it experiences little swelling, is pain-free, and is fully flexible), after an injury it should be taped or braced before engaging in all physical activity. However, therapeutic taping or bracing presents a paradox. Bracing or taping increases support but restricts mobility and impairs performance; not bracing or taping allows better mobility and thus better performance, but it comes at the cost of support. (Neither significantly affects jumping ability.)

Removable therapeutic braces are becoming an increasingly

Guidelines for Buying Shoes

Not all shoes are the same. Shoes may look the same, use the same design and many of the same materials, yet be very different. Different constructions, primarily different midsole designs, produce shoes with remarkably different performance characteristics. Here are some guidelines for selecting the right shoe:

1. Select by fit, not size, which varies according to manufacture and style.
2. Choose a shoe that conforms to the foot's shape.
3. Measure the feet often. It is not uncommon for the left and right foot to be of different sizes.
4. Remember that feet change over time. Pregnancy for women and excessive weight gain by men or women tend to make feet larger. And as one ages, the force of gravity on the body tends to make the feet bigger.
5. Stand up when being fitted and make sure that there is one-eighth to one-half inch of space in front of the longest toe. Do not buy tight shoes hoping they will stretch.
6. Buy shoes designed for the appropriate sport. Replace shoes once they "break down" (lose support or cushioning): if the foot stretches the leather and starts sagging over the side of the sole, support will be compromised. This is especially important for high-impact sports like basketball and volleyball.
7. Motion control is provided by a multidensity midsole. Buy a shoe that provides adequate motion control. If overpronation is a problem, a shoe with harder and denser materials located at the heel and midsole of the shoe, to better stabilize the foot, is required.
8. Finally, it is necessary to analyze the shape of the foot in order to select the right shoe. Check the imprint of the foot (for example, in the sand at the beach) against the three imprints pictured below. They represent the three common foot types, each requiring different shoe stability and cushioning characteristics.

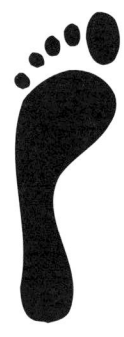

Normal foot. The normal foot usually lands on the outside of the heel and rolls slightly inward (pronates) as it absorbs the shock of landing.

Recommended: Shoes that provide moderate cushioning and support.

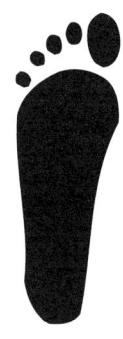

Flat foot. The low arch usually means that the runner's foot markedly rolls inward (overpronates) as it absorbs the shock of landing.

Recommended: Shoes with very firm midsoles and motion control to reduce the degree of pronation. Avoid highly cushioned shoes because they exaggerate the pronation as the heel "sinks" into the innersole surface.

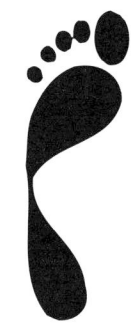

High-arched foot. This foot usually rolls outward or does not pronate enough.

Recommended: Some pronation is needed for effective shock absorbency, so these individuals should use well cushioned shoes with plenty of flexibility to improve foot motion. Shoes that restrict foot motion should be avoided.

common treatment option. These lightweight braces allow one to put weight on the foot soon after an injury. This more rapid return to action helps return mobility to the ankle and maintains muscle strength. The main advantage of braces over tape is that braces do not stretch to any significant extent. As tape stretches, it loses its ability to restrict ankle motion. A study involving collegiate women volleyball players found that tape restricted ankle ROM by 41 percent initially but quickly loosened during activity (after about 20 minutes); by the end of practice it restricted ROM by only 15 percent. In comparison, a therapeutic brace restricted ROM by 42 percent initially and dropped to 37 percent only at the end of 3 hours (Greene, 1990). One study estimated that the better stability provided by a therapeutic ankle brace lowered the risk of reinjury by 40 percent compared with tape (Renstrom, 1993). Furthermore, proponents claim that the use of removable therapeutic braces can cut healing time for severe sprains in half. However, the athlete should not use the brace too long. Prolonged use does not allow the weak leg muscles to strengthen, and this makes the injured ankle even more prone to reinjury.

James R. Holmes, M.D., and John Zumerchik

References

Albright, J. *The Scientific Basis of Orthopaedics*. New York: Appleton, 1987.

Appenzeller, O. *Sports Medicine: Fitness, Training, Injuries*. 3rd ed. Baltimore, Maryland: Urban and Schwarzenberg, 1988.

Arnheim, D. *Modern Principles of Athletic Training*. St. Louis, Missouri: Times Mirror Mosby, 1989.

Bloomfield, J., et al. *Textbook of Science and Medicine in Sports*. Champaign, Illinois: Human Kinetics, 1992.

Chan, C., and A. Rudins. "Foot Biomechanics During Walking and Running." *Mayo Clinic Proceedings* 69, no. 5 (1994): 448–460.

Frankel, V. *Basic Biomechanics of the Skeletal System*. Malvern, Pennsylvania: Lea and Febiger, 1980.

Gamble, J. *The Musculoskeletal System: Physiological Basics*. New York: Raven, 1988.

Greene, T. "Comparison of Support Provided by a Semi-Rigid Orthosis and Adhesive Ankle Taping Before, During, and After Exercise." *American Journal of Sports Medicine* 18, no. 5 (1990): 498–506.

Helminen, J. *Joint Loading: Biology and Health of Articular Structures*. Bristol, England: Wright, 1987.

Renstrom, J. *Sports Injuries: Basic Principles of Prevention and Care*. Boston: Blackwell Scientific, 1993.

Seireg, A., and R. Arvikar. *Biomechanical Analysis of the Musculoskeletal Structure for Medicine and Sports*. New York: Hemisphere, 1989.

Tietz, C. *Scientific Foundations of Sports Medicine*. St. Louis, Missouri: Times Mirror Mosby, 1989.

Body Composition

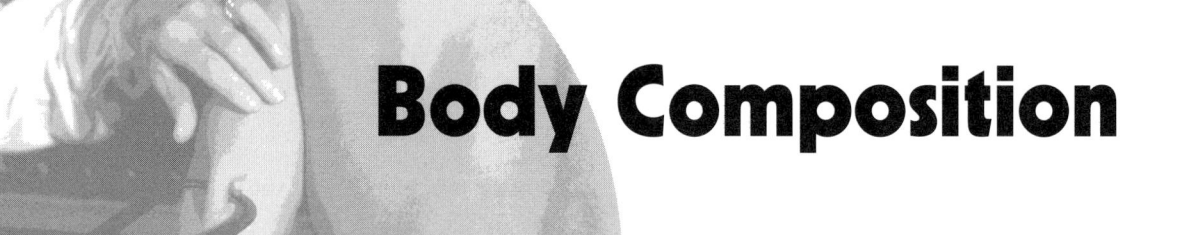

MANY SOCIAL SCIENTISTS believe the United States is one of the most weight-conscious societies in the world. However, obsession with weight is not a recent phenomenon. Society's view of the ideal weight has changed and will continue to change. Throughout history, the number of people considered to be suffering from obesity has risen and fallen as a function of social customs. Obesity has often reflected wealth—only the rich can afford fattening foods, or to eat in great quantities.

Cultural views regarding beauty also affect a society's perception of the ideal body composition. During the baroque period in Europe, for example, the definition of feminine beauty included wide hips and ample proportions. In some agrarian societies, weight has also been considered a criterion for choosing a mate. Because farming requires physical strength and endurance, a thin, frail mate was not thought capable of contributing adequately toward maintaining the household.

Since physical labor has become less and less common as an occupation, and many physically intensive factory jobs have been replaced by computer-operated machines, the number of overweight people in the United States has increased. The increase in recreational eating, such as cookouts, coffee breaks, and dinner parties, has also contributed to obesity—as long as convenience foods and packaged snacks continue to be popular, this trend is likely to continue. Furthermore, household chores continue to require less and less physical work, and the car has replaced the walk or bike ride. Obesity often follows when the use of physical energy declines at home and at work, and when leisure time and food intake increase.

Obesity can be caused by several factors, not simply by eating in excess of the body's needs. Some people begin life with an advantage: they have a genetic predisposition to leanness. This makes weight control easier (*see also* ENERGY AND METABOLISM).

Body weight reflects both the amount of fatty tissue in the body (adiposity) and the body's build (morphology). There is a range of body weights and compositions that experts consider healthy. Understanding the biological basis of body composition (the amount of fat in the body relative to other tissues) helps in forming a healthy conception of ideal weight. This is important, since some psychologists

The Obesity Burden

The National Center for Health Statistics conducted a survey of 30,000 people from 1991 to 1994 and found that, for first time, the overweight outnumber normal-size people. Forty percent of women and 59 percent of men were classified as overweight (National Center of Health Statistics, 1996). Besides the psychological problems caused by being overweight and obese, excess weight is also a factor contributing to many medical problems. Compared with a 20- to 44-year-old person of normal weight, an overweight person of the same age faces more than five times the risk of hypertension, nearly four times the risk of diabetes, and a higher risk of heart failure, gallstones, gout, and carcinoma (Pollack, 1990).

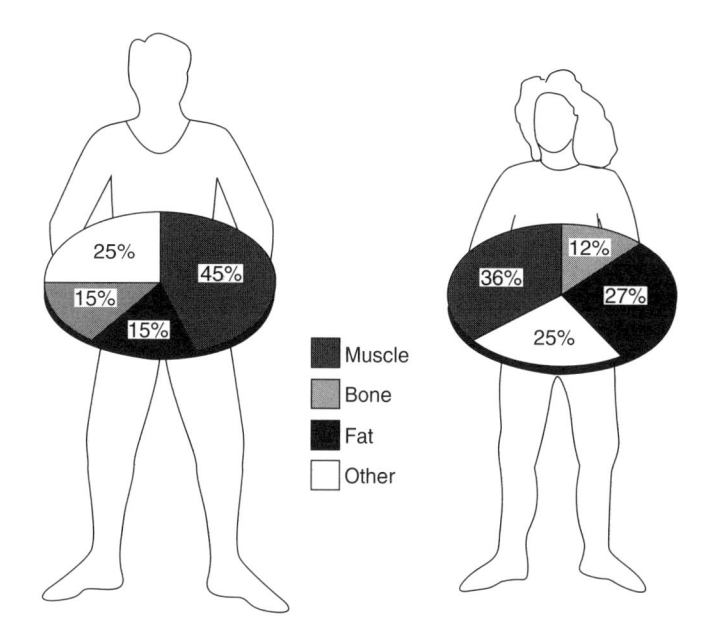

Figure 1. *Body composition of a typical adult male, with height of 175 centimeters (5 ft. 9 in.) and weight of 57 kilograms (154 lb.); and a typical adult female, with height of 163 centimeters (5 ft. 4 in.) and weight of 47 kilograms (125 lb.). (Adapted from Lamb, 1984)*

believe that severe misconceptions about body image may cause eating disorders, such as anorexia and bulimia.

Typical Fat and Nonfat Components

Body composition refers to the proportions of the major tissue components of the body. In particular, fitness professionals are concerned with the ratio of the body's lean tissue to fat tissue. Figure 1 shows typical body composition profiles for adult males and females in the United States. Men on average are a few inches taller, weigh slightly more, and possess a greater muscle-to-fat ratio. The biggest difference between men and women is in essential fat. Fitness professionals define essential fat as the minimum level of fat necessary for the body to maintain itself.

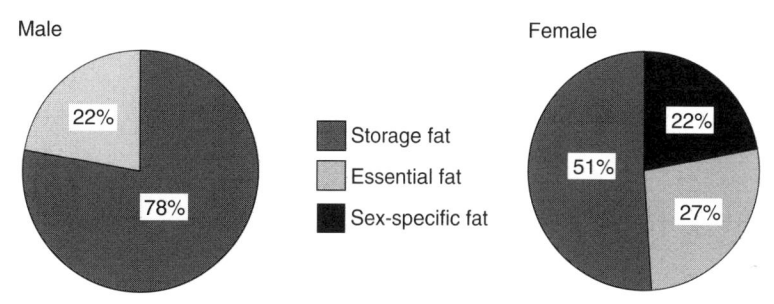

Figure 2. *Although the typical female body contains a higher proportion of fat than that of a male, there is a reason for this. The amount of essential fat, the fat necessary for the body to function, is higher for women.*

Much of the differences in body composition between the sexes can be attributed to the extra essential fat women carry (*see Figure 2*).

A second type of fat, storage fat, is located throughout the body, with major deposits beneath the skin and around major organs, such as the kidneys and heart. While these reserves are not called "essential," they serve some very vital purposes: as energy reservoirs, as insulation against the cold, and as protective cushions against impact to the body. Men and women carry similar percentages of storage fat. Reducing the amount of storage fat is a major goal of diet and exercise plans.

Measuring Body Composition

A Body Fat Advantage?

Swimming is one of the few sports in which an athlete with a higher percentage of body fat may have an advantage. Studies have found that women can swim long distances at for significantly lower energy cost than men. Or stated another way, at any given energy expenditure, women can attain a higher swim speed. Their higher body fat composition gives them more buoyancy. Moreover, the distribution of their fat helps. Since a greater proportion of a woman's body fat lies in the legs, it is easier to maintain them in a horizontal position, reducing speed-robbing drag, and increasing swimming efficiency (*see the essay "Body Fat as a Predictor of Athletic Performance"*).

For most people, the only indications of weight come from stepping on a bathroom scale, and a thorough survey in the mirror. A pinch here, a squeeze there, a quick eyeball examination, and presto: a simplistic and often erroneous interpretation of body composition. Neither the scale nor the mirror is a very scientific approach to body composition analysis. Fortunately, however, a number of scientific techniques are available. When these scientific techniques are administered by trained technicians even in nonlaboratory settings, reliable estimates of body composition can be obtained.

An accurate body composition analysis is important for health as well as for athletic performance. Most medical experts believe that increased body weight in the form of excess fat does pose a health risk. Extra fat may contribute to high blood pressure, high cholesterol levels, and diabetes. Each of these disorders is a primary risk factor for coronary artery disease, one of the leading causes of death for adults in the United States. Because of these concerns, it is necessary to determine the composition of the weight on an individual's frame in addition to the quantity. For example, consider two women of the same height who weigh 47 kilograms (125 lb.) and 54 kilograms (145 lb.), respectively. One cannot necessarily assume that the heavier woman has the higher health risk from excess fat. A better comparison involves determining the proportion of fat mass to nonfat mass (muscle, bone, and other organs) to calculate what percentage of body weight is actually fat, by using one of several standardized body composition measures. Both women may have a body composition of about 20 percent fat, despite their 20 pound difference in weight. This is possible because variations in bone structure, density, and muscle mass may increase weight without adding fat.

Body fat measurements, although only estimates, are useful additional indicators of health, as are regular tests for blood pressure and cholesterol levels. Early and regular checks of body composition can serve as a barometer of health throughout life, as well as a baseline measure to chart changes over time. Currently, there are three common methods available outside the laboratory or clinic for determining body composition: skin-fold tests, hydrostatic weighing, and bioelectrical impedance. Each of the techniques has its advantages and disadvantages.

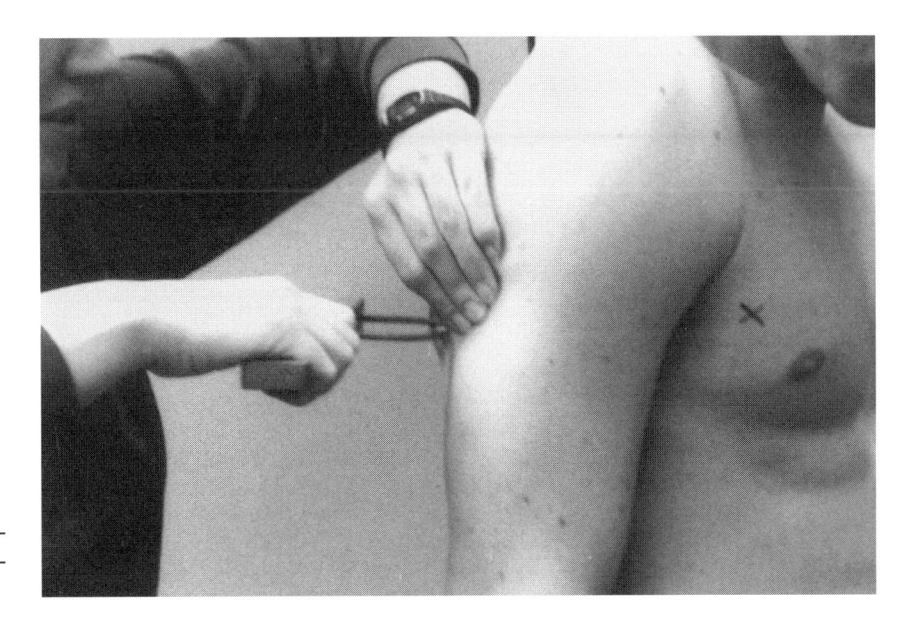

Figure 3. *Common sites of skin-fold measurements include the triceps, abdomen, thighs, and chest.*

Skin-Fold Sum

The skin-fold sum is the most practical and widely used technique for determining percentage of body fat. A skin fold is the thickness of a compressed double fold of skin (the amount of skin that can be pinched between the thumb and forefinger) and the underlying adipose tissue. The principle behind this method assumes that about 50 percent of the fat on the frame is found just below the skin (subcutaneous fat). Folds of skin and underlying fat at specific anatomical sites are measured using special calipers (*see Figure 3*). Measurement sites usually include, but are not limited to, the chest, abdomen, and thigh for men; and the triceps, hips, and thighs for women. These measures are summed and then put into a series of equations to calculate body density and percentage of body fat.

For the most accurate measurement, skin-fold measures should be taken by a technician trained in site determination and the use of calipers. General "adjustment" equations have been developed to account for gender- and age-related differences among the population. However, skin-fold tests have an error rate of about 3.7 percent, or as much as 5 percent if poor measurement techniques are used. This means that a 20 percent body-fat measurement taken by a trained technician reflects a range of 18.3 percent to 23.7 percent. With skin-fold tests, accuracy is not as important as regularity. If they are administered regularly (every 6 months or so), They can be used as a benchmark for comparing health assessments over time and can indicate changes in overall body composition. One advantage of skin-fold testing is that it can track changes in the distribution of body fat.

Hydrostatic Weighing

With an error rate of about 2 percent, hydrostatic, or underwater, weighing is more accurate than the skin-fold method. However, because this technique requires sophisticated equipment and skilled

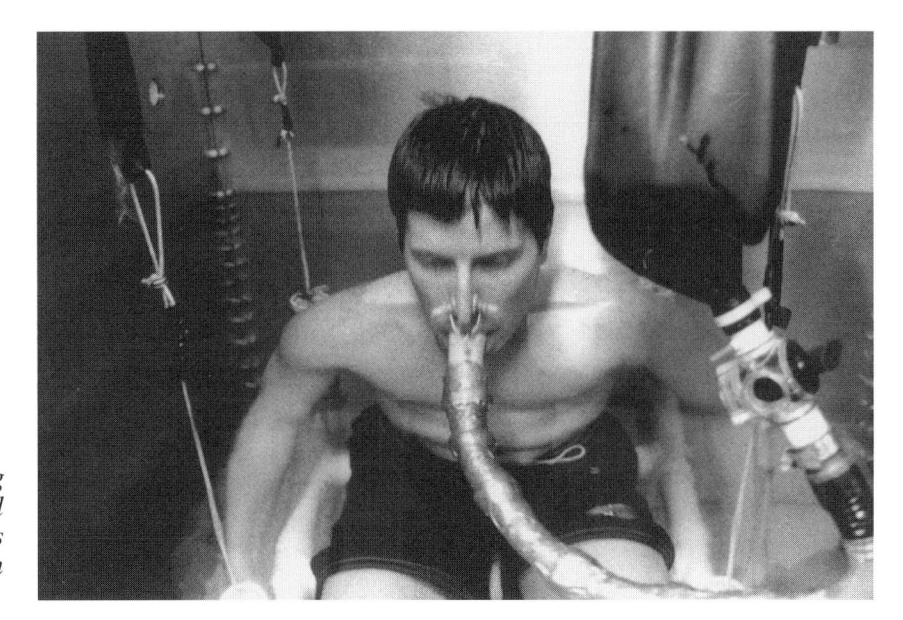

Figure 4. *Hydrostatic weighing requires special equipment, operated by skilled technicians; thus, despite its greater accuracy, it is used less often than the skin-fold method.*

technicians, it is a far less commonly used method of body-fat estimation. Hydrostatic weighing uses densitometry analysis. As the name indicates, it is a measure of the body's density; percentage of body fat is predicted from the amount of water displaced in relation to general formulas developed to account for body density. Because density is a measure of mass per unit of volume—such as kilograms per liter or pounds per gallon—it requires a measurement of body volume in order to attain a body density figure. According to Archimedes' principle, a body submerged in water is buoyed by a counterforce equal to the weight of water it displaces. This buoyant force supports the submerged body against the downward force of gravity. By subtracting the weight of the individual underwater from the weight on a scale, the weight of water displaced can be determined. Dividing this figure by the density of water gives the volume of water displaced.

The principle behind hydrostatic or underwater weighing is that fat mass floats in water because its density (mass per unit of volume) is less than that of water. On the other hand, bone and muscle do not float in water because their densities are greater than that of water. In other words, when submerged in water, a very lean person tends to sink, while an overweight person tends to float. The lower a body's density, the greater the percentage of body fat; the higher a body's density, the lower the percentage of body fat. Body densities range from 0.93 grams per cubic centimeter to 1.10 grams per cubic centimeter (1.0 is the equilibrium density of water; *see also* SWIMMING).

The calculation method for determining body fat percentage by hydrostatic weighing may be expressed as follows:

$$\text{Body density} = \frac{\text{mass}}{\text{volume}} = \frac{\text{body weight} \times \text{water temperature correction}}{\text{body weight} - \text{underwater weight} - \text{residual lung volume} \times \text{water temp. correction}}$$

Since water density varies slightly with temperature (it is denser at lower temperatures), water temperature is recorded to correct for the density of water at the weighing temperature. The amount of water displaced, or the body's volume, is also affected by the volume of air in the lungs. Therefore, before submersion, the participant makes a forced maximal exhalation. Nevertheless, a residual volume of air remains in the lungs and must be measured and factored out of the calculations to predict body fat. Air left in the intestines and other body cavities may also contribute to the error.

Other factors to consider are the race and age of the subject. Bone density varies among different segments of the population. In the formative years, bone density, water content, and potassium content tend to vary, and in the later years the demineralization of bone caused by osteoporosis affects bone mass.

Anxiety also may contribute to an inaccurate estimate. Fear of being submerged can result in irregular breathing and throw off the residual volume measure. To prevent this error, the underwater weighing procedure is repeated several times, to allow the individual to relax and expel as much air as possible from the lungs.

Bioelectrical Impedance

The main advantage of bioelectric impedance is its ease of administration. This method is based on a simple physical principle: percentage of body fat can be calculated by measuring the resistance of fat mass and nonfat body mass to a low voltage electrical current. An electric current is passed through the body through small electrodes attached to the wrists and ankles, and the conductivity of the tissue, its ability to conduct electricity, is measured. Conductivity is higher in lean body tissue, due to its high water content, than fat tissue.

This method provides consistent measurements for an individual, but it is not as accurate as hydrostatic weighing. Bioelectrical impedance is easy to perform, and the potential for error is about the same as with skin-fold tests. However, the error can be greatly increased if normal levels of hydration are not maintained. A dehydrated individual will register a higher fat percentage because the dehydrated nonfat body tissue will register a reading closer to that of fat tissue. Because of this potential for error and the relative expense of the equipment, bioelectrical impedance is a less common method of measurement than skin-fold testing or hydrostatic weighing, though it is growing in popularity.

Other Methods

Skin-fold testing, hydrostatic weighing, and bioelectrical impedance are the three most common measuring methods used in health clubs, fitness centers, sports medicine clinics, and university hospitals. The tests are usually relatively inexpensive, but they all have certain limitations. Therefore, other methods of a more clinical nature are receiving closer attention by experts in the field of body composition. These techniques, which are not yet widely available, require additional study for both reliability and validity.

Body fat as a predictor of athletic performance

Watching an obese person laboriously trying to jog, it is apparent that, in comparison with leaner counterparts, this person must make an added affort to run. No one would dispute the fact that the effect of carrying around "dead" weight, excess storage fat, affects athletic performance. However, many people wonder if there is a correlation between body fat and performance when, say, male collegiate athletes with a very typical 13 to 17 percent body fat are compared with exceptionally lean collegiate athletes with 6 to 9 percent body fat.

A male athlete 178 centimeters (5 ft. 10 in.) tall of average build who measures 17 percent body fat carries 28 pounds of fat, approximately 15 pounds more than a similar athlete with 8 percent body fat. Depending on the person, storage fat may be evenly distributed throughout the body or may tend to be concentrated in certain areas, such as thighs, hips, or waist. Studies have found that when weights are strapped to the body (by backpack, vest, or belt) distribution of the weight has little effect on performance. This seems to indicate that the added body fat hurts performance because it is detrimental to the overall biomechanics of motion, not because it weighs down one particular part of the body. Further, performance differences were smaller between athletes with 13 to 17 percent body fat and those with 6 to 9 percent body fat than between the 13 to 17 percent group and athletes with body fat of about 35 percent.

In prolonged weight-bearing sports, such as distance running, excess body fat decreases performance. For any given level of work performed, greater energy is required the heavier the person. The maximum oxygen uptake (a measure of aerobic capacity) of a heavier person occurs at a lower rate of work, and the pace that can be maintained for any period of time declines. If the added weight comes from muscle, the added energy production necessary is insignificant because greater muscle mass has the potential to generate greater power and energy. But if the added weight comes from body fat, aerobic capacity declines. Body fat reduces the overall oxidative energy (long-term endurance energy) that can be made available to move each pound of body weight. Furthermore, the cardiovascular system reaches capacity at a slower running pace because more work is required to move the body at any given speed.

The narrowing gap between men's and women's world-record times over the last 20 years in many sports can be attributed in part to the narrowing gap in body-fat percentage. The table below shows the body composition and power output for world-class speed skaters. Although there is a 12 percent difference between the power output of men and women, this gap narrows to 3 percent when adjusted for kilograms of body fat. According to this study, the remaining 3 percent difference in power output can be attributed mostly to lower body fat. Women's less efficient knee bend angle was also a minor contributing factor.

Oxygen consumption among male and female speed skaters was also found to be equal when measured relative to body weight. While many experts believe it is unlikely that female athletes will ever perform at the same speeds as their male peers, the gap between men's and women's world-record times may continue to narrow as the differences in percentage of body fat continue to narrow.

John Zumerchik

POWER OUTPUT AS A FUNCTION OF BODY WEIGHT

	Body weight (kg)	Percent fat	Power output (watts)	Power output/ body weight
Male	73.6	9.5	388	5.27
Female	66.3	20.6	340	5.13

The power outputs for male and female skaters were measured for 1,500 meters of skating (about 2 minutes). Although there is a 12 percent difference in power output between males and females, this discrepancy narrows to 3 percent when expressed in terms of kilograms of body weight. This remaining 3 percent difference in power per kilogram of body mass is attributed mainly to the difference in percentage body fat between men and women, with a minor effect from the female skaters' less optimal knee angle position. (Source: van Ingen Shenau, 1989)

These methods borrow tools used in medicine, such as x-rays, computerized tomography (CT), nuclear magnetic resonance (NMR), and ultrasound electromagnetic waves. The CT and NMR scanning procedures may become commonly used tools in evaluating body composition in the twenty-first century. Ultrasound shows promise, too. Using a lightweight ultrasound meter, electromagnetic sound waves are sent into the body to measure the distance between the skin and fat-muscle layer and between the fat-muscle layer and bone. The waves pass through the body until they reach muscle tissue and then echo back to the ultrasound meter. By considering the speed of the waves through different substances, it is possible to determine body-fat composition.

Desirable Weight

No matter which method is used to determine body composition, the result is always an estimate. As yet, there is no way to ensure absolute accuracy in the measurement of body fat in the adult population. Moreover, the measurements obtained tend to be less accurate for individuals with extremely low or extemely high body fat. Using two or more of these techniques may significantly improve the accuracy of estimation.

In determining ideal weight, consideration of body composition is essential. A body composition measure will help identify a weight goal that is realistic and healthy. Quite often individuals have unrealistic expectations of how much they should weigh and are perpetually frustrated by not achieving that weight. Efforts to lose weight tend to be more effective when they focus on changes in body composition rather than changes in overall weight. This strategy offers a more precise means of monitoring overall health.

Recommended ranges of percent of body fat for the average nonathletic adult population are 14 to 19 percent for men and 20 to 24 percent for women. Under the age of 20 and over the age of 60, body fat percentages should be higher. As the body grows, the store of essential body fat is greater, and as the body ages, a drop in physical activity leads to a decline in lean body tissue. Although the body-fat percentages for competitive athletes are highly variable, they are significantly lower than for the general population (see Table 1).

While excessive body fat is a health risk and can hinder performance, essential levels of fat are still necessary for the body to function efficiently. Essential body fat is about 3 to 4 percent for men and 10 to 12 percent for women.

None of the above techniques is perfect, and many assumptions

**BODY FAT IN OLYMPIC ATHLETES
(AS PERCENTAGE OF TOTAL BODY MASS)**

Event	Male	Female
Throwers	29.4–30.9	27–33.8
Jumpers	6.8–8.2	8.4–14.1
Swimmers	9–12	14.5–16.6
Gymnasts	7–9.9	11–14.7

Table 1. *(Source: Lamb, 1984)*

> ## A Desirable Weight
>
> The best way to determine one's desirable weight is not by stepping on a scale, but by determining the ratio of lean body tissue to fat tissue. Here is how a 93-kilogram (250-lb.) man with 30 percent body fat should calculate how to reduce his overall body fat to 20 percent.
>
> Fat weight = 250 lb. × 0.30 = 75 lb.
>
> Lean weight = 250 lb. − 75 lb. = 175 lb.
>
> $$\text{Desirable weight} = \frac{\text{Lean weight}}{1.00 - \text{fat goal (\%)}} = \frac{175 \text{ lb}}{1.00 - 0.20} = 218.75 \text{ lb.}$$
>
> Desirable fat loss = 250 − 218.75 = 31.25 lb.
>
> If he loses 31.25 pounds of body fat, his new body weight of 218.75 pounds results in a fat content equal to 20 percent of body weight.

are made based on the information available on the composition of bone, muscle, fat, and other body tissues. Nonetheless, an individual is far wiser in using professionally administered body-fat measurements than relying on a bathroom scale and mirror. Body composition measures should be viewed as additional information for exercise professionals to employ in fashioning an effective program of diet and exercise.

Nancy Rowland, M.S., and John Zumerchik

References

American College of Sports Medicine. *Resource Manual for Guidelines for Exercise Testing and Prescription*. 2nd ed. Philadelphia: Lea and Febiger, 1993.

Cureton, K., and P. Sparling. "Distance Running Performance and Metabolic Responses to Running in Men and Women with Excess Weight Experimentally Equated." *Medicine and Science in Sports and Exercise* 12, no. 4 (1980): 288ff.

Lamb, D. *Physiology of Exercise: Responses and Adaptations*. 2nd ed. New York: Macmillan, 1984.

Lampman, R., and D. Schteingart. "Moderate and Extreme Obesity." In B. Franklin (ed.), *Exercise in Modern Medicine*. Baltimore: Williams and Wilkens, 1989.

McArdle, W., F. Katch, and V. Katch. *Exercise Physiology: Energy, Nutrition, and Human Performance*. 2nd ed. Philadelphia: Lea and Febiger, 1986.

National Center for Health Statistics. *The National Health and Nutrition Examination Study*. Hyattsville, Maryland: National Center for Health Statistics, 1996.

Pollack, M., and J. Wilmore. *Exercise in Health and Disease*. 2nd ed. Philadelphia: Saunders, 1990.

Sleamaker, R. *Serious Training for Serious Athletes*. Champaign, Illinois: Leisure, 1989.

Stuart, R., and B. Davis. *Slim Chance in a Fat World*. Champaign, Illinois: Research, 1972.

van Ingen Schenau, G. "Speed Skating." In C. Vaugham (ed.), *Biomechanics of Sports*. Orlando, Florida: CRC, 1989.

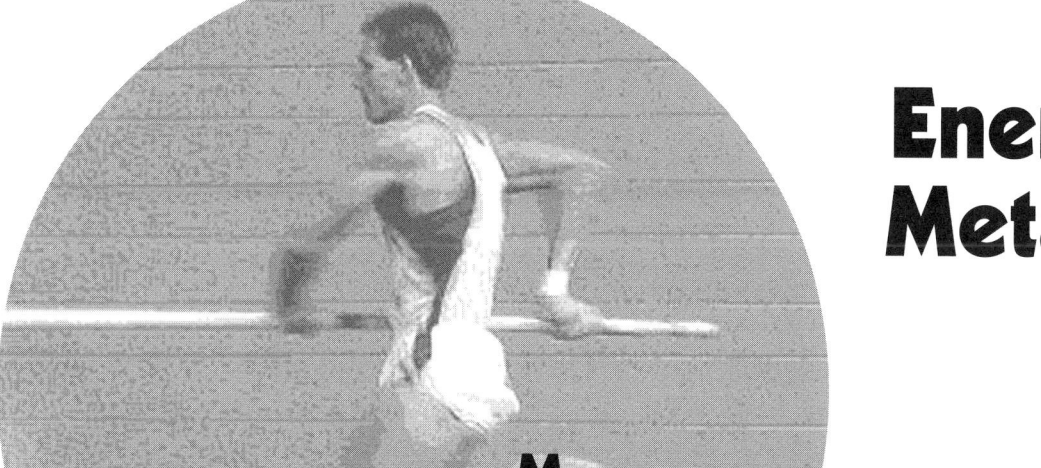

Energy and Metabolism

MANY ATHLETES STRIVE to maintain optimum energy stores, which will allow them to compete at their best. Hikers and cross-country skiers want to be sure to eat enough to power them through a long day in the woods. Marathon runners need enough fuel to allow them to exert themselves nonstop for more than 2 hours. Weight lifters need to replenish their energy stores after a workout. Hockey and soccer players need an energy source that will prevent them from tiring in the middle of a game. And the average fitness enthusiast wants to know whether it is best to eat before or after a workout, what are the best ways to burn fat, and how to improve stamina. To understand the way in which foods power the body and to learn how to optimize energy use for athletic activity, it is essential to understand metabolism.

Whether asleep or at rest, the body is always at work: new tissue is built, old tissue is torn down, substances are moved in and out of cells, food is digested, wastes are excreted. As the body performs the work of living, chemical reactions occur constantly. The term *metabolism* refers to the sum total of these chemical reactions (*meta*, "with"; *bole*, "change"). Metabolism includes anabolism, the buildup of larger molecules from smaller ones (*ana*, "up"); and catabolism, the breakdown of larger molecules into smaller ones (*cata*, "down"). Food molecules—carbohydrates, proteins, and fats—are broken down in the body to release energy that can be used for work. Smaller food molecules, like sugar, are built into larger fuel molecules—fat,

ENERGY USE

Mode	MPH	kcal/mile
Walker	3	70
155-lb. runner	9	120
200-lb. runner	9	140
Cyclist	15	55
Cross-country skier	13	60
Automobile	55	963
Motorcycle	55	481
Executive jet	400	14,467

Table 1. *It requires energy to travel, whether the mode of travel is self-propelled or by vehicle.*

for example—for the storage of energy. *Metabolism* also refers to the constant buildup and breakdown of body tissues and the disposal of waste products.

The amount of energy the body uses in a given time is called the metabolic rate. The rate at which one expends energy depends primarily on one's activity level but is also affected by food consumption, stress, and temperature. The energy cost of maintaining the body at rest is the basal metabolic rate (BMR). A person's BMR depends on age, sex, size, rate of growth, health, and level of fitness.

During exercise, contraction of skeletal muscles is the most significant physiological activity occurring in the body, and it has the most profound effect on the metabolic rate. It takes energy to do work, that is, to move muscles to exert a force. The source of that energy is food, but the body must convert the energy of its food sources to a usable form. This article will discuss the processes through which the body harnesses the energy provided by food.

Chemistry: The Basis of Change

It requires energy to hold the atoms of a molecule together. When a chemical bond is broken, energy is released. When wood burns or gasoline ignites in the cylinder of an engine, the fuel is reacting with oxygen (oxidation), and bonds are broken with a sudden and uncontrolled release of energy. In the body, fuels combine with oxygen in a controlled fashion so that energy is released in small, usable quantities. This process can be expressed as:

$$\text{food} + \text{oxygen} \rightarrow \text{water} + \text{carbon dioxide} + \text{work energy} + \text{heat energy}$$

Heat and work energy are measured in units called calories (*calor*, "heat"): 1 calorie is the amount of heat required to raise the temperature of 1 gram of water 1 degree Celsius. A more useful measure is the kilocalorie (kcal), which equals 1,000 calories. The term *calorie* is commonly used to refer to the energy content of food, but a calorie in this sense actually means 1 kcal.

The first law of thermodynamics states that energy can be neither created nor destroyed; it can only be transferred from one form to another. In most chemical reactions, the energy of the products is not equal to the energy of the reactants; therefore, energy is either taken from or released to the environment in the course of the reaction. A chemical reaction that releases energy is called exothermic (*exo*, "out"; *therm*, "heat"), and one that absorbs energy is called endothermic (*endo*, "in"). For example, when carbonic acid (H_2CO_3) breaks down into water (H_2O) and carbon dioxide (CO_2), 4 kcal of heat energy per mole of carbonic acid is released. (A mole is about 6×10^{23} molecules; because atoms and molecules are so small, it is a very useful unit for the laboratory. One mole of any substance has a mass, in grams, equal to its molecular weight expressed in atomic mass units. For example, 1 mole of carbon-12 has a mass of 12 g; 62 g of carbonic acid constitutes 1 mole.) The breakdown of carbonic acid may be expressed as follows:

$$H_2CO_3 \rightarrow CO_2 + H_2O + 4 \text{ kcal/mol}$$
$$(155 \text{ kcal/mol}) \quad (94 \text{ kcal/mol}) \quad (57 \text{ kcal/mol})$$

The energy content of the reactant (carbonic acid) is higher than the sum of the energy content of the products, water and carbon dioxide (94 + 57 = 151). If the reaction goes in the reverse direction—that is, if carbon dioxide and water combine to form carbonic acid—then 4 kcal/mol of energy must be added.

Sometimes an endothermic reaction is linked with an exothermic reaction, and the energy released by the breaking bonds of one molecule is used for building bonds in another. Instead of being turned into heat, the energy released from the exothermic reaction is in effect "stored" in the bonds of another molecule.

A catalyst is a substance that accelerates a chemical reaction without being used up itself in the reaction. The catalyst interacts with one or more of the reactants to make them more reactive. Because it is not used up in the reaction, the catalyst can be used again and again; a small amount can go a long way. Enzymes are large molecules that act as catalysts in living organisms. They are responsible for facilitating many of the thousands of chemical reactions that occur in plants and animals. In an enzyme reaction, the reactant is called the substrate. The substrate attaches to the enzyme to form an enzyme-substrate complex, which quickly breaks down to release the product (or products) and the unchanged enzyme (*see Figure 1*).

A coenzyme is sometimes necessary for an enzyme to work. The coenzyme helps by shuttling a few atoms between the enzyme and the substrate and, like the enzyme, is used over and over. However, unlike the enzyme, the coenzyme is changed in the reaction and has to be recycled. A single coenzyme can act as both a donor and a recipient. For example, the coenzyme may pick up two atoms of hydrogen from a substrate in one enzyme reaction and deliver it to a different substrate in a different enzyme reaction, returning to its original form (*see Figure 1b*).

Many reactions can proceed both forward and in the reverse direction; these are called reversible reactions. For example, carbonic acid can be broken down into water and carbon dioxide; or, with the addition of heat (energy), water and carbon dioxide can combine to form carbonic acid. Generally, the exothermic (energy-releasing) direction is favored. Consider the reaction A + B ↔ C + energy (energy is released), and suppose that it begins with a mixture of A and B. As the reaction proceeds, the amount of A and B decreases and the amount of C increases. The law of mass action states that the rate of reaction is proportional to the concentration of the reactants. Thus, as the amount

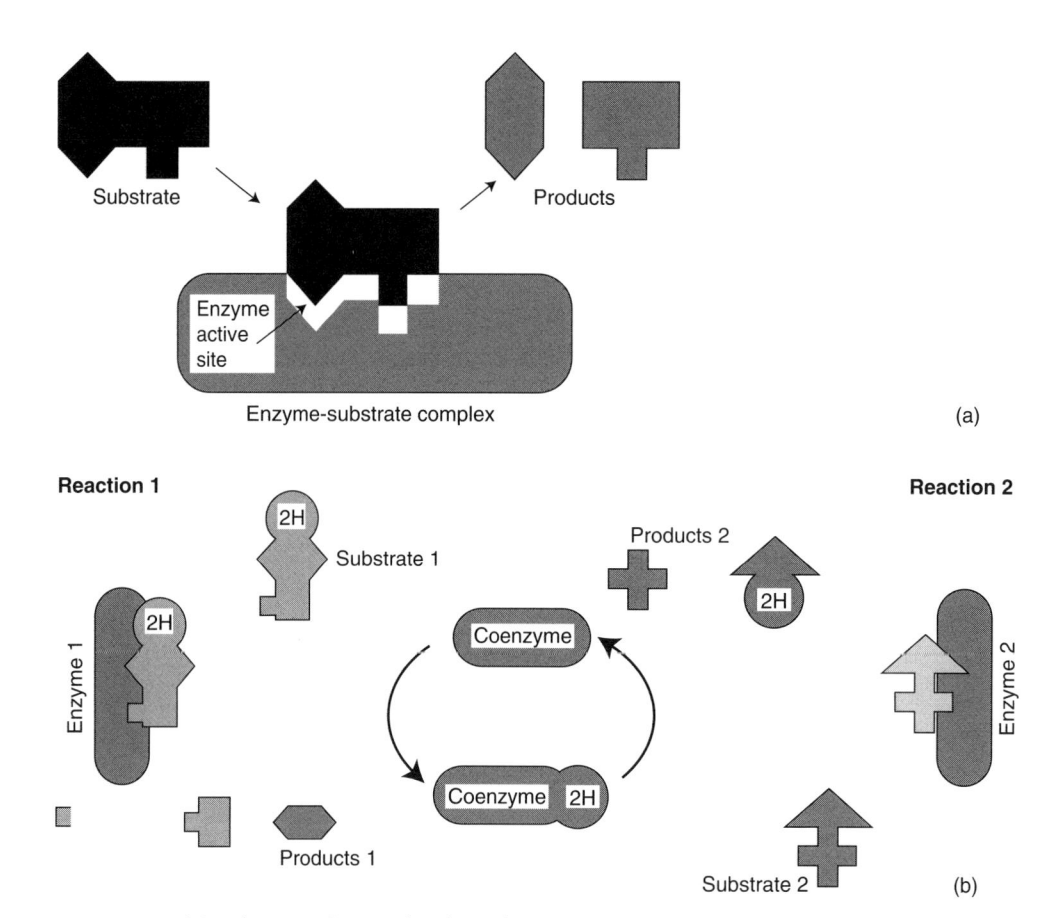

Figure 1. *(a) When a substrate binds to the active site of an enzyme, the enzyme catalyzes the formation of products. (b) A coenzyme assists two different enzyme reactions by receiving (reaction 1) or donating (reaction 2), in this example, a pair of hydrogen atoms.*

of A and B decreases, the rate of the forward reaction slows, and the rate of the reverse reaction increases. When the rates of the forward and reverse reactions are equal—that is, each time a molecule of A combines with a molecule of B to form a molecule of C, a C breaks down into an A and a B—the reactants and products are in chemical equilibrium. Note that at equilibrium, the concentrations of reactants and products are not necessarily equal. Their relative amounts depend on the amount of energy added or released in the reaction. At equilibrium, the concentration of C, being lower in energy than the sum of A plus B, will be higher than that of A and B. If the difference in energy between the products and reactants is very large, the probability that the reaction will go in the reverse direction is very small, and the reaction is said to be irreversible.

Note: The special role of carbon. Carbon is the most versatile of all the elements. Carbon atoms can share chemical bonds with other carbon atoms, as well as atoms of other elements, to form an enormous variety of molecules. The American Chemical Society maintains a register of chemical compounds, and, of the nearly 5 million compounds listed, more than 4 million are based on the carbon backbone.

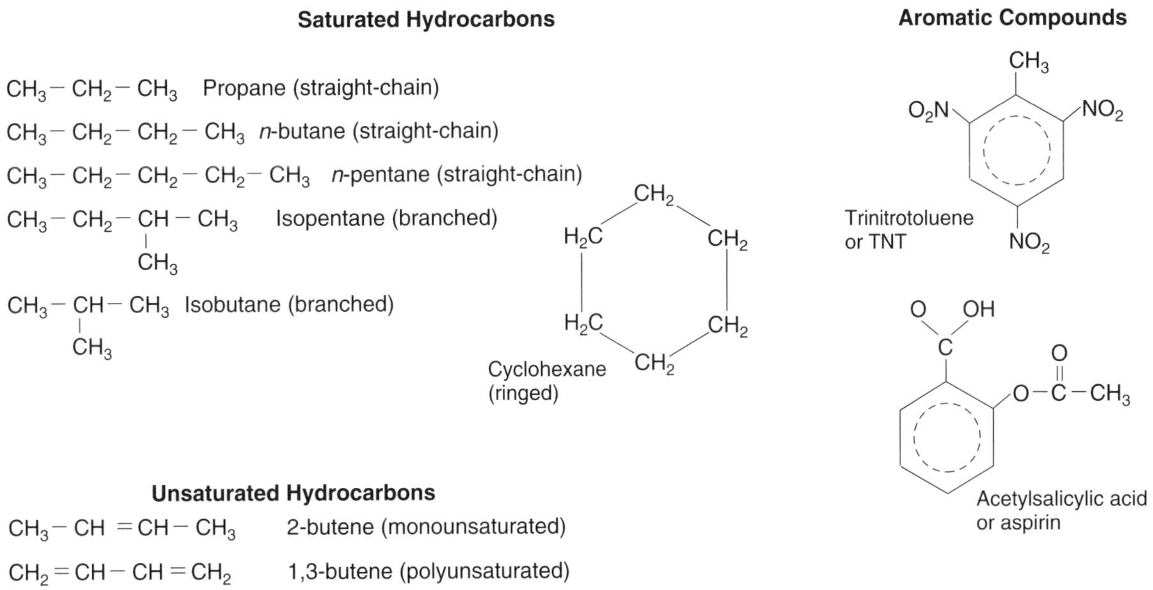
Saturated Hydrocarbons
CH3 – CH2 – CH3 Propane (straight-chain)
CH3 – CH2 – CH2 – CH3 n-butane (straight-chain)
CH3 – CH2 – CH2 – CH2 – CH3 n-pentane (straight-chain)
CH3 – CH2 – CH – CH3 Isopentane (branched)
CH3
CH3 – CH – CH3 Isobutane (branched)
CH3
CH2
H2C
CH2
H2C
CH2
CH2
Cyclohexane (ringed)
Aromatic Compounds
CH3
O2N
NO2
NO2
Trinitrotoluene or TNT
O
OH
C
O
O – C – CH3
Acetylsalicylic acid or aspirin
Unsaturated Hydrocarbons
CH3 – CH = CH – CH3 2-butene (monounsaturated)
CH2 = CH – CH = CH2 1,3-butene (polyunsaturated)

Figure 2. *Some different types of carbon-based molecules.*

Molecules containing carbon are known as *organic* (to signify "living") compounds, because the term initially referred to compounds derived directly from plants and animals (*see Figure 2*). When carbon-containing compounds were first synthesized in the laboratory in the early 1800s, *organic* came to refer to the chemistry of carbon compounds.

The simplest carbon molecules are chains of the unit -CH_2-, one carbon and two hydrogens. Because a single carbon atom can make up to four bonds, it can form branched and cross-linked chains. Carbon can also make multiple bonds with itself and other elements. Because a multiple bond can be converted to a single bond by the addition of hydrogen, multiple-bond organic compounds are called unsaturated. If a carbon chain contains only single bonds, it is said to be saturated. (That is, no more hydrogen can be added.) Compounds that form rings may have special shared bonds, called aromatic bond because many of these compounds have an aroma.

Cellular Metabolism: Breaking Down Fuels for Energy

All the cells in a living organism need energy to function. They obtain this energy from fuels—that is, food. The following sections will describe the specific processes involved.

ATP: The Energy Currency of Living Cells

Cells obtain their energy from the chemical energy stored in the bonds of organic molecules from food. When the bonds break, some energy is released as heat, which the cells cannot harness as usable energy. But some of the energy released in the catabolism of fuel molecules is transferred to another molecule: that is, it is used to form new chemical bonds and increase the energy content of the new molecule. In the cells of all organisms, the molecule used to transfer energy in this way is adenosine triphosphate (ATP), the energy "currency" of living tissue

It is important to remember that the role of ATP is to transfer energy, not to store it. Consider an analogy: If the fare on city buses is $1 but the toll boxes accept "exact change only," a rider might change, say, $5 into quarters for use as bus fare. ATP plays a role similar to the quarters. Energy released from fuels such as sugar or fat comes in quantities too large to be used by cellular machinery, just as a $5 bill or a $1 bill is too large to be used as a fare. Energy released from the breakdown of fuel molecules is transferred to ATP molecules, which are able to transfer just the amount of energy, in small doses, that cell functions require. In brief, just as quarters can be the currency of bus fare, ATP is the currency of cellular work.

ATP is formed from adenosine diphosphate (ADP), and a phosphate group plus 7 kcal/mol of energy (*see Figure 3*). In this way, energy is temporarily stored in the newly created phosphate bond. The chemical reaction in which a phosphate group (abbreviated P_i) is added to a molecule to form a phosphate bond is called phosphorylation:

$$ADP + P_i + 7 \text{ kcal/mol} \rightarrow ATP + H_2O$$

During the catabolism of nutrients, about 40 percent of the nutrients' energy is transferred to form ATP from ADP, while roughly 60 percent is lost as heat (this is the reason why the body stays warm and gives off even more heat during work or exercise). Energy is released from ATP when it combines with water (hydrolysis) and breaks down to form ADP.

$$ATP + H_2O \rightarrow ADP + P_i + 7 \text{ kcal/mol}$$

The energy released by breaking the high-energy phosphate bonds in ATP can power such cell functions as muscle contraction, nerve transmission, building of new tissue, glandular secretion, movement of substances across cell membranes, and digestion.

The total amount of ATP in the body at a given moment is suffi-

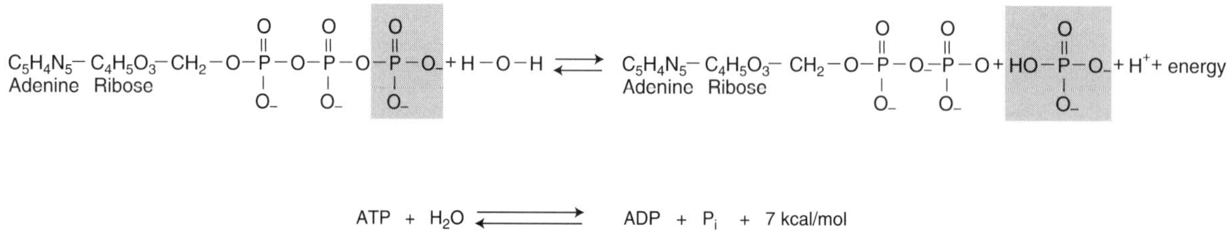

Figure 3. *Adenosine triphosphate, or ATP, releases 7 kcal/mol of energy when it reacts with water and breaks down into ADP, adenosine diphosphate, plus phosphate. This energy can be harnessed to perform cellular work.*

cient to maintain the resting functions of the tissues for only about 90 seconds and can sustain intense activity, such as sprinting, for no more than 10 seconds. Therefore, the body must transfer energy continually from fuel molecules to ATP.

Oxidative Phosphorylation: The Aerobic Pathway

During the entire process of breaking down fuel molecules, hydrogen atoms are stripped away from them and are ultimately passed on to oxygen to form water, H_2O. Along the way, the hydrogen atoms and chemical energy are transferred from the nutrient molecules to coenzymes (molecules derived from the B vitamins niacin and riboflavin).

$$\text{fuel-2H} + \text{coenzyme} \rightarrow \text{fuel} + \text{coenzyme-2H}$$

The energy transferred to the coenzyme with the addition of hydrogen is passed on to ATP in special organelles called mitochondria. Mitochondria, present in most cells and especially abundant in muscle cells, serve as the cells' "energy factories." Along the inner membranes of the mitochondria, special iron-containing proteins called cytochromes (see Figure 4) form the pathway along which the electrons from hydrogen are delivered to oxygen, which then reacts with the hydrogen to form water.

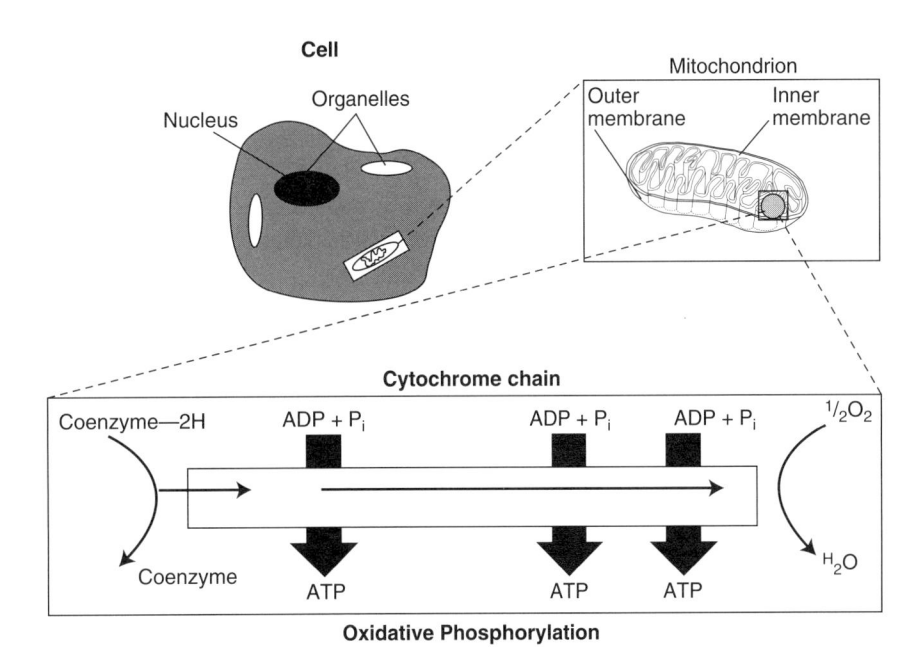

$$\text{coenzyme-2H} + \tfrac{1}{2} O_2 \xrightarrow{\text{cytochrome}} \text{coenzyme} + H_2O + 52 \text{ kcal/mol}$$

Figure 4. *Within the mitochondrion—oxidative phosphorylation—the aerobic transfer of energy, occurs along the cytochromes. Coenzyme-2H donates its two hydrogen atoms, which are passed along the cytochrome chain. As the hydrogen atoms pass through, ATP is formed from ADP. At the end, ionized hydrogen combines with oxygen to form water.*

As the electrons are passed along the cytochrome chain, energy is released in small amounts, and some is transferred to form the high-energy phosphate bonds of ATP from ADP. Each hydrogen pair ultimately results in the formation of two or three ATPs. This process, in which ATP is synthesized during the transformation of oxygen to water, is called oxidative phosphorylation. Because oxygen is required, it is called an aerobic process. Ninety percent of the body's ATP is formed this way, in the mitochondria. Oxidative phosphorylation has an efficiency of roughly 40 percent, forming three ATP (7 kcal/mol × 3 = 21 kcal/mol) from the 52 kcal/mol of energy released in the oxidation of coenzyme-2H (21 kcal/mol ÷ 52 kcal/ mol × 100 = 40 percent). Considering that the steam engine has about 30 percent efficiency, the human body does quite well.

During exertion, one breathes more deeply and rapidly, and the heart pumps faster. This is because the muscles are using a large quantity of ATP to do the work of contraction, and mitochondria in the muscle cells are demanding more oxygen. In strenuous exercise, the rate at which oxygen is used may exceed the rate at which the lungs and heart can deliver it. This creates a bottleneck at the cytochrome chain, and hydrogen (bound to coenzyme) begins to accumulate. When oxygen is lacking, an intermediate of sugar and protein catabolism called pyruvic acid (*discussed below*) can capture a hydrogen pair to form lactic acid and help ease the bottleneck. The buildup of lactic acid is responsible for the burning sensation felt in the muscles during strenuous exercise.

The point at which lactate begins to accumulate in the blood is called the lactate threshold. Trained endurance athletes have a higher lactate threshold than the average person; therefore, they can perform at higher levels of effort before experiencing the fatigue caused by the accumulation of lactic acid in the muscles.

The three different kinds of fuels—carbohydrate, fat, and protein—can all be broken down to supply energy for building ATP from ADP, but each of these three follows a different metabolic pathway; that is, carbohydrates, fats, and proteins each undergo a different chain of reactions to release energy for ATP formation.

Energy from Carbohydrates

Carbohydrates are essentially sugars made of carbon, hydrogen, and oxygen. The simplest sugar is glucose, which has the chemical formula $C_6H_{12}O_6$. The carbon backbone of this molecule is in the shape of a six-membered ring (*see Figure 5*). Two or more simple sugars, such as glucose, fructose, and galactose (there are more than 400 simple sugars found in nature), can be strung together to form more complex sugars. Glucose is a monosaccharide (*mono*, "one"; *saccharum*, "sugar"), meaning that it is made up of a single simple sugar. Common disaccharides (two sugars) include sucrose (glucose plus fructose), or table sugar; lactose (glucose plus galactose), a carbohydrate found in milk; and maltose (glucose plus glucose), the sugar

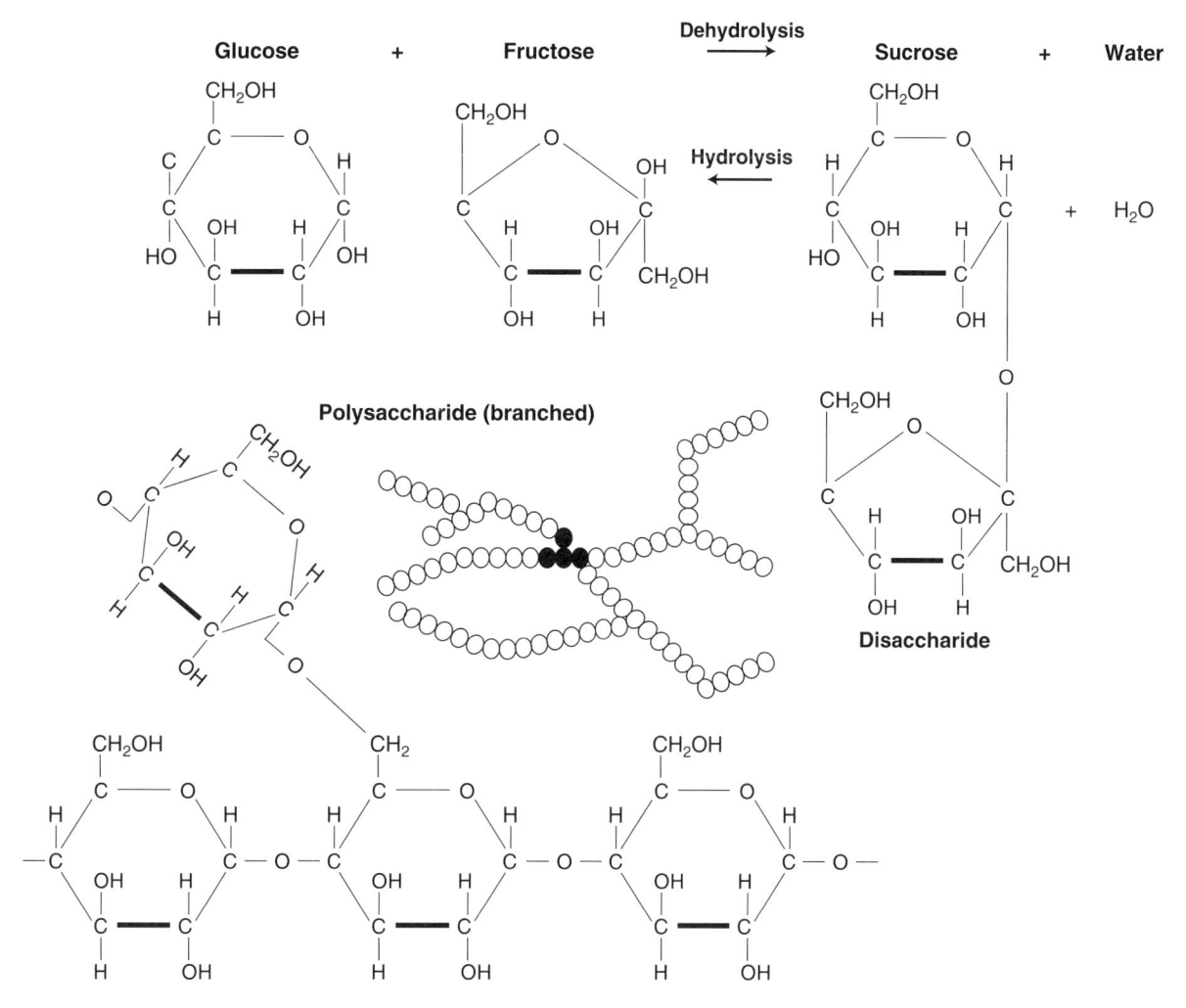

Figure 5. *Carbohydrates are essentially sugars made of carbon, hydrogen, and oxygen. Carbohydrate is the most important nutrient for athletes because it is the main source of energy for working muscles.*

fermented to produce beer. Three or more simple sugar molecules strung together form polysaccharides (*poly*, "many"), which can contain a few to hundreds to thousands of sugar monomers. Common polysaccharides are starch (a good energy source) and cellulose (the indigestible plant carbohydrate known as fiber).

Carbohydrate polymers are broken down in digestion and enter the blood as monosaccharides. Most of the sugar that the body metabolizes is the monosaccharide glucose, though galactose and fructose can also provide energy. For simplicity, this article will refer to fuel monosaccharides as glucose.

The six-carbon molecule glucose is catabolized, or broken down, into two molecules of the three-carbon intermediate called pyruvic acid in a 10-step process called glycolysis (*see Figure 10 later in this article*). Two of these steps require energy, and ATP is converted to ADP to provide the necessary energy. Other steps in glycolysis release energy stored in the carbon bonds of glucose, and that energy is transferred to ADP molecules to produce four ATPs. Glycolysis occurs in the cell's cytoplasm (the fluid that fills the cell), not in the mitochondria, and the transfers of energy to ADP that occur in this process do not require oxygen and are therefore called anaerobic. Oxygen is not required, because energy from bond breaking transfers directly to ADP without the assistance of the cytochromes of the mitochondria. Two pairs of hydrogen atoms are transferred to coenzyme during glycolysis. In all, the glycolysis of one molecule of glucose produces two molecules of pyruvic acid, a net total of two ATP (four are created, but two are used up) and two coenzyme-2H. In the absence of oxygen, coenzyme-2H is recycled into coenzyme in the conversion of pyruvic acid into lactic acid (*again, see Figure 10*). The hydrogen pairs transferred to coenzyme can enter the mitochondria and, through the cytochrome, produce three ATP each through oxidative (aerobic) phosphorylation, as described above. Thus, the glycolysis of one glucose molecule to pyruvic acid leads to the production of eight ATP.

But this is not the end of the potential of glucose for supplying energy. Glycolysis harvests only a small part of the energy available from a molecule of glucose. More energy is gleaned from the product of glycolysis, pyruvic acid, $C_3H_4O_3$, or $CH_3COCOOH$. Pyruvic acid is stripped of one hydrogen by coenzyme and releases the carboxyl group, –COOH, to produce one molecule of carbon dioxide, CO_2. The reamining acetyl group, $CH_3CO–$, combines with a molecule called coenzyme A to form the intermediate acetyl CoA (pronounced *uhseetuhl-coh-ay*). The conversion of pyruvic acid to acetyl CoA is irreversible.

This glucose by-product can provide still more energy; acetyl CoA enters a second stage of carbohydrate breakdown, a series of reactions called the Krebs cycle. In the reactions of the Krebs cycle, the acetyl fragment of acetyl CoA is broken down into carbon dioxide and four hydrogen atom pairs. Along the way, one molecule of ATP is formed, three molecules of water are used, and two molecules of carbon dioxide are released (*again, see Figure 10*). In all, the transformation of one pyruvic acid molecule into acetyl CoA and the passage of acetyl CoA through the Krebs cycle produces five coenzyme-2H and one ATP. The net reaction is as follows:

$$C_3H_4O_3 + 3\ H_2O + ADP + P_i \rightarrow 3\ CO_2 + OH + ATP + CoA + 4\ \text{coenzyme-2H}$$

Because one of the four hydrogen pairs released in the Krebs cycle enters the cytochrome at a point partway down the chain, it produces two, rather than three, ATP. Thus, the transformation of one molecule of pyruvic acid and the passage of acetyl CoA through the Krebs cycle produces 15 ATP.

The complete breakdown of one molecule of glucose, which breaks down into two pyruvic acid molecules, produces 38 ATP (worth 7 × 38 = 266 kcal/mol of energy): 8 from glycolysis, 6 from the conversion of pyruvic acid to acetyl CoA, and 24 from the Krebs cycle. If 1 mole of glucose (180 g) were fully converted to water and carbon dioxide by some other process, 686 kilocalories (kcal) of energy would be released:

$$C_6H_{12}O_6 + O_2 \rightarrow 6\ H_2O + 6\ CO_2 + 686\ \text{kcal/mol}$$

In the body, the complete metabolism of glucose produces 266 kcal/mol of usable energy. Thus, 39 percent of the energy in a molecule of glucose is usable for cellular work, as long as a sufficient amount of oxygen is present to allow oxidative phosphorylation.

When the body is engaged in strenuous exercise, the supply of oxygen cannot always meet demand. During this type of anaerobic exercise, the aerobic, or oxidative, pathways for harvesting energy from glucose are not used to their fullest, and far less than 39 percent of the energy is used. Oxygen insufficiency causes a buildup of coenzyme-2H in the muscle tissue, where oxygen demand is highest. The excess coenzyme-2H reacts with pyruvic acid ($C_3H_4O_3$) to form lactic acid ($C_3H_6O_3$), as shown here:

$$C_3H_4O_3 + \text{coenzyme-2H} \rightarrow C_3H_6O_3 + \text{coenzyme}$$

The conversion of pyruvic acid to lactic acid frees up coenzyme and allows anaerobic glycolysis to proceed. Glycolysis, which harvests only 5 percent of the available energy in glucose, is an inefficient pathway, and it cannot keep up with the energy demand for long. Fatigue soon sets in. When the intensity of the exercise is decreased, sufficient oxygen again becomes available. Lactic acid converts back to pyruvic acid (with the formation of coenzyme-2H), which can then enter the Krebs cycle to produce more energy. Extra lactic acid diffuses into the bloodstream and is converted to glucose by the liver. Thus, lactic acid is not a metabolic waste product but a diversionary molecule that helps the body maintain the proper glucose balance.

When extra glucose is available in the blood, the glucose molecules can be strung together to form a glucose polymer called glycogen. A small amount of glucose is stored this way in muscle tissue and in the liver to provide a readily available energy reserve. When less glucose is available, glycogen breaks down to release glucose. The body stores about 1,500 kcal worth of energy in the form of glycogen, enough to keep the body going at a moderate level of activity for 1 to 2 hours.

Energy from Fats

There are three major classifications of fats, or lipids: triglycerides, phospholipids, and steroids. Triglycerides serve as fuel stores, phospholipids form cell membranes, and steroids are found in cholesterol and the sex hormones (*see Figure 6*).

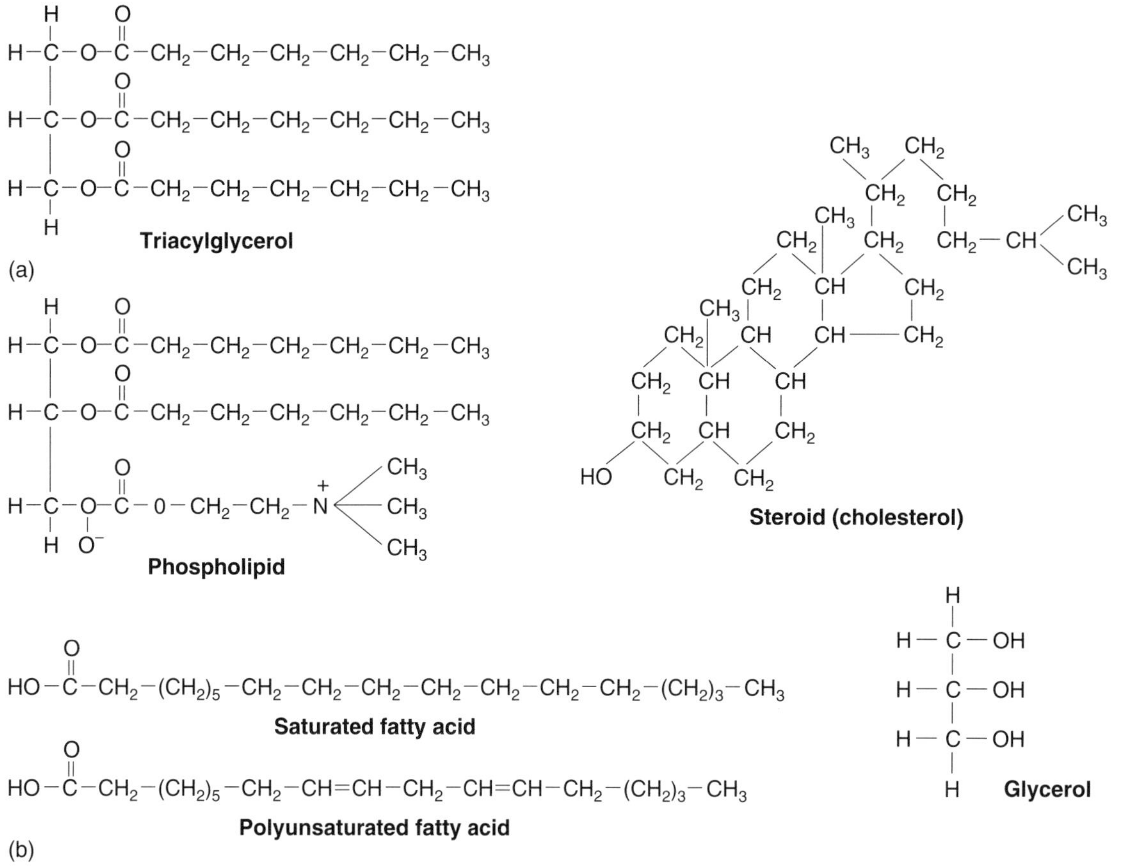

Figure 6. (a) Three types of fats are used by the body: phospholipids form cell membranes, steroids are found in cholesterol and the sex hormones, and triglycerides serve as fuel stores. (b) Triglycerides are made up of glycerol (a carbohydrate) and three long-chain fatty acids.

Why Limit Your Fat Intake?

Fat is a highly concentrated source of energy—that is, a very efficient way to store energy. In one fat molecule, there is more than 12 times as much energy as in one carbohydrate molecule. The phenomenal energy efficiency of fat is underappreciated, and fat is disdained by many people. But if energy were stored as carbohydrates rather than fats, the body would have to carry at least 30 percent more weight in fuel reserves. Still, because most people have plenty of storage fat and eat meals regularly, it is wise to limit fat intake. One exception might be mountain climbers. Several weeks of all-day climbing in frigid conditions may require the use of energy from the body's fat supply (*see also* NUTRITION and RESPIRATION).

About 80 percent of the body's energy reserve is stored as fats. The potential energy of the body's fat stores, around 100,000 kcal (compared with 2,000 kcal in carbohydrate stores), is virtually limitless. At rest, fat metabolism meets about half of the body's energy needs. This changes during moderate aerobic exercise, when a higher proportion of energy comes from burning fat. Many types of cells store some fat, but most fat resides in special storage cells called adipocytes. Adipocytes cluster together to form adipose tissue, found primarily just under the skin.

Just after a meal, when the blood glucose level is high, adipocytes synthesize and store triglycerides. The triglyceride molecule is formed by linking one glycerol, a three-carbon carbohydrate, to three fatty acids, which are long hydrocarbon chains.

Between meals, when blood glucose is low, and during exercise, when glucose is in high demand, the adipocytes break down the triglycerides, releasing free fatty acids and glycerol into the blood. Glycerol, a three-carbon carbohydrate, is converted to pyruvic acid, which can enter the Krebs cycle. The total metabolism of glycerol produces 22 ATP. The fatty acid portion of triglyceride produces even more energy. In the mitochondria, fatty acid molecules combine with coenzyme A (this reaction costs two ATP). In a series of reactions called beta oxidation, a molecule of acetyl CoA splits off from the fatty acid–coenzyme A derivative, stealing two carbons from the long hydrocarbon chain. Then another coenzyme A attaches (no ATP is used this time) to the end of the fatty acid, which is now two carbons shorter. This process is repeated until all the carbon atoms have been transferred to molecules of coenzyme A, two carbons at a time. Each beta oxidation produces enough coenzyme-2H to build five ATP through oxidative phosphorylation. The acetyl CoA molecules can enter the Krebs cycle, where each two-carbon fragment ultimately produces 2 carbon dioxide molecules and 12 ATP (*see Figure 7*).

Thus, a typical 18-carbon fatty acid yields 146 ATP ($9 \times 12 = 108$ ATP created from the resulting nine acetyl CoA molecules; $8 \times 5 = 40$ ATP created from the eight beta oxidation steps; and two ATP used up in the first CoA-fatty acid reaction). Because a triglyceride molecule is made of three fatty acids and a glycerol, one fat molecule produces, on average, 460 molecules of ATP ($[3 \times 146] + 22$), more than 12 times the amount from one molecule of glucose (38 ATP). Fat is thus a very efficient way to store energy.

The body's fat stores are made through reactions that are nearly

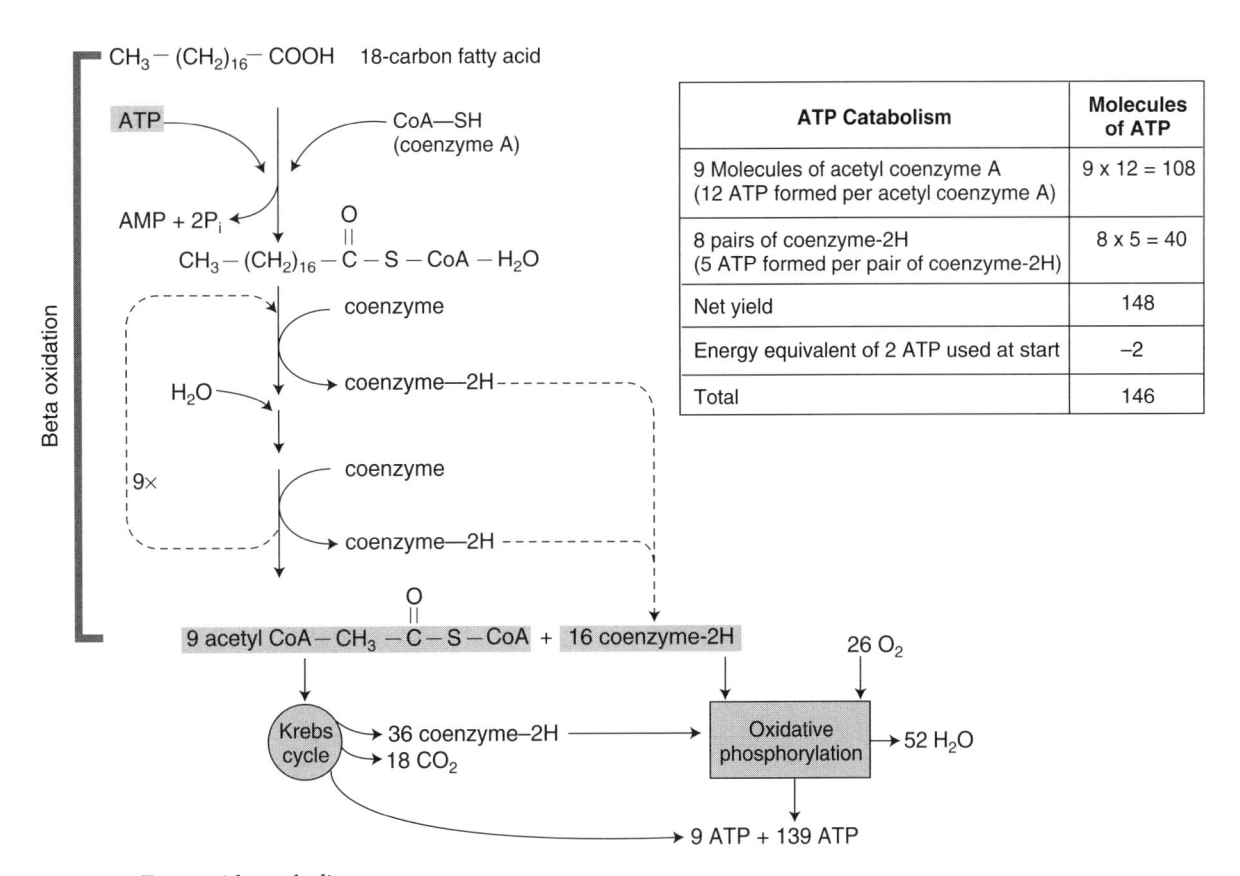

ATP Catabolism	Molecules of ATP
9 Molecules of acetyl coenzyme A (12 ATP formed per acetyl coenzyme A)	$9 \times 12 = 108$
8 pairs of coenzyme-2H (5 ATP formed per pair of coenzyme-2H)	$8 \times 5 = 40$
Net yield	148
Energy equivalent of 2 ATP used at start	−2
Total	146

Figure 7. *Fatty acid catabolism.*

the reverse of fatty acid catabolism; the long fatty acids are built up two carbons at a time in the cytoplasm of the adipocytes (fat cells). Three completed fatty acids are then linked to glycerol to form a triglyceride. The starting material for the buildup of fatty acids is acetyl CoA. Just after a meal, when glucose is plentiful, a large amount of acetyl CoA is formed. The body usually does not need to use all the carbohydrate energy available from the meal for work. So rather than enter the Krebs cycle to produce unneeded ATP (which is for immediate energy use, not for energy storage), excess acetyl CoA is converted to fat and stored in the adipose tissue for use when more immediate supplies are low.

Glucose can be converted into fat, but the reverse is not true. Fatty acids cannot be used to synthesize glucose, because the formation of acetyl CoA from pyruvic acid is irreversible: acetyl CoA cannot be turned into pyruvic acid (the glycerol portion of the triglyceride can, however, be built up into glucose). While carbohydrates, proteins, and fats can all be stored as fat, fats are put into storage most efficiently. Thus, people who are trying to shed pounds are well advised not just to cut calories, but to cut the proportion of fat in their diets.

Energy from Protein

Proteins, which account for roughly 50 percent of the organic matter in the body, provide important building blocks for the formation of tissues and cell components, particularly during periods of rapid growth, as in infancy, childhood, or adolescence. Hair, skin, nails, tendons, and ligaments are all made of protein. Muscle cells are filled with contractile proteins. Enzymes, critical catalysts for nearly all body functions, are proteins. Proteins in the blood carry oxygen and are involved in clot formation.

Proteins contain carbon, hydrogen, oxygen, and nitrogen, along with small amounts of other elements, such as sulfur and phosphorus. Proteins are very large molecules, or macromolecules, that can contain thousands, or even hundreds of thousands, of atoms (by comparison, glucose has 24 atoms). They are essentially chains, or polymers, of units called amino acids, all of which (except one, called proline) have an amino group, $-NH_2$, and a carboxyl group, $-COOH$, attached to one end of a short carbon backbone. These strings of amino acids are called polypeptides. The polypeptide chain tends to form coils, like the cord on a telephone, and those coils fold and bend to form a "globular" structure (*see Figure 8*).

Ingested proteins are broken down in the gastrointestinal tract into amino acids, which are absorbed into the blood at the small intestine. These amino acids are incorporated into new proteins to build a huge array of important molecules and structures in the body. Amino acids also can be broken down to provide energy for ATP synthesis.

Before they can transfer energy to ATP through glycolysis and the Krebs cycle reactions, the amino acids must be stripped of their nitro-

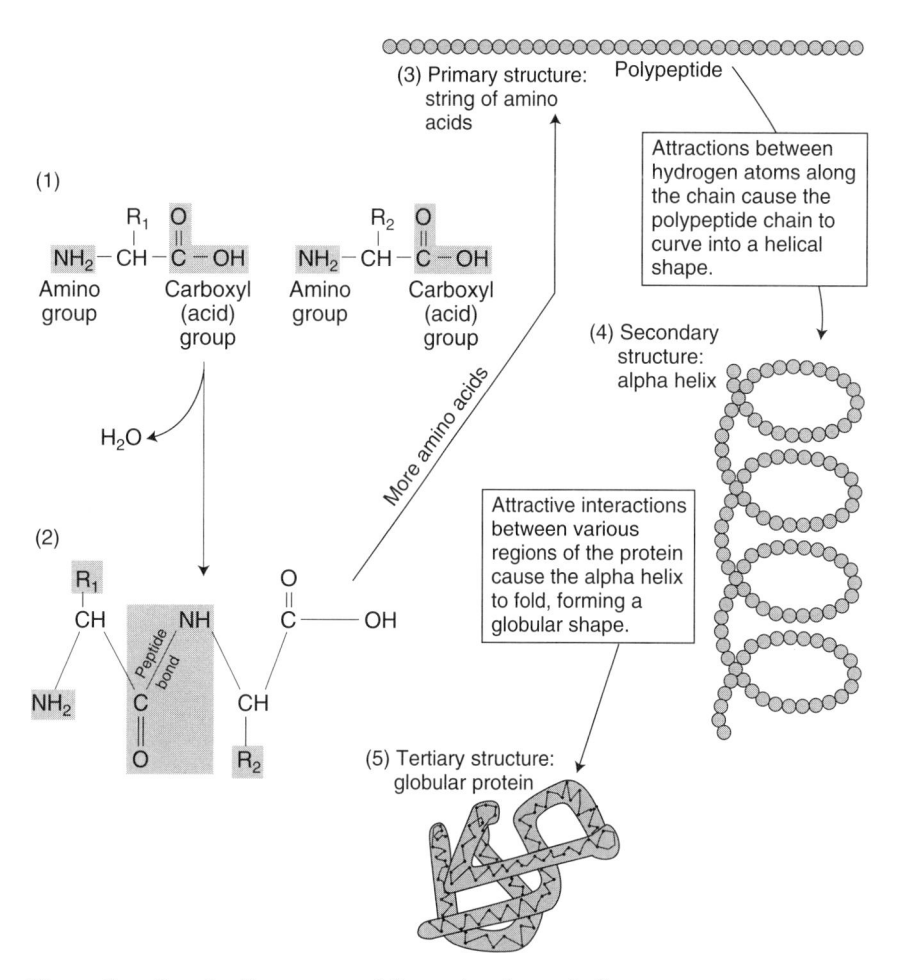

Figure 8. *Protein: Structure and formation (steps 1–5).*

gen atoms. The removal of nitrogen produces a waste product, ammonia (NH_3, the same substance as the common household cleaning agent). The remaining carbon skeleton forms a type of molecule known as a keto acid. Keto acids can be metabolized to produce ATP and CO_2, built up to form glucose, or built up to form fatty acids. Ammonia, which can be toxic at high concentrations, enters the blood and finds its way to the liver, where it combines with CO_2 to form urea, which is far less toxic (*see Figure 9*). The kidneys filter urea from the blood and excrete it into the urine.

In Summary: Three Fuels, One Body

Organic compounds produced by the breakdown of any of the three types of fuel molecules—carbohydrates, fats, and proteins—can enter the Krebs cycle to produce energy for the creation of ATP. In addition, the three types of fuels can be converted from one to another to make up for imbalances. Glucose can be converted to fat and some of the amino acids. Some amino acids can form glucose and fat. Fatty acids cannot be used to build glucose, but they can be used in the synthesis of some amino acids (*see Figure 10*).

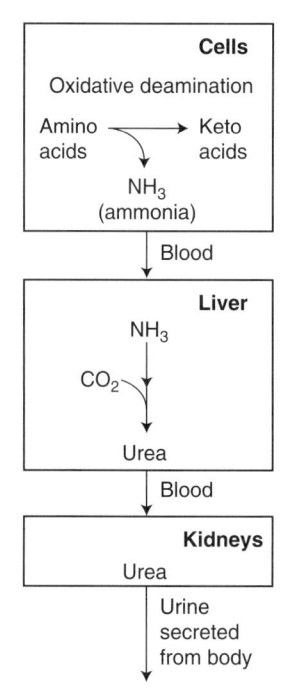

Figure 9. *The catabolism of protein results in the formation and elimination of urea.*

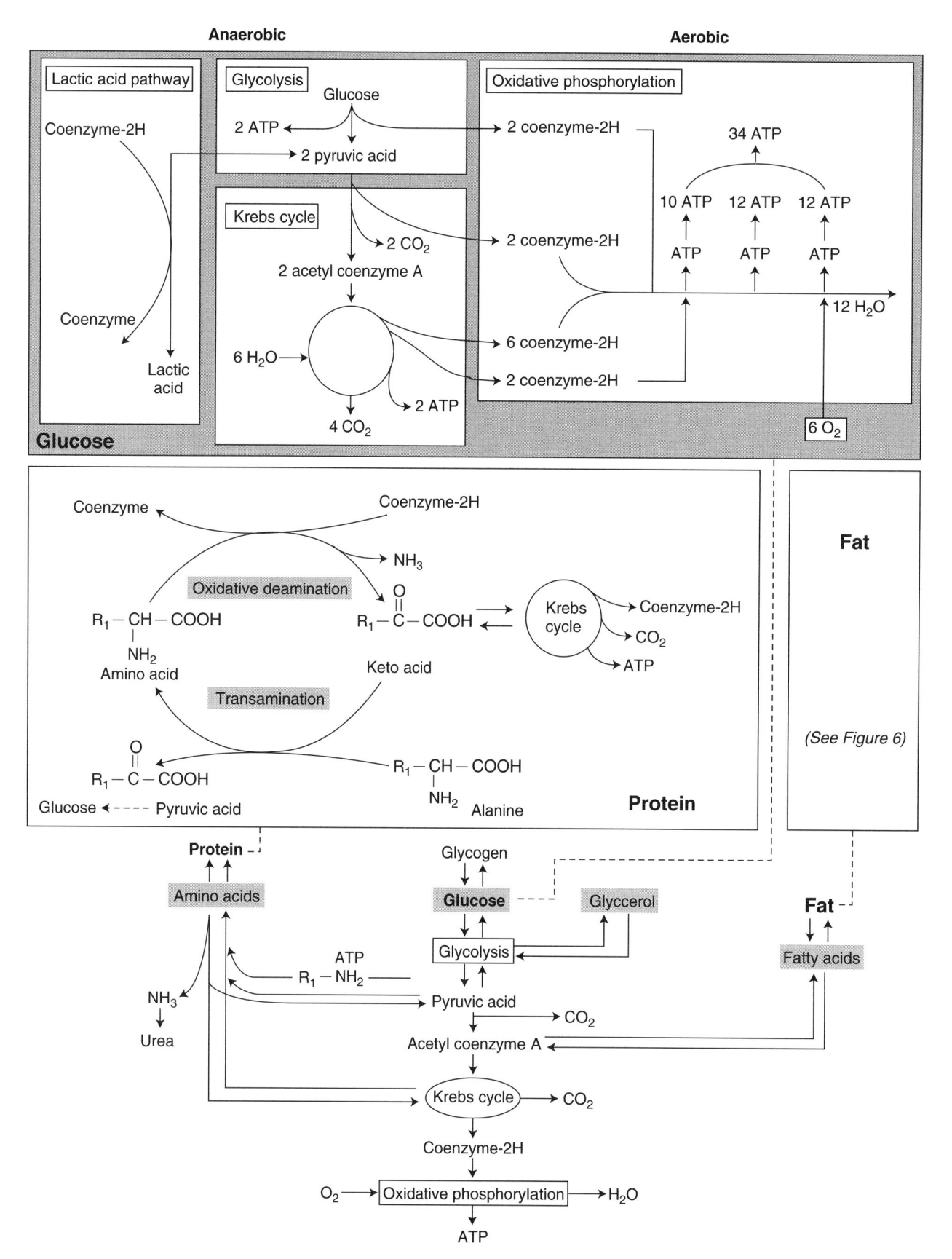

Figure 10. *The chemical conversion of the three fuels—carbohydrates, fats, and proteins—for energy.*

Whole-Body Metabolism

Given this background in cellular metabolism, significant aspects of whole-body metabolism can be better understood. This section considers metabolism and body weight, compares and contrasts "fueling" and "fasting" metabolism, examines the crucial role of insulin, and discusses the use of fuel during exercise.

Metabolism and Weight

Some of the energy released from the metabolism of food is released as heat (about 60 percent). The rest is either used to perform work or stored. A person who wants to lose weight is trying to decrease his or her energy stores (fat), and this can be done by taking in less food (dieting) or expending more energy (exercising) or both, to achieve a negative energy balance. However, studies have shown that there is an additional, hidden factor in this equation: when the level of food intake or the level of activity changes, the body adapts by making adjustments in the metabolic rate. People who decrease their caloric intake find that despite dieting, they eventually stop shedding pounds. Volunteers fed high-calorie diets in metabolism experiments observe that they do not gain as much weight as expected. These people's bodies compensate for the change in their diets by readjusting their basal metabolic rates, higher if they eat more or lower if they eat less.

To offset a decrease in metabolic rate, therefore, it is crucial that, in addition to cutting calories, a person trying to lose weight exercise regularly. Not only does exercise burn calories; it also raises the metabolic rate slightly, offsetting the decrease in metabolic rate triggered by cutting calories. Another important consideration is that a low-calorie diet will cause the body to burn protein as well as fat when blood glucose is low, and therefore to lose lean tissue. During aerobic exercise, fat (rather than protein) tends to be burned, so lean tissue is spared while the fat disappears.

Most people find that their metabolism—and, therefore, the number of calories they require—slows as they age. Muscle mass often decreases with age, and because muscle demands more energy than fat, a decrease in muscle mass translates into a decrease in required calories. Many people find themselves gradually gaining weight in middle age, because their caloric intake does not drop as rapidly as their caloric requirement is dropping.

Absorptive and Postabsorptive Metabolism

Most people eat three meals a day, in between periods of work, play, and rest. Thus, the body alternates between periods of fueling and fasting, known respectively as the absorptive and postabsorptive periods. In the absorptive period, nutrients from food enter the blood through the gastrointestinal (GI) tract; this period lasts about 4 hours after a meal. In the postabsorptive period—late morning, late afternoon, and overnight—the GI tract is empty, and fuel nutrients are

Boosting Your Metabolism?

One cannot drastically alter one's metabolic rate, which is largely determined by genetics. But the metabolic rate may remain elevated for as long as 24 hours following exercise, and so the medical community recommends daily exercise for people trying to lose weight. Also, research suggests that moderate long-term increases in metabolic rate can be accomplished with good habits—regular exercise and eating the right foods at the right time. Athletes should eat smaller meals and not exercise on an empty stomach; this ensures that the body will not cut its metabolic rate to compensate for a lack of fuel (*see also* NUTRITION and WRESTLING).

METABOLIC CHARACTERISTICS OF THE ABSORPTIVE AND POSTABSORPTIVE STATES

Absorptive state (right after a meal)

Energy supplied mainly by absorbed carbohydrates.
Net uptake of glucose by the liver.
Net synthesis of body proteins.
Storage of excess carbohydrate, fat, and protein, mainly as fat but also as glycogen.

Postabsorptive state (between meals)

Cessation of glycogen, fat, and protein synthesis.
Net breakdown of glycogen, fat, and protein.
Liver releases glucose, made from glycogen, amino acids, lactate, and pyruvate—all used as energy sources.
Glucose utilization reduced in most tissues (glucose sparing).
Increased availability of fatty acids for energy production.

Table 2.

not entering the body. During these times, the body turns to its fuel stores for energy. Thus there are differences in metabolic activity between the absorptive and postabsorptive states (*see Table 2*).

When the body is in the absorptive state, monosaccharides, amino acids, and fatty acids enter the system. With the scales tipped to the supply side, there is a net intake of all three nutrients by the cells. During this absorptive period, glucose is the major source of energy for most cells. In the cells of the liver and skeletal muscle, some of the glucose is converted to glycogen for later use. Excess glucose is converted to fat in the adipose (fat) tissue and the liver. Most of the ingested fat is stored in the adipose tissue, and a small fraction is used to provide energy during the absorptive period. (Light exercise after a meal, such as a brisk walk, will burn some of the fuel just eaten, leaving less available for storage as fat.) Most of the amino acids are taken up by the cells for protein synthesis. Excess amino acids are not stored as proteins but converted to carbohydrate or fat. Thus, eating extra protein will not, by itself, add lean tissue and may even add fat. However, while the body is growing, or when it is building muscle through strength training, it does need extra protein.

After a meal is digested and the supply of nutrients slows, there are no longer extra glucose, fat, and amino acid molecules available in the blood plasma for storage as glycogen and fat or for the synthesis of proteins. Instead, during the postabsorptive period these stored substances are broken down and enter the bloodstream to supply energy. Because the brain requires glucose to function, the level of glucose in the blood must be maintained in the postabsorptive period even though none is being supplied from outside. The level of glucose is maintained in two ways: (1) glucose is created from the breakdown of glycogen, fat, and protein; and (2) glucose is spared when certain tissues rely on fat, rather than glucose, for fuel. This glucose sparing occurs through an increase in the release of free fatty acids from fat

WARNING SIGNS OF ABNORMAL BLOOD SUGAR LEVELS

Hypoglycemia (low blood sugar)	Hyperglycemia (high blood sugar)	Ketoacidosis (severe insulin deficiency)
Double vision	Increased thirst	Stomach pain
Headache	Increased urination	Dehydration
Fatigue	Drowsiness	
Trembling	Fruity breath	
Increased heart rate	Nausea	
Excessive hunger		
Sweating		

Table 3.

cells into the blood plasma. The fatty acids can then be picked up by working cells (in tissues other than the brain) to create energy via the Krebs cycle.

Exercise seems to enhance glucose sparing. In other words, during moderate aerobic exercise, fat supplies a higher proportion of the body's energy needs than does glucose. During strenuous anaerobic exercise, more carbohydrates than fats are burned. However, because the carbohydrate store is limited, a person cannot sustain this type of exertion for very long.

In the absorptive and postabsorptive periods, the body's metabolic activities seem to have opposing goals: overall synthesis, net uptake, and glucose utilization in the absorptive state; and overall catabolism, net release, and glucose sparing in the postabsorptive state. Yet these metabolic swings are necessary to maintain a relatively constant level of glucose in the blood to fuel the central nervous system. The hormone insulin (*discussed below*) is the key to the body's ability to balance two sets of goals in the absorptive and postabsorptive states.

Metabolism and Insulin

The concentration of glucose in the blood acts as the signaling mechanism between the absorptive and postabsorptive states. The switch is signaled by the lower level of blood glucose that occurs as the body enters the postabsorptive state, or by the higher level of glucose in the absorptive state. An increase in blood glucose triggers special cells in the pancreas (a small organ that lies underneath the liver) to secrete the hormone insulin.

Insulin affects metabolism in two ways: it increases the ability of many cells to take up glucose and amino acids; and it stimulates the synthesis of glycogen and fat in the liver, adipose tissue, and skeletal muscle. When the amount of sugar in the blood rises immediately after a meal, these processes remove glucose from the blood, keeping blood sugar stable. As the glucose level decreases, the secretion of insulin decreases, and metabolism shifts to the postabsorptive state: synthesis stops, glucose is conserved, and fat is used as fuel. During exercise, insulin secretion is inhibited, and fat utilization is increased.

Some people's bodies are unable to manufacture insulin. They suffer from the disease diabetes mellitus (type 1 diabetes) and must have injections of insulin to prevent blood glucose levels from getting dangerously high (hyperglycemia; *see Table 3*). Short-term symptoms of hyperglycemia are increased thirst and urination. In the long term, high levels of glucose in the blood can lead to kidney failure, low blood pressure, blindness, and vulnerability to infection in the extremities. Without insulin, the body thinks it is always in the postabsorptive state, marked by lean tissue (protein) wasting, fat mobilization (rather than fat storage), and high blood glucose levels. Severe insulin insufficiency can lead to a potentially fatal condition called ketoacidosis, caused by an excess of keto acids, the by-products of protein catabolism.

Some people have a reduced sensitivity (hyposensitivity) to glucose, meaning that although they produce insulin, their bodies do not respond to it. This disease, called type 2 diabetes, is found mainly in overweight, sedentary adults. Type 2 diabetes can often be reversed by decreasing caloric intake. Exercise can also increase sensitivity to insulin.

Regular exercise can reduce insulin requirements and provide other benefits to people with diabetes. However, diabetic athletes must take precautions to prevent not only hyperglycemia but also hypoglycemialow blood sugar—which can be brought on by an excessive dose of injected insulin. These precautions include monitoring blood sugar levels before, during, and after exercise; adjusting the diet to compensate for the extra energy expended during activity; and eating 2 to 3 hours before and then after exercise. While exercise is particularly beneficial for controlling type 2 diabetes, it can lead to complications for people with type 1.

Use of Fuel during Exercise

This final section will consider several aspects of metabolism and exercise: fuel requirements, pathways of energy supply, recovery, and metabolic training.

Fuel requirements. As mentioned above, the body has large fuel requirements during exercise, with the metabolic rate increasing by as much as tenfold, or even more. Glucose, fatty acids, and glycogen supply much of the energy needed in exercise. During activity, blood glucose is supplied by the liver, which breaks down its own glycogen stores and also synthesizes glucose from pyruvic and lactic acids (formed during glycolysis), glycerol (from the breakdown of triglycerides), and amino acids in the blood. The blood glucose level does not change with moderate exercise for short periods of time and may even increase briefly with short-term strenuous exercise, as glycogen and the products of anaerobic glycolysis are converted to glucose. However, as the duration of exercise increases beyond 1 hour or so, glucose levels fall.

Fatigue and Energy

A common complaint—among Americans, at least—is "I don't have any energy." It is often assumed that there must be an association between chronic fatigue, or tiredness, and glycogen depletion, which occurs when the body has used up its supply of quickly available energy. For most people, however, glycogen depletion is rarely a cause of fatigue, because glycogen is depleted only after several hours of strenuous activity. For instance, a marathon runner often "hits a wall" at about 18 to 22 miles (29–35 km), that is, after 2 to 3 hours of running; and this sudden onset of fatigue can be attributed to depletion of glycogen in the muscles. Most people never exercise this strenuously.

The fatigue experienced under more common circumstances, during exercise and in ordinary everyday situations, can have various causes.

Causes of Fatigue during Exercise

- Accumulation of metabolic by-products, such as lactic acid.
- Breakdown in transmission of nerve impulses to muscle fiber membrane (see SOCCER).
- Central nervous system (CNS) reaction: sensing pain, the CNS may slow the pace of exercise to a tolerable level, to protect the body.

Causes of Everyday Fatigue

- *Sleep disturbances*. During sleep, many changes take place in bodily functions, including muscular tension, blood pressure, heart rate, respiratory rate, and chemical patterns in the brain. Thus some physiologists believe that insufficient sleep impairs the body's restorative functions. There is some evidence for this: many people who are chronically tired return from, say, a week's vacation fully refreshed—perhaps an indication that their daily routine prevents them from getting enough sleep.
- *Lack of exercise*. Many people feel that they do not have enough energy to exercise; they arrive home from school or work mentally exhausted. This can lead to a vicious circle: because they are tired, they don't feel like exercising; and because they don't exercise, they feel more and more tired.
- *Anemia*. About 20 percent of American women are anemic, meaning that they have a deficiency in hemoglobin molecules: the carriers of oxygen to the cells (see FEMALE ATHLETES and NUTRITION). Usually, dietary supplements of iron, vitamin B_{12}, or folic acid are an adequate treatment.
- *Clinical depression*. Clinical depression is the most common condition treated by psychotherapists, accounting for about 30 percent of all patients seen. It is characterized by pervasive sadness, loneliness, loss of interest or pleasure, and a sense of worthlessness; and it is thought to be caused by abnormally low levels of neurotransmitters in the brain that affect mood and behavior. (Neurotransmitters are chemical messengers that allow neurons to communicate with each other.) For some people, regular exercise helps to moderate the effects of clinical depression.
- *Hypothyroidism*. When the thyroid gland malfunctions, it can produce an abnormally low level of hormones, leading to a metabolic slowdown, muscle aches, and a significant decline in mental functioning. To completely reverse these effects, lifelong hormone supplementation is usually required.
- *Chronic fatigue syndrome*. This is an abnormal level of exhaustion, with no underlying organic or psychological cause, following regular activities. Symptoms are often vague and nonspecific; they include muscle pain, muscular weakness, headaches, joint pain, sore throat, low-grade fever, sleep disturbances, difficulty concentrating, and forgetfulness. Doctors are uncertain about the cause or causes of chronic fatigue syndrome; but some believe that it is caused either by a genetic defect in the immune system, or by a failure of the immune system to slow down—that is, resume its steady state—after fighting a virus, stress, or trauma. Although there is no completely effective treatment, doctors recommend an improved diet, a reduction of stress, plenty of rest, and regular aerobic exercise.

During exercise the cellular machinery works to keep the level of blood glucose high enough to meet the needs of working muscles and to fuel central nervous system function, just as it does during the postabsorptive state. There is, however, one important difference; while insulin secretion is low during exercise, glucose uptake by cells remains high. The reason for this remains unknown. Normally, insulin helps cells absorb glucose, but exercise somehow reduces the body's need for insulin by increasing glucose absorption.

During exercise the body obtains energy from fatty acids and glucose. Protein is also available if other energy sources run low. However, physically fit people burn relatively more fatty acid during moderate exercise than unfit people. This metabolic adaptation is beneficial to endurance athletes, such as marathon runners and cyclists, because it helps to conserve carbohydrates during prolonged exertion.

Overall, with the exception of long-distance activities (such as marathon running, bicycle touring, and backpacking), most athletic events require a small number of calories relative to the total number burned daily, about 2,500 calories (that is, 2,500 kcal). A 1-hour aerobic workout or cycling at 10 miles per hour (16.1 KMH) burns only about 400 kcal. In a contact sport, such as football, a player may burn 400 to 800 kcal in 1 hour.

When their muscle glycogen has been depleted, athletes experience a feeling of being unable to continue. Marathon runners at this point say they have "hit the wall." At 60 to 80 percent maximum exertion (as in a long-distance running race) glycogen is depleted after 90 to 180 minutes (often around mile 20 for a marathon runner). Other activities also can also deplete the body of stored glycogen. During activities performed at very high, intermittent intensities of 90 percent or higher maximum exertion (as in a hockey or lacrosse game), glycogen is depleted in 15 to 30 minutes. It takes 20 hours to fully replenish depleted glycogen stores. Frequent meals of complex carbohydrates and a period of rest help restore muscle glycogen.

Carbohydrate loading, or "carbo-loading," helps increase muscle glycogen stores in preparation for an event (*see also* NUTRITION). This strategy is effective only if an athlete has trained intensively for his or her sport. In carbohydrate loading, the athlete tapers off the intensity of training and increases the percentage of complex carbohydrate in the diet 5 or 6 days before the event. Then, the day before the event, the athlete rests and takes 70 to 80 percent of calories in the diet as complex carbohydrate.

Aerobic and anaerobic pathways. Different kinds of exercise elicit different modes of ATP production. Activities of high intensity and short duration—such as sprinting, weight lifting, and fast breaks in basketball or hockey—require immediate and rapid energy. In such concentrated activity, which often lasts less than 10 seconds, energy is supplied to the working muscles solely from the high-energy phosphate molecules that are present in the muscle cells. After about 7 seconds of such activity, this energy source is depleted. In a 100-meter dash, for example, the available store of muscle ATP is gone before the race is over.

For prolonged, strenuous exercise, ATP must be synthesized rapidly. The main route for ATP synthesis during strenuous exercise is the anaerobic process of glycolysis, which uses glucose and stored

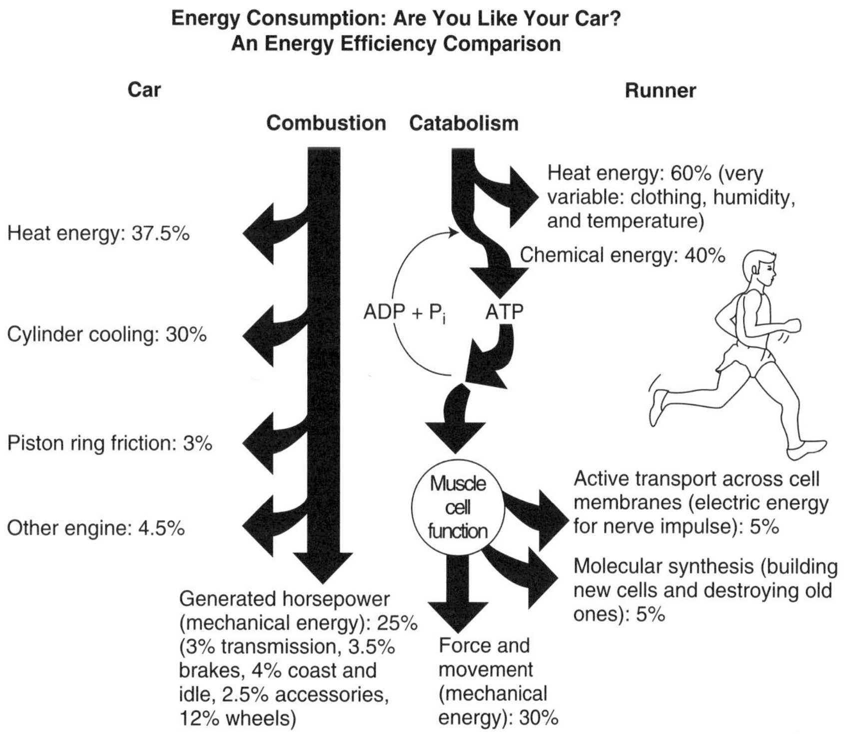

Energy Consumption: Are You Like Your Car?
An Energy Efficiency Comparison

Car	Runner
Combustion	Catabolism

Heat energy: 37.5%

Cylinder cooling: 30%

Piston ring friction: 3%

Other engine: 4.5%

Generated horsepower (mechanical energy): 25% (3% transmission, 3.5% brakes, 4% coast and idle, 2.5% accessories, 12% wheels)

Heat energy: 60% (very variable: clothing, humidity, and temperature)

Chemical energy: 40%

ADP + P_i ⇌ ATP

Muscle cell function

Active transport across cell membranes (electric energy for nerve impulse): 5%

Molecular synthesis (building new cells and destroying old ones): 5%

Force and movement (mechanical energy): 30%

Figure 11. *In terms of energy consumption, the body can be compared to an automobile. The body uses energy much as a car does: both require fuel; both convert chemical energy to mechanical energy; both need to be cooled; and both need oxygen to run over extended periods of time. Shown here is an "energy efficiency" comparison. (Howes, 1991)*

glycogen as fuel and produces lactic acid. (About 20 percent of the energy comes from the aerobic pathway, oxidative phosphorylation.) The formation of lactic acid from pyruvic acid allows for the synthesis of ATP when the oxygen supply is insufficient, but the lactic acid pathway is really a short-term, stopgap measure. If the rate of lactic acid buildup exceeds the rate of removal, a feeling of fatigue will force the athlete to slow down or stop. After 2 or 3 minutes of activity, aerobic ATP synthesis becomes relatively more important. Table 4 shows the relative contribution of aerobic and anaerobic metabolic systems for exercise of different intensity and duration. In most cases, both the anaerobic and the aerobic metabolic systems are operating during exercise.

Recovery. After exercise, muscle cells need time to replenish depleted high-energy phosphates and glycogen—up to 20 hours if glycogen stores have been fully depleted. Recovery time for moderate, or submaximal, exercise is fairly rapid, because moderate activity, which is largely aerobic, does not deplete muscle ATP. It takes longer to recover from strenuous activity: ATP is replenished through oxidative phosphorylation, lactic acid is converted into glucose, and

RELATIVE CONTRIBUTIONS OF THE AEROBIC AND ANAEROBIC SYSTEMS IN SEVERAL SPORTS

Type	Time (seconds or minutes)	Example	% Anaerobic/ % Aerobic
All-out	< 10 sec.	Snatch (Olympic lifting)	100/0
<All-out	10 sec.	100-m sprint	90/1
Intense	1 min.	400-m sprint	70/30
Intense	2 min.	200-m swim	50/50
Intermittent	1-min. bouts	Hockey, soccer, basketball	20/80
Endurance	60 min.	20-mi. (32-km) bicycle race	2/98
Endurance	120 min.	Marathon	1/99

Table 4. *At one extreme, Olympic snatch weight lifters raise the barbell from ground to overhead in less than 1 second; here, the contribution is solely anaerobic. At the other extreme, marathon runners need more than 2 hours to cover the 26-mile (42-km) course. Here, the contribution is almost entirely aerobic. (Adapted from McArdle, 1986)*

muscle glycogen is restored. Eating after exercise is the best way to supply carbohydrate for restocking depleted glycogen stores. Studies have found that recovery from strenuous anaerobic exercise is facilitated when followed by light aerobic exercise in a "cool-down" period. This process is not fully understood, but some physiologists posit that this mild exercise stimulates the flow of blood to the muscles, which delivers oxygen and washes away the excess lactic acid that causes fatigue.

Training for metabolic excellence. The purpose of training is to produce adaptations in the body that lead to improved performance of a specific task. Running out of energy is, obviously, a sure way to diminish athletic performance. As explained above, different sports utilize different means of ATP production; it is possible, however, to train for the improvement of specific energy delivery systems.

Fitness training facilitates several beneficial adaptations for the whole body. The heart is enlarged and pumps more blood with each stroke, heart rate and blood pressure drop, and lung capacity increases. All these changes increase the delivery of oxygen to the muscles. The ratio of muscle to fat tissue also increases. At the molecular level, anaerobic training (weight lifting or sprinting) produces changes in the short-term energy delivery systems: increased resting levels of high-energy phosphates and glycogen, a greater number of the enzymes involved in anaerobic glycolysis, and an increased tolerance of lactic acid in the blood. Aerobic training (running, swimming, or cycling) improves all the processes—both whole-body and cellular—related to the use and transport of oxygen. Aerobic training increases the number and size of muscle mitochondria, the capacity of mitochondria to produce ATP by oxidative phosphorylation, the amount of stored muscle glycogen, the ability of muscle to mobilize and burn fat, and the capability of the muscles to oxidize carbohydrate.

Maximizing Energy Delivery

Regular exercise improves the body's ability to convert fuel to do work.

Anaerobic training improves short-term energy delivery by: increasing the levels of high-energy phosphates and glycogen; producing more of the enzymes involved in anaerobic glycolysis; increasing tolerance of blood lactic acid.

Aerobic training improves oxygen transport by: increasing the number and size of muscle mitochondria; improving the capacity of mitochondria to produce ATP by oxidative phosphorylation; increasing the amount of stored muscle glycogen; improving the ability of the muscle to burn fat and oxidize carbohydrates.

Benefits from aerobic training vary with the frequency, intensity, and duration of exercise. Many experts recommend exercising at an intensity of 70 percent of the maximum heart rate to improve aerobic capacity. A slightly lower intensity, about 60 to 65 percent, is best for those beginning an exercise program. Trained athletes may benefit from a higher level of intensity, about 80 percent of maximum heart rate (*see also* HEART AND CIRCULATORY SYSTEM). The recommended duration of exercise depends on the level of intensity. Working out at lower intensity does not expend as much energy as possible, but the shortfall can be offset by increasing the duration of exercise. Exercising 20 to 30 minutes at 70 percent of maximum heart rate is sufficient for an active person; competitive athletes need longer workouts. There are no conclusive data on the optimum frequency of workouts, but most experts recommend exercising 3 or 4 days a week. To lose weight, a person should exercise more often, 5 to 7 days a week for 30 minutes, or long enough to burn about 300 kcal. The mode of training is not of primary importance, as long as large muscles exert force in a rhythmic way. Even a daily 30-minute walk has been found to confer significant health benefits.

One type of anaerobic training involves bursts of all-out effort for 5 to 10 seconds, as in weight lifting or in a track-and-field throwing event. This type of exertion allows the use of high-energy phosphates with little production of lactic acid. Another type of anaerobic exercise trains the lactic acid system by overloading the anaerobic glycolysis pathway. This type of training is physically and psychologically difficult and requires motivation. Performing cycles of 1-minute bouts of intense exercise to near exhaustion followed by a few minutes of rest does not allow full lactic acid recovery, so lactic acid builds up—to a level that could not be achieved in a single intense bout of exercise to exhaustion (for example, a fast run of 1 mi., or 1.6 km). The intermittent nature of some sports makes it particularly important for participants to improve their lactate threshold (*see also* SOCCER, HOCKEY, and BASKETBALL). These players stretch their lactate threshold by incorporating interval sprints as a main part of their training regimen.

There are several methods of aerobic training. Aerobic training for a world-class 1,500-meter runner or a long-distance cyclist would include some interval training. Interval training involves repeated cycles of intense and moderate activity, allowing the athlete to accomplish more work before tiring than could be completed through continuous intense activity. The "intense" interval should be close to the athlete's competition level, performed to early fatigue. The duration of the "moderate" interval should be about 1 to 1.5 times that of the "intense" interval. To produce greater aerobic stress, it is critical to resume the "intense" interval before complete recovery.

Continuous training is steady exercise at moderate or high intensity for a sustained period of time. Marathon runners train in this way. Surprisingly, it is also the training routine recommended for a sedentary person just beginning to exercise. A 40-minute walk, jog, swim, or aerobics class—at a moderate pace—is a safe and effective way for untrained people of any age to start exercising (*see also AGING AND PERFORMANCE*).

Ellen J. Zeman

References

Coleman, Ellen. *Eating for Endurance*. Palo Alto, California: Bull, 1988.

Howes, R., and A. Fainberg. *The Energy Sourcebook: A Guide to Technology, Resources, and Policy*. New York: American Institute of Physics, 1991.

McArdle, W. D., et al. *Exercise Physiology: Energy, Nutrition, and Human Performance*. Philadelphia: Lea and Febiger, 1986.

Vander, J., et al. *Human Physiology*. 6th ed. New York: McGraw-Hill, 1994.

Female Athletes

THE 1960S WERE A TIME of social upheaval. The struggle for civil rights and the protests against the Vietnam War divided American society and became a catalyst for broader changes, causing many people to question traditional structures and institutions. One group involved in the pressure for change was by no means a minority of the population but was in many ways hindered from taking full part in civil, business, political, or military life. That group was women.

During the early 1970s one sportswoman, the tennis player Billie Jean King, became a symbol of the struggle for gender equality. In 1973, in a match highly publicized as a "battle of the sexes," King defeated a male opponent, Bobby Riggs, in straight sets. Despite the fact that King was in her prime and Riggs was well past his, this outcome was unexpected: the assumption had simply been that a woman could not beat a man in tennis. Not only did King's match with Riggs overturn this assumption; it was widely taken as conveying a more important message: that the time had come to start transforming male-dominated gymnasiums and playing fields.

In 1972, a bill signed into law by President Richard Nixon contributed to greater participation by females in athletics: Title IX of the Education Amendments of 1972 refined the Civil Rights Act of 1964 by prohibiting discrimination by sex in all educational institutions that receive federal funding. While the law covers all aspects of education, Title IX has perhaps had its largest impact on high school and college sports. The law does not require that equal numbers of male and female students participate in sports, or even that sports programs for male and female students be funded equally, but it does mandate that students of both sexes have an equal opportunity to participate in sports. This was an important change, because traditionally, boy's and men's athletics received hugely disproportionate funding. By the early 1990s, Title IX, although it was still far from being fully implemented, had substantially increased the opportunities for girls and women to play organized sports, to improve their physical fitness, and to learn skills and techniques from trained coaches.

Through the 1970s and 1980s, participation of American girls and women in organized sports skyrocketed. In the early 1970s—before

Title IX—only 7.4 percent of high school athletes (about 300,000) were girls; in 1976, this figure had risen to 28.6 percent, or more than 1.6 million. In 1995, more than 2 million girls participated in high school athletics, representing about 38 percent of high school athletes. And by the mid-1990s nearly half of all athletes at the college and university level were women.

There has been an equally significant change in knowledge and attitudes. Until relatively recently, many people believed that women and girls were too frail to engage in many forms of athletics. For instance, it was not until 1984 that the women's marathon was included as an Olympic event. The accomplishments of a number of individual athletes have shown that women can meet the physical demands of athletics as well as men—and in some cases better. In 1990 in New York City, Ann Transon (at age 29) became the first woman to win a mixed-gender national championship: the TAC/USA 24-hour, 143-mile (230-km) ultraendurance run. In 1992, Paula Newby-Fraser set the course record for a 400-mile (640-km) bicycle race from San Francisco to Los Angeles, with a time of 19 hours 49 minutes. In 1993, the jockey Julie Krone won the Belmont Stakes, a "triple crown" event in thoroughbred horse racing; that year she was also the third most-winning jockey, male or female. Shelley Taylor-Smith won many mixed-gender marathon swimming events throughout the early 1990s. Susan Butcher won the Iditarod, a grueling 1,100-mile (1,760-km) dogsled race in Alaska, four times (*see also STATISTICS*).

Still, even though the notion of female frailty has been debunked, there are some physiologic differences between men and women that do have a bearing on athletic performance. On average, women tend to be smaller than men: shorter, smaller-boned, and with less muscle mass. Women's capacity for childbearing and breast-feeding is also a factor. Thus while women may be able to compete on a par with men in events based primarily on ultraendurance or precision of technique, it seems reasonable, because of differences in size and strength, to have the top male and female athletes compete separately in events for which size and strength confer a significant advantage. And as more and more girls and women compete in sports and place higher and higher demands on their strength, stamina, and willpower, it is useful to understand the physiological factors that female athletes may need to consider.

Body Composition and Strength

Before puberty, there are no obvious differences between boys and girls in strength or athletic performance. But during adolescence, when boys begin to outpace girls in body size, skeletal structure, and muscle mass, differences become apparent. At puberty, girls do not generally experience an increase in relative muscle mass, and their

Findings on Sports, Fitness, and Women's Health

High school girls who participate in sports are less likely to have an unwanted pregnancy, less likely to take drugs, and more likely to graduate from high school.

As little as 2 hours of exercise a week may reduce a teenage girl's risk of developing breast cancer (which may afflict as many as 1 of every 8 women).

Girls who play sports have higher confidence and self-esteem and a lower incidence of depression.

Exercise in the teens and twenties contributes to bone density later in a woman's life and thus can help prevent osteoporosis (which is estimated to affect 1 of every 2 women over age 60).

Women who exercise have a lower incidence of weight problems than women who do not exercise, lower levels of blood sugar and cholesterol, and lower blood pressure. They also report being happier, feeling more energetic, and missing fewer days of work. (Compiled by the Women's Sports Foundation)

---

hips widen relative to shoulders and waist; boys do experience an increase in muscle mass, and their shoulders broaden relative to hips and waist. Height also begins to differ, so that by adulthood the average male will be 5 feet 9 inches tall and the average female 5 feet 5 inches tall. These differences have some implications for athletics.

With regard to muscle mass, average body fat (in adults) is about 12 percent for men and 26 percent for women; thus men have a greater muscle mass for a given height than women. It should be emphasized, though, that these figures are averages: an individual woman may be leaner than an individual man or than the average man. (This is equally true with height, of course: any given woman may be taller than a given man or taller than the average for men.) Also, most trained female athletes have a lower percentage of body fat than the average woman, and some female athletes—especially runners and gymnasts—have a lower percentage of body fat than the average college-age man (less than 20 percent; see BODY COMPOSITION).

Moreover, if absolute strength is calculated as strength relative to lean body weight (body weight minus fat weight), there is no significant difference between men and women: per unit lean body size, elite female athletes have upper-body strength virtually equal to that of their male counterparts. Differences in strength, then, are due mainly to difference in muscle size: the total cross sectional area of muscle in women is on average only 60 to 85 percent that of men. These differences in strength between men and women tend to be greater for the upper body than for the lower body. However, while women cannot achieve the same increase as men in overall muscle mass (and hence in strength) through resistance training, women are able to achieve the same relative strength gains (see STRENGTH TRAINING).

With regard to the size of hips, shoulders, and waist, men are usually wider at the shoulder relative to the hips; women, on average, are wider at the hips relative to the shoulders. One might suppose that this difference would result in a lower center of gravity for women and would therefore give women an advantage in sports that require balance, such as figure skating and gymnastics. In fact, however, differences in center of gravity depend more on individual body types than on gender. Studies have found that center of gravity varies more among women than between men and women because there is so much variation among women in the shape of the pelvis. In general, though, a woman does tend to have a wider, shallower pelvis than a man, resulting in a greater angle of the femur from the vertical, which could lead to an increased risk of knee injuries. Most injuries are sport-specific rather than gender-specific, but there does appear to be a slightly greater incidence of intra-articular knee injuries in women basketball players than men basketball players (*see KNEE and PELVIS, HIP, AND THIGH*).

An addtional factor in body composition has to do with the bones. Women have thinner, lighter bones than men; therefore, as they age, women are more likely to develop osteoporosis, a condition that causes bones to lose minerals—mainly calcium—and become thinner and weaker, sometimes to a point where they can easily break. The female sex hormone estrogen (and the male sex hormone testosterone) helps to preserve bone density by aiding the absorption of calcium and its incorporation into bone tissue (*see SKELETAL SYSTEM*). After menopause, when a woman's estrogen level drops, calcium is depleted from bone. Small, thin-boned women, women who smoke, women who have a light complexion, and women who are deficient in vitamin D are at particular risk of osteoporosis.

Osteoporosis is to some extent preventable. For women, prevention should begin at adolescence and continue throughout life. Beginning in the preteen years and continuing throughout their lives, they should strengthen their bones through adequate nutrition and exercise. They should have a diet that includes sufficient calcium and vitamin D for healthy bones and should engage in physical activity to stimulate bone deposition. Regular menstrual periods also contribute to healthy bones: an irregular menstrual cycle can lead to insufficient estrogen and, hence, to problems with absorbing and utilizing calcium. Physicians may treat irregular menstrual periods by prescribing oral contraceptives. Postmenopausal women might want to consider estrogen-replacement therapy or other drug treatment—along with adequate calcium intake and weight-bearing exercise—to prevent bone loss (*see also SKELETAL SYSTEM*).

Some young female athletes are at particular risk of premature osteoporosis, that is, premature bone loss. A very high level of training combined with inadequate nutrition can lead to oligomenorrhea (irregular menstrual cycle) or amenorrhea (the absence of three to six consecutive menstrual cycles in a woman who has already begun menstruating), with concomitant low levels of estrogen. At an age when they should be building up bone to minimize the effect of losses after

Gender and Metabolism

Myth—Because women have more essential body fat than men, this physiological difference has long been used to explain the ability of some women to compete at a par with men in ultraendurance events. The additional fat is said to predispose women to burn fat for fuel and "spare" glycogen, so that they can keep going longer. *Reality*—Studies suggest that performance in long-distance events is related to the body's ability to consume more fat than carbohydrate to fuel the muscles, and that a person's ratio of fat to glycogen metabolism—along with other physiological and psychological traits important in endurance events—is unrelated to testosterone. Through training, an athlete—male or female—can improve this ratio. However, some individuals may just be born to burn fat, and those individuals may turn out to be women more often than men.

menopause in the fifties and sixties, athletes who experience long episodes of amenorrhea suffer bone loss and inadequate bone formation, which can lead to stress fractures or more debilitating fractures of the hip and spine (*see the essay "The 'Female Athlete Triad'"*).

Physiological Functions

One important physiologic factor is metabolism. The basal metabolic rate is the rate at which the body burns fuel for energy when at rest. For women, on average, this rate is 5 to 10 percent lower than it is for men. This is because, generally, women have a higher percentage of fat whereas men have a higher percentare of muscle, and fat tissue is metabolically less active—that is, it uses less energy—than muscle tissue. (Gender differences in resting metabolic rate largely disappear when the rate is expressed relative to fat-free mass; *see also BODY COMPOSITION and ENERGY AND METABOLISM.*)

Resting metabolism accounts for 60 to 85 percent of an individual's daily energy expenditure. Exercise is the most variable component of energy expenditure, varying from 15 percent for a sedentary person to 30 percent for a person who exercises regularly. The energy cost of a particular activity depends on body weight: the more a person weighs, the more energy it takes to walk a mile or pedal a stationary bike for half an hour. Also, the greater the amount of muscle tissue activated, the larger the energy expenditure. Because women generally have a higher percentage of body fat and lower muscle mass, they may expend far fewer calories than men for exercise of the same duration and intensity. However, regular moderate aerobic exercise seems to increase the resting metabolic rate. (This rise can be a boon to women, and men, who are trying to lose weight by restricting their caloric intake; *see NUTRITION and ENERGY AND METABOLISM.*)

Oxygen capacity is another significant physiologic factor. Adult women tend to have a lower oxygen-carrying capacity than men. This is because, in comparison with women, men generally have higher plasma concentrations of both red blood cells and hemoglobin—the molecule in red blood cells that carries oxygen in the blood and delivers it to working cells. Women have a greater risk of anemia (insufficient concentration of red blood cells) because their iron stores are lower than men's, and they lose more iron through menstruation.

Iron-deficiency anemia impairs the ability of blood to carry oxygen. Thus all women should be sure to obtain sufficient dietary iron, and some may be advised by their physicians to take iron supplements. There is also a condition called "sports anemia" in which blood volume is expanded with no corresponding increase in red blood-cell count: that is, the count of red blood cells remains normal, but the red cells are effectively "diluted" because the blood volume is

The "Female Athlete Triad"

The term *female athlete triad* refers to three interrelated disorders seen in athletic women: (1) disordered eating, (2) amenorrhea, and (3) osteoporosis. Pressure to excel in a sport, coupled with the desire for a certain body type, can dispose a female athlete to disordered eating, which in turn can lead to menstrual dysfunction and premature osteoporosis. Any one of these disorders alone is serious; when the three are combined, they represent an even more severe risk to health.

Disordered eating is a spectrum of abnormal eating behaviors including bingeing alternated with purging; food restrictions; voluntary starvation; use of diet pills, diuretics, and laxatives; preoccupation with eating; fear of gaining weight; and a distorted body image. At the extreme end of the spectrum are two serious eating disorders: anorexia nervosa and bulimia nervosa. These are compulsive patterns that can lead to metabolic, skeletal, endocrine, and psychiatric problems and—in the case of anorexia—to death.

Menstrual irregularities among female athletes also form a spectrum. At one end are occasional long menstrual cycles. In the middle is oligomenorrhea—menstrual cycles longer than 36 days—which is probably due to lack of ovulation caused by a low level of progesterone. At the extreme is amenorrhea—defined as the absence of at least three consecutive menstrual cycles—which is characterized by low levels of estrogen. Menstrual dysfunction can be caused by malnutrition, a by-product of disordered eating.

Low estrogen in young, amenorrheic women can lead to premature bone loss, or osteoporosis, and inadequate bone formation. This creates an increased risk of stress fractures and other bone injuries.

The most serious immediate consequence of this "triad" of disorders is premature death from anorexia: studies have reported a 10 to 18 percent mortality rate among *treated* anorectic women. The long-term effects on health, though, are also very serious. To avoid these dangers, prevention, early detection, and treatment are vital.

All female athletes seem to be at risk of the "female athlete triad," but those whose sport demands a lean body for either biomechanical or aesthetic reasons are particularly susceptible. Athletes in individual sports are at a higher risk than those in team sports. These individual sports include figure skating, gymnastics, distance running, and cross-country skiing. (Though ballet is not a sport, it is worth mentioning that the problem is especially acute among ballet dancers.)

Because denial and secrecy are characteristically associated with disordered eating, it is difficult to estimate the actual prevalence of the "female athlete triad." However, studies of the incidence of disordered eating and amenorrhea provide a clue. Various studies have estimated the prevalence of disordered eating at anywhere between 15 and 62 percent of female athletes. In the general female population, by contrast, the prevalence of anorexia nervosa is estimated at 1 percent and the prevalence of bulimia nervosa at 1 to 3 percent. (The incidence is higher among adolescents and young women who are white, are of higher socioeconomic status, and have a family history of eating disorders.) Another clue comes from the prevalence of amenorrhea among female athletes. The lowest estimate of amenorrhea is 3.4 percent; other estimates range as high as 66 percent. In the general female population, by comparison, the incidence is 2 to 5 percent.

It should be noted that male athletes in sports with weight classifications, such as wrestling, often practice inappropriate weight reduction and are therefore also at risk of eating disorders (*see* WRESTLING). However, these male athletes often seem to resume normal eating patterns when the season ends—possibly because men feel less pressure to base their self-worth on their appearance. Whatever the reason, women with eating disorders outnumber men by a margin of 9 to 1.

Ellen J. Zeman

---

greater. Sports anemia is probably not detrimental to performance, but iron-deficiency anemia is.

Certain other physiologic differences between men and women, mainly resulting from differences in size, also reduce oxygen intake and delivery. Women, because of their smaller thoracic cage, have less lung volume than men. Women also have a smaller heart, and thus a smaller stroke volume and a lower cardiac output (*see* HEART AND CIRCULATORY SYSTEM).

Reproductive Function

A woman's hormonal environment changes over a lifetime, from puberty through the reproductive years (during which she may experience conception, pregnancy, childbirth, and lactation) and eventually into menopause—the cessation of her menstrual cycles. This section will examine the menstrual cycle, pregnancy, and menopause with regard to female athletes.

Menstrual Cycle

For much of her life, a woman experiences the periodic variation of hormones that occurs during the menstrual cycle. During a normal menstrual cycle, in which an egg is produced by and released from the ovaries (ovulation), a specific chain of events occurs. Hormones from the pituitary gland at the base of the brain signal the release of female sex hormones. These hormones—estrogen and progesterone—cause the lining of the uterus to thicken and ovulation to occur. During the first half of the cycle, called the follicular phase, an egg develops in one of the ovaries, while the levels of the sex hormones estrogen and progesterone remain low (*see Figure 1*). At midcycle, there is a surge of estrogen accompanied by the release of the egg (ovulation). For

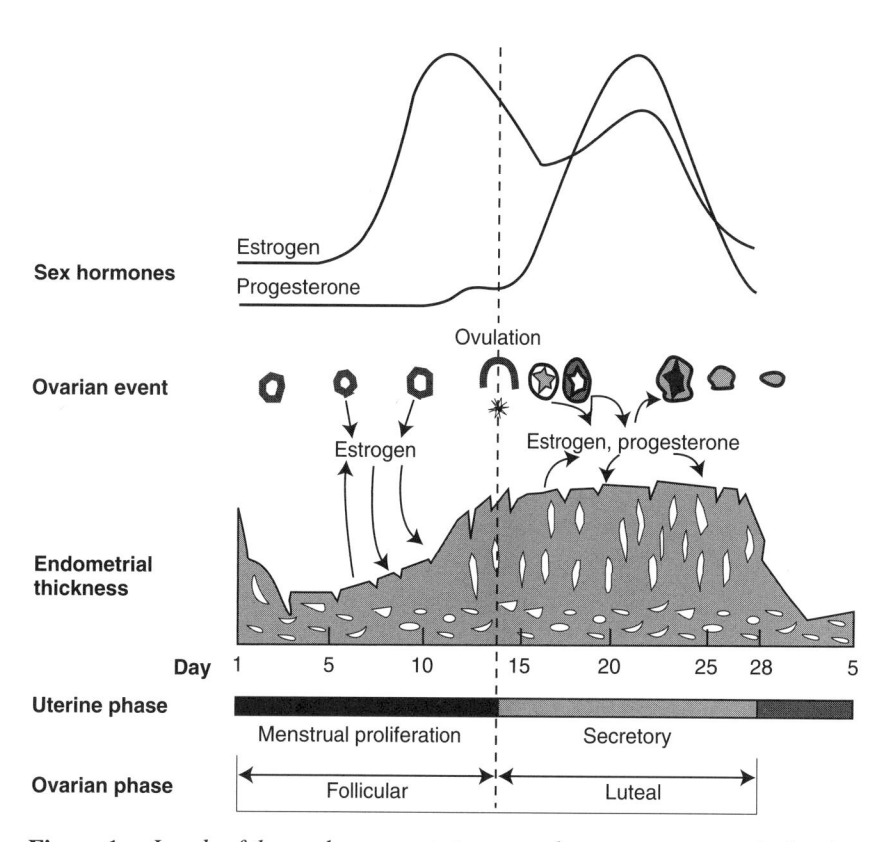

Figure 1. *Levels of the sex hormones estrogen and progesterone vary during the reproductive cycle.*

the remainder of the cycle, the luteal phase, estrogen levels remain high and progesterone levels begin to rise, causing a buildup of the lining of the uterus, the endometrium. If the egg is fertilized, it begins to divide, forming a zygote. The zygote makes its way to the uterus and settles (or "implants") into the spongy lining, which is designed to nourish it during its early development into an embryo. However, if the egg is not fertilized (as is most often the case), a drop in the levels of estrogen and progesterone causes the endometrium to deteriorate, with bleeding, or menstruation, resulting. After menstruation, the cycle begins anew.

The sex hormones have other, secondary, effects on the body besides the primary reproductive effects. Estrogen has several secondary effects. One such effect is that estrogen promotes fat deposition around the breasts, buttocks, and thighs. A second effect is that estrogen holds down the levels of total cholesterol and low-density-lipoprotein (LDL, or "bad") cholesterol, while increasing the level of high-density-lipoprotein (HDL, "good") cholesterol. These hormonal effects on cholesterol can help protect against heart disease and are probably the main reason that premenopausal women have a much lower incidence of coronary artery disease than men of the same age (*see also NUTRITION*). Third, estrogen seems to cause an increased utilization of fat (rather than carbohydrate) for fuel. This carbohydrate-sparing effect could theoretically have a positive impact on a woman's performance in endurance sports. And, fourth, as mentioned above, estrogen facilitates the incorporation of calcium into bone.

Progesterone also has a number of significant effects on the body. During the luteal phase the rise in progesterone is responsible for a rise in basal metabolic rate and an increase in core body temperature (about 0.5° F, or 0.27° C—this rise is an excellent indicator that ovulation has occurred). Some researchers believe that progesterone can cause slight hyperventilation and an increased response to high carbon dioxide or low oxygen levels in the blood, which might make an athlete perceive training as slightly more difficult during the luteal phase of her cycle. Progesterone, like estrogen, can cause a shift away from burning carbohydrates and toward burning fat; this could possibly lead to lower lactate formation during exercise and, hence, to better endurance. It should be emphasized, however, that these effects of estrogen and progesterone on athletic performance are theoretical and have not been proved scientifically.

The changes in hormone levels over the course of the menstrual cycle can cause a number of systemic effects, though their impact varies widely among women. Common effects in the luteal phase include fatigue, fluid retention, breast tenderness, and swings in appetite and mood. For most women, these effects are mild and simply signal the normal functioning of the menstrual cycle. However, for some women they are heightened to the point of becoming troublesome or even debilitating—a condition known as premenstrual syndrome (PMS). Although it is difficult to scientifically evaluate the effects of PMS on athletic performance, it seems logical that symptoms like fatigue and depression could be detrimental. However, for many women regular exercise seems to lessen the severity of PMS. During menstruation itself, some women experience pain—dysmenorrhea—probably caused by contractions of the uterus. Dysmenorrhea may interrupt training or competition, but it is often successfully treated with over-the-counter pain relievers such as aspirin or ibuprofen. Again, regular exercise seems to help reduce menstrual pain for many women.

Whether the menstrual cycle has any significant impact on athletic performance is debatable. There have been many studies of this issue, but the findings are often contradictory. The physiological changes that might be supposed to affect performance—such as changes in metabolism, blood volume, and ventilation—are subtle and do not actually appear to alter performance to any measurable degree. Although anecdotal evidence indicates that some women may perform worse during the premenstrual phase or during menstrual flow, most women report no noticeable detriment at these times.

Oral contraceptives regulate the menstrual cycle, but there is no clear evidence that oral contraceptives—any more than the unregulated cycle—diminish athletic performance. In fact, oral contraceptives, while they may have negative side effects, are often prescribed to treat amenorrhea, dysmenorrhea, and PMS. (They may also lower the risk of endometrial and ovarian cancer, and they have a protective effect against premature osteoporosis.) In any attempt to sort out the impact of the menstrual cycle on athletic performance, it is important to realize that women—both those taking an oral contraceptive ("the pill") and those taking none—have won Olympic medals and set records in all phases of the cycle.

Athletes and coaches sometimes wonder whether intense athletic training can affect the menstrual cycle. There is in fact a higher incidence of amenorrhea among athletes than in the general population: it has been estimated that 3 to 5 percent of sedentary women are amenorrheic; but depending on the sport, anywhere from 12 percent (collegiate swimmers) to 25 percent (competitive runners) of athletes are amenorrheic. (The incidence is even higher among ballet dancers: 44 percent.)

Until quite recently, many doctors and trainers believed that amenorrhea was caused by or related to a very low percentage of body fat—which can result from training hard. Studies have shown no link between low body fat and irregular menstrual cycles, so simply being thin as a consequence of training intensely will not necessarily have an adverse affect on a woman's reproductive health. "Athletic amenorrhea," though, may still be a consequence of intense training. There are two theories about the cause of athletic amenorrhea: (1) There may be a suppression of the reproductive organ–stimulating hormones released from the hypothalamus (the brain region largely responsible for regulating the body's internal environment) that signal the release of estrogen and progesterone; this suppression may be caused by an increased secretion of endorphins during intense training (*see RUNNING*); (2) There may be a "calorie drain," or negative calorie balance, caused by low caloric intake and high energy expenditure. On the basis of this second theory, "athletic amenorrhea" may indeed be "nutritional amenorrhea."

All in all, then, the effect of exercise itself on the menstrual cycle is unclear. Other factors probably have an impact—for example, diet, psychology, the environment, and predisposition to reproductive disorders. Women with "athletic" or "nutritional" amenorrhea often resume menstruating after cutting back exercise only slightly (as little as 5 to 15 percent) and increasing their intake only slightly (100 to 300 additional calories per day, the equivalent of two glasses of milk). Severe dieting or weight "cycling" (a repeated pattern of losses and gains), erratic eating patterns, and a diet low in protein and high in fiber all seem to be predisposing factors for amenorrhea. One factor should be noted especially: there appears to be a strong link between amenorrhea and eating disorders (*see the essay "The 'Female Athlete Triad'."*).

The most adverse consequence of amenorrhea is its effect on bone calcium deposition. Without sufficient estrogen, bones lose calcium. Premature bone loss can lead to stress fractures, which can bring an athlete's training regimen to a halt. Even more troubling, this early bone loss appears to be irreversible in many cases; thus the efficacy of treatment—calcium supplements, decreased training, estrogen replacement, and nutritional counseling—is uncertain. Low estrogen may also put a woman at higher risk of heart disease.

On the other hand, excessive exercise and disordered eating are not the only possible causes of amenorrhea. One very simple (and common) explanation is pregnancy: in diagnosing amenorrhea in a young athlete, a physician should consider a pregnancy test. Other diagnostic steps would include tests for hypothyroidism or a pituitary tumor, evaluation of numerous hormones, and examination of the pelvic area for polycystic ovarian disease.

Pregnancy

Moderate exercise during pregnancy can mitigate some of the unpleasant side effects of pregnancy, such as morning sickness. Exercise can also help prepare a woman for labor, and it reduces the risk of complications during childbirth. In addition, exercise can help the mother recover more quickly after the baby is born. However, while most athletic women are eager to maintain a reasonable level of physical activity during a pregnancy, questions often arise about how much exercise can be done at the various phases of pregnancy without harming the pregnant woman or the growth and development of the fetus.

In 1985, the American College of Obstetricians and Gynecologists issued a set of guidelines for exercise during pregnancy that encountered a storm of controversy. These guidelines delimited a strict "zone of safety" for exercise: 15-minute sessions in which the heart rate would not exceed 140. This seemed too conservative for women who were highly active before pregnancy, so the question remained: what is safe for active pregnant women?

One basis for concern is that exercise during pregnancy may place competing demands on the cardiovascular system by diverting blood flow from the uterus and placenta to muscle tissue and skin. Another concern is that exercise can raise the core body temperature, and this can, theoretically, endanger the fetus—especially early in a pregnancy, when the fetus's central nervous system is being formed. A third concern has to do with the fact that later in a pregnancy, a woman gains weight, her ligaments relax (in preparation for childbirth), and her center of gravity changes: these factors could increase her susceptibility to injury. These theoretical considerations, then, have raised some doubt about the safety of vigorous exercise during pregnancy.

In practice, however, the results of many studies indicate that a healthy woman can maintain or even begin a regular exercise program during pregnancy without harming the outcome. For example, exercise in itself does not lead to miscarriage (loss of the pregnancy), although caution, or possibly complete restriction, is suggested if certain maternal or fetal factors indicate a heightened risk of miscarriage or fetal distress.

Following are some commonly recommended guidelines for exercise during pregnancy:

• Determine whether there are any preexisting or obstetric risk factors (such as cardiac disease, high blood pressure, multiple pregnancy, multiple previous miscarriages, or diabetes) that would preclude exercise.

• Enlist regular prenatal medical supervision to ensure adequate weight gain and fetal development and to detect any medical complications. Any athlete wishing to maintain a serious training program during pregnancy (more than 7 hours per week) should be monitored frequently to ensure that there is no risk to fetal development. During the third trimester, the intensity of training should be decreased.

• Cease exercise immediately at the first sign of any unusual symptom such as dizziness, bleeding, uterine pain, shortness of breath, heart palpitations, back pain, pubic pain, or difficulty walking.

• Exercise regularly rather than intermittently, with warm-up and cool-down periods that include gentle stretching. Measure heart rate at times of peak activity, and do not exceed the heart rate limits established in consultation with a health-care provider. (Usually, this limit is around 140 beats per minute.) Vigorous exercise should last no more than about 30 minutes, unless the pregnant woman is in very good physical condition and has received the approval of a health care provider. Serious competition involving all-out effort should probably be avoided.

• To prevent dehydration, drink plenty of liquids before and after exercise, and take water breaks if necessary. Avoid vigorous exercise in hot, humid weather. Core body temperature should not exceed 38 degrees C (about 100° F).

• After the first trimester, avoid contact sports and sports that pose a risk of abdominal trauma (ice hockey, football, horseback riding, downhill skiing).

• During the last trimester, exercise should not be performed in a supine position (lying on the back), because the weight of the uterus may interfere with blood flow to the heart. Avoid exercises that use the Valsalva maneuver (holding one's breath during isometric exercise; see STRENGTH TRAINING).

• Throughout a pregnancy, avoid any activity that takes place in a high- or low-pressure environment (scuba diving, mountain climbing, high-altitude skiing).

Some physicians simply trust a pregnant patient to monitor her own bodily responses to exercise and to train within a reasonable zone of comfort. However, others are more cautious and prefer to have their patients follow set guidelines. In either case, though, it is important to realize that no upper limit has yet been established for safe exercise. An exercise regimen therefore needs to be tailored to the individual, preferably in consultation with a physician or a nurse-midwife; and the athlete herself should be flexible and willing to adjust her routine to the changes that occur during pregnancy.

Menopause

At about age 50, women's menstrual cycles become less regular as their production of estrogen begins to decrease. Eventually the menstrual cycle ceases altogether; this phenomenon is called menopause. The climacteric, a broader phenomenon that includes menopause and may begin at around age 45, encompasses the gradual change from the beginning of menstrual irregularities through the postmenopausal stage, around age 60, when estrogen levels become quite low. (Men also experience reproductive changes after about age 40, as their testosterone levels drop, but the changes men undergo are more gradual and less dramatic.)

Although women produce some residual estrogen after menopause, the level of this hormone is too low to maintain estrogen-dependent tissue: thus breasts and genital organs atrophy, and there is an increase in bone resorption—removal of calcium from bone, with a consequent decrease in bone mass (see SKELETAL SYSTEM). This sometimes results in osteoporosis, as discussed above. A menopausal woman may experience hot flashes: episodes of sweating and feeling warm, as a result of dilation of blood vessels in the skin (although it is not known why low estrogen levels cause this phenomenon). The incidence of heart disease and high blood pressure rises rapidly for postmenopausal women.

Some women take supplemental estrogen to reduce these symptoms. However, exercise is probably most beneficial for women entering menopause. Exercise can reduce the risks of heart disease and osteoporosis and can mitigate the mood swings that may also accompany menopause. Not long ago, there was widespread doubt that older people could benefit from exercise. However, by now any number of studies have shown that exercise—even simply walking—can improve cardiorespiratory endurance, reduce body fat, increase strength, reduce fatigue and depression, and contribute to an overall feeling of well-being.

Older women who want to embark on an exercise program should first be evaluated for coronary risk factors and should have a complete physical exam, including a stress test. The minimum activity level to maintain fitness is 20 minutes of aerobic activity (walking, low-impact or water aerobics, swimming, or bicycling) three days per week. Women are also advised to do exercises to strengthen the pelvic floor; this can help prevent or correct urinary incontinence, which may accompany menopause. To prevent bone demineralization, strength training should supplement aerobic activities (*see AGING AND PERFORMANCE*).

Eating Disorders

Participants in some sports feel that they ought to have a certain body type or weight. There are various reasons for this, some biomechanical and some aesthetic. Sports such as figure skating, diving, and gymnastics are judged subjectively, and appearance can affect the score. In some other sports, such as competitive running and cross country skiing, leanness is a physical advantage. In sports that involve weight classifications—such as wrestling, rowing, weight lifting, and taekwondo—a weigh-in before a match becomes of primary importance. In sports like body building, in which the body is displayed, the athlete's attention is focused almost exclusively on appearance and body image.

In general, too, physical training increases a person's consciousness of how the body moves, looks, and feels; thus athletes tend to be sensitive to their own body image. Added to this is the fact that athletes are often "high achievers": strong-willed, competitive, and goal-oriented. Also, through rigorous training athletes may learn to endure and ignore pain.

Although many of the factors just described represent positive conditions or characteristics for an athlete, these same factors can predispose athletes to disordered eating. Another factor predisposing individuals to disordered eating—in fact, the strongest factor—is gender: women with eating disorders outnumber men 9 to 1. Thus, female athletes are vulnerable to eating disorders to begin with, not only by virtue of being athletes but also by virtue of being female. In addition to their initial vulnerability, many young female athletes are under special pressure to be thin—from coaches, parents, peers, and society, and simply from themselves—because there is so much emphasis in their sports on appearance and winning.

Not surprisingly, then, there is a high prevalence of disordered eating among female athletes. In an effort to optimize performance and meet criteria for weight or body fat, they may undergo inappropriate weight loss or weight cycling (gaining and losing weight throughout the season or between seasons; see *ACROBATICS*). Studies have found that 15 to 62 percent of female athletes may develop compulsive eating behaviors. By the early 1990s, several famous athletes—including the gymnast Cathy Rigby, the diver Jenifer Magnum, and the runner Patti Catalano—had begun to talk about their own experiences with eating disorders.

Disordered eating is not a single behavior but a spectrum of behaviors (*see also the essay "The 'Female Athlete Triad'"*). These behaviors range from moderate—skipping meals, occasionally taking laxatives, fad dieting—to extreme. At the extreme end of the range, disordered eating becomes an "eating disorder," a clinically diagnosed psychiatric condition. This extreme end of the spectrum includes anorexia nervosa and bulimia nervosa. Anorexia is characterized by voluntary starvation coupled with excessive exercise; bulimia is characterized by habitual binge eating followed by a sense of guilt and self-induced vomiting or purging. Each of these disorders is diagnosed on the basis of criteria established in the *Diagnostic and Statistical Manual of Mental Disorders* (abbreviated DSM-IV; see Table 1).

Many athletes show signs of disordered eating at various stages in their careers, even if they do not meet the DSM-IV criteria for anorexia or bulimia. Full-fledged eating disorders are obviously dangerous to health and even to life. However, it is important to realize that disordered eating patterns, although they are more moderate conditions, also increase the risk of a number of serious health problems: skeletal damage, impaired endocrine functioning, infertility,

SIGNS OF ANOREXIA NERVOSA AND BULIMA NERVOSA

Anorexia

Weight: 15 percent or more below what is considered normal for height and age.
Intense fear of gaining weight, even when thin.
Distorted body image; undue influence of body weight or shape on self-image; denial of weight.
Vigorous exercise to prevent weight gain.
Amenorrhea (in women).

Bulimia

Recurrent episodes of binge eating (at least twice a week for 3 months).
Habitual use of self-induced vomiting, diuretics, or laxatives.
Sense of being out of control during binges.
Self-image unduly influenced by weight and shape.
Vigorous exercise to prevent weight gain.

Table 1.

RECOGNIZING DISORDERED EATING

Signs of disordered eating

Preoccupation with food, appearance, and weight; criticism of one's body.
Eating in secrecy; stealing food.
Consumption of large amounts of food, inconsistent with weight.
Bloodshot eyes, swollen parotid glands; mood swings.
Rapid weight flucuations; use of laxatives; excessive dieting.
Compulsive exercise beyond what is necessary in a training regimen.
Continuous drinking of diet soda.
Trips to the bathroom after large meals; odor of vomit in bathroom.

Table 2.

and psychiatric and psychological difficulties. Additionally, if the health consequences of disordered eating or an eating disorder become severe enough, an athlete will be forced to drop out of training and competition.

If treated early, disordered eating can be overcome, and eating disorders can usually be overcome or at least controlled. Treatment typically consists of nutritional counseling along with psychiatric evaluation and possibly some form of psychotherapy. Hospitalization may be necessary if other treatement has failed, or if the patient's weight is 30 percent below normal, because at that point cardiac function is compromised, blood pressure falls, the patient becomes severely dehydrated, and electrolyte balance is abnormal. Athletes with eating disorders often bring positive attributes to treatment: they may be able to apply the discipline and motivation developed through training. But they do require some special consideration with regard to treatment, since therapeutic measures should not further impair a patient's athletic career.

The most important approach to dealing with disordered eating, however, is not treatment but prevention. Education is crucial here. Both coaches and athletes should learn to recognize the signs of disordered eating (*see Table 2*). Coaches should be educated about how their expectations and demands might influence their athletes' self-image and eating behaviors. Athletes should be taught proper nutrition and safe methods of weight control (*see NUTRITION*) and should be made aware that disordered eating is detrimental to their health and their performance.

Unfortunately, in the United States in the 1990s, anyone who tries to implement these preventive measures is swimming against the tide. Americans are constantly bombarded with messages that equate thinness with beauty, sexuality, success, and power, and American society has become obsessed with appearance in general and thinness in particular. One indicator of the obsession with thinness is the simple fact that more than 75 percent of people with eating disorders have never been overweight. Thus until society—and the sports establishment—changes its emphasis, prevention of disordered eating will be difficult at best.

Ellen J. Zeman

References

Clinics in Sports Medicine: *The Athletic Woman* 13, no. 2 (1994).

Costa, D., and R. Guthrie. *Women and Sport: Interdisciplinary Perspectives*. Champaign, Illinois: Human Kinetics, 1994.

Hargarten, K. "Menopause: How Exercise Mitigates Symptoms." *Physician and Sportsmedicine* 22, no. 1 (1994): 49ff.

Noble, E. *Essential Exercises for the Childbearing Year*. 2nd ed. Boston: Houghton Mifflin, 1982.

Shangold, M., and G. Mirkin. *Women and Exercise: Physiology and Sports Medicine*. 2nd ed. Philadelphia: Davis, 1994.

Wichmann, S., and D. Martin. "Eating Disorders in Athletes." *Physician and Sportsmedicine* 21, no. 5 (1993): 126ff.

White, J. "Exercising for Two: What's Safe for the Active Pregnant Woman?" *Physician and Sportsmedicine* 20, no. 5 (1992): 179ff.

Heart and Circulatory System

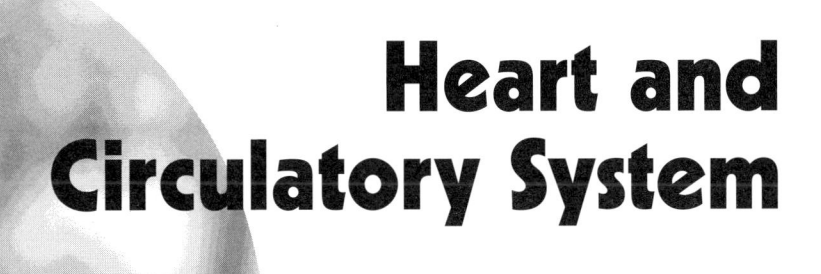

AS THE MARATHON RUNNERS enter the stadium for the final lap of their 26.2-mile race, lungs heaving and hearts pounding, they are pushing themselves to their physical limit. Their leg muscles, working to propel them forward, are using oxygen and producing carbon dioxide at a high rate. Blood is coursing through their hardworking muscles, delivering oxygen and removing carbon dioxide. The blood is being pumped by the heart through a system of tubes that pass into every part of the body.

In this scenario, it is obvious that work is being done. Even when a person is completely at rest, though, each cell in the body is performing some sort of work. To use fuel energy (that is, energy from food) to perform work, a cell consumes oxygen and creates carbon dioxide, a waste product that must be disposed of. During exercise, both the need for oxygen and the production of carbon dioxide rise to very high levels. But regardless of whether the body is at work or at rest, a continuous supply of blood rich in oxygen is essential to the survival of all bodily tissues, and the removal of the waste products of working cells is equally important. The cardiovascular system—which consists of the heart and the blood vessels—meets these vital needs.

Circulation: The Basic Pattern

To understand the cardiovascular system, it is necessary to keep the basic pattern of circulation in mind (*see Figure 1*). At the lungs, oxygen is added to the blood while carbon dioxide is removed. At the tissues, oxygen is removed from the blood while carbon dioxide is added. Blood rich in carbon dioxide but poor in oxygen returns from the body tissues to the right side of the heart. The chambers of the right side of the heart pump this blood out to the lungs, where carbon dioxide is removed and oxygen is added. This oxygen-rich blood returns to the left side of the heart, which pumps it out to the body tissue. At the body tissues, oxygen is removed from the blood and carbon dioxide produced by the tissues is added.

Given this information, a drop of blood can be traced as it travels around the circulatory system. The circulatory system (as the term

Figure 1. *The basic pattern of the cardiovascular system is shown here. The pulmonary system carries blood through the lungs; the systematic system carries blood to the other body tissues. Blood rich in carbon dioxide but poor in oxygen (light shading) returns from the body tissues to the right side of the heart. The chambers of the right side of the heart pump this blood out to the lungs, where carbon dioxide is removed and oxygen is added. This oxygen-rich blood (dark shading) returns to the left side of the heart, which pumps it out to the body tissue. When blood passes through the lungs, oxygen is added to the blood as carbon dioxide is removed. The reverse process occurs at the body tissues: oxygen is removed as carbon dioxide is added.*

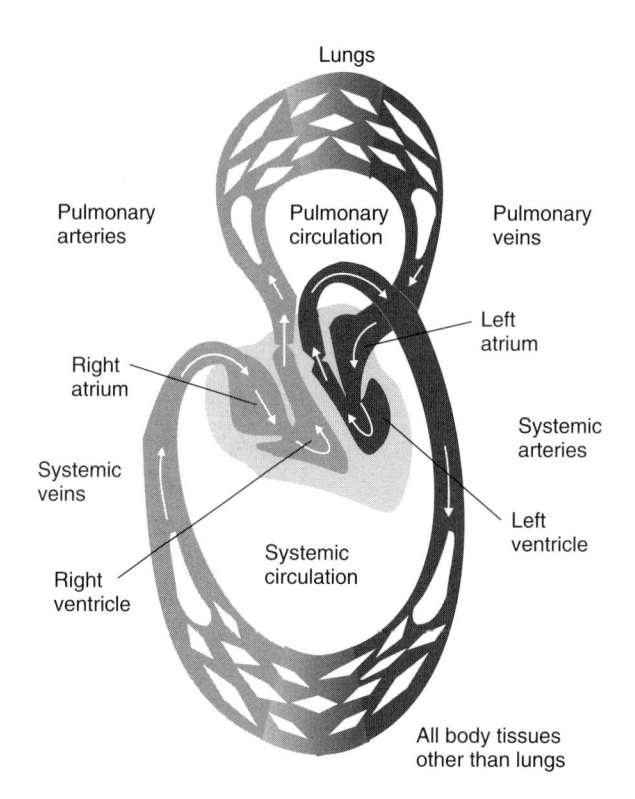

The Importance of Oxygen

The body's need for oxygen has been demonstrated, tragically, in a relatively new sport: snowboarding. A snowboarder's feet are both lashed to the board with non–release bindings. Snowboarders who ride "out of bounds" on ungroomed slopes sometimes fall headfirst into deep, powdery snow, and because they cannot release their feet from the board, they are unable to get up. As a snowboarder lies buried, the hearts slows because of the cold, depriving the body tissues—most importantly, the brain—of oxygen. Soon, the heart stops, and death follows from lack of oxygen. The snowboarder has literally drowned. Mountaineers know that a climber buried in a snow avalanche for more than 30 minutes has less than a 50 percent chance of survival. Thus a snowboarder trapped upside down in deep snow for several hours is not likely to be revived after being rescued, even with the best medical treatment. Obviously, preventive measures are important, such as better education for snowboarders, release bindings, and bright-colored snowboard bottoms.

implies) is a continuous loop with no beginning or end, but for convenience this tracing can start at the right side of the heart.

The heart consists of two pumps: the right side pumps blood to the lungs; the left side pumps blood to the tissues. Each side of the heart, in turn, is made up of two chambers, an atrium and a ventricle (*see Figure 2*). Blood from the body (low in oxygen, high in carbon dioxide) returns to the right atrium. This blood then passes to the right ventricle, which pumps it out to the lungs by the pulmonary artery. From the pulmonary artery the blood enters the pulmonary capillaries, where oxygen is added to the blood and carbon dioxide is removed from it. The blood, now oxygen-rich, flows through the pulmonary vein to the left atrium. Next it enters the left ventricle, which pumps it through the largest artery, the aorta. The aorta branches into smaller arteries that lead to every body tissue.

At the body tissues, the arteries divide into the smallest blood vessels, the body capillaries. Here oxygen leaves the blood for the tissues while carbon dioxide enters the blood from the tissues. The body

Figure 2. *Blood from the body (low in oxygen, high in carbon dioxide) returns to the right atrium of the heart. When the blood passes to the right ventricle, it is pumped out to the lungs through the pulmonary artery. From the pulmonary artery the blood enters the pulmonary capillaries, where oxygen is added to the blood and carbon dioxide removed. The blood, now oxygen-rich, flows through the pulmonary vein to the left atrium. Next it enters the left ventricle, which pumps it through the largest artery, the aorta. The aorta branches into smaller arteries that lead to every body tissue. At the body tissues the arteries divide into the smallest blood vessels, the body capillaries. Here oxygen leaves the blood for the tissues while carbon dioxide enters the blood from the tissues. The capillaries join together into larger and larger veins, returning to the right atrium and thereby completing the cycle.*

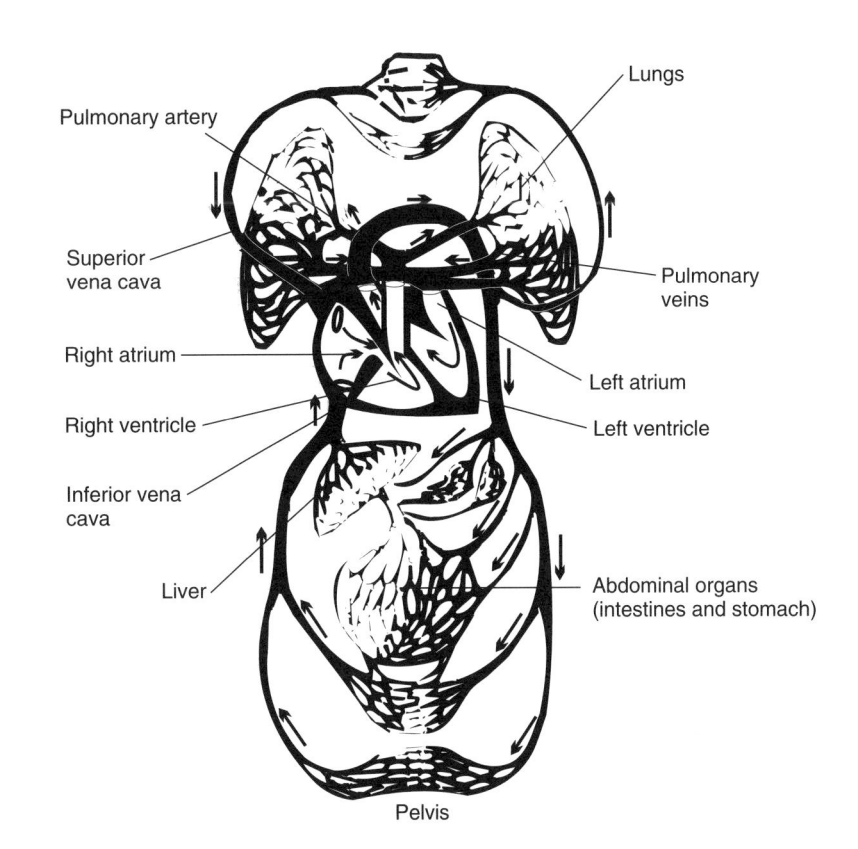

capillaries join together into larger and larger veins. The veins from the lower part of the body converge into the inferior vena cava while those from the upper body converge into the superior vena cava. These two large veins return blood from the body (now oxygen-poor) to the right atrium.

Note that what distinguishes arteries from veins is simply direction—toward or away from the heart. Any vessel that carries blood away from the heart is called an *artery*; any a vessel that carries blood toward the heart is called a *vein*. The arteries from the left ventricle to all body tissues carry high-oxygen blood; but the pulmonary artery, from the right ventricle, carries low-oxygen blood. The veins that lead to the right atrium from all body tissues carry low-oxygen blood; but the pulmonary vein, which leads to the left atrium, carries high-oxygen blood.

Oxygen, of course, is not the only molecule the body tissues need for energy. All body tissues also need carbohydrates, fats, proteins, vitamins, and minerals (*see ENERGY AND METABOLISM*). The arterial blood that flows to the stomach and intestines picks up nutrients from food. The veins that carry blood away from these organs go first to the liver through the portal vein (*again, see Figure 2*) before returning to the right atrium in the inferior vena cava. The liver has several vital functions: it extracts food molecules absorbed from the intestines, converts them for storage, and destroys any toxic substances absorbed into the blood with food.

Just as oxygen is not the only molecule the tissues need for energy, carbon dioxide is not the only waste product they produce. The breakdown of proteins creates ammonia, a highly toxic substance that the body must dispose of. This disposal is also accomplished by the liver, in conjuction with the kidneys. In the liver, ammonia is removed from the blood and converted to a less toxic form called urea. The urea is released back into the blood, where it circulates to the kidney. The kidneys, which act as the body's filters, receive as much as one-fourth of the blood pumped by the left ventricle and extract the urea from this blood. The urea is then excreted in urine.

The Heart

The basic structure of the heart has already been described as part of the pattern of ciculation. This section will examine some other important aspects of the heart and its functioning.

Heart Valves

Functioning of the valves. For blood to circulate, it is vital that the chambers of the heart pump blood only in the correct direction. This is ensured by the presence of four valves guarding the outflow from each chamber of the heart (*see Figure 3*). The right and left atrioventricular (A-V) valves are located between the atrium and ventricle on the two sides of the heart and open into the ventricles. The pulmonary valve is located between the right ventricle and the pul-

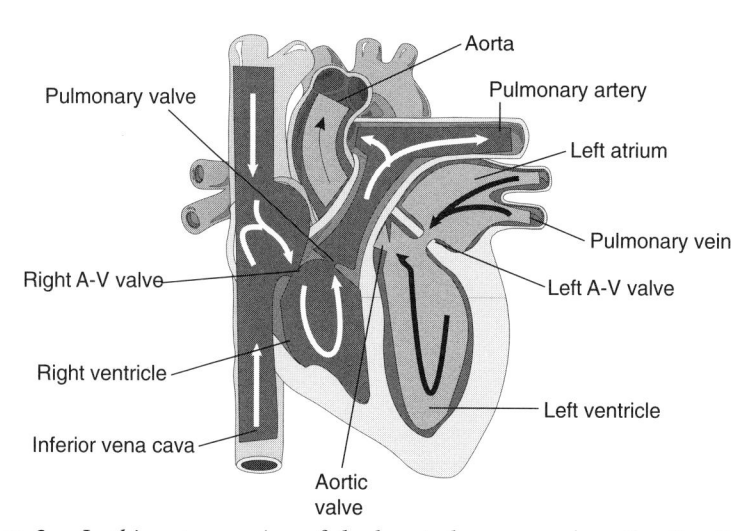

Figure 3. *In this cutaway view of the heart, the arrows show the direction of blood flow. For blood to circulate, the chambers of the heart must pump it only in the proper direction; this is regulated by the four valves of the heart: right A-V, left A-V, aortic, and pulmonary. Each valve acts to prevent outflow from its chamber.*

SYSTOLE

Isovolumetric ventricular contraction

Atrium, Ventricle, Relax, Contract

Ventricular ejection (blood flows out of ventricle)

Relax, Contract

A-V valve:	closed	closed
Aortic and pulmonary valves:	closed	open

DIASTOLE

Isovolumetric ventricular relaxation

Relax, Relax

Ventricular filling (blood flows into ventricle)

Relax, Relax, Contract, Relax

A-V valve:	closed	open	open
Aortic and pulmonary valves:	closed	closed	closed

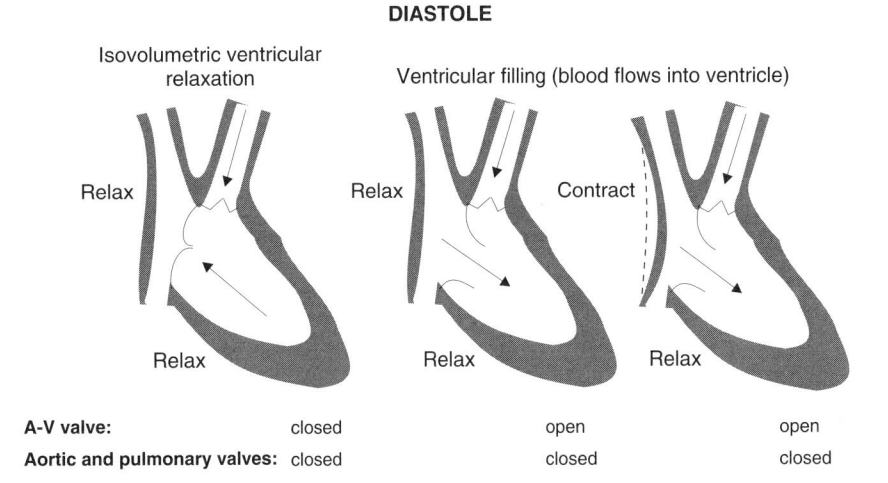

Figure 4. *The valves of the heart open and close in response to pressure changes in the heart chambers. (Adapted from Vander, 1994)*

monary artery, opening into the pulmonary artery. The aortic valve is located between the left ventricle and the aorta, opening into the aorta.

These valves function like a one-way swinging door. They open and close in response to changes in pressure in the heart chambers (*see Figure 4*). When the ventricles contract, blood pressure in the ventricles rises. This pressure closes the A-V valves and opens the pulmonary and aortic valves; thus blood is pushed out into the arteries rather than backward into the atria. When the ventricles relax, the pressure in the ventricles falls; then the aortic and pulmonary valves snap shut, and the A-V valves open. This configuration allows the blood to circulate in only one direction. The ventricles fill with blood from the atria—not with blood moving backward from the arteries.

It is the closing of the heart valves that causes the well-known "lub-dub" sound heard through a stethoscope. The first heart sound ("lub") is caused by the closure of the A-V valves and thus marks the

The Fragile Liver

The importance of the liver and its fragility were illustrated by the illness and death of the baseball star Mickey Mantle in 1995. For many years, during his baseball career and after his retirement, Mantle had been a heavy drinker—in fact, an alcoholic. Alcohol is absorbed into the blood in the stomach and intestines and transported to the liver, which recognizes it as a toxic substance and breaks it down. To break down alcohol, the liver must use cellular mechanisms normally reserved for the breakdown of sugar. Thus, when sugar enters the liver, this cellular machinery is already in use, and so the sugar is not broken down but instead is stored as fat. If enough alcohol is consumed over a long enough time, these fatty deposits in the liver will eventually destroy it, causing blood to back up in the portal vein. The veins that carry blood away from the stomach and intestines to the liver then bulge and may burst; the resulting bleeding is life-threatening. In the case of Mickey Mantle, although he was finally able to confront his alcoholism and stop drinking, his liver had already been irreparably damaged and had to be replaced with a donor organ. Liver transplants can be successful (though success is by no means certain); but Mantle died a few months later from lung cancer, which had not been detected earlier.

beginning of ventricular contraction. The second heart sound ("dub") is caused by the closure of the pulmonary and aortic valves. It marks the beginning of ventricular relaxation.

The heart valves and heart murmurs. Abnormal heart valves are a common cause of a heart "murmur," an abnormal sound in addition to the normal "lub" and "dub." Narrowed (stenosed) valves cause abnormally high resistance to the flow of blood. The blood becomes turbulent as it is forced through the narrow opening, producing a swishing sound—the "murmur." If the left A-V valve is stenosed, this will produce a murmur during ventricular relaxation. Valves may also bend backward (prolapse), allowing blood to leak through the valve in the wrong direction (regurgitation). This too produces a murmur. If the left A-V valve is prolapsed, a murmur will be produced during ventricular contraction. Abnormal openings between the two atria (atrial septal defects) or between the two ventricles (ventricular septal defects) can also cause heart murmurs.

Young people, including young athletes, can have a heart murmur. Some murmurs are entirely normal, but some are caused by congenital heart defects—that is, heart problems present from birth—or by childhood infections, such as rheumatic fever. Murmurs can indicate significant medical problems, including some conditions that may lead to sudden cardiac death. For this reason, a physical examination given as a prerequisite for a young person's participation in an athletic program often includes listening to the heart with a stethoscope.

The symptoms that accompany heart murmurs depend on the severity of the problem causing the murmur. Severe heart-valve abnormalities and large septal defects can cause extreme shortness of breath and greatly reduced tolerance for exercise. Small valve and septal abnormalities may be benign, posing no danger and not limiting activity in any way. Unfortunately, however, there is one exceptional condition in which a small and otherwise benign septal defect can pose a threat to health: the presence of even a small septal defect can make a scuba diver more susceptible to a serious complication known as "the bends" (*see also* RESPIRATION). Thus any athlete who has a heart murmur should consult a physician, especially before becoming involved with underwater sports, which involve high pressures.

Electrical Activity of the Heart

The heart is made up of millions of individual muscle cells. Each cell contracts when it is stimulated by an electrical current. For the heart to pump blood effectively, the cells must all contract in coordination. For example, a contraction cannot be effective if half of the left ventricle contracts while the other half relaxes. To prevent this kind of uncoodinated activity, heart muscle has a built-in electrical system that starts each heartbeat and stimulates all the cells to contract cooperatively.

The electrical impulse responsible for each heartbeat is begun in a small piece of specialized tissue in the right atrium called the sinoatrial (SA) node (*see Figure 5*). The SA node starts heartbeats at regular intervals; it usually works at a rate of about 70 beats per minute but can speed up or slow down when it receives directions from the brain to do so.

The part of the nervous system responsible for matching the heart rate to the body's needs is the autonomic nervous system. The autonomic nervous system has control centers in the brain and nerves which extend out to the heart and other organs. This system is made up of two divisions: the sympathetic and parasympathetic systems. Exercise stimulates the sympathetic nervous system, which sends messages to the SA node instructing it to increase the heart rate. Resting after a large meal stimulates the parasympathetic nervous system, which commands the SA node to slow the heart down. Even without input from the brain, however, the SA node will continue to initiate heartbeats at regular intervals. This is illustrated by the fact that a heart being transplanted from one person to another continues to beat even though it no longer has nerves connecting it to the brain.

Once the SA node has initiated an electrical impulse, the impulse spreads through the atria and causes them to contract. The contraction of the atria pushes blood into the ventricles, filling them and priming them for contraction. The electrical impulse then spreads from the atria to the ventricles via the atrioventricular (A-V) node. The A-V node delays the electrical impulse long enough for the atria to finish contracting and filling the ventricles with blood. Then the A-V node passes the electrical activity down specialized conduction pathways called "bundle branches" to the right and left ventricles. The ventricles then contract, pumping blood out to the lung (right ventricle) and the body (left ventricle). Finally, the heart cells ready themselves to receive another electrical impulse and to contract again.

The electrocardiograph (EKG) is a familiar and useful tool that measures the electrical activity of the heart from the body surface. Its output is a tracing called an electrocardiogram (also abbreviated EKG; *see Figure 6*). The different parts of this complex electrical pattern are caused by the electrical impulse initiated by the SA node passing through the various parts of the heart and are designated by different letters. The P wave is caused by the electrical impulse pass-

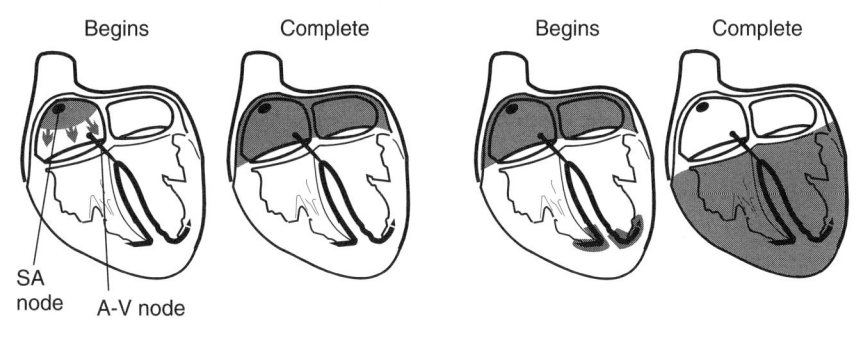

Figure 5. *Contractions begin in the contractile cells in the right atrium and spread to the left atrium. Left: Beginning and completion stages of atrial contraction. Right: Ventricular contraction.*

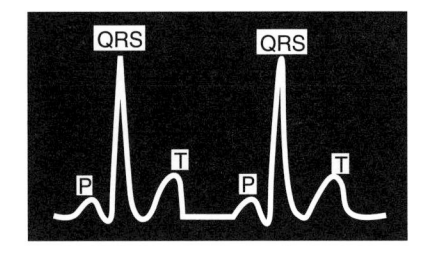

Figure 6. *A normal electrocardiogram is shown here. The first upward deflection is the P wave. Next comes QRS, the upward spike. The cycle is complete with the T wave. P is caused by the electric impulse passing through the atria; QRS is caused by the impules passing through the ventricles; the T wave is caused by the ventricles preparing for the next impulse.*

ing through the atria; the QRS complex is caused by the electrical impulse passing through the ventricles; the T wave is caused by the ventricles preparing for the next impulse.

Some minor irregularities in an EKG are normal. For instance, in many young people the SA node slows down slightly with an inhalation and speeds up slightly with an exhalation. However, other irregularities may be significant, and thus an EKG can help diagnose heart disease. For instance, diseases of the A-V node that delay the electrical impulse between the atria and the ventricles can widen the gap between the P wave and the QRS complex. In a disease called Wolff-Parkinson-White (WPW) syndrome, an abnormal band of conducting tissue connects the atria and ventricles so that the electrical impulse can bypass the delay of the A-V node. In WPW syndrome, therefore, the gap between the P wave and the QRS complex is abnormally brief. (WPW can affect young people; and even in a highly trained young athlete, it can cause episodes of extremely rapid heartbeat during exercise, producing palpitations—an alarming pounding in the chest. It can usually can be treated with medication, however, and a person with WPW can often continue to participate in athletics.)

Because the EKG provides so much useful information about the function of the heart, an athlete who seeks a physician's advice about symptoms that may be heart-related will often be given this test.

The Cardiac Cycle

The direction of blood flow through the heart, the opening and closing of the heart valves, and the spread of electrical activity are all part of the complete picture of how the heart contracts (*see Figure 7*, which shows the electrical and mechanical, or pressure, activity of the

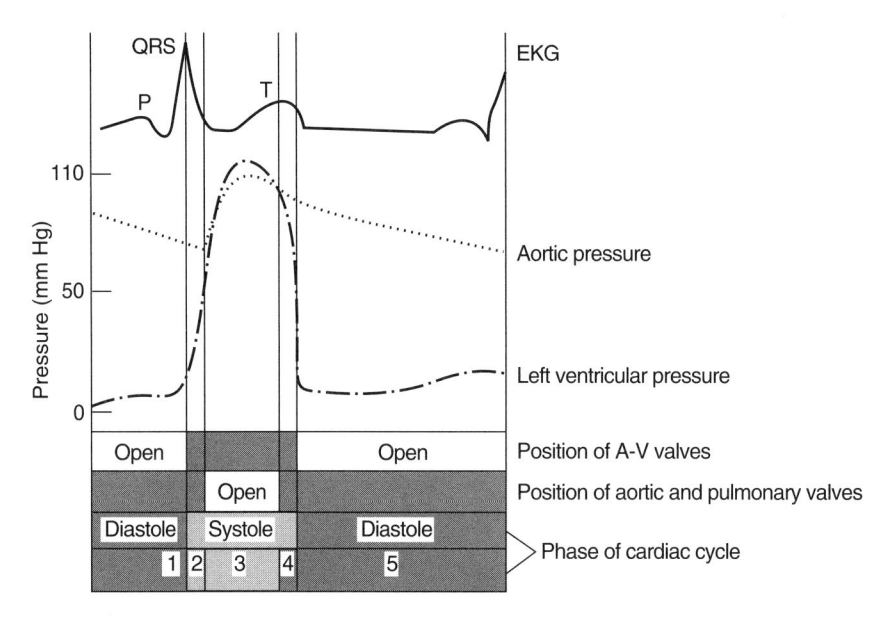

Figure 7. *The chronology of the cardiac cycle is as follows: (1) ventricular filling; (2) isovolumetric ventricular contraction; (3) ventricular ejection; (4) isovolumetric ventricular relaxation.*

heart from the left side; *and refer back to Figure 4*, which shows a single heart contraction).

The cardiac cycle (like the circulatory system, discussed earlier) is continuous, with no beginning or end. For convenience, this description will begin with the left ventricle full at the end of its relaxation period (diastole).

As the left ventricle begins to contract (systole), ventricular pressure exceeds atrial pressure and the A-V valve closes. Since ventricular pressure is less than aortic pressure, the aortic valve is also closed. The ventricle continues to contract with both valves closed. Since both the inflow and the outflow tracts of the ventricle are blocked by closed valves at this point in the cardiac cycle, the ventricle is contracting at a constant volume (isovolumetric contraction). During isovolumetric contraction, ventricular pressure rises rapidly until it exceeds aortic pressure. At this point, the aortic valve opens and the left ventricle pushes blood out into the aorta. The period during which the aortic valve is open and blood is being pumped into the aorta is called the ventricular ejection phase of systole.

Once ventricular ejection is complete and the ventricle begins to relax, ventricular pressure falls quickly. As soon as ventricular pressure falls below aortic pressure, the aortic valve closes. Now both valves are closed again. The ventricle continues to relax at a constant volume and ventricular pressure falls during the period of isovolumetric relaxation. Finally, ventricular pressure falls below atrial pressure and the A-V valve opens. Blood flows from the atria to the ventricle during the period of ventricular filling. At the end of ventricular filling the atria contracts, completing the process of delivering blood to the ventricle. The next cardiac cycle begins as the ventricle, now filled with blood, begins to contract again.

The Heart during Exercise

Benefits of exercise.
Most people are aware that exercise is "good for the heart." This section examines why.

The amount of blood pumped by the heart each minute—called the cardiac output—is found by multiplying the volume pumped with each beat (stroke volume) times the number of beats per minute (heart rate):

$$\text{Cardiac output} = \text{stroke volume} \times \text{heart rate}$$

In this equation, approximate normal values for an adult male at rest are as follows:

$$\text{Stroke volume} = 70 \text{ milliliters/beat}$$
$$\text{Heart rate} = 70 \text{ beats/minute}$$
$$\text{Cardiac output} = 4{,}900 \text{ milliliters/minute}$$

During exercise, the oxygen demands of the skeletal muscles increase as the work done by the muscles increases. As cardiac output

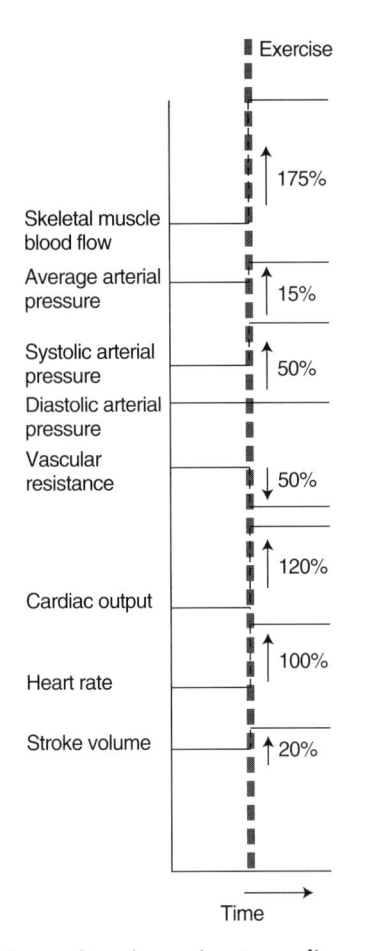

Figure 8. *Approximate cardiovascular changes that occur during exercise are shown here.*

increases to meet this increased demand for oxygen—to deliver the extra blood needed by the muscles—the heart is forced to work harder. Most of the increase in cardiac output comes from an increase in heart rate. Stroke volume increases to a lesser extent (*see Figure 8*).

Thus exercise puts additional stress on the heart, but for a normal heart, this is beneficial: it makes the heart stronger. Endurance athletes are a striking example of this beneficial effect. An endurance athlete's heart has a larger, stronger left ventricle, with thicker walls. Because of this physiologic adaptation, a trained athlete—in comparison with a sedentary person—has a slower heart rate at rest and a greater capacity to increase both heart rate and stroke volume with exercise. In consequence, the heart of an endurance athlete can deliver more blood, and thus more oxygen, to the muscles.

In terms of actual numbers, this difference can be dramatic. A sedentary person may reach a heart rate of about 195 beats per minute, with a stroke volume of about 113 milliliters (ml) per beat, for a cardiac output of 22,000 ml per minute. By contrast, during maximum exercise, at the same heart rate (195 beats per minute), a trained athlete can have a stroke volume of 179 ml per beat, for a cardiac output of 35,000 ml per minute. The difference is 37 percent.

Sudden death during exercise. In the early 1990s, a number of athletes died of during exercise because of cardiac problems; they included the volleyball star Flo Hyman; two basketball stars, Hank Gathers and Reggie Lewis; and the Russian skater Sergei Grinkov. These deaths led many people associated with sports to consider how physicians could identify athletes at risk. This is an important point, although to put the matter in perspective, it should be noted that for young people the risk of sudden cardiac death during exercise is actually very small: in the United States, where 25 million young athletes participate in various sports each year, there are fewer than 100 cases of sudden cardiac death. On the other hand, with improvements in safety equipment the number of deaths from sports-related trauma has declined so much that for high school and college athletes, cardiovascular disease is now the leading cause of death during sports activity.

The major cause of sudden cardiac death in young athletes is a poorly understood disease called hypertrophic cardiomyopathy (HCM)—meaning a disease of the heart muscle (*cardio*, "heart"; *myo*, "muscle"; and *pathy*, "disease") which involves abnormal thickening of the heart wall (*hyper*, "increased"; and *trophy*, "growth"). HCM usually runs in families, but its exact cause is not known. What is known is that during exertion a person with HCM may experience shortness of breath, fatigue, chest pain, dizziness, and fainting. HCM can be diagnosed with an echocardiogram, a simple test that uses sound waves to determine the size and shape of the heart. HCM can be treated with medication and, in some cases, surgery. However, people with HCM are at increased risk of sudden cardiac death and are generally advised to avoid extreme competitive exertion. For this reason, it is important for people who experience the symptoms of HCM during exercise to seek medical advice.

HCM is not the only disease of the heart muscles that poses a threat to athletes. Reggie Lewis's death, for example, was probably due to the fact that his heart had been enlarged and damaged by a common virus that causes respiratory infections. (Lewis, who was captain of the Boston Celtics, died in July 1993 at age 27.) The boxer Evander Holyfield, a heavyweight champion, retired in April 1994 at age 31 after being diagnosed with a heart disease unrelated to HCM. He returned to the ring, though, in 1996, defeating Mike Tyson and regaining his heavyweight title.

Drugs can represent another threat. Interactions between drugs taken concurrently—such as antifungal agents and antihistamines—can occasionally cause arrhythmias. Also, the abuse of stimulants such as cocaine can create a risk of heart damage and sudden death because these drugs act to produce sudden, extreme stimulation of the heart. Every athlete should be aware that drugs and sports are a potentially lethal combination.

When a young athlete has symptoms during exercise that may be related to the heart, an examination by a doctor is important. However, even the most dramatic symptoms, such as fainting, are rarely serious. Fainting, for instance, most commonly results from a drop in blood pressure and heart rate brought on by an overstimulation of the part of the nervous system that slows the heart (the parasympathetic nervous system; *see "Electrical Activity of the Heart," above*). This is called a vasovagal reaction, and it is related to the dizzy feeling most people have at some time experienced on standing up quickly from a lying or sitting position. Such dizziness is made worse by overheating, dehydration, and low blood sugar; thus adequate food and fluid intake during exercise may help prevent it.

Despite the occasional sudden death, then, getting regular exercise is one of the most "heart-healthy" lifestyle factors a young person can adopt. One important reason why a young athlete who is experiencing symptoms that may be heart-related should see a doctor, therefore, is simply to get a clean bill of health and resume activity.

The Arteries

The function of the heart is to supply blood rich in oxygen and nutrients to all the body tissues. This section will consider the arteries, which are the first part of the process in which blood moves from the heart to the body tissues—the process that allows the heart to meet the demands of the body. (The capillaries, which complete the process, are discussed later.)

The arteries function as conduits (analogous to pipes) that carry blood pumped by the heart to every organ of the body. Arteries are muscular, thick-walled tubes able to carry blood at high pressure; blood flows through them in waves every time the heart contracts.

The Arteries and Blood Pressure

When any fluid flows through a pipe, the pressure of the fluid within the pipe is the product of volume of flow through the pipe multiplied by the pipe's resistance to flow. For the cardiovascular system, this relationship can be expressed as follows: blood pressure (BP) equals cardiac output (CO) times vascular resistance (VR):

$$BP = CO \times VR$$

As this equation indicates, blood pressure (BP) will increase if either cardiac output (CO) or vascular resistance (VR) increases.

Cardiac output (CO) increases when the heart is stimulated by the sympathetic nervous system to contract more forcefully. For this reason, it can be expected that blood pressure will be increased by stress, fear, and anger, even if these emotional states are not accompanied by excessive muscle activity. Vascular resistance (VR) is determined by the arteries themselves. Exercise can cause the arteries to the skeletal muscles to dilate (increase in diameter), lowering vascular resistance and thus lowering blood pressure. A high-fat diet can cause the walls of the arteries to become stiff and incapable of dilating; this condition raises blood pressure.

As noted earlier, blood flows through the arteries in waves with each contraction of the heart. Therefore, blood pressure reaches a maximum value while the left ventricle is ejecting blood into the aorta—this is called systolic blood pressure. Blood pressure falls to a low value—this is called diastolic blood pressure—just before the next beat.

When blood pressure is measured, both systolic and diastolic pressure are recorded. Systolic pressure is noted first and diastolic pressure second, separated by a slash (/):

Systolic blood pressure / diastolic blood pressure.

The most common way to measure blood pressure is with a blood pressure cuff and a stethoscope (*see Figure 9*). The cuff is used to create pressure on the artery, and the stethoscope to listen to the flow of blood. The flow of blood is audible—that is, the blood makes a noise—only when it is passing through a narrowed artery. Obviously, there will be no sound if blood is not flowing through an artery at all; but it may be less obvious that blood flows silently—there is no sound—when it is passing through an unconstricted artery.

In measuring blood pressure, first the cuff is wrapped around the subject's upper arm. Then the stethoscope is placed over the brachial artery, which is located on the inner aspect of the arm in the crease of the elbow's bend (anticubital fossa). At this point, no sound will be heard from the blood flowing through this artery, because the artery

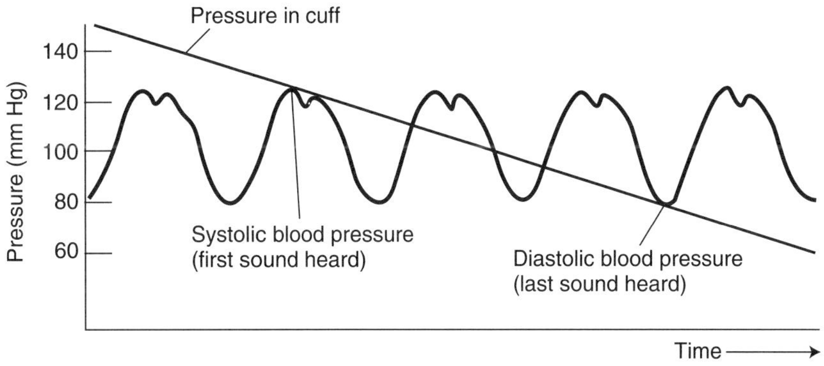

Figure 9. *Blood pressure changes in relation to cuff pressure. Blood makes a noise only if it is flowing through a narrowed artery. If it is flowing smoothly through an unconstricted artery, it will not make any noise.*

is unconstricted. Next, the cuff is pumped up with a handheld squeeze bulb until its pressure exceeds the subject's systolic blood pressure. If the subject is young and healthy, 150 mm Hg pressure (the amount of pressure needed to support a column of mercury 150 milimeters high) should be more than enough. At this point there is still no sound to be heard through the stethoscope: with cuff pressure greater than systolic blood pressure, no blood will flow through the brachial artery. Next, the pressure in the cuff is slowly relaxed. When the cuff pressure falls below the systolic blood pressure, blood will begin to squeeze through the artery under the cuff each time the heart beats. Now a swishing noise will be heard through the stethoscope as the blood moves through the artery, because the artery is partially compressed by the cuff. The pressure at which the "swishing" sound is first heard is systolic blood pressure. Next, the pressure in the cuff continues to be lowered. At the point where cuff pressure falls below diastolic blood pressure, the artery will no longer be compressed at all and the swishing sound will stop. This pressure is diastolic blood pressure. There is a range of normal values for systolic and diastolic pressure; however, one commonly reported "normal blood pressure" for adults is systolic = 120 mm Hg, diastolic = 80 mm Hg, or simply 120/80. For young people, blood pressure values of 90/60 or even slightly lower may be normal.

Blood Pressure during Exercise

Even before a person begins exercising, the anticipation of exertion causes the sympathetic nervous system to stimulate an increase in cardiac output. This will cause the blood pressure to rise. How the blood pressure responds when exercise actually begins depends on the activity.

Resistance exercises, such as weight lifting, stimulate the sympathetic nervous system but use only a relatively modest number of muscles for any given lift. In this kind of exercise, cardiac output increases with little decrease in vascular resistance. In fact, vascular resistance may even be elevated because the arteries carrying blood to the exercising muscles are compressed by the high, sustained force the muscles are generating. As a result, blood pressure may be as high as 225/150 during weight lifting.

> ## Off-Season Training
>
> Ideally, athletes should maintain cardiovascular fitness during the off-season. But in case they do not, coaches should make a preseason assessment of fitness before rigorous training resumes. It is best to test athletes often, to establish benchmarks. Following are some common tests for cardiovascular fitness:
>
> - Timed distance run, usually two or three miles.
> - Interval sprint run. A number of sprints of various distances (e.g., 10 to 400 yd. or m) over a half-hour period.
> - Treadmill run. This is particularly useful because it is easy to maintain a targeted heart rate. As athletes' fitness improves, they will perform more "work" at the same heart rate.

In aerobic exercises, the situation is quite different. Multiple intermittent contractions of large-muscle groups, such as the leg muscles during running, increase the oxygen demands of these muscles. The muscles respond to this increased oxygen demand by sending signals that cause their arteries to dilate. This allows more blood, carrying more oxygen, to flow to the working muscles. As an effect of this dilation of the muscle arteries, the vascular resistance is reduced. This reduction in vascular resistance partially balances the increase in cardiac output, so that blood pressure increases very little (*refer back to Figure 8*).

The increase in blood flow to the skeletal muscles during strenuous exercise can be as much as tenfold. This dramatic increase is accompanied by an increase in blood flow through to the coronary arteries—the arteries that supply oxygen to the heart muscle itself—because of the increased workload of the heart. Skin blood flow also increases, as the body tries to keep itself cool (*see ENERGY AND METABOLISM*, in which temperature control is discussed). At the same time, there are modest decreases in blood flow to organs not directly needed for exertion, such as the intestines and kidneys. However, the overall effect is that exercise increases the total blood flow to the body—the cardiac output.

The interplay of cardiac output and vascular resistance in determining blood pressure was illustrated in a rather dramatic experiment. The subjects were young, healthy athletes who were told to exercise to maximum exertion on an exercise bicycle in a temperature-controlled room. After a while, the temperature in the room was slowly increased. The higher temperature caused the athletes to overheat. Their skin arteries dilated to bring blood to the surface, in an attempt to cool it. The simultaneous maximum dilation of the muscle arteries and the skin arteries caused the subjects' peripheral resistance (the resistance to blood flow through the arteries) to fall very low. Despite their high cardiac output, their vascular resistance was so low that their blood pressure dropped. The experiment had to be abruptly stopped when the subjects' blood pressure fell so low that they fainted.

High Blood Pressure

High blood pressure—hypertension—is elevated blood pressure that can be caused by an increase in cardiac output, an increase in peripheral resistance, or both. Hypertension can often be treated successfully (*see below*), but if left untreated it can lead to heart failure, stroke, and kidney failure. Screening for hypertension is extremely important because in its early stages hypertension causes few if any symptoms.

Hypertension is sometimes considered a disease only of middle-age and elderly people. This is a misconception. It is true that over half of Americans over age 50 have hypertension, but this is also true of nearly 10 percent of people between ages 18 and 24. In fact, hypertension can occur in people of any age, and it can occur in athletes, including competitive athletes of high school and college age.

Some 85 percent of hypertension is of unknown origin (this is called essential hypertension); most of the remaining cases result from kidney disease. Hypertension seems to run in families, although environmental factors are also significant. It can be triggered by a variety of medications, including hormones (anabolic steroids and birth control pills), appetite suppressants, cold medicines, caffeine, the nonsteroidal anti-inflammatory drugs often prescribed for sports injuries, and illegal drugs. (Patients diagnosed with hypertension should discuss their use of drugs—even illegal drugs—with the physician.)

Hypertension, plaques, and coronary artery disease. People with hypertension often have fatty deposits called plaques on the inside walls of the arteries. These plaques narrow the arteries, increasing vascular resistance thus aggravating hypertension. Plaques also produce roughened areas on which blood clots can form, and a blood clot can further narrow or even completely block an artery. As an artery narrows, blood flow to the organ the artery supplies is restricted, with consequences that depend on the organ affected. For instance, a narrowing of the renal arteries, which supply blood to the kidneys, can destroy the kidneys; a narrowing of the arteries that supply blood to the brain can cause a stroke; plaques in the arteries leading to the penis can cause erectile dysfunction (impotence), because an erection is hydraulic—that is, accomplished by a large inflow of blood.

Plaques in the coronary arteries—the arteries that supply high-oxygen blood to the heart muscle itself—can have particularly serious consequences. It might be supposed that the heart extracts the oxygen it needs as it pumps blood through its chambers, but this is not the case: heart muscle, like any other muscle, is supplied with high-oxygen blood through its own arteries. These coronary arteries branch off from the aorta soon after this huge artery leaves the left ventricle; they run along the surface of the heart and then send off futher branches, deep into the muscle mass of the heart (*see Figure 10*). If the coronary arteries become blocked by plaques or blood clots (a condition known as coronary artery disease, abbreviated

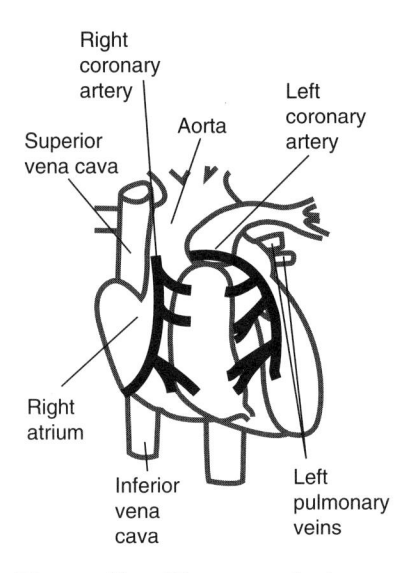

Figure 10. *Heart muscle is supplied with high-oxygen blood by its own arteries, the right and left coronary arteries. If the coronary arteries become blocked by plaques or blood clots, blood flow to the heart muscle is interrupted, the heart muscle becomes starved for oxygen, and a heart attack can ensue.*

CAD), blood flow to the heart muscle is interrupted, the heart muscle becomes starved for oxygen, and a heart attack can ensue. The technical term for a heart attack, *myocardial infarction*, is very descriptive of this process: *myocardium* means "heart muscle" and *infarction* means tissue death from lack of oxygen.

One warning sign of a heart attack is angina—the sharp, crushing chest pain that comes on during exertion. In young people, and even in middle-age athletes, most chest pain is not an indicator of a heart attack. In young athletes, chest pain is more likely to be caused by a muscle strain or a blow to the chest, though it may also be a result of a lung disorder such as asthma or pneumonia. Nevertheless, angina should never be ignored; the possibility that chest pain is caused by a heart attack or another heart problem may be remote, but the potential consequences are serious enough to warrant medical attention.

Treatment of hypertension and CAD. Typically, the initial treatment of hypertension involves weight loss, increased exercise, and a low-sodium (low-salt) diet. If these measures do not work, medication may be required. Many people advocate exercise as a treatment for hypertension, particularly mild hypertension. It has been found that people who are physically fit are less likely to develop hypertension. Thus, exercise may work directly to lower blood pressure, perhaps by encouraging the expansion of the muscle arterial network and thus decreasing vascular resistance. Exercise also may work indirectly to lower blood pressure: that is, a person who takes up exercise may be less likely to smoke or drink, may lose weight, may sleep better, and may react more positively to stress, and all these lifestyle factors can help decrease blood pressure.

To gain the most benefit from exercise, people with hypertension should design workouts for the specific goal of lowering blood pressure. For this purpose, aerobic exercise is much more beneficial than weight training; in fact, for a person with hypertension, weight lifting may be inadvisable because it is known to involve additional increases in blood pressure. People who are out of shape may find it difficult to begin an exercise program, but to be beneficial exercise does not need to be extremely strenuous. The usual guidelines for a person with hypertension are moderate exercise (55–70% of maximum heart rate) for 30 to 40 minutes five to six times per week. This schedule differs from the usual guidelines for aerobics: the exercise sessions recommended for hypertension are somewhat more frequent, somewhat longer, and somewhat less intense. A person who has just been diagnosed with hypertension and has not previously been active should discuss any proposed exercise program with the doctor before beginning.

Changes in lifestyle can also benefit people with coronary artery disease (CAD); such changes can actually help clean out their arteries. A low-fat diet combined with exercise and measures to reduce stress not only can keep CAD from getting worse but can even reverse it. Moreover, these lifestyle changes also alleviate angina and thus contribute to a more pleasant life.

The Capillaries

When the arteries reach their target organs, they divide into smaller and smaller vessels. Finally the arteries flow into the smallest blood vessels, the capillaries. The blood pressure in the capillaries is much lower than that in the arteries, and the capillaries have much thinner walls. These thin walls are necessary for oxygen to leave the blood and enter the cells and for carbon dioxide to leave the cells and enter the blood.

The capillaries differ from the arteries in another important way. Arterial walls do not allow any fluid to pass through them. However, capillary walls have gaps, called fenestrations, through which water and salt—though not blood cells or large protein molecules—can pass (*see Figure 11*). As the blood moves through the capillaries, some fluid is pushed out of the capillaries by the blood pressure. This fluid enters the interstitial space, that is, the space surrounding the body cells. However, the fluid that leaves the capillaries is protein-free, so the proteins that remain in the blood act as a sponge to pull this fluid back into the capillaries. The result is a constant balanced movement of fluid out of the capillaries into the interstitial space and from the interstitial space back into the capillaries. This fluid movement aids in the movement of nutrients and waste products between the blood and the body cells.

The fragile nature of the capillary walls and the dynamic balanced movement between the blood and interstitial fluid through those walls are of vital interest to the athlete. Skiers and mountain climbers at high altitudes commonly experience shortness of breath. After a few days at the high altitude, this usually goes away; but a few people develop a potentially life-threatening condition called high altitude pulmonary edema, abbreviated HAPE (*see also RESPIRATION*). The low oxygen levels at high altitudes cause the blood vessels of the lung to constrict. This increases the resistance to blood flow through the lung and increases the blood pressure in the lung capillaries. When

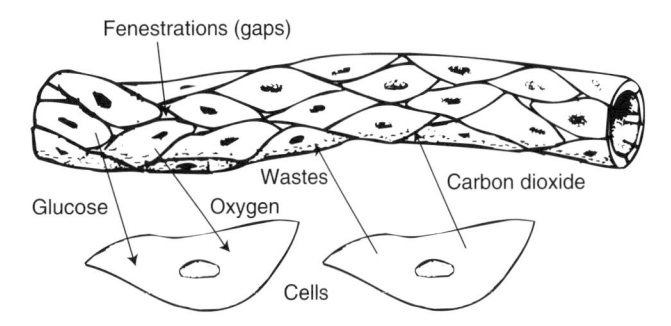

Figure 11. *Capillary action. The capillary walls have gaps (fenestrations) through which water and salt can pass (the gaps are small enough so that neither blood cells nor large protein molecules can pass through). Capillaries bring glucose and oxygen to the cells, and the cells send back carbon dioxide and wastes.*

this pulmonary capillary pressure rises, the force pushing fluid out of these capillaries increases and more fluid moves from the blood to the interstitial space of the lungs than can return. The lungs fill up with fluid—hence the term *pulmonary edema* (*pulmonary*, "of the lungs"; *edema*, "excess fluid")—and the person is unable to breathe. HAPE is a medical emergency; the victim must be given extra oxygen and evacuated to a lower altitude as soon as possible.

Another example of a disturbance in the balance of fluid movement between the capillaries and the interstitial fluid is seen with starvation: starving people, especially children, have stick-thin extremities and a swollen abdomen. Usually, a person who is starving continues to consume just enough calories to stay alive, but protein intake is no longer adequate. In this situation, a disease called kwashiorkor develops. Without sufficient protein intake, the body first breaks down muscle tissue; this leads to the wasting of the limbs (*see also* ENERGY AND METABOLISM). Next, the level of proteins in the blood begins to fall. When the blood protein level is low, the spongelike effect that pulls fluid back from the interstitial space into the capillaries is weakened. Fluid collects outside of the capillaries, particularly in the abdomen; this leads to the abdominal swelling referred to as nutritional edema.

The Veins

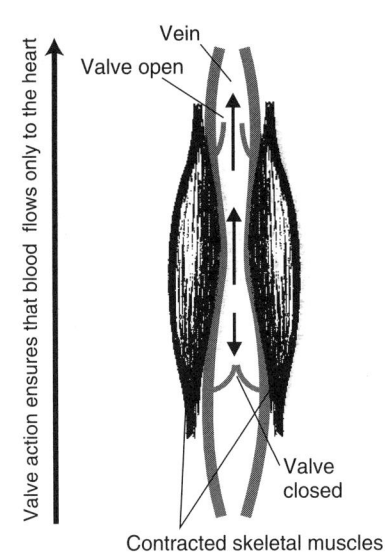

Figure 12. *Venous blood flow is so sluggish that the veins have one-way valves to keep the blood moving toward the heart. Contractions of skeletal muscles pump the blood, and the valves prevent it from flowing back as the skeletal muscles relax and prepare for the next contraction.*

The veins carry blood from the capillaries back to the heart. The smallest arteries and capillaries present a large resistance to blood flow. This resistance reduces the blood pressure as the blood moves from the arteries to the veins, much as a narrow section in a garden hose reduces water pressure in the part of the hose beyond the narrowing. Since the veins carry blood moving slowly and at a low pressure, their walls can be much thinner than the walls of arteries of similar size. Also, because the blood flow through the veins is so sluggish, the veins need one-way valves to keep the blood moving toward the heart (*see Figure 12*). One important force that pushes blood back through the veins to the heart is the contraction of skeletal muscles. When skeletal muscles contract, they raise the pressure in nearby veins. This contraction causes a local increase in venous pressure and pushes blood through the one-way valves back toward the heart.

The importance of skeletal-muscle contraction to the venous blood flow can be illustrated by a simple example: people with sedentary jobs may have problems with their veins. Commonly, the blood flow through the leg veins is so sluggish that eventually the blood backs up, causing the veins to bulge—varicose veins. People who have jobs where they remain sitting or standing in one spot are particularly prone to varicose veins because their leg veins do not experience the frequent muscle contractions needed for good venous flow. People who walk around on the job are somewhat less likely to have these problems. (For this reason, people with sedentary jobs should take the time to get up and walk around for a few minutes at regular intervals during the workday.)

One consequence of the slow blood flow through the veins that concerns athletes is the possibility of blood clots. Clots can form in the slow-moving blood of leg veins, and these clots are made more likely by dehydration and by minor trauma, which are both common during exercise. Dehydration can lead to clotting because fluid loss concentrates red blood cells, thickens the blood, and thus slows venous circulation. Trauma can trigger the beginning of the clotting mechanism. Common symptoms of blood clots in the leg veins are tenderness, swelling, and pain in the calves. It is important to recognize these signs as indicators of clots rather than simply attribute them to a pulled muscle. It is common to rub sore muscles, but rubbing an area with a vein blood clot could cause the clot to break off and travel to the heart or lungs.

High-altitude mountaineers are at particular risk of vein blood clots because they are exposed to the cold and subject to dehydration. These two factors combine to make blood flow in the leg veins sluggish, and that leads to blood clots. If these clots break loose and travel to the lungs (a lung clot is called a pulmonary embolism), they can partially block the pulmonary artery and decrease the efficiency with which the blood picks up oxygen. This serious problem is worsened by the low oxygen levels in the thin air at high altitudes. Pulmonary emboli have killed many expert mountaineers.

Bleeding

Since blood is such an important liquid, it is hardly surprising that the body has a complex and effective way to keep from losing it. When a small blood vessel is cut, specialized blood cells called platelets set off a series of chemical reactions within the blood that end with the formation of a clot which blocks the hole in the blood vessel. Pressure over the site of a cut can slow bleeding, making it easier for a clot to form. Once a clot has formed, no more blood is lost.

This process works well for cuts in small blood vessels. However, disruption of large blood vessels—which can occur as a result of sports trauma—are a serious matter. A healthy body will try to compensate for blood loss by increasing heart rate and vascular resistance in order to keep blood pressure and cardiac output from falling dangerously low (*see Figure 13*). This response can work until the blood loss becomes too severe. Adults have a blood volume of about 70 milliliters of blood per 1 kilogram (2.2 lb.) of body weight—or about 5 quarts (5 L) for a person weighing 150 pounds (68 kg). Loss of one-third of this amount (say, more than 1.5 qt.), even in a healthy athlete, can cause a serious drop in blood pressure, leading to circulatory shock and even death.

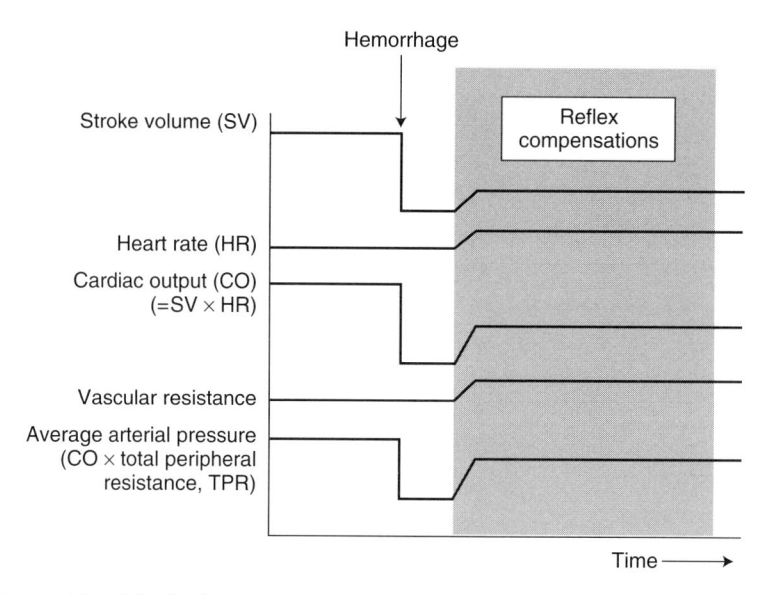

Figure 13. *The body tries to compensates for blood loss. To prevent blood pressure and cardiac output from falling dangerously, a healthy body will increase heart rate and vascular resistance.*

A person who is losing a significant amount of blood needs to have that loss stopped by a skilled surgeon, and to have the lost blood replaced. Salt solutions given intravenously can replace the volume of blood lost. However, virtually all of the oxygen in blood is carried bound to a protein within the red blood cells (this specialized protein is called hemoglobin). Thus, a person who has experienced extensive blood loss may require a transfusion of blood to restore the ability of the blood to transport oxygen.

Even when it does not involve a large amount of blood, bleeding may be life-threatening if it occurs in the wrong place. In the mid-1990s, this point was illustrated by two deaths. The first case occurred in the winter of 1993–1994 in the western United States, when a young skier fell into a steep, narrow mountain chute. He hit his chest hard enough, possibly against the rocks which bordered the chute, so that he dislocated a shoulder, fractured a rib, and severed the subclavian vein, a large vein in the chest. The bleeding from this vein collected in his chest, between the lung and the chest wall, collapsing one lung (and probably dispacing the contents of the chest toward the opposite side so that the remaining lung was compressed); unable to breathe, he died just before being rescued. The second case was that of the boxer Jimmy Garcia in the spring of 1995. During a fight, Garcia received multiple blows to the head, of such ferocity that they ruptured blood vessels supplying his brain. The bleeding that resulted was not massive, but because it was in the head it created enough pressure to compress and then destroy his brain. (Garcia died in May 1995. His death and similar recent events have renewed calls for protective headgear; *see also* BOXING.)

David E. Harris

References

Bernhardt, D., et al. "Chest Pain in Active Young People: Is It Cardiac?" *Physician and Sportsmedicine* 20, no. 4 (1994): 70ff.

Daniels, S., and J. Loggie. "Hypertension in Children and Adolescents." *Physician and Sportsmedicine* 20, no. 4 (1992): 97ff.

Guyton, A., and J. Hall. *Textbook of Medical Physiology*. Philadelphia: Saunders, 1994.

Maron, B. "Hypertrophic Cardiomyopathy in Athletes." *Physician and Sportsmedicine* 21, no. 9 (1993): 83ff.

McArdle, W., et al. *Exercise Physiology: Energy, Nutrition, and Human Performance*. Philadelphia: Lea and Febiger, 1986.

Van Camp, S. "What Can We Learn from Reggie Lewis's Death?" *Physician and Sportsmedicine* 21, no. 10 (1993): 73ff.

Vander, J., et al. *Human Physiology*. New York: McGraw-Hill, 1994.

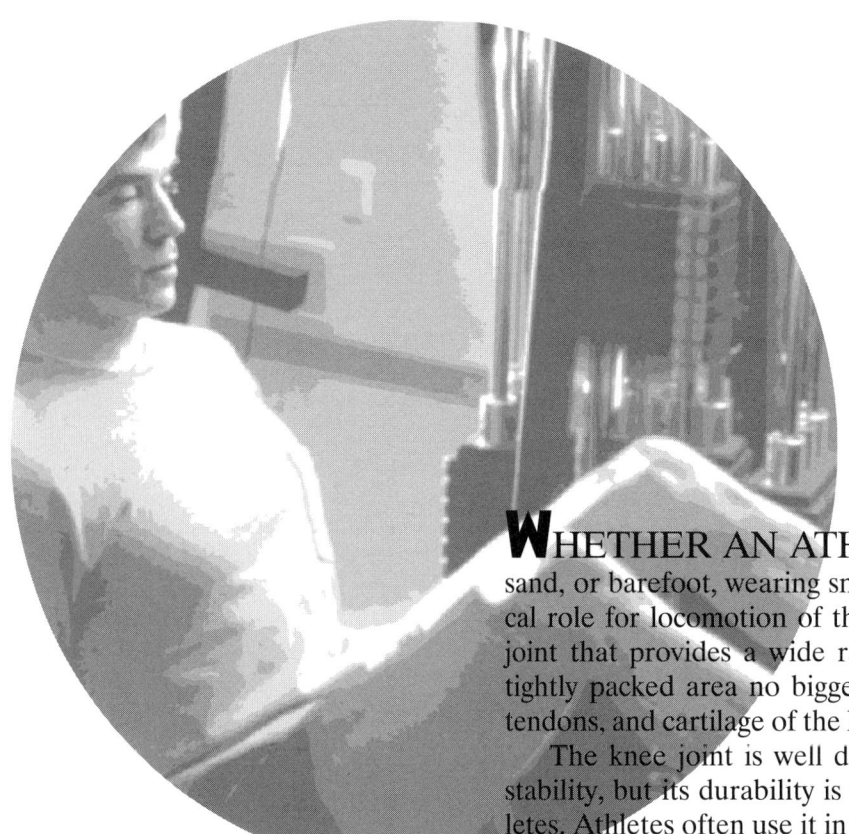

Knee

WHETHER AN ATHLETE is playing on grass, pavement, sand, or barefoot, wearing sneakers or on skis, the knee plays a critical role for locomotion of the human body. It is an efficient, stable joint that provides a wide range of motion and mobility. Within a tightly packed area no bigger than a softball, the bones, ligaments, tendons, and cartilage of the knee accomplish a variety of movements.

The knee joint is well designed for providing functionality and stability, but its durability is tested by the demands put on it by athletes. Athletes often use it in ways that place great stress on the joint. Some sports require repetitive twisting and turning movements that overuse the knee. Other sports, such as football, basketball, volleyball, and marathon running, force the knee to continually absorb impact from running, jumping, and collisions. Damage to the knee occurs when rigorous participation in these sports tests the outer limits of its ability to withstand stress.

Knee injuries are the most frequent serious extremity injuries in sports. According to the American Academy of Orthopedic Surgeons, knee injuries account for 26 percent of all sports-related injuries. They account for more time lost from competition than any other injury, and they end more athletic careers than any other injury. Many athletes retire from their respective sports with chronic pain in the knee joint or other knee dysfunction, chronic pain that can make the simplest tasks of everyday life difficult.

Functional Anatomy

The knee joint is the bridge linking the femur (thighbone) to the tibia (shinbone) and patella (kneecap). A group of strong, thick fibrous ligaments work like rubber bands to hold the joint together. They support and stabilize the joint against the forces moving it from side to side and back and forth. Figure 1 shows the ligaments surrounding the knee. The anterior patellar ligament and lateral and medial ligaments (collateral ligaments) provide external support, while internal support is provided by the anterior and posterior cruciate ligaments and the medial and lateral menisci.

The knee is one of the largest and most complicated joints in the body. Unlike a hinge joint, which allows movement only along one

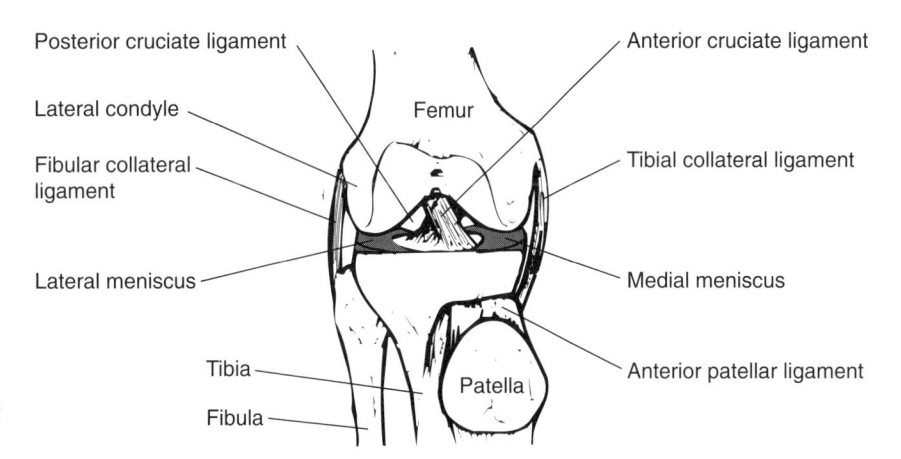

Figure 1. *Frontal view of the right knee with the patella flipped down.*

axis, the knee permits movement by bending (flexion) and straightening (extension), as well as rotating. When the knee is bent, the knee joint allows both inward (internal) and outward (external) rotation of the lower leg. Rotation is a vital part of many sports skills, such as kicking in soccer, twisting in ice skating, and turning in skiing. None of these actions would be possible without bending the knee slightly.

When the leg is fully extended, or locked, it not only restricts twisting motions but also becomes more vulnerable to injury from a blow to the leg. In this position, the ligaments in the knee are unable to effectively absorb the energy of a blow.

The knee joint, like the wrist, is able to bend, or flex, in different ways. Figure 2 shows that it can either roll along the back of the shinbone (a), or turn over the same spot of the shinbone (b). Although the end position (c) is the same in both cases, the knee starts out bending in different ways. In (a) the anterior cruciate ligament is fully stretched first, whereas in (b) the anterior cruciate ligament is stretched in unison with the other ligaments in the leg.

The crisscrossing anterior and posterior cruciate ligaments are extremely strong internal joint ligaments. The anterior cruciate liga-

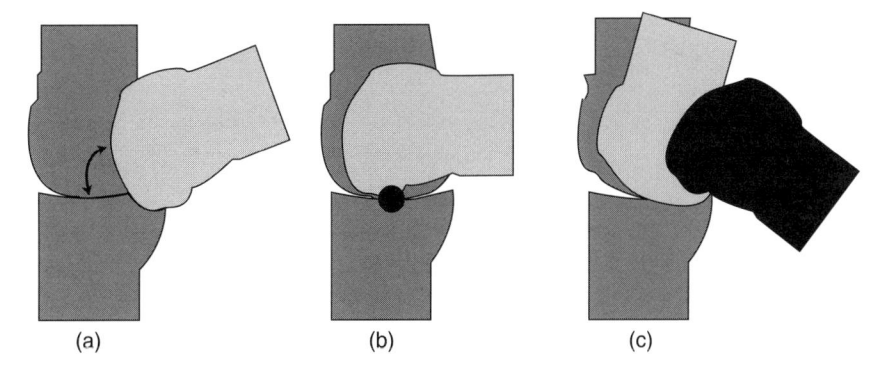

Figure 2. *In theory, the knee can flex in two different ways. The femur can roll along the tibia (a), or the femur can hinge or pivot off the same spot on the tibia (b). In practice, (b) usually follows (a). Once the femur rolls along a given distance, the anterior cruciate ligament becomes fully stretched, which then allows the second, hinge-like movement—during which the femur glides on the tibia (b). In combination, the knee bends about 135 degrees, to position (c).*

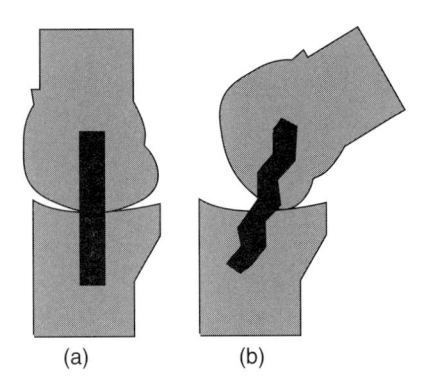

Figure 3. *During side-to-side bending, as one lateral ligament stretches (a), the ligament on the opposite side slackens (b). The lower leg rotates farther inward than outward because outward movements cause the anterior and posterior cruciate ligaments to twist about each other.*

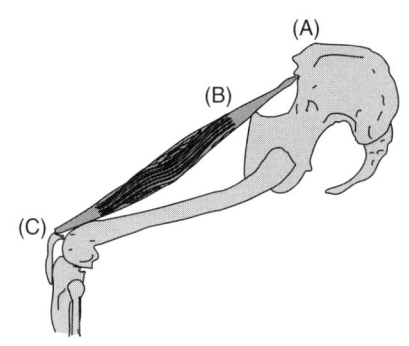

Figure 4. *The four muscles responsible for straightening the knee joint are called, collectively, the quadriceps femoris. They all have different insertion points. The rectus femoris (A) originates in the iliac (upper region of the pelvis). This muscle must be completely shortened to extend the leg in a horizontal plane. The other three thigh muscles that straighten the knee originate at the thigh bone ridge (B). All these muscles are attached to the patella by tendons, except for the internal thigh muscle, which is inserted directly into the patella.*

ment stabilizes the knee joint against movement of the lower leg forward in relation to the thigh, and the posterior cruciate ligament stabilizes the knee against a backward movement of the lower leg in relation to the thigh. A posterior cruciate ligament injury, although rare, can occur through certain impact injuries, as when a skier runs into the back of the lower leg of another skier, or when a soccer or hockey player collides with a stationary goalpost.

The two collateral ligaments prevent the knee from bending too far to either side. Of the two, the tibial collateral ligament is the longer and wider ligament, and it provides greater stability. The tibial collateral ligament also attaches to the medial meniscus (knee cartilage). Sideways bending makes these lateral ligaments taut on the stretched side and slack on the bending side (*see Figure 3*). Sideways movement is limited primarily by how far the collateral ligaments can stretch. As a backup, secondary lateral restriction occurs from the other ligaments. For example, the lower leg usually cannot rotate as much inward as outward because the cruciate ligaments restrict movement by twisting about each other during inward rotation (Wirhed, 1989).

The action of the knee joint is also dependent on how the femur sits on the tibia. The ellipsoid-shaped bottom of the femur sits on the rather flat upper end of the tibia. The two do not fit neatly together; a thick layer of cartilage on top of the shinbone fits between them around the end of the femur. Two crescent-shaped pieces of cartilage, the menisci, increase joint stability. The menisci are loosely anchored to the joint, which allows them to slide while the knee is straightening or bending. They move forward as the knee straightens and glide backward as the knee bends. Because the medial meniscus is attached to the medial collateral ligament, off-balance landings and collisions can put more load on one part of the meniscus and thus cause injury. Outward rotation on a bent knee can tear the meniscus by trapping it between the thigh- and shinbones. Inadequate integrity, caused by prior damage to the anterior cruciate ligament, contributes to the high incidence of meniscus tears.

A secondary function of the menisci is to distribute the load on the knee. The underside of each meniscus is shaped to evenly distribute the stress that the knee receives over the large surface area atop the tibia. When the shock-absorbing ability of the menisci deteriorates, the knee of an athlete involved in sports with excessive jumping, such as volleyball and basketball, may become more prone to injury.

While the ligaments and menisci are responsible for stability, muscles generate movement. A group of four muscles, known as the quadriceps femoris, is responsible for straightening the knee. It is considered a four-headed thigh muscle because each muscle in the group has a different point of origin near the hip joint (*see Figure 4*). Besides powering the straightening of the knee, the quadriceps femoris assists the ligaments in stabilizing the joint, so the femur glides within the concavity of the joint.

The muscles responsible for bending the knee are the three ham-

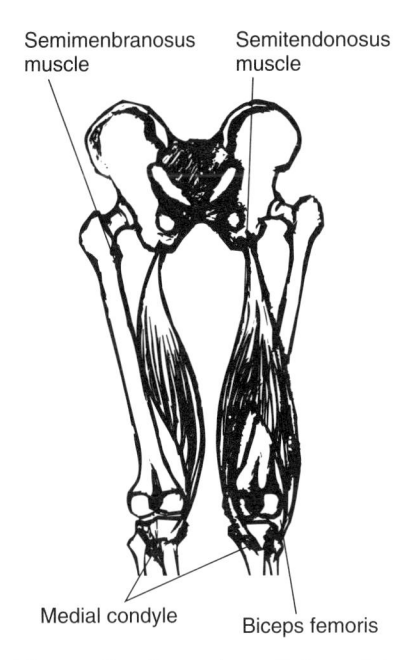

Figure 5. *Rear view of the pelvis showing, the three hamstring muscles responsible for bending the knee.*

string muscles: biceps femoris, semitendinosus, and semimembranosus (*see Figure 5*). The hamstring muscles work two joints. They serve as both knee flexors (bending muscles) and hip extensors (straightening muscles). This means that the way they function depends mainly on the position of the hip and knee joints. The biceps femoris inserts into the fibula, which allows it to rotate the lower leg so that the foot points outward. The other two muscles insert into the medial condyle of the tibia and allow the leg to rotate inward. A hurdler uses this inward rotating action to pull his lead leg inward as he clears a hurdle.

The hamstring and quadriceps muscles are the primary drivers of locomotion and are crucial to sprinting. As the body ages, these muscles do not necessarily lose their functionality, but the functionality of the joint itself declines. Some doctors believe that the knee is capable of withstanding only 35 to 40 years of use (Brody, 1989). The knee joint begins to deteriorate as the ligaments and tendons weaken and stretch and as the shock-absorbing menisci deteriorate. Thus, as the body ages, movement of the knee may become limited and cause pain. This 35- to 40-year span of functionality may be even shorter for athletes. The stress caused by years of flexing, rotating, pivoting, extending, shifting, running, jumping, and landing may damage the knee and prematurely end an athlete's career. The average career for players in the National Football League is about four years long, and few professional basketball players remain in the National Basketball Association longer than 10 years.

Pathophysiology and Treatment

An injury involving the knee is one of the most debilitating and most feared injuries for most athletes. Knee injuries can cause not only impairment in sports but also an inability to carry out everyday activities. However, proper treatment and therapy may lessen the severity of many knee injuries.

Despite some loss in functionality, collateral ligament sprains and tears usually heal satisfactorily. Healing of a sprained or torn ligament depends largely on the response of the tissue to injury. Sprains and tears alter the matrix structure (building blocks) of the ligaments, damage blood vessels, and injure cells. Hemorrhaging, or internal bleeding, starts a process of inflammation, repair, and rebuilding. Ligament injuries trigger a quick physiological response from the fibroblasts (tissue builders and binders) which quickly migrate to the injured tissue and clot. They replace the clot and the injured tissue with a loose fibrous matrix, which becomes progressively denser as it aligns along the lines of stress. The ability of the repaired ligament tissue to withstand pulling apart, known as tensile strength, increases as its collagen content increases.

Collateral ligaments heal quickly, but the interior cruciate ligaments that cross each other inside the knee joint heal more slowly and are more difficult to repair once torn. This difficulty is caused by limited blood supply to the internal anterior cruciate ligament relative to the external ligaments. When the anterior cruciate ligament ruptures, it often fails to heal properly. This may result in an unstable knee joint that requires a ligament reconstruction (insertion of dense fibrous tissue such as a tendon graft) at the site of injury.

Although ligament tears are common, repairing a torn meniscus accounts for about 90 percent of all knee surgeries. Problems occur when the meniscus becomes trapped in one area of the joint, restricting the movement of the joint as if one had lodged a pencil in the hinge of a door. The meniscus begins to deteriorate and impairs movement. The outer third of a healthy meniscus receives an active blood supply that helps grow new tissue in response to wear and tear, but its regeneration is slower than that of muscles. Though the quadriceps and hamstring muscles may gain mass and strength quickly through training, the connective tissue in the knee responds more slowly. Different tissues in the body adapt to the stress of exercise at different rates, and the meniscus happens to be one of the slowest (*see also* BODY COMPOSITION). Thus, rehabilitation from a meniscus injury can take a considerable amount of time.

Because cartilage heals poorly, a damaged meniscus is difficult to save, and surgeons did not usually attempt corrective surgery until the late 1970s. Instead, they would make a large incision into the knee and remove all or part of the meniscus. Unfortunately, taking out all the meniscus is like taking out the shock absorbers in a car. Moreover, the loss of the shock-absorbing capability of the meniscus hastens the onset of arthritis, and may eventually necessitate a total knee replacement. Arthritis usually follows a severe meniscus injury, but the rate of onset depends on the amount of cartilage removed. Patients undergoing less invasive partial excision usually can go many years without before the onset of arthritis, while complete meniscus removal may result in the onset of arthritis in a much shorter time frame.

In the 1970s and 1980s, a less invasive procedure, called arthroscopic surgery, was developed and refined, which allows surgeons to retain as much cartilage as possible. The arthroscope is several inches long and resembles a pencil. Designed like a telescope, with a series of lenses aligned above one another, it has optic fibers that give off a concentrated and directed source of light. Inserting an arthroscope into the joint requires only a very small incision. Another small incision is made to shave off and reshape the damaged areas and then remove the shaved cartilage. To enhance surgical precision, a camera attached to the end of the arthroscope projects an enlarged image of the internal knee joint onto a screen.

Doctors have found that in the long run, repair rather than removal is the most successful procedure, and partial removal is more effective than total removal. Because of the limited blood supply to the joint (nourishment comes from synovial fluid), surgeons in the

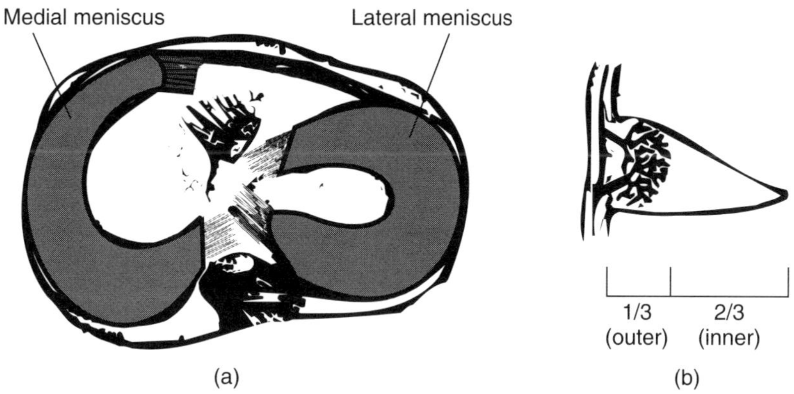

Figure 6. *The crescent shaped menisci from above (a) and viewed as a cross-section (b). Because of its less abundant blood supply, healing of the inner two-thirds of the meniscus is more difficult.*

Water on the Knee

Complicating most injuries to the knee is the synovium, the protective lining of the joint. It lubricates the joint by secreting a fluid with a viscosity, or resistance to flow, similar to olive oil. Loose pieces of meniscus or inflamed ligaments trigger the synovium to produce excess amounts of lubricant as a defensive mechanism. This causes stiffness and swelling in the joint, a condition often referred to as water on the knee. The skin around the knee swells outward and can be treated in most cases with ice, compression, and rest.

1970s believed that torn cartilage could never heal. In the 1990s, it is common for surgeons to perform repairs on the outer third of the meniscus, where the blood supply is plentiful and can support some healing (*see Figure 6*). The success rate for this type of surgery is about 80–90 percent, though it is lower for tears to the inner two-thirds of the meniscus. With some tears, after repairing the meniscus, surgeons may leave a small partly clotted drop of blood on top of the tissue. This clot contains natural "growth factors" that help healing by attracting progenitor cells (immature cells) to help close up the tear.

Despite the surgeons' best efforts, healing in the inner two-thirds of the meniscus is rarely achieved. In some cases, doctors have tried experimental techniques, such as meniscus transplants. Results have been generally positive because compared with many other types of tissue, cartilage is not as susceptible to rejection by the body's immune system after a transplant. Another alternative involves grinding up and re-forming the Achilles tendons of cows to create a fibrous sponge made up mostly of collagen, a naturally occurring protein, to replace the damaged meniscus. Other researchers have had some success in growing cartilage by isolating cells from healthy cartilage and taking cultures from these cells to produce new tissue. In one study (Hecht, 1994), results after 2 years ranged from good to excellent for 14 of 16 patients treated, including one professional hockey player and one bowler.

Prevention of Injuries

Experts estimate that about 600,000 people each year undergo arthroscopic surgery to diagnose and repair knee injuries, 68,000 have ligament reconstruction surgery, 30,000 undergo procedures to realign the joint, and 75,000 undergo knee replacement surgery. Many of these injuries are the result of injuries received in sports. Unlike most other sports-related injuries, knee injuries are not as easy to prevent through strength and flexibility training. The knee joint benefits from such training to a point, but beyond that, the pre-

Common Knee Injuries

The knee, one of the most frequently injured parts of the body, accounts for more time lost from competition than any other injury. It can be difficult to diagnose the severity of a knee injury, but advances in arthroscopic and ligament reconstructive surgery have significantly improved surgeons' ability to treat knee injuries.

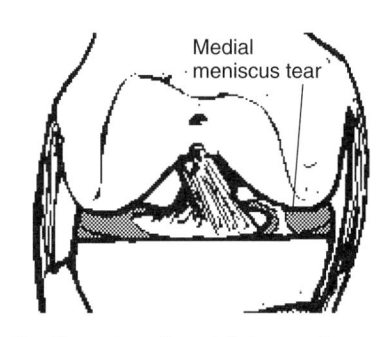

Cartilage (meniscus) injury. A tearing of the medial or lateral meniscus can cause the knee to give way, snap, or sometimes lock up. Twisting or rotations are the usual causes of this injury. A pencil-sized device called an arthroscope is inserted through a small incision to remove or repair the damaged cartilage. This relatively noninvasive technique causes minimal damage to the joint. This has cut rehabilitation time down from several months to a few weeks.

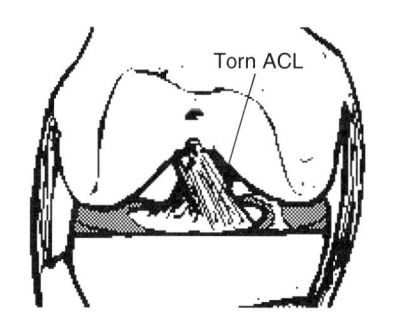

Anterior cruciate ligament (ACL) tear. Any type of ligament tear is a severe injury, but the ACL is perhaps the most severe. Despite recent advancements in surgical techniques, an athlete who experiences an ACL tear may never be quite the same, because the ACL is a key ligament in a healthy, athletic knee. This injury strikes athletes of every size, strength, and weight, from the 90-pound gymnast to the 300-pound football tackle. Although strength training helps some athletes, this injury is not preventable. Quick plants, pivots, blows, and awkward landings all can "pop" this ligament.

---

ventive effect is negligible. In fact, improper or excessive training poses a much greater risk than insufficient training. Exercise can be looked at as a double-edged sword: vital to strengthen the knee, hazardous if done incorrectly or in excess.

Excess weight is another risk factor for knee injury. Whether a person weighs 200 pounds or 300 pounds, the anatomical structure of the knee joint is about the same, but a 300-pound person inflicts a much greater gravitational force over approximately the same given area than a 200-pound person.

Strength and Flexibility Training

To prevent injuries to the knee, athletes should engage in exercises that strengthen the soft tissues surrounding the knee and the quadriceps and hamstring muscles that straighten and bend the knee. Whether for prevention or rehabilitation, it is best to construct an exercise program that concentrates on putting the greatest stress on the leg while it is fully extended. Deep knee bending exercises can be dangerous because the force pulling the kneecap over the thighbone can be four to five times body weight (Wirhed, 1984). But, though

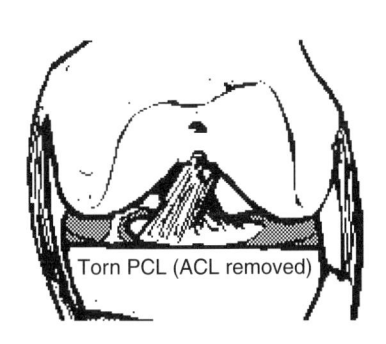

Posterior cruciate ligament (PCL) tear. This ligament, located in the back of the knee joint, is much less likely to sustain injury than other ligaments. It occurs most often in sports such as football, soccer, and skiing, and can occur in conjunction with a tear of one or more of the other three ligaments.

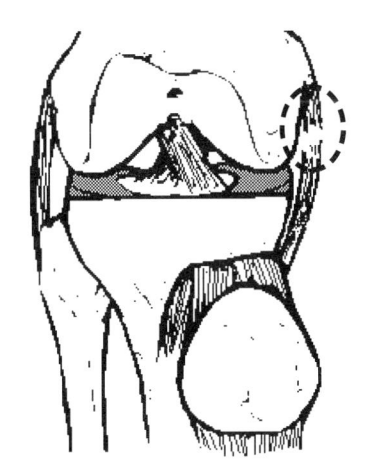

Medial collateral ligament (MCL) tear. Because the MCL is vulnerable to impact and the stresses put on it during quick lateral movements, medial collateral ligament (MCL) tear is a common injury. The tear can occur near the thighbone, near the joint, or along the shinbone. When doctors refer to knee sprains, they mean the stretching of the medial or lateral collateral ligaments. It is often difficult to diagnose whether an injury is a tear or a sprain.

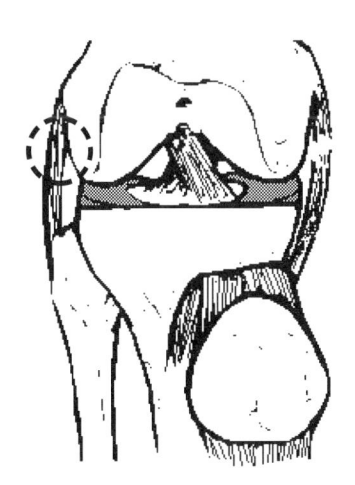

Lateral collateral ligament (LCL) tear. This ligament is located along the outside of the leg. Although tears to it are not as frequent as tears to other ligaments, they can result in permanent nerve damage, a partial paralysis called "drop foot." The ligament is less frequently injured because it is not as vulnerable to impact and stretches less when "cutting" off the outside foot than the MCL.

even a moderate bending of the knees can create a significant force pulling the kneecap over the thighbone, half-squat exercises have proven to be very effective for strengthening the muscles, tendons, and ligments surrounding the knee (*see Figure 7 and STRENGTH TRAINING*).

Strength training can help prevent both traumatic and overuse injuries. About 30 percent of the 15 to 30 million joggers in the United States suffer from overtraining syndrome, also known as runner's knee. This condition is most common in athletes who increase their level of exertion too quickly. Overtraining occurs when the rate of stress exceeds the rate of adaptation and may seriously injure the knee. By incrementally increasing stress loads, athletes may be able to condition the connective tissue in knees to the stress. The knee is a much more complex joint than the elbow. It must do more, too. It bears more weight and withstands collisions when the leg is planted.

Because repair and rehabilitation of a serious knee injury can cost from $20,000 to $50,000, many Rocky Mountain ski resorts require leg-strength tests before hiring ski instructors and ski patrollers. Leg-strength testing involves not only testing for total leg

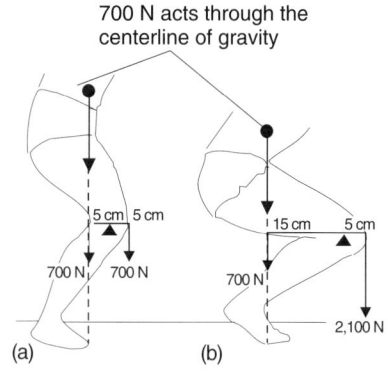

Figure 7. *For a minimum knee bend (a), the center of gravity lies 5 centimeters behind the axis of motion of the knee joint. This requires the quadriceps muscle to create a contracting force to prevent the athlete from sitting down. The quadriceps muscle's lever arm and the gravitational lever arm both lie 5 centimeters from the pivot point, the joint's center. The quadriceps therefore must exert a force equal to the gravitational force acting through the center of gravity (700 newtons) to keep the body in balance. In the moderate knee bend (b), the gravitational lever is 15 centimeters from the joint while the quadriceps' lever arm remains 5 centimeters from the joint. A lever arm three times shorter requires the quadriceps muscle to exert a contracting force three times as great (2,100 newtons). Because of these dynamics, half-squat exercises are a very effective way to strengthen the muscles, tendons, and ligaments surrounding the knee. (Adapted from Wirhed, 1984)*

strength and endurance, but also for strength balance between the legs, and between the quadriceps and hamstring muscles. In a 1983 preseason test, 491 of the 623 employees at Vail, Colorado, showed adequate strength and endurance for skiing. Out of the 132 who showed deficiency, it was usually in one leg. At the end of the season, only 0.8 percent of the employees judged to possess adequate strength experienced a knee injury, while 18.9 percent of those with deficiencies experienced injuries (Nelson, 1989).

Recreational athletes, as well as professionals, benefit from proper strength and flexibility training. Forgoing it increases the risk of secondary and more serious injury. Orthopedic surgeons recommend the athletes return to action only after building up the strength and endurance of quadriceps and hamstring muscles. They also recommend that athletes wait until the injured leg has attained about 90 percent of the uninjured leg's strength before returning to play.

Stretching and warm-up exercises also play a crucial role in preventing knee injury because they prepare the muscles and joints for a high level of stress. Warm-up exercises raise the temperature of muscles and joints and make them more pliable, conditioning the muscles and connecting tissue. Muscles work best at their maximum length. For example, a runner with tight or shortened muscles experiences a restricted stride length and a decline in fluidity, which forces the knee joint to do more of the shock-absorbing work. Ten to 15 minutes of pre- and postcompetition stretching can significantly reduce injuries.

Knee Braces

Knee braces are designed to absorb some of the force that would otherwise stress the knee ligaments, and braces have become common among both recreational and professional athletes in the 1990s. Myriad versions of knee braces and supports are worn on football fields, basketball courts, and ski slopes (*see Figure 8*).

Tests of the effectiveness of knee braces have been largely inconclusive, however. Designing studies is difficult because of a wide range of extraneous variables affecting rates of injury, such as physiological conditioning, conditions of use, preexisting physical problems, and congenital predisposition to injury. Another major variable is the wide variety of playing surfaces and playing conditions.

Though there have been conflicting data on the topic, the American Academy of Orthopedic Surgeons reached a consensus in 1994 that the use of prophylactic braces has not been proved effective in reducing the number or severity of knee injuries. Nonetheless, most doctors recommend the use of braces in rehabilitation. These braces allow for physical therapy involving controlled joint motion after surgical and nonsurgical treatment of knee injuries. Once sufficient knee strength develops, therapy can proceed without the brace.

The experts have not reached a consensus on the merits of functional knee braces. Like the prophylactic braces, functional braces are designed for use while playing. Except for the psychological ben-

Jumper's Knee: Pain That Comes with the Territory

Probably the most common chronic injury among basketball and volleyball players is patellar tendinitis, commonly called jumper's knee. Continual jumping takes its toll, and over time, many players complain of persistent pain in the knees. Because National Basketball Association (NBA) players participate in more than 100 games a year, and twice as many practices, almost every player experiences this condition to some degree. Its prevalence has led players to humorously refer to jumper's knee as the official injury of the NBA. Volleyball players are perhaps even more prone to the injury because "blocking" and "spiking" entail hundreds of jumps a game. Patellar tendinitis is the result.

When a basketball or volleyball player jumps, the musculoskeletal structure of the body must absorb tremendous impact, a force five to six times the jumper's body weight. An average player jumps 20 to 30 times a game, plays over 100 games a season, and practices 200 or more times a year. The resulting wear and tear leads to injury. Additionally, the airborne player often lands in an off-balance position (e.g., on one foot), so the force of impact often must be absorbed over a smaller area.

The patellar tendon acts as one of the most important shock absorbers for the body, absorbing much of the impact of the jumper's landing. When a player jumps repeatedly, the impact of landing creates oscillations (vibrations) of the patellar tendon, which eventually result in jumper's knee. Fatigue plays a part, too. When the fatigue of competition sets in, muscles do a poorer job of absorbing shock, leaving more work for the tendons and ligaments.

The first sign of the condition is pain and tenderness below the kneecap and over the patellar tendon. Continual stress on the knee causes micro-tearing of the attachments of the tendon to the bone. Although the symptoms of jumper's knee usually subside with rest, surgery is performed in severe cases to remove calcification and scar tissue, or to increase the blood supply to the tendon. This corrects circulatory impairments that may prevent proper healing.

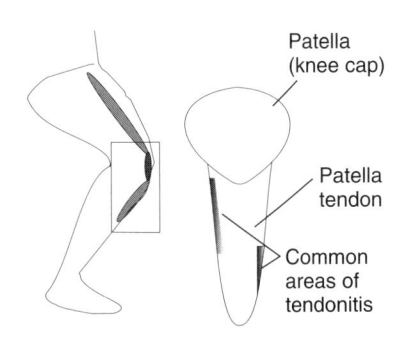

To prevent the onset of jumper's knee, athletes must improve their strength and conditioning, perfect their landing technique, and stretch adequately prior to activity. During the off-season, the injury should be treated with ice and, more important, rested. During the season, many athletes choose to play with this injury. Players who decide to play with the pain should ice down their knees after play and limit their anti-inflammatory medications to over-the-counter drugs such as acetaminophen or aspirin. Continuing to play with pain can lengthen recovery time if further damage to the tendon occurs.

Some experts believe that a different playing surface or subfloor may help prevent knee injuries. Most arenas' hardwood floors are laid over ice or sit on a concrete base. Like the "tuned" tracks now used by runners, a better "tuned" basketball and volleyball surface may reduce the incidence of patellar tendinitis. Of course, to change to a floor with a different surface compliance (the coefficient of restitution or rebound ability) also could affect how the basketball bounces. Either players would have to adjust to a different bounce, or the ball's pressure would need to be adjusted.

Replacing hardwood floors may end a basketball tradition, but a similar change was a boon to the sport of tennis. High-tech composite rackets significantly improved the performance of most players and contributed to a significant drop in the incidence of tennis elbow (overuse tendinitis). A materials science solution may not eliminate jumpers' knee injuries, but it may curtail them.

efits, such as fostering a feeling of confidence, there is limited scientific evidence that functional knee braces help the healing process by preventing further injury. Strengthening the muscles that hold the knee together is far more important in preventing knee injuries.

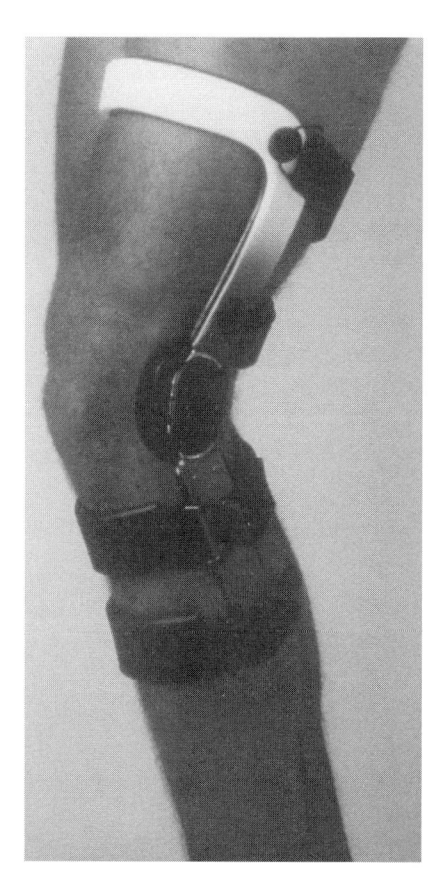

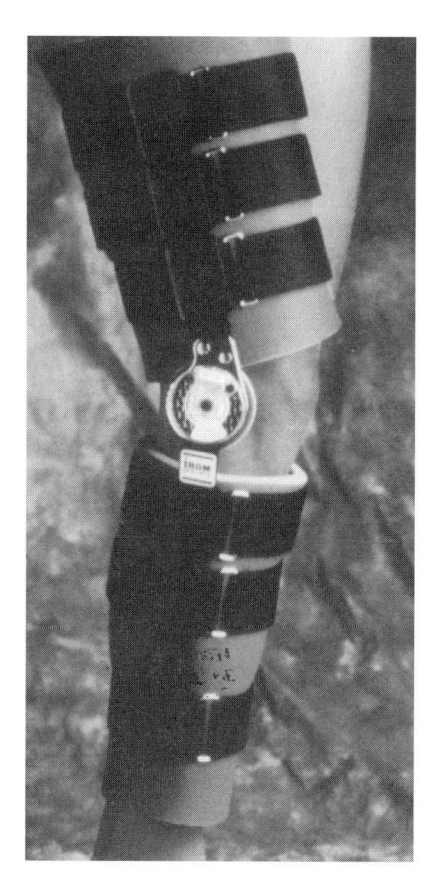

Figure 8. *Two types of knee braces used in rehabilitation and during sports are pictured here. Left: A functional brace is designed to protect damaged knee ligaments from stress. Sturdy bands around the thigh and calf hold it in place and prevent rotation of the knee. It is particularly helpful in protecting the medial collateral ligament. Right: A rehabilitative brace is used to restore mobility after injury or surgery. It has very wide bands around the thigh and calf, and the hinges can be gradually loosened during healing. (Photo courtesy of Smith & Nephew Don Joy, Inc.).*

An athlete's choice of knee brace should depend on the following variables: speeds, loads, and instability encountered while participating in the sport (because some braces offer more lateral support while others are better for anterior-posterior control); comfort, durability and ease of use; and correct fit, because slippage decreases the effectiveness of the brace and might even cause injury elsewhere.

Many athletes opt for a custom brace, but a custom-designed brace does not guarantee avoiding slippage. The cost of a custom-fit functional knee brace ranges from $400 to $1,000, not including the physician's services. In many cases, physical therapy to strengthen the knee may be a better investment because it treats the cause of injury rather than the effect. It provides prevention at the point of weakness, the source of the problem.

John Zumerchik and David H. Janda, M.D.

References

Baker, B. "Prevention of Ligament Injuries to the Knee." *Exercise and Sport Science Review* 18 (1990).

Brody, J., "The Human Knee Is Not Built to Last as Long as the Rest of the Body, but Its Life Can Be Extended," *New York Times*, 28 September 1989, sec. 2, p. 15.

Brown, E. "Transplants May Offer Help for Knee Injuries." *AMA News,* 16 March 1990, 17.

Duff, J. *Youth Sports Injuries: A Medical Handbook for Parents and Coaches*. New York: Macmillan, 1992.

Hecht, J. "Cartilage Culture Mends Damaged Joints." *New Scientist* 144 (29 October 1994): 25ff.

Nelson, J., "Care and Heeding of Knee Injuries," *New York Times*, 4 December 1989, sec. 3, p. 13.

Rosenthal, E., "Mending and Replacing Torn Cartilage in the Knee," *New York Times*, 11 November 1992, sec. C, p. 14.

Wirhed, R. *Athletic Ability and the Anatomy of Motion*. New York: Wolf Medical, 1984.

Zueler, W. "Knee Bracing." In R. Bushbacher and R. Braddom (eds.), *Sports Medicine and Rehabilitation*. Philadelphia: Hanley and Belfus, 1994.

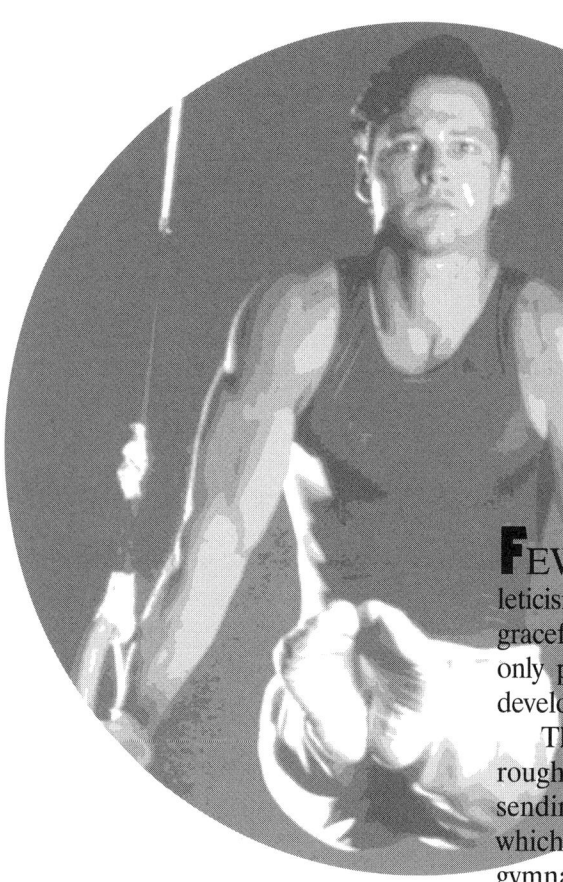

Motor Control

FEW ATHLETES IN ANY SPORT can match the sheer athleticism of gymnasts. A gymnast flips, twists, curls, and swings through a graceful routine that has been perfected through years of practice—and only practice can lead to such perfection, because only practice can develop the necessary motor control.

The gymnast's movements are controlled by the brain, which is roughly half the size of a football. The brain controls movement by sending signals throughout the body through the nervous system, which in turn controls the muscles. When all goes well, this allows the gymnastic maneuvers to be executed flawlessly.

Of course, not everything always goes according to plan. When movements diverge from a plan, feedback mechanisms come into play. Sensory signals from the eyes (visual signals), ears (auditory), skin (tactile), and vestibular system (inner-ear balance and orientation) provide information to the brain so that it can in turn send back a signal for a "recovery strategy." Thus in the motor control system, traffic flows in two directions: the brain sends signals to the muscles, and the muscles send feedback to the brain. For example, if the hands start to slip from the uneven parallel bars, the gymnast can recover by adjusting body movements—compensating for the unbalanced position—in order not to fall. Every movement, then, is a result of numerous control systems that interact continuously and extensively.

Motor control includes all the internal and external signals and feedback mechanisms that result in body movement. It is often studied in the context of a particular motor activity, in which there are two areas of primary concern: speed and precision. Speed is often useful and sometimes crucial, as when a boxer must quickly raise an arm to block a punch. Precision is essential when, for instance, a golfer needs to sink a 60-foot (18-yd.) putt. Often, athletes need both speed and precision: a batter, for example, needs speed to get the bat around in time to react to a fastball, and precision to get the bat in the right place to make contact.

To understand a movement—which is a result or an end—it is first necessary to understand the nerve action involved: the means necessary to achieve the end. Thus, after a brief introductory description of theories of motor control, this article gives a basic description of the nervous system in general. Next it discusses the central nervous system and motor control; then, the sensory system and motor con-

Motor Control: Speed and Precision

Mark Wohlers, a pitcher for the Atlanta Braves, could throw a blazing fastball—it was clocked at 99 MPH (nearly 160 KPH). After such a fastball left Wohlers's hand, the batter had less than 0.2 second to decide whether or not to swing. This illustrates the fact that to be effective, the nervous system must not only exert precise motor control over the muscles and joints but also must act extremely quickly.

trol. Finally, it offers some insights into the developmental learning processes involved.

Theories of Motor Control

Unless an injury or a disease affects our ability to move, most of us take movement for granted. In fact, motion is so much a part of life that it was long believed to define life; the seventeenth-century scientist Blaise Pascal once wrote: "Our nature consists in motion; complete rest is death." Still, many people have been curious about what makes movement possible. To understand the nature and cause of movement, neurophysiologists and others have been investigating the mechanisms of motor control for over a century. Today, there are a number of approaches to motor control, but two widely accepted theories—"ecological theory" and the "systems approach"—are at the core of most research.

Ecological Theory

The ecological theory of motor control focuses on our perception of the environment and what is necessary to carry out a particular motor task in a particular environment. This theory is based on the idea that motor control evolved so that animals and humans could move effectively to find food and shelter, to flee predators, and even to play. Ecological theory stresses how a person uses information from the environment and processes this information in order to initiate, modify, and control movement.

Ecological theory has widened our understanding of how the nervous system functions to influence our perception of the environment in which we are operating (such as a basketball court, a soccer field, or a ski slope) in order to perform a given task effectively.

Systems Approach

The systems approach, or systems theory, is based on the idea that human movement results from the interaction of a person, a particular motor task, and the environment within which the task is performed. Its premise is that movement is a result of highly integrated interactions among body systems. These body systems have perceptual, cognitive, and action components, and they include the neuromuscular and musculoskeletal systems. A neurophysiologist who takes the systems approach, for example, might examine how a soccer player's motor control over the legs and feet is affected when the player is kicking a ball on a wet, poorly lit field.

The Nervous System

The nervous system is the foundation for—the basis of—motor control. Whenever an athlete somersaults, hits a tennis ball, fires off a jump shot, or clears a hurdle, a tremendous amount of muscle coordination is taking place, and it is the nervous system that must provide the messages needed to coordinate muscular activity for such complex movements.

Divisions of the Nervous System

The nervous system, the coordinator of complex movement, is a network of cells extending from the brain throughout the body (*see Figure 1*). This system is the means by which information is communicated within the body, in the form of electrical impulses that travel back and forth between the brain and the periphery of the body.

The nervous system has two main divisions: the central nervous system (CNS) and the peripheral nervous system (PNS). The central nervous system includes the spinal cord and brain. The peripheral nervous system extends from the spinal column and innervates the body and extremities.

The peripheral nervous system consists of two subdivisions: the somatic nervous system and the autonomic nervous system. The somatic nervous system is concerned with voluntary movements of the skeletal muscles and communication to and from the sense organs. Sensory information is carried from the eyes, ears, joints, and skin to the CNS by the afferent nerves; information is carried back from the CNS to the skeletal muscles through the efferent nerves. Thus, the somatic nervous system plays a major role in voluntary actions such as throwing a ball or walking up a flight of stairs.

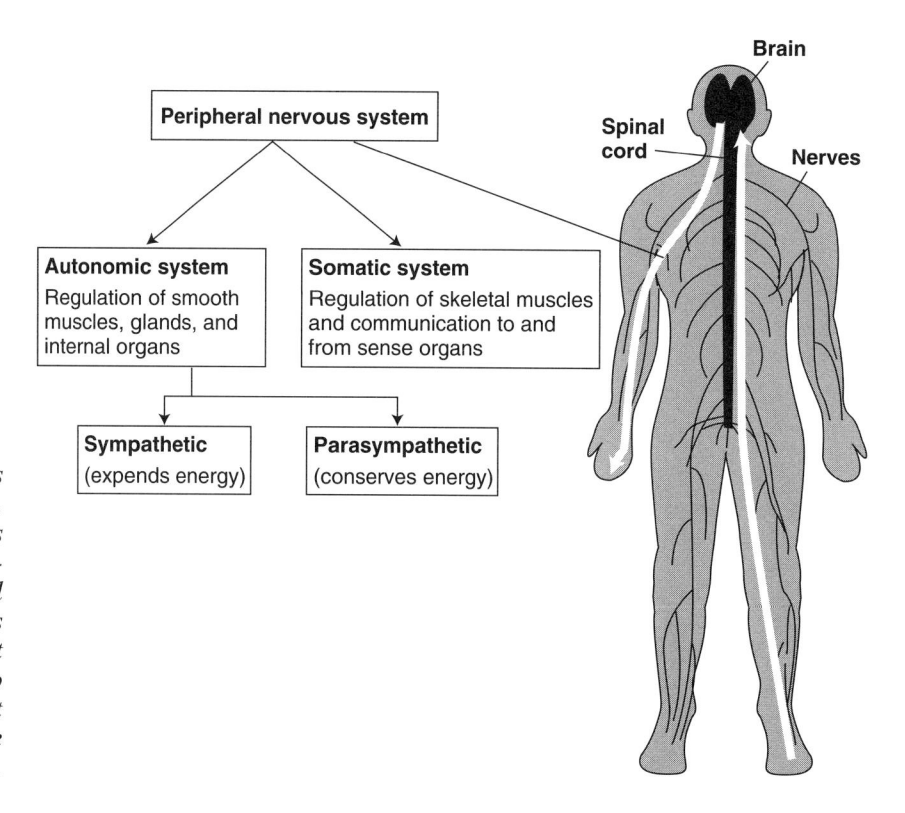

Figure 1. *The nervous system has two divisions: central and peripheral. The central nervous system includes the brain and spinal cord; the peripheral nervous system extends outward from the spinal cord and innervates the body and extremities. Afferent nerves carry sensory information to the central nervous system; efferent nerves carry information from the central nervous system to the muscles.*

The autonomic nervous system regulates the body's internal environment: for example, it controls the smooth muscles, the glands, and the internal organs such as the heart and lungs. Nerves of the autonomic nervous system carry information from the organs to the CNS.

The nerves carrying information back from the CNS are further subdivided into the sympathetic division and the parasympathetic division. Sympathetic nerves prepare the body to respond to threatening situations; this is sometimes called the "flight or fight" response. The sympathetic nervous system carries the signals from the brain that cause the heart to beat faster, breathing rate to increase, blood pressure to rise, digestion to slow, pupils to dilate, and adrenaline to be pumped into the blood. For early humans, this sympathetic arousal would have occurred when, for example, a predator was confronted. Modern humans more commonly experience this reaction in situations like public speaking and, of course, in sports—before tipping a jump ball in a basketball game, or before starting down a slalom course in skiing. In short, the sympathetic nervous system mobilizes the body for action. By contrast, the parasympathetic nervous system serves to conserve bodily energy; therefore, in many ways its functions are opposite those of the sympathetic division. For example, the parasympathetic nerves serve to slow heart rate and breathing, lower blood pressure, and promote digestion.

When discussing the nervous system, physiologists often divide the system into two distinct parts that work in concert: the motor system and sensory system. The motor system controls contraction of muscles throughout the body, everything from simple reflexive movements to very complex skilled movements. The sensory system helps guide those movements: it provides a means by which the nervous system can interpret the world.

Anatomy of the Neuron

The nervous system—both the motor system and the sensory system—is composed of billions of tiny nerve cells called neurons. Neurons have some of the same characteristics as other cells in the body, but they also have unique characteristics that allow them to carry out specialized functions. The basic neuron consists of a cell body (including nucleus, mitochondria, and ribosomes), which is common to most cells; and of dendrites and axons, which are unique to neurons (*see Figure 2*). The entire neuron—cell body, dendrites, and axons—is housed within a cell membrane that is semipermeable: that is, some substances can pass through it.

Branching out from the cell body are the dendrites, which serve as the receptors of incoming nerve impulses. The axons—long, thin, tubelike extensions—carry the nerve impulse away from the cell body toward the dendrites of other neurons. The area of the neuron where the axon branches off from the cell body is called the axon hillock.

Around the exterior of the axon is found an insulating material consisting of glial cells, which are specialized cells of fat and protein. This insulating material, called myelin or the "myelin sheath," serves

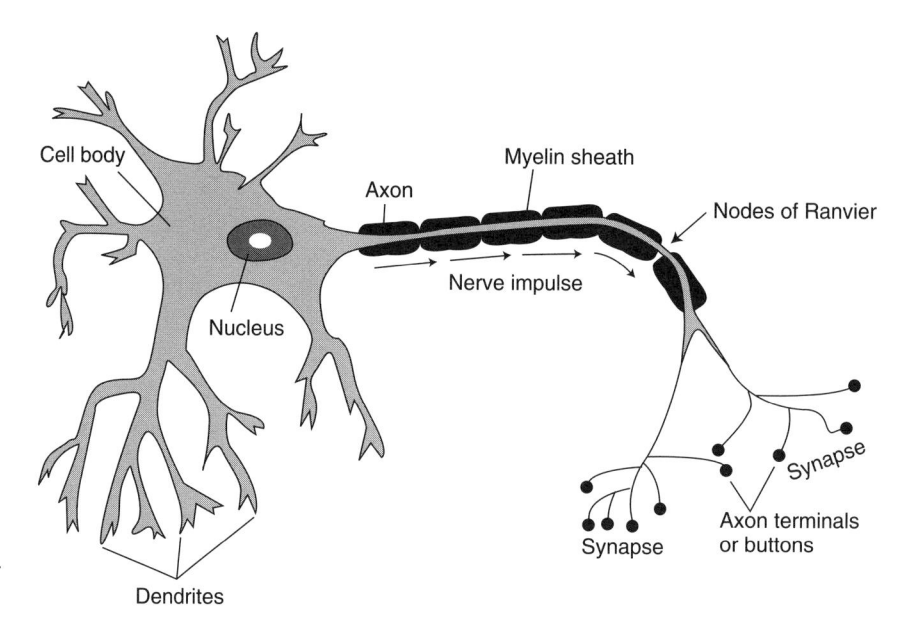

Figure 2. *The anatomy of a neuron is shown here.*

to speed nerve conduction. (In demyelinating diseases, such as multiple sclerosis, the myelin sheath deteriorates or is destroyed, with the result that nerve conduction is greatly slowed. When a number of neurons slow conduction, the cumulative effect is functional impairment. For example, people with multiple sclerosis often need to walk with a cane because of the weakness caused by this demyelinization process.) The myelin sheath does not completely cover the axon. The uncovered spaces where there are separations between myelin-forming cells are called the nodes of Ranvier.

At the tip of the axon is the axon terminal, aptly called the "button" because of its shape. It is through the button that messages are produced and stored in synaptic vesicles.

Nerve Impulses

Neuron electric impulses travel in two ways: by conduction and by synaptic transmission. Conduction is the process by which the electric impulse is received by and transmitted through a single neuron. Synaptic transmission is the propagation of electric impulses between neurons.

The conduction of an electric charge has been likened to shooting a rifle, because a neuron either "fires" or does not fire; there is no "semi-firing." Also, a neuron is either off or on, that is, in a resting state or an active state; it cannot be "partly off" or "partly on." Physiologists call this the "all or none" principle.

The fluid inside and outside of the cell membrane of the neuron contains electrically charged particles, or ions. Ions inside the membrane are negatively charged and those outside are positively charged; thus the neuron is like a miniature battery. In a resting state, the neuron typically carries an electrical charge of –70 millivolts. This charge changes during the firing of the neuron. The elements that play the

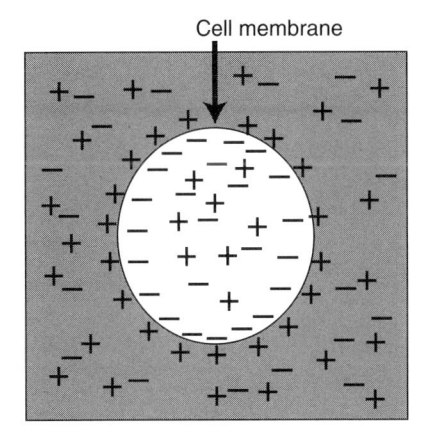

Figure 3. *Polarization: Excess positive charges outside the cell membrane and excess negative charges inside the cell membrane collect near the membrane.*

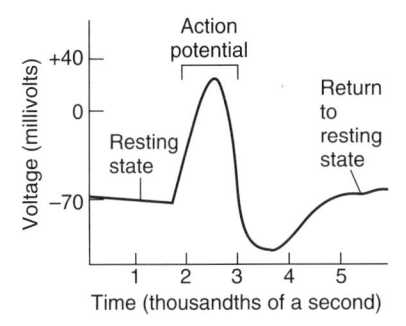

Figure 4. *Shown here are changes in the electrical charge from resting state to action potential, and then back to resting state. In the resting state, the neuron has an electric charge of –70 millivolts. The triggering of the action potential causes the charge to become positive: about +40 millivolts. After the action potential passes, the charge becomes even more negative than it is during a typical resting state. Only when the action potential again returns to resting state can it be fully ready to be triggered again.*

most significant role in neuronal conduction are potassium (K+) and sodium (Na+), which have a positive electrical charge, and chloride (Cl–), which has a negative charge. When an area of the cell membrane is at resting potential, there are high concentrations of potassium ions in the cell and high concentrations of sodium and chloride outside the cell. It is because of this distribution of ions that the fluid inside the cell has a negative electrical charge relative to the fluid outside the cell. This is called polarization (*see Figures 3 and 4*).

A nerve impulse is conducted through the neuron when the cell membrane at the axon hillock receives a signal from the dendrites and cell body that is sufficient to trigger a change in the polarization of the cell membrane. The electrical charge changes from negative to positive and back to negative. This "flipping" back and forth is called an action potential. It occurs when the concentration of sodium, potassium, and chloride inside and outside of the cell change. When an action potential occurs in a region of the cell membrane, it acts as a stimulus, causing the nearby areas of the membrane to undergo a change in electrical charge. Therefore, an action potential triggered at the axon hillock will be conducted down the length of the axon, setting off a chain reaction of changes in the polarization pattern of the cell membrane. The movement of the action potential along the length of the axon is called a nerve impulse; this is what is referred to as the "firing" of the neuron.

Nerve impulses travel at different speeds: conduction velocity can vary from less than 1 meter (3.3 ft.) per second up to 100 meters (33 ft.) per second. Some of this variation in speed is due to the myelin sheath covering the axon, which (as noted above) is broken up by the nodes of Ranvier. Because the myelin insulation is resistant to conduction, the impulse is speeded along when it jumps from node to node—this is called saltatory conduction.

After the action potential or firing occurs, the neuron cannot immediately be fired again. It is like a rifle that has to be reloaded after every shot. The time after an action potential during which the nerve cannot fire, or depolarize, is called the absolute refractory period. In other words, if a second stimulus is received by a nerve during the absolute refractory period—say, within 0.4 millisecond—that stimulus is ineffective. The duration of the absolute refractory period varies from nerve to nerve and is dependent on the diameter of the nerve. Soon after this absolute refractory period, the ability of the nerve to depolarize gradually returns; the time of this gradual return is called the relative refractory period. During the relative refractory period, a stimulus that is greater than normal will cause the nerve to depolarize. The existence of these refractory periods may be the reason behind the "coordination fatigue" experienced by sprinters. World-class sprinters reach their top speed around the 50- to 60-meter mark but find it extremely difficult to maintain their top speed from the 60-meter mark onward. Although this phenomenon is still being investigated, it seems plausible that the refractory periods of the neurons involved could affect prolonged maximum-intensity sprinting

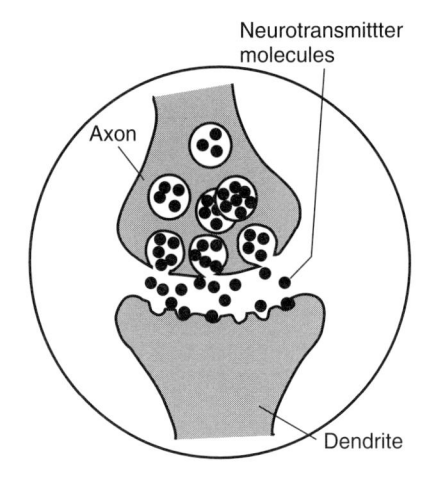

Figure 5. *Neurotransmitters bridge the synapse between the axon and dendrite.*

Communication between Neurons

Neurons are separated by a space called a synapse (*refer back to Figure 2*). In order for a nerve impulse to travel from one neuron to another, the synapse must be "bridged" or "connected." Neurons release chemical messengers called neurotransmitters into the synapse so that neuron-to-neuron communication takes place (*see Figure 5*). When the nerve impulse reaches the end of an axon of the presynaptic neuron, neurotransmitters are released into the synapse. These neurotransmitters spread across the synapse and interact with specialized receptor sites on the dendrites and cell body of the postsynaptic neuron. The effect of this interaction is that the electrical charge of the membrane at the postsynaptic site changes in one of two ways: it either depolarizes (becomes less negative) or hyperpolarizes (becomes more negative). When the incoming hyperpolarization or depolarization of the membrane reaches the axon hillock and causes the membrane charge to change from –70 to –65 millivolts, the neuron fires, thus releasing neurotransmitters into the synapse, contributing to the chain reaction of firing neurons which is communication in the nervous system.

Acetylcholine, found in the synapses between motor nerves and skeletal muscles, is a primary neurotransmitter that signals muscles to become active. Two other potent neurotransmitters, epinephrine and norepinephrine, are central to functioning during sports because they are found in the adrenal glands and sympathetic nervous system, which produce arousal and alertness.

Endogenous opioids, also called endorphins, are another group of well-known neurotransmitters. Endorphins interact with a neuron called an opiate receptor, and they are produced by the body in order to suppress pain. However, it is thought that in some cases endorphins not only reduce pain but can also produce a feeling of well-being; in fact, many people believe that endorphins are responsible for the phenomenon known as "runner's high." Some long-distance runners do report a sense of euphoria—or intense happiness—during and just after a run; but it is still hotly debated whether endorphins are responsible for this "high," and if so, whether the release of endorphins is triggered by a certain amount of exercise as such or rather by a certain degree of pain (*see also RUNNING AND HURDLING*).

The Central Nervous System and Motor Control

Movement is the end result of a number of control subsystems within the nervous system as a whole. All activity—from very simple motor activities such as walking and breathing to very complex activities, such as a double somersault with a full twist—is directed by the central nervous system (CNS), which is made up of the spinal cord and the brain. The CNS is the command and control center that directs muscles to move through a large range of motion to accomplish many tasks. Neurophysiologists characterize the activities of the central nervous system by their functions.

The Spinal Cord

The spinal cord consists of nerve cells encased by the bony spine. It helps to control movement of the arms, legs, and trunk; and it receives (and processes) information from the neurons located in the muscles, joints, and skin. The upper spinal cord, called the brain stem, is specialized to receive sensory information from the eyes, neck, and face and is responsible for vital functions like breathing, control of heart rate, and digestion. It conveys information regarding movement from the cerebral hemispheres to the cerebellum.

Damage to the spinal cord can result in temporary or permanent dysfunction. Temporary dysfunction, from which recovery is possible, can take the form of transient weakness in the arms or legs (*see the sidebar*). Permanent dysfunction takes the form of partial or near-total paralysis; as of the 1990s, recovery from such loss of function was not possible. (A famous case was that of the actor Christopher Reeve, who was paralyzed after falling from a horse in 1995.)

The Brain

If the spinal cord is like a telephone line or modem for messages sent from the brain, the brain itself is the computer in which motor function is controlled.

Parts of the brain. The brain, which is above or adjacent to the brain stem, consists of the cerebellum, diencephalon, and cerebral hemispheres (*see Figure 6*). The cerebellum is important in modulating or helping to control the amount of force that is required for a given activity. Additionally, the cerebellum helps control the amount of motion needed to accomplish a given task. For example, in a soccer kick the player is concerned with how "hard" to kick the ball. The amount of force imparted by the foot to the ball is a function of the controlled action of the hip, knee, and ankle. These activities are modulated by the cerebellum. In other words, it assists in the acquisition of motor skills.

The diencephalon processes much of the information that reaches the cerebral cortex from other parts of the CNS. The diencephalon also helps regulate autonomic function (such as heart rate, blood pressure, dilation of the pupils of the eyes, sweating, and shivering); visceral function (such as digestion and bowel movements); and endocrine function (such as the secretion of adrenaline and insulin). During running, the diencephalon is extremely active: it increases the heart rate, increases respiration (breathing) rate, cools the body by sweating, decreases digestive activity, and regulates insulin production.

The cerebral hemispheres participate in the regulation of motor

---

Temporarily Disabling Spinal Cord Injuries

1. A football player who makes a shoulder block sometimes experiences a "stinger"—tingling and weakness shooting into one arm. The team physician makes a diagnosis of "spinal cord bruise" to the neck.
2. A diver who hyperextends the lower back during a full gainer may temporarily or permanently lose the use of the legs, owing to weakness. The team physician makes a diagnosis of "spinal cord injury—lumbar spine."

The Brain and Exercise

Just as muscles respond to strength training by becoming larger and stronger, evidence accumulating from research seems to suggest that mental facilities also improve from exercise. Aerobic exercise increases the brain's supply of oxygen and the density of the brain's blood vessels, and these effects in turn increase the flow of nutrients to the brain so that it can function optimally. Skilled exercise—like playing tennis or dancing—increases the number of brain synapses, improving the brain's ability to process information quickly. Exercise may also slow effects of aging on the brain (*see also AGING AND PERFORMANCE*).

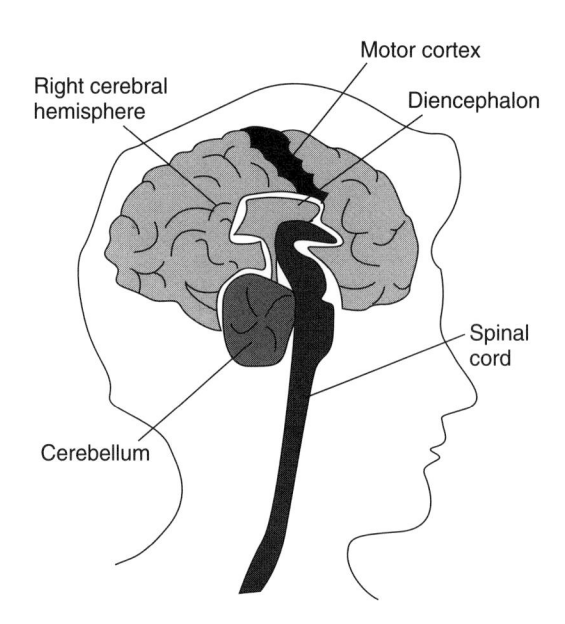

Figure 6. *The central nervous system consists of the brain—cerebral cortex, cerebellum, and diencephalon (shown here)—and the spinal cord (upper end shown here).*

performance, in sensation and the processing of information (which includes memory of past motor performance), in autonomic and endocrine responses, in the emotions, and in cognition (thinking). Each cerebral hemisphere is primarily involved with processing sensations and motor activity on the opposite (contralateral) side of the body. Thus sensations that enter via the spinal cord from the right side of the body cross over to the left side of the nervous system before being conveyed to the cerebral hemisphere. Similarly, motor control exerted by one cerebral hemisphere influences, in most cases, movements on the opposite side of the body. Not uncommonly, then, when a person sustains a head injury affecting one side of the brain, motor control of the opposite side of the body will be changed.

Specialization in the brain: left and right hemispheres. The two cerebral hemispheres are specialized for many different functions. As noted earlier, each hemisphere is primarily involved with motor and sensory function on the opposite (contralateral) side of the body. For example, motor areas in the left hemisphere will have control over movement of the right arm and leg. Similarly, the outer area of the cerebral hemispheres—the cortex—will receive sensory information, such as temperature, pain, and the position of the joints, from the opposite side of the body.

Although the cerebral hemispheres look nearly identical, their structure and, more important, their function are not. Interestingly, neurophysiologists have found that areas of motor control are often much more highly developed in one cerebral hemisphere—this is called the "dominant" hemisphere—than the other. In fact, it is estimated that in at least 90 percent of people, the left hemisphere is dominant. Obviously, this helps to explain why 90 percent of people throw with the right hand and kick with the right foot. In left-handers, by contrast, the right hemisphere is dominant; and it is sometimes argued that this is the reason why left-handers are so prominent in many sports (see the essay "Are Left-Handers Inherently Superior Athletes?").

The left and right hemispheres communicate with each other through a structure called the corpus callosum, a large pathway of nerve fibers and neurons that interconnect the two.

Sensation and Motor Control

The function of the sensory system is an enormously important and underappreciated aspect of motor control. The correct moment-to-moment activities of the motor system are dependent on constant input from the sensory system. Hearing the firing of the starter's pistol, seeing the seams of the pitcher's curveball, and rotating a basketball in the hands before shooting a free throw (touch) provide information about where an individual is in space and where other objects are relative to that position. Also, sensory receptors in the joints and muscles, called proprioceptors, provide information to the motor system about the position of the joints and how much tension is being exerted by the muscles.

Motor Programs

The activity the motor system is capable of carrying out can be broadly divided into three overlapping types of movements: (1) reflexes, (2) voluntary movements, and (3) rhythmic motor patterns. Reflexes—the first type of activity—are more or less automatic motor responses that are quick and involuntary. One example is the tendon reflex, which a doctor tests by tapping the large tendon below the patient's patella (kneecap). Another example of a reflex is "unweighting" an ankle as one begins to feel it sprain: there is no need to think about lifting the foot—it is an automatic (involuntary) response.

The second broad area of motor function is called voluntary movement. Throwing or catching a ball or riding a bicycle represents the more complex functions of the motor system and can be considered a skill. These movements are purposeful and goal-directed. As voluntary movement is practiced, the performance has the potential to improve greatly; there is no question that great athletes are great because of practice. As voluntary movements are practiced and mastered, little (and often no) conscious attention needs be paid. For example, once people have mastered the skill of riding a bicycle or ice skating, they do not necessarily have to think about it—it has become automatic.

When a series of movements have been mastered to the point

Are Left-Handers Inherently Superior Athletes?

Left-handedness is one of the most readily identifiable physical traits. In sports, there is considerable fascination with left-handers (or "lefties," or "southpaws"). This is in part simply because their execution of certain movements is completely different from, and often opposite to, that of right-handers; but it also has to do with persistent speculation about whether left-handedness improves, worsens, or has no effect on athletic performance.

Out of the total population, over 90 percent of individuals are right-handed, with the remaining 10 percent primarily left-handed, though a few are ambidextrous. Since only 1 person out of 10 is left-handed, the question arises: Why are there so many left-handers in sports? To put this another way: Does left-handedness give some innate advantage, or does it represent simply a strategic advantage specific to certain sports? In considering this question, it is helpful to know something about left-handedness in general.

Historically, the left side has typically had negative connotations. The English word *left*, for instance, comes from the Anglo-Saxon *lyft*, which means "weak" or "broken," and the Oxford English Dictionary lists several unflattering synonyms for *left-handed*, including *defective*, *doubtful*, and *illegitimate*. In recent years, research has suggested that left-handedness is much more than a minor physiological difference: doctors and social scientists have found both subtle and substantial differences between left- and right-handers (Geshwind and Galaburda, 1985; Coren, 1993). In comparative studies, for instance, each group seems to show a higher rate of certain talents and disabilities than the other group.

One interesting aspect of left-handedness is how it originates. There is little evidence to suggest that handedness is learned; however, it does not seem to be entirely a matter of inheritance either, for at least three reasons. First, in numerous studies of inherited traits, parents' handedness had less effect on siblings than genetic theories would suggest; it is true that 90 percent of children born to right-handed parents grow up to be right-handed, but less than half of the children of two left-handed parents are lefties. Second, identical twins often have opposite dominant hands (Shute, 1994). Third, until about age 2, children frequently use both hands interchangeably; it is when they begin to perfect fine motor skills that a dominant hand emerges. Thus scientists are coming to the conclusion that handedness is not strictly inherited. There is wide agreement that genetic factors play a very important part in handedness, but during the course of development—both prenatal and postnatal—several other factors affect the direction and magnitude of these genetic differences. Evidently, all humans carry the genetic code for right-handedness, but then something happens to make some people left-handed.

Another significant aspect of left-handedness is what it may imply about the brain. The brain of a left-handed person is widely acknowledged to be different in certain respects from that of a right-hander. In particular, lefties show less left-hemisphere and right-hemisphere specialization, that is, there is more crossing over between the hemispheres. Because their hemisphere specialization is less, left-handers have a much better chance of fully recovering from the concentrated death of brain cells that occurs with a stroke. Such differences in the brain might be a factor in improving motor control (spatial skills), and thus in helping left-handers to excel at athletics.

Still another aspect of left-handedness has to do with its possible implications for other body systems. Some scientists believe that the same factors that modify brain organization and structure to create left-handedness in the first place also affect other bodily functions. If so, this might explain the controversial statistics suggesting that left-handed people have a higher rate of learning disabilities and health-related problems, and a shorter life expectancy. But, as with the brain, such considerations might also suggest possible advantages in athletics.

Why are left-handers overrepresented in sports? For example, if only one person in ten is left-handed, why have six of the ten best baseball players of all time been left-handed? Left-handed hitters include Ty Cobb, Babe Ruth, Ted Williams, and Lou Gehrig; left-handed pitchers include Sandy Koufax, Lefty Grove, and Steve Carlton. In the 1990s, two of the most dominant hitters were left-handed: Ken Griffey, Jr., and Barry Bonds. The presence of left-handers in baseball is so impressive that some observers have been led to overstate the case. For example, in his book *The Natural Superiority of the Left-Hander*, James De Kay says that "over half of the major league batting stars, and at least half of the major league pitching stars, are left-handed"—a considerable exaggeration. Left-handers actually account for about 30 percent of the total baseball roster (Brancazio, 1984); but the point remains that 30 percent is enormously out of proportion for a group constituting only 10 percent of the general population. Of course, there are some obvious factors that give lefties certain advantages in baseball. First, most pitchers are right-handed, and it is easier for a left-handed batter to hit a breaking ball from a right-handed pitcher—the ball breaks toward (rather than away from) a left-handed batter. Second, a left-handed batter has a split-second advantage in "beating out" a hit, because the batter's box for a lefty is a few feet closer to first base. Third, most major league teams keep left-handed relief pitchers on the roster even though they may be relatively ineffective; these lefties serve one purpose: very short relief appearances. (A left-handed reliever may pitch to one or two left-handed batters and then be promptly yanked and replaced by a star reliever.) These advantages do inflate the number of lefties in the major leagues; still, a countereffect must also be noted: there are several positions major league managers do not allow lefties to play because of difficulties with throwing fast and accurately: second base, third base, shortstop, and catcher.

The issue of left-handers in baseball is further complicated by definitional problems. For instance, consider Wade Boggs of the New York Yankees, a superstar who threw right-handed and batted left-handed; would Boggs be considered left-handed or not? In this regard, it is generally agreed that batting handedness is a poor predictor of general handedness.

Another complication is that superiority in batting seems to be related less to left-handedness as such and more to "cross-sidedness" of hand and eye dominance. (Although everyone is familiar with handedness, eye dominance is not so well known. In the general population, 66 percent of individuals are right-eyed, 25 percent "ambi-eyed," and 9 percent left-eyed; *see also VISION.*) A list of the greatest average hitters of all time would probably reveal that most were "cross-sided" with respect to hand and eye. The greatest batters in recent baseball history—Pete Rose, Rod Carew, George Brett, and Wade Boggs—all threw right but batted left, and this pattern is generaly an indication of cross-sidedness.

Actually, to evaluate the relationship between handedness and athletic performance, it may be more useful to consider tennis—another sport in which left-handers have been overrepresented. The proportion of lefties at the elite level of professional tennis seems to always be greater than the 9 or 10 percent found in the general population; even more interesting is the fact that the percentage of lefties increases at the very highest level—among the top 100 tennis professionals (Annett, 1985). Outstanding left-handed tennis players over the years include Rod Laver (in the 1960s), Jimmy Connors (1970s), John McEnroe (1980s), Martina Navratilova (1980s), and Monica Seles (1990s). Again, the question is whether left-handedness is an innate advantage in tennis or simply a strategic advantage.

One slight strategic advantage for left-handed tennis players is that right-handed opponents must reverse their usual tactics: for instance, a deep chip shot to a right-hander's relatively weak backhand would be a shot to a left-hander's strong forehand. However, it is argued that this cannot account for the large—and increasing—proportion of left-handers at the top of the rankings. The very best tennis players spend more hours practicing (they practice more than 4 hours a day) and playing against left-handed opponents; thus the percentage of left-handers who can reach the top and stay there would be expected to decline, not increase.

Of all sports, the percentage of left-handers is greatest at the top levels of boxing and fencing. Left-handers have dominated in both these sports—again, especially among the elite. In fencing, for instance, at the Olympics in Moscow in 1980, the top eight fencing places were all taken by lefties. In the same year, twelve of the top twenty-five ranked fencers (48 percent) were left-handed. In fencing and boxing, the explanation may have to do with the importance of anticipation and reaction. Apparently, left-handers are better at anticipating and reacting, and that would be a decided advantage in these sports. To avoid a punch or foil, the athlete needs fast reflexes; but studies of reaction times have found that it is not possible for a world-class boxer to avoid a punch on the basis of reaction time alone—an elite boxer avoids punches with a combination of reaction time and antcipation. A fencer must, clearly, have to do the same.

Anticipation and reaction would represent an innate advantage; but some observers feel that the advantages of left-handedness in boxing and fencing are primarily strategic. It is claimed that left-handed boxers have a tactical advantage because they use unfamiliar stances and their punches come from unfamiliar angles and directions, which a right-handed boxer is unaccustomed to seeing. Moreover, a right-handed fighter who is unfamiliar with left-handed opponents cannot anticipate these punches. This strategic advantage—the opponent's unfamiliarity with the left-hander's tactics—might be a plausible explanation for the high proportion of left-handed boxers; but it cannot be extended to fencing, where nearly 50 percent of world-class players are left-handed. In fencing, obviously, all the world-class competitors must be familiar with opposite-handed opponents.

Neurologists at the Harvard Medical School have proposed a theory that may explain the high proportion

---

LEFT-HANDED PITCHES
Randy Johnson, a left-hander on the Seattle Mariners, was perhaps the most feared pitcher of the 1990s. Most major league veterans believe that a left-hander's curveball moves much more unpredictably than a right-hander's. This belief is plausible, but there is no biomechanical theory to support it.

(continued)

Are Left-Handers Inherently Superior Athletes? (continued)

of left-handers in sports (Geshwind and Galaburda, 1985): they believe that the neurological differences seen in left-handers give superior motor control. These researchers found that the brain of a left-hander had a relatively larger right hemisphere, presumably as a result of prenatal retardation in the growth of the left hemisphere. As a consequence, they suggest, functions heavily dependent on the right hemisphere, like eye-hand spatial ability, become sharper.

It should be noted that left-handers excel disproportionately only in sports in which quick eye-hand reaction is essential; that is, left-handers are not overrepresented in other sports. For example, one study confirmed the greater proportion of left-handers in tennis but found that for goalkeepers in soccer the percentage of left-handers was the same as in the general population. Goalkeeping in soccer is a position where hand dominance does not matter, because both hands are used equally (Wood, 1989). Although only a few studies exist, these statistics seem to indicate that left-handers' advantage in sports heavily reliant on quick reflexes is innate. Further statistical studies may provide more evidence of innate superiority; but even so, it may take a long time before we can explain this, because knowledge of the neurological processes of the brain is still in its infancy.

John Zumerchik

LEFTIES AT THE TOP
In sports that are highly dependent on reaction time, there is often a high percentage of left-handers at the elite level.

Fencing: At the 1980 Moscow Olympics, the top 8 fencing places were all taken by lefties; that year, 12 of the top 25 fencers (48 percent) were left-handed.

Basketball: All coaches stress fast reaction time, to "read and react" or for the quick first step. Of the 5 playing positions, the point guard depends particularly on quick reflexes. During the 1995–1996 NBA season, 8 of 29 starting point guards—27 percent—were lefties. This is almost three times the percentage of lefties in the general population.

that they are automatic, the movements are called a rhythmic motor pattern. This is the third broad area of motor function. Examples are running, walking, and riding a bicycle. Once the movement has begun, the repetitive movements that are being carried out can continue almost automatically, much like a reflex, until the movement is stopped. Joggers, for example, do not have to think about moving their arms and legs—they move their limbs automatically.

Most skilled motor activity relies on all three areas of motor function: reflex, voluntary movement, and rhythmic motor patterns. Most sports depend on a preplanned pattern of approach to nervous system activity; such planned patterns are called motor programs. During the performance of a motor task in a sport, the role of the sensory system is to help control movement in the present, in addition to influencing future motor activity by upgrading the athlete's motor programs. Thus, the sensory system is not isolated from the motor system but instead is an integral part of the whole and is vitally important for skilled motor control.

The Somatosensory System

According to present-day research in neuroscience, the sensory system carries out many varied functions during sports activity. First the sensory system stimulates reflex movement organized in the

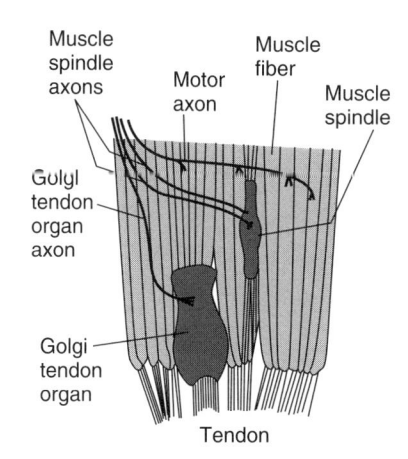

Figure 7. *Shown here are the muscle spindle and Golgi tendon organ in a typical muscle.*

spinal cord. Second, the sensory system plays a crucial role in regulating rhythmic motor patterns, as discussed previously. A third important function of the sensory system, in regard to motor control, is carried out via neuron connections ascending from the extremities and trunk to the spinal cord and brain; this function contributes to motor control in many complicated processes.

Specialized sensory receptors throughout the body are considered part of the somatosensory system. The somatosensory system is responsible for receiving input from sensory receptors in the skin, joints, and muscles, and transmitting information to the brain via the nervous system. Two sensory receptors that are vital to motor control during sports are the muscle spindle and the Golgi tendon organs (*see Figure 7*).

Muscle spindles. Muscle spindles are sensory receptors that inform the CNS about changes in the length of muscles throughout the body. Most of the muscle spindles are found within the skeletal muscles, that is, muscles that cause movement of a joint. Anatomists have determined that the muscles containing the greatest number of muscle spindles are those of the neck, eye, and hand. To athletes in many sports, this would not be surprising, since they are well aware of the skill required to kick, hit, catch, or shoot a ball effectively: that is, a high degree of eye-head, eye-hand, and eye-foot coordination is necessary for these activities.

When a skeletal muscle is stretched, the muscle spindle is stretched as well. Information about the speed and amount of stretch, sensed by the muscle spindle, is then transmitted to other parts of the nervous system for processing. For example, when a volleyball player crouches and then jumps before hitting the ball, the muscle spindles in the player's gastrocnemius muscles (calves) sense the stretch and become excited. Through their connections, via other neurons, to the gastrocnemius muscles, they excite the motor neurons, which in turn cause the gastrocnemius muscle to contract.

Golgi tendon organs. The Golgi tendon organs (GTOs) are typically located where a muscle and its tendon connect together. Many GTOs are connected in series to a group consisting of many muscle fibers. A Golgi tendon organ functions to sense change in tension in a muscle as the result of the muscle's being stretched or contracted. The GTO continually monitors tension within the muscle and is sensitive to both large and small changes in tension. It is thought that the GTO also has an influence on muscle tone when the muscle becomes fatigued. Thus, the GTO has the ability both to excite and to inhibit muscle contraction (Shumway-Cook and Woollacott, 1995).

The muscle spindles and Golgi tendon organs work in concert to convey complementary information regarding the condition of the muscle. The muscle spindles convey information about muscle length while the tendon organs convey information about changes in muscle tension.

Stay on Your Toes?

No. Instead, stay on the balls of the feet. In many sports, coaches extol the virtues of getting body weight off the heels and concentrating it fully on the balls of the feet. The purpose is to improve reaction time. This is a good idea because as the athlete centers body weight on the ball of the foot, the muscle spindles in the leg muscles become excited. Evidence from research suggests that the strong, propulsive muscles of the legs (the gastrocnemius, quadriceps femoris, and gluteal muscles) become stretched when the weight of the athlete is concentrated on the ball of the foot. When these muscles are stretched, the muscle spindles within them become excited and prepare them to contract rapidly, improving reaction time (*see also RUNNING AND HURDLING*).

For instance, because the length of a muscle changes as the angle of the joint it acts on changes (as when an athlete jumps for a rebound), the muscle spindle will deliver sensory input to the brain to determine the positions of segments of the legs. At the same time, sensory input from the Golgi tendon organs will deliver information about the tension provided by the muscles (for example, the amount of tension needed in the hand muscles to maintain grip on the ball).

Development and Motor Control

This section will consider two aspects of development as it pertains to motor control: first, the phases or stages involved in acquiring motor skills; and second, the concept of plasicity and the early athletic training of young people.

Stages in Developing Motor Control

According to a widely accepted scheme, the typical development of motor control has four major stages: (1) mobility, (2) stability, (3) controlled mobility, and (4) skill. With regard to early infancy, *mobility* (stage 1) refers to erratic motion of the arms and legs that often has no particular purpose. In the adult, mobility is influenced by range of motion (ROM) of the joints and muscles as well as reflex behavior. *Stability* (stage 2) refers to the ability of postural muscles to maintain the joints of the body in a stable position. This is necessary for the body to maintain an upright position against gravity and for holding a joint steady against some physical resistance. In *controlled mobility* (stage 3), motion is added to a stable posture. In other words, the person has the ability to hold one part of the body still while moving another part of the body, under control, through space. *Skill* (stage 4), the highest degree of motor control, is based on the three

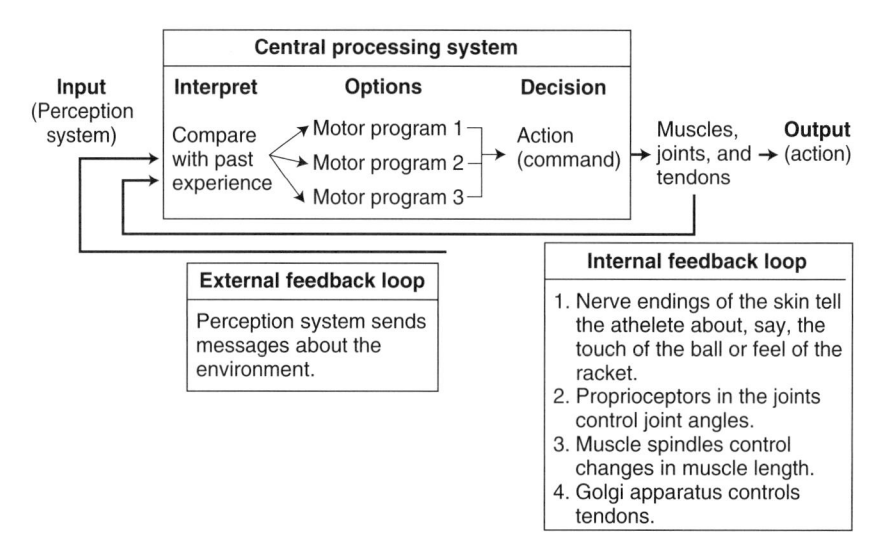

Figure 8. *This flowchart shows the human motor control system in action.*

previous stages—mobility, stability, and controlled mobility. At the point when a skill is developed, all four stages are integrated. Major requirements for skill development also include normal balance, equilibrium, and postural reflexes.

Independent locomotion is a good example of motor development early in life. This is actually an extremely complex motor skill, although at first glance it may seem simple and automatic. The typical sequence of development progresses from erratic movement to crawling or creeping to walking and finally to running. These motor skills are essentially cumulative in nature, that is, each skill builds on the preceding skill: "Crawl, walk, then run."

Alpine skiing can serve as an example of the development of motor control in an adult. First, mobility—such as the length of the hamstring muscles or the knee ligaments—must be adequate. (Of course, control of erratic movements is also necessary, as can be seen by watching beginning skiers on the slopes.) Second, stability allows beginning skiers to remain upright while standing on the ski slope, getting used to balancing on the skis. Third, the controlled mobility that follows allows the skiers, with practice, to move the skis back and forth while holding the upper body still as they descend the slope. Fourth, when mobility, stability, and controlled mobility have been integrated, the skill necessary for Alpine skiing has been learned.

Plasticity and Early Athletic Training

How soon should youngsters become involved in sports? In most sports, precise motor control is necessary not only for skillful performance but even for overall enjoyment; for example, in watching an experienced gymnast or golfer, it becomes obvious that accurate, exact motor control is essential. In this regard, many coaches believe that to have any hope of excelling at a sport—any hope of eventually becoming a champion—a person must begin at a very young age. They reason that acquiring motor control skills through the development of motor memory (a physiological process) is the equivalent or counterpart of learning another language (a cognitive process); and, as with learning a language, the earlier you start, the better. Research in motor learning does lend some support to this belief, because the nervous system of a young person has greater plasticity.

Plasticity can be defined as the ability of the nervous system to be modified. To say that a younger person's nervous system has more plasticity means that it is more readily able to change—in particular, to change the efficiency and strength of the connections between neurons. For instance, with repetitive, continued practice, the nervous system develops greater concentrations of neurotransmitters; and in general, as the concentration of neurotransmitters increases, nervous system activity becomes more efficient. Further, structural changes in the synapses make the nervous system more effective at carrying out precise motor activities (Shumway-Cook and Woollacott, 1995).

Plyometrics: Exercise to Enhance Motor Control

Plyometric exercise has been used to train many types of athletes to improve their quickness, speed, strength, and power, which in many cases serve to improve vertical jumping height. What distinguishes plyometric exercise from traditional weight training is that it overloads the muscles in a different way. In comparison with weight training, plyometric exercise has been found to provide a twofold benefit (Chu, 1992). First, it utilizes the force and velocity attained by accelerating body weight against gravity; this exceeds the force and velocity weight training can provide. Second, it simulates many sports activities—such as jumping, sprinting, and throwing—more closely than weight training does. This leads to a specificity of training that can produce more power and speed. Researchers are still investigating how plyometric exercise produces more force and velocity.

Plyometric exercise has enabled athletes to improve their force, speed, and strength primarily through a cycle of stretching and shortening. The stretch-shortening cycle is a functional contraction of a muscle which involves a concentric (shortening) contraction that is immediately preceded by an eccentric (lengthening) contraction. When an elastic muscle is stretched, it stores potential elastic energy, which can be reutilized during the following concentric contraction. This type of contraction enables the muscle to generate higher torque than concentric contraction alone (Helgeson & Gajdosik, 1993). The mechanism behind this effect is still unknown, but there are a number of theories explaining how the higher torque is produced (*see also* WEIGHT LIFTING).

One theory is that an eccentric contraction immediately preceding an concentric contraction will increase the force generated concentrically, because of the storage of elastic energy. During the stretch-shortening cycle, the muscle can increase the concentric force by utilizing the force produced by the series elastic component and the contractile component. Stretching a muscle causes elastic energy to be stored in the series elastic component—thought to be located in the tendons and in the cross-bridges between actin and myosin filaments (Bosco & Komi, 1979). The actin and myosin filaments are the proteins that do the work of the muscle by causing it to contract. The storage of elastic energy may occur by rotating the myosin heads backward against their natural tendency to a position of higher potential energy. The series elastic component generates a force when it is stretched, during either a concentric or an eccentric contraction. The series elastic component is stretched more and produces more force during an eccentric contraction. The ability to utilize the series elastic component is affected by time, the magnitude of the stretch, and the velocity of the stretch. The concentric contraction is increased by the greatest amount if the preceding eccentric contraction is of relatively small amplitude and is performed rapidly with no delay between the eccentric and concentric contraction.

A second theory is that the stretch-shortening cycle influences the muscle

Although youngsters have greater plasticity, the principles of effective training for motor memory and motor control are essentially the same for children and adults. These principles cover several areas: specificity, intensity, frequency, duration, and progression (*see also* STRENGTH TRAINING). Still, there are some points to consider regarding the training of children.

With young children, training for motor control and coordination should always have an element of fun, in order to maintain their interest. In fact, children's attention span is probably the major consideration in developing a training program: the component of "play" should never be omitted. This does not mean, of course, that children's training must be limited to simple skills: even children of elementary school age can succeed at a fairly sophisticated training program—as long as the coach does not actually call it "motor skills spindle lying within and parallel to the muscle fibers. The muscle spindle serves as a stretch receptor as it transmits sensory information via afferent axons to the central nervous system. It then informs other neurons in the spinal cord and brain about the length, and the rate of change in length, of the muscle. Also, the muscle spindle is composed of contractile elements that are innervated by gamma efferent neurons—neurons that regulate the sensitivity of the spindle (Voight & Draovitch, 1991). When the muscle is stretched in an eccentric contraction, the muscle spindle increases its firing rate and sends an impulse to the spinal cord, which in turn sends motor impulses back to the muscle and the synergistic muscles, signaling them to contract. At the same time, the spinal cord sends a motor impulse to antagonistic muscles to relax. This is called the myotactic stretch reflex. This impulse can cause the muscle to contract with greater force. The greater the load applied to a muscle, and the more quickly it is applied, the greater the firing frequency of the muscle spindle, which results in a correspondingly stronger muscular contraction. This can be thought of as maximizing the contracting potential of any given muscle. It should be noted, though, that investigators have disagreed about the theory that myoelectric activity or utilization of the myotactic stretch reflex can play a role in plyometric exercise.

During the stretch-shortening cycle, the Golgi tendon organ (GTO) inhibits the production of force. Golgi tendon organs are in series with the muscle and act as a protective mechanism to limit the amount of force that can be produced in the muscle. When muscular tension is high, the GTO generates a neural impulse that reduces the excitation of the muscle and causes it to relax. With stressful, explosive training the GTO may become desensitized. Desensitization of the GTO allows more muscular force to be produced: that is, inhibiting the GTO itself allows greater loading of the muscle in the eccentric phase of contraction. This increases the stored elastic energy that can be reused in the concentric contraction immediately following it.

However, the amortization phase—the time between the lengthening and shortening contractions—must be short, or the stored energy will be lost through heat production. In fact, the shorter the amortization time, the greater the release of stored energy. Komi (1984) reported that with a delay of even 0.9 second, all the stored elastic energy that was expected to increase force production (and thus to improve performance) instead simply escaped as heat.

There is greater muscle fiber recruitment and neuromuscular efficiency following a prestretch of the muscle. The speed at which an athlete can perform an activity is limited by neuromuscular coordination. Regardless of how strong the muscular system is, the body can move only within a range of speeds set by the nervous system. Plyometric exercise may enable muscle groups to be better coordinated as a result of changes in the nervous system. Training with an explosive prestretch improves neural efficiency; and this improved neural efficiency increases neuromuscular coordination and leads to improved neuromuscular performance—including increased speed, strength, power, and vertical jumping height. (*See also* VOLLEYBALL, "Plyometric Training: Can Jumping Ability Be Improved?")

Bruce Hauger

development." Young children, for instance, need to relate to a mental image, such as a frog jumping off of a lily pad or a kangaroo jumping over a fence; and they can readily understand the skill and ease with which a horse can bound over a hurdle. In other words, "motor skills development" needs to be placed in an appropriate context for young children. A child will always be far more receptive to the idea of "playing leapfrog" than to the idea of "plyometric exercises," though leapfrog is actually in essence a plyometric exercise (*see the essay "Plyometrics: Exercise to Enhance Motor Control"*).

Once young athletes approach pubescence (ages 8–12), they are better able to benefit from direct sport-specific training by coaches and other adults. At this age, young athletes are better able to undertand the connection between training activities suggested by their coach and their own eventual performance in a particular sport. Also,

718   THE BODY

there are effective sequential strategies for improving the performance of youngsters of this age; in other words, the development of motor skills should be approached as a continuum rather than as discrete stages. The coach or instructor needs to precisely identify the stages in the acquisition of a fundamental motor skill, select appropriate learning activities and environments, and—most important—provide accurate feedback so that these young athletes will be able to improve sequentially.

Following is an example of sequential strategies in teaching the overarm throw to children:

1. Stepping forward as they throw the ball while at the same time rotating the pelvis forward.
2. Rotating the upper back while swinging the upper arm to throw the ball.
3. Rotating the shoulder inward while straightening the elbow to throw the ball.

Throwing a ball is no easy task, but with a sequential strategy the development this skill—and many other complex sports skills—can begin as early as age 8 (or possibly even age 7) and can be improved on into adulthood. (For more details and sequential strategies for other skills, see Haywood, 1993.)

There is no question that tremendous advances in motor skills can be made during preadolescence, and in adolescence. At this stage, skills learned earlier, during young childhood, can be dramatically improved. Coaches and parents often note that in some sports world-class athletes seem to be younger and younger, and this makes them anxious or even discouraged at the slower progress of their own youngsters. But coaches and parents are wise to defer final judgment regarding a child's long-term potential and eventual athletic ability—in other words, this judgment should not usually be based on ability in late childhood or, for that matter, in early adulthood. Many top athletes did not begin until late adolescence, and some did not excel until they reached their thirties.

Do Athletes Need to Begin Training as Children?

Some coaches believe that in order to master the fine motor skills of some sports, athletes must start at a very early age. This is not necessarily true, however. Although many superstars do start at a very early age, there are always exceptions.

Kenny Rogers, an all-star pitcher for the Texas Rangers in 1995, started playing baseball in high school. During his senior year, while he was playing the outfield, a baseball scout noticed his tremendous arm strength. He was sent to rookie camp to learn how to pitch.

Hakeem Olajuwon was voted Most Valuable Player in the National Basketball Association Championship in 1995. Hakeem had been a top soccer player in high school, but he had not begun playing basketball until the year before he entered college.

In Conclusion

In essence, the study of motor control is the study of interaction between a body in motion and the environment in which the movement is taking place. The work of the Greek philosopher Aristotle (384–322 B.C.E.) and other early investigators led to a largely correct view of human movement and motor control as an intimate interplay of the neuromusculoskeletal system and external forces imposed on it by the environment.

Everyone, of course, can admire the sheer athleticism of a skier or the sheer aesthetics of a triple somersault with a one-and-a-half twist, but it is an entirely different matter to understand the precision and coordination of the underlying motor control. There is still much to be learned about the interconnections among neurons and between neurons and the brain, and about their overall influence on movement. If athletes are to continue to improve, present and future scientists will need to continue explaining what is known and exploring what is unknown.

Bruce Hauger and Angela Rosenberg

References

Albert, M. *Eccentric Muscle Training in Sports and Orthopaedics*. New York: Churchill Livingstone, 1991.

Annett, M. *Left, Right, Hand and Brain: The Right Shift Theory*. London: Erlbaum, 1985.

Bosco, C., and P. Komi. "Potentiation of the Mechanical Behavior of the Human Skeletal Muscle through Prestretching." *ACTA Physiologica Scandinavica* 106, no. 467 (1979).

Brancazio, P. *Sport Science*. New York: Simon and Schuster, 1984.

Chu, D. *Jumping into Plyometrics*. Champaign, Illinois: Leisure, 1992.

Coren, S. *Left-Handedness: Causes and Consequences*. New York: Random House, 1993.

De Kay, J. *The Natural Superiority of the Left-Hander*. New York: Evans, 1979.

Ekblom, B. *Football (Soccer)*. Boston, Massachusetts: Blackwell Scientific, 1994.

Enoka, R. *Neuromechanical Basis of Kinesiology*. Champaign, Illinois: Human Kinetics, 1988.

Geschwind, N., and A. Galaburda. "Cerebral Lateralization: Biological Mechanisms, Associations, and Pathology." *Archives of Neurology* 42 (1985): 428–459.

Goldstein, T. *Functional Rehabilitation in Orthopaedics*. Gaithersburg, Maryland: Aspen, 1995.

Haywood, K. *Life Span Motor Development*. Champaign, Illinois: Human Kinetics, 1993.

Helgeson, K., and R. Gajdosik. "The Stretch-Shortening Cycle of the Quadriceps Femoris Muscle Group Measured by Isokinetic Dynamometry." *Journal of Orthopedic and Sports Physical Therapy* 17, no. 17 (1983).

Kandel, E., J. Schwartz, and T. Jessell (eds.). *Principles of Neural Science*, 3rd ed. New York: Elsevier, 1991.

Komi, P. V. "Physiological Biomechanical Correlates of Muscle Function: Effects of Muscle Structure and Stretch Cycle on Force and Speed." *Exercise Sport Science Review* 12, no. 81 (1984).

Montagne, G., and M. Laurent. "The Effects of Environmental Changes on One-Handed Catching." *Journal of Motor Behavior* 26 (1994): 237ff.

Shumway-Cook, A., and M. Woollacott. *Motor Control: Theory and Practical Applications*. Baltimore, Maryland: Williams and Wilkins, 1995.

Shute, N. "Life for Lefties: From Annoying to Downright Risky." *Smithsonian* (December 1994).

Sullivan, P., P. Markos, and M. A. Minor. *An Integrated Approach to Therapeutic Exercise: Theory and Clinical Application*. Reston, Virginia: Reston, 1982.

Voight M., and P. Draovitch. "Plyometrics." In M. Albert (ed.), *Eccentric Muscle Training in Sports and Orthopaedics*. New York: Churchill Livingstone, 1991.

Wood, C., and J. Aggleton. "Handedness in 'Fast Ball' Sports: Do Left-Handers Have an Innate Advantage?" *British Journal of Psychology* 80 (1989): 227–240.

Nutrition and the Athlete

THE STUDY OF NUTRITION—what we eat and drink and how it affects health and performance—may be important to everyone, but it is vital for the athlete. The body cannot perform at its best without appropriate fuel and raw materials. A good understanding of nutrition allows the athlete to adapt her diet to adjust for the different needs of various activities and for peak performance on the day of competition.

Nutrition is a relatively new science, appearing as a distinct field of study only since 1934, when the American Institute of Nutrition was founded. There are thus many unanswered questions about nutrition. Though science has largely answered the question of what constitutes an adequate diet, there is still no consensus in the scientific community on what constitutes the ideal diet for the average person, let alone for the athlete. Athletic performance is a function of muscle power, coordination, and endurance. Every time a muscle cell contracts, that muscle uses fuel; if the fuel is not available, the muscle cannot contract. The fuel to power skeletal muscle comes from the food we eat and is stored in a variety a forms that can be accessed as needed. Both diet and training can maximize fuel storage for a particular event.

Terminology

Nutrients are substances, obtained from food, that the body needs for maintenance, growth, and repair. There are six classes of nutrients: carbohydrates, fats, proteins, vitamins, minerals, and water. Nutrients that the body can create from other components are called nonessential nutrients. For example, the body can make almost all of the fats it needs by converting proteins and carbohydrates to fats; these fats are thus called nonessential fats. Other nutrients must be included in the diet because the body cannot make them; these are the essential nutrients. Vitamin C, for example, is a substance the human body needs but cannot manufacture and is, therefore, an essential nutrient for human beings.

Some nutrients are measured in grams or milligrams (thousandths of a gram). Other nutrients are measured in calories, and still others are measured in international units. Grams are units of measurement used to describe how much mass a substance has. (Mass and weight are often used interchangeably, although they are not precisely equivalent.) A steak weighing 180 grams (about 6 oz.) might contain 38 grams of fat, 42 grams of protein, and 100 grams of water.

That same steak can also be measured in calories. Calories measure how much energy is contained in a substance. A calorie (as it is used in relation to food energy) is the amount of energy needed to raise the temperature of 1,000 grams of water by 1 degree Celsius. Energy may be defined as the ability to do work. The body requires fuel to move around and to maintain body functions.

Many foods contain combinations of nutrients. Some nutrients can be used by the body for fuel and some cannot. If they can be used for fuel, they have a caloric value; if they cannot, they have no caloric value. The steak mentioned above may be used as an example. The water in the steak cannot be used for fuel and thus provides no calories. The protein, on the other hand, can be used for fuel. Each gram of protein contains 4 calories of energy; thus the 42 grams of protein in the steak will provide 168 calories. Each gram of fat contains 9 calories of fuel; the steak's 38 grams of fat will provide 342 calories. The steak therefore contains a total of 510 calories—enough fuel to do very vigorous exercise for an hour. It is also enough fuel to sustain an average female through a night of sleep. Grams, milligrams, and calories are the most common ways to measure nutrients. Other measures are used when these units prove inadequate.

Every 6 or 7 years, a committee of nutritional experts in the United States sets Recommended Dietary Allowances (RDAs) for protein, vitamins, minerals, and energy (calories). These recommendations represent daily averages only and do not imply that one will get sick if one does not consume the RDA of every vitamin and mineral every day. These recommendations are also meant to include 98 percent of the healthy population. Because no two people are exactly the same, nutritional needs vary. Taking into account size, age, and gender, most people require less than the recommendation. Thus, there is a considerable safety margin.

Historically, the RDAs were designed to prevent deficiency diseases. By eating the RDA of any given nutrient, a person could be reasonably assured that he or she would not develop the deficiency disease associated with a lack of that particular nutrient. If one averages 60 milligrams of vitamin C every day, it is highly unlikely that one will get the deficiency disease scurvy. This does not mean, however, that the RDA is the optimal amount of that nutrient. Some people believe that 250 milligrams of vitamin C can prevent colds and cancer; other researchers recommend even more. Thus, the minimum amount of vitamin C required to prevent deficiency disease is known, while the amount needed to optimize health is not. This is true for all of the vitamins and minerals, as well as for protein. Much information on nutrient requirements is still unknown; this is the reason for ongoing study and periodic revisions of the RDAs.

The RDA for energy intake is calculated differently from those for nutrients. If the committee set the RDA for calories at a point that ensured an adequate caloric intake for 98 percent of the population, then the recommendation for 97.9 percent of the population would be too high. Because excess caloric intake is a significant problem in this country, the RDA for calories is set at the mean, or average. For a female between the ages of 15 and 18, for instance, the RDA for calories is 2,200.

Because RDAs vary by gender, age, and size, it is impossible to list the RDAs for every group on food labels. In an attempt to simplify the nutritional labels on the foods we buy, the USRDA was born. This figure represents the highest RDA in each gender and age group for a given nutrient. For example, the RDA for iron for adult men is 10 milligrams, while for women it is 15 milligrams. Thus, the USRDA for iron is 15 milligrams. The RDA for vitamin B6 for men and women is 2 milligrams and 1.6 milligrams, respectively; the USRDA is the higher value, 2 milligrams. Nutritional labels, now required on all food packaging in the United States, list the percentages of the USRDAs that a typical serving of that food provides. For example, if a breakfast cereal provides 5 milligrams of iron, the label would say that it provides 33 percent of the recommended daily amount of this nutrient, even though it would provide 50 percent of the recommended amount for men.

The Caloric Nutrients

The nutrients that can be measured in calories are the fuel nutrients: carbohydrates, protein and fat. Only these can be used to provide energy for the body's working tissues. A person's total daily caloric consumption is the sum of the ingested protein calories, carbohydrate calories, and fat calories. Experts cannot fully agree on the optimal relative amounts of each of these three nutrients, and recommendations often vary. The purpose of this section is to provide the athlete with an understanding of the fuel, or caloric, nutrients so that he or she will be able to make dietary decisions based on research and individual needs. How these nutrients enter the body will be discussed in the section on digestion.

Carbohydrates

The carbohydrates are a class of nutrient that can be used for fuel and can therefore be measured in either grams or calories. Carbohydrates are the favorite fuel of exercising muscle cells and are the only fuel brain cells can use. These molecules consist of rings of carbon atoms with hydrogen and oxygen. Rings may exist singly, coupled, or in chains. Single rings are known as monosaccharides (*mono,* "one"; *saccharide,* "sugar"). There are three common monosaccharides in our foods. Fructose is a monosaccharide found in fruits and honey. It is also added to sodas and other prepared foods as a sweetener. Galactose is a monosaccharide associated with milk products. Glucose is a monosaccharide seldom found by itself in nature; rather, it is usually found linked by chemical bonds to other glucose molecules to form long chains of glucose. These long chains are known as polysaccharides (*poly*, "many"). Monosaccharides can also link up in pairs through chemical bonds to form disaccharides (*di*, "two"). Sucrose (table sugar) is glucose and fructose linked together. Lactose, the carbohydrate found in diary products, is glucose and galactose linked together. Maltose is two glucose molecules linked together. The monosaccharides and disaccharides are often referred to as either sugars or simple carbohydrates. All of the sugars dissolve in water and have a sweet taste.

Polysaccharides, the long chains or sheets of monosaccharides linked together to form very large molecules, are the structural components of plants. Most commonly, all of the monosaccharides in a polysaccharide are glucose molecules. The physical arrangement of the molecules and the types of chemical bonds between the glucose molecules determine the nature or particular properties of polysaccharide. The polysaccharides are known as complex carbohydrates.

The human digestive system can absorb monosaccharides but not disaccharides or other more complex carbohydrates. The disaccharides and polysaccharides that we eat must be broken down into their monosaccharide subunits before these molecules can be transported to the blood. The body has the digestive enzymes to break some types of polysaccharide bonds to release the single glucose subunits. These digestible polysaccharides are known as starch. Other polysaccharides contain chemical bonds that humans cannot break because we lack the proper enzymes. These indigestible polysaccharides are called fiber. Even though fiber never gets into the blood and therefore is not used by the body for fuel, it serves very important functions in maintaining health. High-fiber diets help with weight control by providing bulk, which makes one feel full on fewer calories. Fiber reduces the cholesterol in the blood by trapping cholesterol from bile in the intestine so that it is eliminated from the body. Lowering the amount of absorbed cholesterol reduces a person's chances of developing atherosclerosis (the deposition of fat in arteries). Fiber slows the rate of absorption of carbohydrates, providing the cells with a more steady fuel supply. It also helps prevent constipation and hemorrhoids and may reduce the risk of colon cancer.

The fate of carbohydrates, once they enter the body, varies depending upon the type of carbohydrate eaten and the needs of the body at the time. All of the carbohydrates that go from the intestines to the blood are in the form of one of the three monosaccharides. Galactose and fructose are converted to glucose by the liver, and glucose is commonly converted to energy in the body, leaving behind the waste products of carbon dioxide and water (*see also METABOLISM*). Some cells (those of the central nervous system) can use only glucose for energy, and many cells, though they can use other substances such as fat for fuel, prefer glucose. Because brain cells can use only glucose for energy, there must be a steady supply in the blood to keep the brain functioning. Because people eat intermittently, some glucose is stored in the liver and in skeletal muscle in a polysaccharide form known as glycogen. When one eats a carbohydrate-rich food, some of the glucose that is in excess of immediate needs by the cells may be converted by the liver into glycogen and stored for later use. Unlike the brain, muscles can use many compounds for fuel. Most commonly, they prefer fat (at rest) or glucose (at work). Muscle cells cannot burn any fat without burning some glucose as well. Each muscle cell can store a small amount of glucose in the form of glycogen. Muscle glycogen stores are limited to approximately 400 grams or 1,600 calories and, once full, will not accept more glucose. If, after glycogen stores are full, there is still an excess of glucose in the bloodstream, the body will convert it to fat for storage. Fat stores are unlimited. A lean young man may carry 15 pounds (6.8 kg) of fat, which amounts to over 50,000 calories.

If a person is exercising and uses up all of her glycogen, the skeletal muscles will simply stop working. Endurance athletes need to maximize the amounts of glucose available to their muscle cells both in the bloodstream and stored in the cell. During competition or training, hard exercise of over 90 minutes' duration will deplete glycogen stores. Unless those stores are replaced, performance will suffer. To maximize glycogen stores, 60 to 70 percent of the calories an athlete eats should be in the form of complex carbohydrates.

Eating before a workout or competition can provide a steady supply of glucose that will spare glycogen reserves. The before-exercise meal should consist of easily digestible carbohydrates that will have time to leave the stomach before competition or training. Solid foods such as pasta, rice, bread and fruit should be consumed at least 3 or 4 hours prior to exercise, but liquids may be consumed within 2 hours of a workout. The athlete should experiment with pregame fueling during training because the optimal time for pregame meals varies considerably from person to person.

Proteins

Proteins form another important class of nutrients. Because it can be used as an energy source, the quantity of protein can be measured in calories as well as grams. Proteins are usually large complex molecules (which look like tangled telephone cords) made up of strings of smaller molecules, called amino acids, bonded together. There are only 20 different kinds of amino acids. Just as all the words of the English language are composed of the same 26 letters in a variety of arrangements, so are different proteins created by changing the arrangement of the 20 amino acids. Over 30,000 different proteins are manufactured within the body. These proteins form structural components, as in bone, hair, muscle, and tissue. Enzymes that facilitate reactions are proteins, as are many hormones (chemicals made by one cell that travel in the bloodstream and affect the activities of

Carbohydrate Loading: Is It Worthwhile For You?

The need for large glycogen reserves is so critical to endurance performance that athletes have tried various diet and exercise regimens to "carboload," to force the body to stuff glycogen into skeletal muscle cells. The classic carbohydrate loading technique involves these steps: One week prior to competition, a high-intensity workout helps the athlete achieve glycogen depletion. Glycogen stores stay reduced during the three following days if the athlete consumes a low-carbohydrate diet (60 g) while continuing modest exercise. On the fourth day, carbohydrate loading begins when the athlete switches to a high-carbohydrate diet (500 g per day) and performs light workouts. Finally, 3 or 4 hours prior to competition, the athlete consumes a high-carbohydrate meal. Though it has been shown to increase glycogen stores, this method has not proved to enhance performance, and athletes often complain of stiff muscles. The loss of lean tissue during the days of low carbohydrate intake and the inability to train hard because of glycogen deficiency causes muscle detraining and atrophy (shrinking), which counterbalance any gains made by enhancing glycogen stores. Most endurance athletes currently use the less stringent, modified carbo-loading procedure. The high-intensity, glycogen-depleting workout is eliminated. The athlete gradually tapers off exercise during the 6 days prior to competition. During the first 3 days, a diet consisting of 50 percent carbohydrates is eaten; this is followed by 3 days of a 70-percent carbohydrate diet.

Carbohydrate loading techniques are useful only for events lasting more than 75 minutes. Otherwise, normal levels of muscle glycogen are more than adequate. Bodybuilders often use the classic technique even though their endurance needs are minimal. A glycogen-loaded muscle is a plump muscle.

Eating or drinking carbohydrates during exercise may be beneficial to endurance athletes. The need for fluid during exercise, however, is more critical than the need for fuel. Carbohydrates in the stomach delay gastric emptying, which may cause discomfort as well as delaying fluid transport.

Eating after exercise is crucial to replace glycogen stores. During the first 2 hours after exercise, carbohydrates are much more likely to be converted to glycogen than to fat. Athletes should consume 50 grams of carbohydrate as soon as is practical after exercise.

---

other cells). Antibodies are proteins that are made to fight off infectious diseases.

A single protein molecule can consist of as few as 10 amino acids or as many as 100,000. Each amino acid has a similar structure consisting of at least one nitrogen atom. Neither carbohydrates nor fats contain nitrogen. If every amino acid contains nitrogen, then every protein contains nitrogen. To construct the proteins the body needs, the cells must have all the necessary raw materials. One essential raw material is thus nitrogen.

Just as with the carbohydrates, the intestinal cells cannot absorb these large protein molecules. The digestive tract is designed to split proteins into their amino acid subunits and then absorb the amino acids. The body can put the absorbed amino acids together in new ways to make new proteins. If one eats more protein than is needed for tissue building, the liver cells can take the amino acids apart and convert the carbons and hydrogens to glucose, if needed, or to fat. The liver cells combine the discarded nitrogens to form a compound called urea, which is then excreted into the urine by the kidneys.

Of the 20 amino acids, the body can make 12, as long as enough carbon, hydrogen, oxygen, and nitrogen are present. The carbons, hydrogens, and oxygens can come from carbohydrates, fats, or proteins, but nitrogen is available only from the proteins that are consumed. Eight of the amino acids used to make proteins cannot be made by the body and must be eaten in food. These eight are called essential amino acids. If the body is constructing a protein, it requires a certain amino acid in a certain place; if the body cannot manufacture that amino acid and it has not been consumed, that protein simply will not be made.

Not only must one eat enough protein to supply the nitrogen one needs to make amino acids; one must also eat enough of the right kind of protein to supply enough of the essential amino acids. Exactly how much protein is needed in the diet is a controversial issue. What is not disputed is that most Americans eat too much protein. Protein in excess of need is converted into glucose and fat, and the conversion process is hard on the liver and the kidneys. A steady protein consumption of more than double one's needs may cause disease in these organs.

A person who eats animal products is likely to be eating proteins that contain all the essential amino acids. Proteins containing all of the essential amino acids are called complete proteins. Because plants use different proteins from those used by animals, most plant proteins do not contain all of the amino acids; thus, their proteins are incomplete. Different plants supply different amino acids, and a knowledgeable consumer can, by eating the right combination of plant proteins, get all of the essential amino acids without eating animal products at all (*see the box "Vegetarianism: Is it Safe?"*).

The body uses a priority system. Maintaining adequate energy to keep the tissues functioning is the top priority. If energy production from carbohydrates and fats is adequate, only then will amino acids be used for making proteins. If these energy sources are inadequate, amino acids will be used for fuel rather than for building new tissue.

Protein requirements vary from person to person. Obviously, a large person needs more than a small person. A growing person needs more than an adult. The RDA for adults is 0.8 milligram for every kilogram of body weight. Though generous, this RDA assumes that the person is at or near ideal body weight and that the diet contains enough carbohydrates and fat so that the ingested protein is not needed to provide energy. If an obese person and a very muscular person weighed the same, the more muscular person would need more protein. An underweight person needs to make all the hormones, enzymes, and antibodies a normal-weight person does. By using actual instead of ideal body weight for the calculations, an underweight person would underestimate his or her protein needs. Another assumption in setting the RDA for protein is that the person is healthy. A sick person needs more protein, not only to repair damaged tissues, but also because her ability to absorb protein might be compromised.

It is tempting to think that an athlete needs much more protein than a nonathlete, but this is simply not true. The athlete usually needs more calories for fuel, not more protein. Even a person in a strength training program (which is comparable to growing) does not need much additional protein. Muscle is three-fourths water; therefore, every pound of muscle contains 12 ounces of water and less than 4 ounces of protein. If a person in a weight training program puts on 10 pounds of muscle in 20 weeks (which would be quite a feat), in each week the gain would be 8 ounces of muscle. Because an ounce is 30 grams, each day would add 34 grams of muscle. Only 8 grams of that 34 is actually composed of amino acids, the rest being water. A person in this program may wish to add an extra 8 or 9 grams of protein to his diet each day, which can be done easily by drinking an extra glass of skim milk. Protein supplements are not only unnecessary but can even be detrimental to one's health. Protein intake in excess of double the RDA has been implicated in osteoporosis, liver and kidney disease, and zinc deficiencies.

On the other hand, eating too little protein has drastic consequences. If one does not eat enough protein to supply the body with enough nitrogen and essential amino acids to construct the enzymes and hormones needed for day-to-day activities, the body will start to use the protein in its own muscle. Though most people in the United States eat more protein than they need, many young women, in an ill-advised attempt to be underweight, often restrict the amounts they eat. By severely restricting calories, they may not get enough protein. Subtle deficiencies produce vague symptoms, such as apathy, that are hard to ascribe to a specific disease. A protein-deficient person might get sick more easily, as her body cannot manufacture all of the necessary disease-fighting proteins. Subtle protein deficiencies could affect the athlete in many ways. An athlete cannot build muscle if protein needs are not being met. Apathy might show up as a lack of motivation for training. Severe protein deficiencies can, in addition, cause swelling of the extremities and abdomen, diarrhea, and liver and heart failure.

Recent research indicates that endurance athletes may need more protein per unit of body weight than sedentary people or even bodybuilders. When glycogen stores are low, the body breaks down skeletal muscle to use the amino acids for energy. Exercise of long duration, like a marathon, is the kind most likely to deplete glycogen stores. Endurance athletes need to have an adequate amount of carbohydrate in their diets to minimize the use of protein for fuel. There is no evidence, however, that a person undertaking a resistance training program requires any more protein in the diet than does a sedentary person.

How much protein is enough? The RDA for adults is 0.8 gram/kilogram/day. (For every kilogram of body weight, an adult should ingest 0.8 gram of high-quality protein.) A 70-kg (154-lb.) male would require 56 grams of protein a day. A 50-kg (110-lb.) woman would require 40 grams of protein a day. This is a generous allowance and is usually more than adequate. Endurance athletes and adolescents might need a bit more, perhaps 0.9 to 1.0 gram/kilogram/day. A growing endurance athlete might need even a little more. Someone who is overweight should base the calculations on ideal rather than actual weight.

Another way to calculate protein intake is as a percentage of total calories. Of the total caloric requirement, 12 to 15 percent should be protein. If a person eats 2,000 calories per day, she should ingest 240 calories, or 60 grams, of protein. Endurance athletes have high caloric requirements. These caloric requirements may give a better estimate of their needs than would body weight.

A high-quality protein not only contains all the essential amino acids, it contains them in ideal ratios. Animal foods such as meat, milk, eggs, and cheese are excellent sources of protein, and animal protein is of high quality. The highest-quality protein is contained in the egg. However, the egg, like other animal protein sources, also contains a fair amount of fat and cholesterol, neither of which is desirable. Lean meats, skim milk, low-fat yogurt, and fish, which are lower in fat and cholesterol, are all good protein choices. An ounce of fish or lean meat contains roughly 7 grams of protein, as does an ounce of hard or firm cheese. Milk contains 1 gram in every ounce, regardless of the fat content. Thus it is quite easy to get large amounts of protein through the typical American diet: one quarter-pound hamburger with cheese offers 29 grams of protein; and the addition of a milk shake brings the total to 40 grams (the fat content, however, is quite high).

Fat

In U.S. society, fat has a bad reputation—a reputation that is not entirely accurate. Many people in the United States do consume too much fat, and the consequences of a high-fat diet include an increased incidence of heart attacks, strokes, and cancer. Because a high-fat diet raises these and other health risks, some people try to eliminate all fat from their diets. This extreme approach is not only unnecessary, but also unwise, because some fat in the diet is essential to good health. How much fat to include, and in what form, is open to question. Not all fats are created equal; some carry higher risks than others. This section will explore the chemistry of fats and what happens to ingested fat in the body.

Scientists refer to fats as lipids. Lipids are a class of compounds composed primarily of carbon and hydrogen that do not dissolve in water but will dissolve in organic solvents such as alcohol, ether, or gasoline. Most of the lipids that are consumed and most of the lipids in the body are in a form called triglycerides. Triglycerides are formed by adding three fatty acids to a glycerol molecule (*see Figure 1*). Glycerol is a three-carbon molecule, and a fatty acid is a chain of carbons (usually 6–24 carbons long). All of the body's storage fat (the fat under the skin) is in the form of triglycerides, and this is the type of fat the body uses for fuel. Each gram of triglyceride can yield at least 9 calories of energy, which is more than twice the caloric content per

Vegetarianism: Is it Safe?

Plants, like animals, require protein to function. Plant proteins differ from animal proteins in that they may lack a few essential amino acids. With a little planning, however, one can fulfill the body's protein requirements without eating any animal products.

Bean and rice are staples for many people of the world. Beans (not green beans, but the legumes: pinto beans, navy beans, chickpeas, and so on) are an excellent food. Each cup contains about 15 grams of protein (about 230 calories), 15 grams of fiber, and less than 1 gram of fat. Beans have little sodium but are high in potassium and folic acid. Combined with rice or other grains, beans provide all the amino acids necessary for tissue growth and repair.

There are many advantages to a vegetarian or low-meat diet. Compared with people who eat a "typical" American diet, vegetarians have lower cholesterol levels and a lower incidence of cardiovascular disease, cancer and many common intestinal disorders, and they are less likely to be obese. Vegetarians also live longer; however, they do have several areas of special concern:

1. Vigilance is necessary to ensure that protein intake is adequate in quantity and quality.
2. Calcium intake may be inadequate.
3. Vitamin B12 and iron intake may be suboptimal.

The vegetarian diet is usually so low in fat that vegetarian endurance athletes may have difficulty eating enough calories to match their energy output. The addition of dairy products to an otherwise all vegetarian diet usually solves the problem of calories, protein, B12, and calcium. Many champion athletes are vegetarians. Diversity is the key to a healthy vegetarian diet, with a plentiful variety of vegetables, whole grains, and legumes.

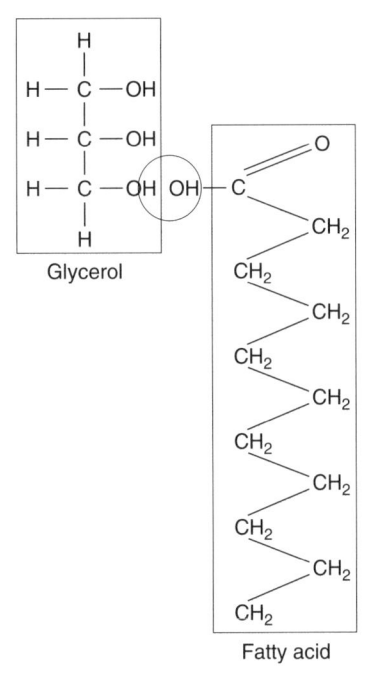

Figure 1. *Triglycerides are formed by adding three fatty acids to a glycerol molecule.*

gram of proteins or carbohydrates. Some cells actually prefer to use fatty acids for fuel—notably heart muscle but also skeletal muscle at rest or at low levels of work (*see also* ENERGY AND METABOLISM). Some cells cannot use fatty acids for fuel at all. Brain cells, for example, lack the enzymes needed to utilize fatty acids for energy. The body is constantly depositing triglycerides into fat cells for energy storage and removing fatty acids from fat cells for use as fuel. The amount of body fat one carries around reflects whether one is making more deposits or more withdrawals. If a person eats more calories than he needs—whether carbohydrate, protein, or fat—the liver and the fat cells convert the excess to triglycerides, which are stored in fat cells.

Not all fatty acids are the same. They can vary in length as well as the amount of hydrogen relative to each carbon. A fatty acid that contains all the hydrogen it can hold is saturated; a triglyceride made of all saturated fatty acids is called a saturated fat. If more hydrogen can be added, it is an unsaturated fat. If hydrogen can be added to only one place, it is a monounsaturated fat. If hydrogen can be added to more than one place, it is a polyunsaturated fat. Saturated fats, like butter, tend to be solid at room temperature. Unsaturated fats, such as vegetable oil, tend to be liquid at room temperature. Chemists can add hydrogen to a liquid unsaturated fat in a process called hydrogenation. This process is done to make vegetable fats more solid, as is done in products like margarine. It is unlikely that a person would get up in the morning, pour oil over her toast, salt it, and eat it. Yet

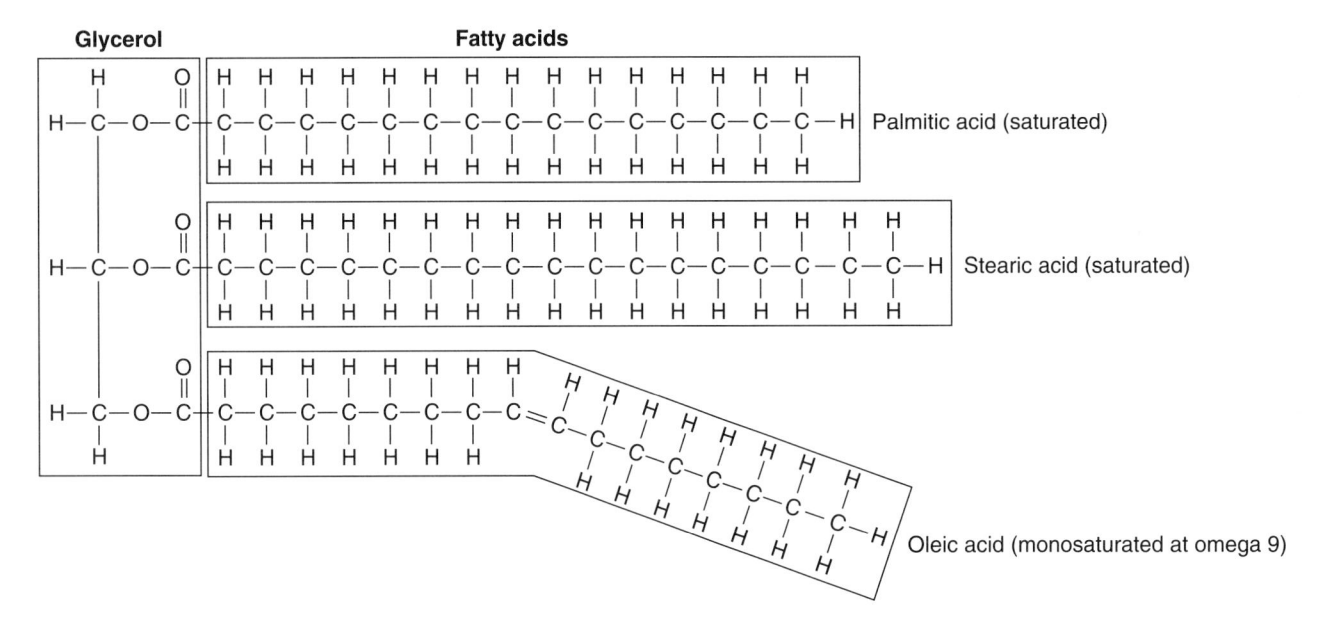

Figure 2. *A triglyceride molecule (neutral fat).*

spreading margarine on toast is essentially the same thing, except that the vegetable oil has been hydrogenated to make it firm.

Not only can fatty acids vary by length and hydrogen saturation, but they also vary by the location along the molecule at which they are unsaturated. These empty sites are referred to as omega positions. An omega-9 fatty acid is unsaturated at the ninth carbon from the right (*see Figure 2*). The degree of saturation and the position of the unsaturated segment are both thought to have health consequences (which will be discussed later).

Not all lipids are triglycerides. Phospholipids constitute another important lipid class. These molecules are similar to triglycerides except that one fatty acid has been replaced by a phosphate group (PO_4). Every single cell in the body is enclosed by a thin membrane, which is composed primarily of phospholipids. Without these phospholipid membranes to hold the cells together, they would disintegrate. Therefore, this kind of fat is necessary to life itself. The body can make most, but not all, of the fatty acids necessary to form these membranes. The two fatty acids that the body cannot make, called essential fatty acids, are abundant in plant and fish oils. Diseases caused by deficiencies of these fatty acids are rare but do occur. Obtaining essential fatty acids is one important reason that some fat must be included in the diet.

The last class of lipids to consider is the sterols. Sterols have an entirely different structure from the other two classes of lipids (*see Figure 3*).

The sterols differ from each other by the atoms attached to various places in this same basic multiring structure. Included in this group are the sex hormones testosterone and estrogen, adrenal hormones, and cholesterol. Cholesterol is a necessary component of animal cell membranes, providing structural integrity. The body also

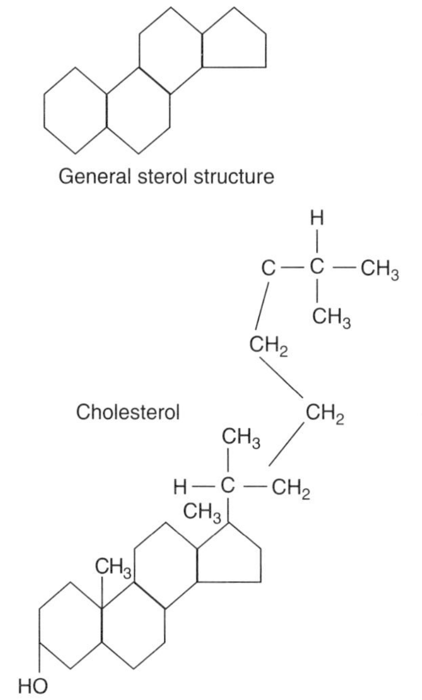

Figure 3. *Sterols include the sex hormones testosterone and estrogen, adrenal hormones, and cholesterol.*

needs cholesterol to make bile, which aids in digestion. Because all animals have cholesterol in their cell membranes, whenever one eats animal products, one consumes cholesterol. The liver can make all the cholesterol the body needs and more, so it is not necessary to consume any. Foods from plants can have no cholesterol but may still be high in total fat content.

Another reason that the human diet requires some fat is that the digestive system can absorb certain vitamins (K, E, and A) only if they have a chance to "ride along" with some fat molecules. These vitamins dissolve in fat rather than in water. One does not need to eat very much fat to supply these needs, and one does not need to eat animal fats at all.

Fat provides 35 to 40 percent of calories consumed by most people in the United States. A diet containing this much fat is a known health risk. The current recommendation from the American Heart Association is to limit fat calories to no more than 30 percent of the total. Many experts believe that this amount of fat is too high and would like to see fat calories limited to 20 percent. Other experts believe it is healthier to eat even less fat, although most feel that consuming less than 15 percent of total calories as fat may cause deficiencies in essential fatty acids and fat-soluble vitamins. In a typical U.S. diet, if a person eats 2,000 calories a day, 800 of those calories would be fat. A 20 percent fat diet would limit fat calories to 400. Fat calories add up quickly. A quarter-pound hamburger with cheese and a bag of fries contains a total of 740 calories, of which 369 are derived from fat. A salad may have no fat, but the salad dressing may have 70 calories of fat in every tablespoon. One hot dog may easily have 150 fat calories.

Not all fats are metabolized by the body in the same way. Some fats carry higher health risks than others. Although the research in this area is not yet conclusive, there are enough data to support some general recommendations. Both saturated fatty acids and transfatty acids, which have straight chains, should be limited to no more than 30 percent of total fat calories. The straight-chain fatty acids appear to be more likely to lead to clogging of the arteries by fat deposits, a condition known as atherosclerosis. When arteries get clogged, the heart has to work harder to pump the blood, which carries oxygen and nutrients, through the body to nourish the cells. If blood flow to a tissue is diminished by arterial blockage, cells cannot work properly and might even die. A heart attack (myocardial infarction) is the death of heart muscle cells, usually caused by atherosclerosis in the arteries that bring oxygenated blood to the heart muscle. Evidence shows that atherosclerosis starts in childhood. Autopsies done on U.S. soldiers during the Vietnam war showed that many American teenagers had visible fatty streaks in their arteries. The Vietnamese soldiers did not. Americans at that time had even more saturated fat in their diets than they do now. The Vietnamese have a low-fat diet with very little saturated fat.

Monounsaturated fats seem to be protective against heart disease. In cultures where dietary fat intake is high but the fats ingested are of the monounsaturated type, people have a lower incidence of cardiovascular disease than do Americans. Fats that are unsaturated at the third position (omega-3 fatty acids), found in fish oils, appear to be especially protective.

Cholesterol is the substance found in the plaques clogging up arteries. People who have high levels of cholesterol in their blood have a greater chance of developing atherosclerosis. It was once thought that the more cholesterol one ate, the higher one's blood cholesterol levels and the greater the chance of clogged arteries. It is now known that the liver makes all the cholesterol the body needs, mostly in response to the total amount of fat in the diet, particularly saturated fat. The more fat one eats, the more cholesterol the liver makes to carry it around (*see the box "Cholesterol: Is the News All Bad?"*).

Except for very young children, it is recommended that the total amount of fat in the diet not exceed 30 percent of total caloric intake. It would probably be best to reduce that to 20 percent. To eliminate all fat from the diet would be harmful and is not recommended. Of the fats eaten, saturated fats should be limited to no more than a third and monounsaturated fats should be at least a third, with the rest polyunsaturated. How does this translate into eating habits? Sausage and red meats have the highest saturated fat content and should be eaten sparingly. Desserts high in animal fats, such as premium ice cream, can still be enjoyed as long as they are eaten sparingly. Foods made with transfatty acids, like margarine, should be limited in the same way that saturated fats are limited or avoided altogether until more is known about them. Substituting oils that are high in monounsaturated fats would not hurt and could be beneficial. For example, olive oil and canola oil can be used in cooking instead of corn or safflower oil to increase the intake of monounsaturated fats without increasing overall fat intake. Low-fat or no-fat dairy products are excellent foods for the athlete, yielding high-quality protein and calcium with very few fat calories. Eating lots of vegetables and grains while limiting meat has been shown not only to prolong life but to improve the quality of life. It is important to remember that usual eating habits are what determine health. If one eats well most days, an occasional splurge will not hurt one's overall health. On the other hand, six days a week of unwise eating cannot be compensated for by one day of smarter choices.

Vitamins and Minerals

People have known for thousands of years that eating habits have a significant impact on health. That specific foods could prevent or treat disease has been known for hundreds of years, though the specific chemicals in the foods have been known only since World War I. The term *vitamin* was coined in 1912 by Dr. Casimir Funk, who was attempting to find the chemical in rice bran that cured beriberi, a disease characterized in its extreme form by severe muscle wasting,

Cholesterol: Is the News All Bad?

Cholesterol is a firm, waxy substance contained in all animal cell membranes. Whenever one eats animal products, one consumes cholesterol. The body makes cholesterol all the time as an essential component of cell membranes and of bile, which aids in digestion.

When one eats fats in the form of triglycerides, these molecules are too big to be absorbed into the body through the intestinal wall. Intestinal enzymes break up the triglycerides into smaller units: fatty acids and glycerol. These smaller compounds are then absorbed by the cells that line the small intestine, where they are reassembled into triglycerides. However, triglycerides do not dissolve in water, and it would not do to have blobs of fat floating around in the blood. To handle this problem, the intestinal cells build a package made up of protein, cholesterol, and triglyceride that allows the fat to travel in the blood as if it were dissolved. This fat and protein combination made by the intestinal cells is called a chylomicron. The chylomicrons travel through the body in the blood. When a chylomicron approaches a cell that needs fat for fuel, an enzyme allows fatty acids to enter the cell. The chylomicrons also deliver triglycerides to fat cells for storage. The more fat that is eaten, the more chylomicrons are made.

When circulating chylomicrons come in contact with liver cells, or when the liver converts excess glucose or protein to fatty acids, the liver cells build a slightly different package to carry the fats around. This package has relatively more cholesterol than the chylomicron. The cholesterol used to make this package is manufactured by the liver. These fat, cholesterol, and protein packages are called lipoprotein. The lipoprotein made by the liver from free fatty acids or chylomicrons is called very low density lipoprotein (VLDL). The VLDLs deliver triglycerides to fat cells for storage. After the delivery, what remains is called a low density lipoprotein (LDL). The role of the low density lipoprotein is to deliver cholesterol to the cells. Cells that need cholesterol put out a signal. If a cell has signaled for a delivery, cholesterol is deposited into the cell by the LDL. Once the cell has an adequate supply, it stops making the signal and no further deliveries are made. If there is more cholesterol in the blood in the form of LDLs than needed, this excess tends to be deposited along the walls of arteries. Again, the more fats that are eaten, the more cholesterol is made.

There is another class of lipoproteins called high density lipoprotein (HDL). These are manufactured by the liver from chylomicron remnants. This lipoprotein can actually pick up cholesterol from the blood and tissues and bring it back to the liver. The liver then can recycle the cholesterol instead of making more. Because excess LDL can clog arteries, it is known as the "bad" cholesterol, while HDL is known as the "good" cholesterol.

A doctor often measures total cholesterol as part of a routine physical. The higher a person's total cholesterol, the more at risk he is of having cardiovascular disease. An even more powerful predictor is the ratio of total cholesterol over HDL. People with ratios of 4.5 or greater are considered at high risk of cardiovascular disease, while ratios of 3 or less are considered low risk.

The development of atherosclerosis is not quite so simple as "the good versus the bad" cholesterol. There are subclassifications of these lipoprotein classes, and research shows that not all LDLs and HDLs are created equal. Diet is not the only factor that affects the ratio of total cholesterol to HDL. Heredity plays an important role. Sex hormones also influence the rate at which the different types of lipoproteins are made. Estrogen promotes a more favorable ratio of HDL to LDL, and testosterone promotes an unfavorable ratio. This effect explains why men have a higher rate of heart attacks than premenopausal women and why postmenopausal women, who produce little or no estrogen, have rising rates of heart disease. Cardiovascular exercise has a very significant and favorable effect on HDL levels. Smoking sharply reduces HDL levels. While we cannot pick our parents or our gender, we can choose what foods to eat and how regularly to exercise. We can also choose not to smoke.

---

including wasting of heart muscle. This disease is caused by vitamin B1 deficiency. A vitamin is now defined as a chemical that is vital for tissue growth, maintenance, and repair and that has no caloric value. Vitamins are also organic compounds; they come from living things. Though vitamins themselves cannot be used for energy, many are essential in facilitating the burning of food fuels. Other vitamins are needed to facilitate different reactions throughout the body. The list of vitamins is fairly standard, and although some references may claim that other, additional substances are vitamins, the provided list is well accepted.

Until very recently, the study of vitamins was undertaken to prevent and treat deficiency diseases. The U.S. government sets standards for the amount of each vitamin needed to prevent deficiency diseases. However, how much of each vitamin is optimal for health is largely unknown, and new data are published daily.

Vitamins have traditionally been split into two categories: water-soluble and fat-soluble (*see Table 1 and 2*). Water-soluble vitamins are stored in the body in small quantities. Having a dietary deficiency of these vitamins for a few days will not cause illness if the diet usually contains adequate amounts. If eaten in excess, water-soluble vitamins are excreted in the urine. Fat-soluble vitamins are dissolved in the fats of foods. When one eats the fat, one consumes the vitamins. If eaten in excess of requirements, these vitamins can be stored in body fat. Because the excess is stored and not excreted, a person can get vitamin toxicities from these compounds by ingesting too much of them in either food or vitamin supplements.

One of the most common misconceptions about vitamins is that if some is good, more is better. This simply is not true. For example, some of the B vitamins are involved with the aerobic conversion of energy, acting as coenzymes in the fuel burning process (*see also ENERGY AND METABOLISM*). A lack of these vitamins causes energy utilization to be inadequate, which is bad for anyone but disastrous for the athlete. However, having an excess of these vitamins will not make energy utilization any more efficient. Taking vitamin B supplements is therefore worthwhile only if the diet is deficient. Megadoses of these vitamins at worst, are dangerous to the health and, at best, produce very expensive urine.

Subtle vitamin deficiencies may not cause overt illness but certainly can impair athletic performance. One of the most common is a deficiency in folic acid, a vitamin found in fresh vegetables and legumes. It can be destroyed when foods are canned, overcooked, or otherwise processed. The wilted iceberg lettuce on a hamburger does not provide much in the way of vitamins. Teenagers often avoid foods that contain folic acid, and the symptoms of deficiency are subtle; early signs are general feelings of fatigue and irritability. Most teenagers, because of less than optimal eating habits, have inadequate stores of this vitamin. In addition, serious birth defects can occur when a woman who is folic acid–deficient becomes pregnant.

Thiamine deficiencies are also fairly common in people who consume a lot of empty-calorie foods such as soda, chips, and candy. Subtle thiamine deficiencies can cause fatigue, sleep disturbances, and personality changes. Severe thiamine deficiency can cause death.

Fat soluble vitamins can be stored in large quantities in the body; this can lead to toxicity. It is unusual to get dangerous amounts through the diet (though explorers and hunters eating polar bear livers have done it). Supplements of these vitamins should be taken with care.

Vitamin A deficiency is the most common cause of blindness in children worldwide. Many people in the United States suffer night vision problems because of deficiencies of this vitamin (*see also* *VISION*). It also presents the most common vitamin toxicity problem, because toxic doses are only slightly higher than therapeutic doses. A vitamin A precursor called beta-carotene is found in many plant foods, especially dark green and orange vegetables. This compound is converted to vitamin A in the body. If an excess of beta-carotene is eaten, the body simply does not convert it; the excess beta-carotene is harmless.

Various minerals are essential to health and well being. Minerals are inorganic compounds that come from the earth's crust. Minerals and their functions are even less well understood than the vitamins. Again, these substances have no caloric value and cannot be used for energy. Some minerals, such as calcium, are needed structurally in the body. (Vitamins are never needed in this capacity.) Other minerals are enzyme facilitators, as are some vitamins, and still others perform different functions. The functions of some minerals are very obscure, such as the role of chromium in glucose transport.

WATER-SOLUBLE VITAMINS

Vitamin	Function	USRDA	Deficiency	Excess	Sources
B1 Thiamine	Assists in ATP formation from carbohydrates	1.5 mg	Muscle weakness, mental confusion, impaired growth	Irritability, headache, sleep disturbances	Legumes, meat, whole or enriched grains
Riboflavine	Assists in ATP formation from carbohydrates, fats, and proteins	1.7 mg	Skin problems around nose and mouth	None reported	Dark green vegetables, milk, meat, whole-grain or enriched breads and cereals
Niacin	Assists in transfer of electrons from Krebs cycle to electron transfer chain	20 mg	Skin, mucous membrane, nervous system, and gastrointestinal (GI) deterioration	Low blood pressure, itching, flushing, headache; may cause death	All protein-rich foods, including legumes as well as meat, dairy, nuts, and eggs
B6	Helps in amino acid and fat metabolism	2 mg	Retarded growth, convulsions, skin, rashes, muscle weakness	Fatigue, headaches, depression; can cause death	Green leafy vegetables, legumes, whole grains, meat, and bananas
Folate	Protein metabolism, cell division	0.4 mg	Poor growth, anemia, nerve degeneration, paralysis	None reported	Green leafy vegetables, legumes
B12	Maintains nerve cells, blood formation, synthesis of genetic material	6 mg	Anemia, nerve degeneration, paralysis	None reported	All animal products, nutritional yeast
Pantothenic acid	Assists in making ATP	10 mg	Retarded growth, sleep disturbances, fatigue	None reported	Widespread in foods
Biotin	Assists in making ATP, needed for fat and glycogen synthesis	0.3 mg	Weakness, fatigue, rash, nausea, muscle pain	None reported	Widespread in foods
C	Needed for connective tissue, antioxidant	60 mg	Frequent infections, anemia, bruising, loss of teeth, poor wound healing	Nausea, diarrhea, kidney stones	Citrus foods, cabbage family, vegetables, potatoes dark green vegetables

Table 1.

Calcium is the most abundant mineral in the body. Most of the body's calcium is located in the bones, which act as a calcium bank (*see also* SKELETAL SYSTEM). The amount of calcium dissolved in the blood needs to be kept steady for normal nerve and muscle function (*see also* SKELETAL MUSCLE). If the level in the blood drops, calcium is taken from the bones to restore the normal concentration. Simply eating more calcium than one needs will not cause the excess to be deposited in the bone bank, however. Excess calcium is excreted in the feces and urine. If a person does not eat enough calcium, her bones will become thin and break easily. Many older American women lose so much calcium from the bones that they become weak enough to break during normal activities such as coughing. This condition of calcium-depleted bone, called osteoporosis, will affect 1 out of every 3 women in the United States and 1 out of every 10 men. The best time to prevent this disease is in the teen years, when a person's ability to lay down thicker bones is at its peak. Making bone is not simply a matter of taking in adequate amounts of calcium. There are many other factors involved. One very important factor is strength. The body makes strong bones where they are needed; the incentive for bone deposition is stress on the bone. If the diet is adequate, where there are strong muscles, there will be thick bones. The other factor is hormonal. The sex hormones, testosterone and estrogen encourage bone deposition. Testosterone's effects are stronger, so men have thicker bones than women. During menopause, ovarian production of estrogen ceases, causing bone loss. Men, on the other hand, make testosterone to the end of their days; osteoporosis is thus much more common in women than in men. Adequate calcium and exercise are essential to women of all ages if they are to maintain bone quality.

Very strenuous exercise, especially when coupled with calorie

FAT-SOLUBLE VITAMINS

Vitamin	Function	USRDA	Deficiency	Excess	Sources
A	Forming visual pigments, hormone synthesis, epithelial repair	1.0 mg	Night blindness, impaired growth, skin deterioration	Central nervous system damage, nausea, irritability, and vomiting; skeletal abnormalities	Orange and dark green leafy vegetables; fortified dairy products
D	Needed for normal bone mineralization.	400 mg	Soft bones, rickets, abnormal growth	Abnormal bone deposition	Sunlight on exposed skin; fortified foods; eggs, liver, fish
E	Stabilization of cell membranes	10 mg	Anemia and skin disorders (rare)	None known	Vegetable oils, whole grains, nuts, seeds
K	Synthesis of blood clotting proteins	80 mg	Abnormal bleeding and bruising	Liver abnormalities	Leafy green vegetables, and vegetables in the cabbage family; bacterial synthesis in the colon

Table 2.

restriction, may cause ovarian dysfunction in some women. This may cause abnormal lowering of estrogen levels, putting a woman at risk of developing osteoporosis even though she might have strong muscles and adequate calcium intake (*see also* FEMALE ATHLETES). Low estrogen levels may be signaled by menstrual irregularities. If a female athlete starts missing periods, this may be an indication that her ovarian function is compromised. She should be evaluated by a physician or health practitioner experienced in this area.

The mineral iron is needed to make hemoglobin, which is the molecule that carries oxygen in the blood. It is also necessary for the electron transport chain in energy utilization (*see also* ENERGY AND METABOLISM). An iron deficiency will make a person feel tired because he cannot make adequate amounts of hemoglobin. Inadequate hemoglobin means inadequate oxygen in the bloodstream, and without enough oxygen, one cannot utilize fuel to make energy. A mild iron deficiency, too subtle to cause anemia, can make one tired and has been implicated in learning disorders in children. Because menstruating women lose blood every month, they lose iron. This iron must be replaced through the diet. Because men do not menstruate, their need for iron is less. The RDA for iron for men is 10 milligrams every day. Because the average diet in industrialized nations contains 5 milligrams of iron for every 1,000 calories, dietary iron deficiency is not a problem for men. Women should get 15 milligrams of iron daily. To get adequate amounts of iron, a woman would have to eat 3,000 calories every day, which is far more than most women need. Many women may be marginally iron deficient without knowing it. The female athlete needs to be especially vigilant as her performance could suffer from this deficiency. Many of the minerals listed in Table 3 have no established RDA. Research is too scanty at the present time to allow a recommendation.

Antioxidants are compounds that prevent the harmful effects of free radicals. Free radicals are chemicals that raid cell walls looking to grab electrons. Antioxidants donate electrons to free radicals without forming harmful substances. Though researchers are not certain, it appears as though free radicals are involved in the development of in atherosclerosis and some cancers. Even more sketchy is the research showing that antioxidants such as vitamins A, E, C, and D can prevent these diseases. Still, the early studies are promising and the currently recommended dosages have no known harmful effects. Some of the research shows that taking vitamin supplements is not quite as good as getting the nutrient from foods naturally. This may be because of a class of chemicals called phytochemicals. There are thousands of these chemicals found in foods, and they are abundant in vegetables and especially in vegetables of the cabbage families. These chemicals are being studied by the National Cancer Institute as part of a multimillion dollar project. Early studies in animals show that they have cancer inhibiting effects.

Research indicates that it is best to eat a variety of foods, including five or six servings of vegetables every day. Legumes and whole

MINERALS

Mineral	Function (needed for)	USRDA	Deficiency	Excess	Sources
Calcium	Bone structure; normal muscle and nerve function	1 g	Bone loss, retarded growth	Kidney stones	Dairy, tofu, legumes, small fish eaten with the bones, greens
Phosphorus	Constantly needed by every cell	1 g	None known	Can create relative calcium deficiency	All animal products
Magnesium	Nerve transmission and muscle contraction; normal mineralization of bones	400 mg	Weakness, confusion, muscle spasms	Unknown	Seafood, whole grains, chocolate
Sodium	Normal fluid and acid-base balance		Weakness, muscle cramps	May contribute to high blood pressure	Processed and pickled foods, soy sauce
Chloride	Normal fluid and acid-base balance		Disturbed acid-based balance (usually caused by vomiting)	Growth failure, apathy, muscle cramps	Same as sodium
Potassium	Fluid balance, nerve transmission, muscle contraction		Cardiac rhythm disturbances, muscle weakness	Slowing and stopping of the heart	Fruits and vegetables
Sulfur	ATP production; essential part of many proteins		None known, illness from protein deficiency occurs first	Not reported in humans	Protein-containing foods; all meats, dairy, legumes
Iodine	Essential component of thyroid hormones	0.150 mg	Enlarged thyroid; hormone deficiency slows metabolism	Extreme intake can interfere with normal thyroid function	Seafood and iodized salt
Iron	Component of hemoglobin and myoglobin; needed in the electron transport chain	18 mg	Anemia; learning disorders	Liver toxicity, may increase risk of cancer and heart attacks	Meat, legumes, dried fruits
Zinc	Part of many enzyme systems	15 mg	Poor wound healing; infertility in men	Unknown	Protein-containing foods
Copper	Hemoglobin formation; component of the electron transport chain.	2 mg	Anemia (extremely rare)	Unknown except in a rare hereditary disorder	Meats, liver, fish
Fluoride	Necessary for bone and teeth		Weakening of bones; tooth decay	Pigmented teeth	Drinking water, seafood
Selenium	Antioxidant	0.07 mg	Anemia	Gastrointestinal disorders	Seafood, meats, grains, garlic
Chromium	Insulin effectiveness in transport of glucose into cells		Inability to use glucose normally	Unknown	Brewer's yeast, wine, meat, some brands of beer, whole grains
Molybdenum	Enzyme reactions		Unknown	Unknown	Legumes, whole grains, organ meats
Manganese	Enzymatic reactions	5 mg	Unknown in humans	Unknown in humans	Wide distribution in foods
Cobalt	Hemoglobin formation and nerve function		Unknown except in B12 deficiency	Unknown	Meat and dairy products

Table 3.

grains also are very nutrient-rich and important for their caloric content. Some animal products are needed for vitamin B12 and dairy products are needed for calcium. It requires some planning to obtain all of the needed nutrients from food, but it is certainly worth the effort and for the athlete, doubly so. Not only does the real food supply the nutrient in the intended form, but it provides fiber and phytochemicals. However, if one has optimized one's diet as much as possible and is still coming up short in some areas, it would make sense to supplement. All of these choices must be tailored for the athlete individually—the ideal being to obtain all nutrients from food. Vitamin megadoses have not been shown to be beneficial to anyone except the sellers of these products and will not enhance athletic performance.

Water

Water is an essential nutrient even though it has no caloric value and it contains no vitamins. The body is a sea of water with a variety of substances dissolved and suspended in it. If all water were removed from a man who weighed 150 pounds, his dry weight would be only 50 pounds. The water in the body is divided into three categories: the water inside the cells (intracellular fluid), the water that sloshes around and in between the cells (extracellular fluid), and the water in the blood (blood plasma). Each of these three environments has a different chemical composition of salts and proteins. The water moves freely from one environment to another obeying basic laws of physics, with dissolved gases and salts moving from areas of higher concentration to areas of lower concentration. The arterial blood has a higher concentration of dissolved oxygen and nutrients than does the extracellular fluid and the intracellular fluid. The abundant oxygen and nutrients diffuse naturally from the blood environment into the extracellular environment. Now the extracellular fluid has a higher concentration of these substances than does the fluid inside the cells, so the oxygen and nutrients move from the extracellular fluid into the cells. Cellular wastes move in the opposite direction to diffuse from the interior of the cell into the blood (*see Figure 4*). In order for this transfer of oxygen, nutrients, and wastes to occur, all must be dissolved in water (*see also RESPIRATION*).

Water is lost through sweat, urine, and each exhaled breath. This lost water must be replaced. In a sedentary adult, the water that needs to be replaced amounts to roughly 2 quarts (or liters) a day. During heavy exertion, athletes can lose 2 quarts every hour. Even mild fluid deficits can affect athletic performance adversely: a fluid deficit prevents the exercising body from cooling efficiently, and the brain responds with a feeling of fatigue. Humans take in water through the fluids they drink and through the water content of the foods they eat. Fruits and vegetables have a high water content; breads, pastas, and many fast foods do not.

If one does not ingest enough water, the body will try to slow down the rate of water loss by reducing urine and sweat output. Although the water content of urine can decrease markedly, some urine will still be made—even in conditions of dehydration—to rid the body of waste chemicals. If sweating is impaired, the athlete

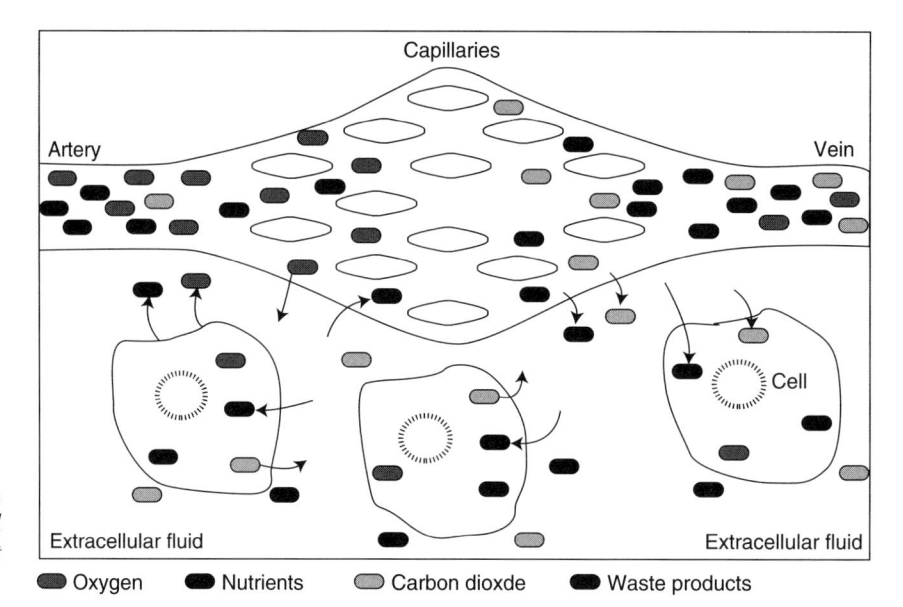

Figure 4. *Flow of oxygen, carbon dioxide, nutrients, and waste in and out of the capillaries and in and out of the cells.*

becomes overheated. Most often this translates to fatigue, and the athlete slows down or stops. Heat-induced fatigue obviously interferes with performance, not only during competition but also during training. Keeping hydrated during training is just as important as on the day of an athletic event.

Lack of water can also be dangerous. An athlete may lose enough fluid through sweating to reduce blood volume, and blood pressure can drop. Low blood pressure may cause dizziness or even fainting. If a person stops sweating completely, heat builds up inside the body to very high temperatures (105° F or more). These temperatures may cause brain damage, seizures, or death.

Thirst is an unreliable indicator of the need for fluid. The sensation of thirst ceases long before the fluids one drinks actually get into the blood, let alone the cells. How much fluid one takes in is largely a matter of habit, and the astute athlete not only trains the muscles but trains the mind to develop healthy habits. As much as half of a person's water intake comes from the foods she eats. The intelligent athlete avoids fast foods and highly salted snack foods for many reasons, their low water content being but one. The body can compensate for overhydration more easily than it can underhydration, so it is far better to drink too much than too little.

How much one should drink depends on the weather and the type of exertion or activity undertaken. Water losses are greatest in hot weather, and likewise, endurance activities require more fluid replacement than power activities. The pole vaulter does not need to think about fluids over and above daily needs on the day of the event, but certainly needs to replace fluid losses that occur during a tough training session. The distance runner, on the other hand, needs to be very conscious of fluid intake. Athletes may think they do not need to replace fluids during cool, dry weather because they do not feel sweaty;

on a cool, dry day the sweat evaporates and cools the body very efficiently. In hot, humid weather, the sweat rolls off the body; because the humidity in the air slows evaporation, less sweat evaporates and the body's cooling is less efficient. The body then gets hotter, causing one to sweat even more. Only the sweat that evaporates cools. Under extreme conditions of heat and humidity, it may be too dangerous to exercise at all. Clothing is also a factor. The football player in uniform, pads, and helmet will sweat much more than someone who is doing the same amount of work but is dressed in shorts and singlet.

It is a good idea for everyone to drink eight glasses of water a day to cover the daily losses that occur without exertion. Cold water leaves the stomach faster than tepid or warm water. Overhydration just prior to exertion delays dehydration and reduces the rise in internal body temperature; drinking two cups of cold water before exercising thus improves performance. Fluids must be taken frequently during exercise to avoid dehydration. However, the stomach can empty only about three cups every hour. Because sweat losses may exceed this rate on hot, humid days, care must be taken to reduce activity to safe levels. Drinking cold fluids at 20-minute intervals appears to work the best. Adequacy of fluid replacement can be assessed by the simple practice of weighing before and after exercise after one has dried off. The difference in weight is lost water. One pint of water weighs 1 pound. If postexercise weight loss is 1 percent of body weight or more, more hydration is needed.

For replacement of ordinary fluid losses, nothing is better than plain water. Endurance exercise may be limited by both fluid losses and carbohydrate depletion. It would appear to be a simple matter, then, of drinking fluids with carbohydrates in them, thereby satisfying both needs. The problem is that the presence of sugars in fluids slows stomach-emptying time. Water replacement is more important than carbohydrate replacement, so solutions delaying water absorption should be avoided. However, if carbohydrate in fluids is provided in the form of large molecules made of many glucose subunits (polysaccharides) instead of in the form of monosaccharides or disaccharides, gastric emptying appears not to be impaired.

A small amount of salt in the fluid enhances intestinal absorption. No more than one-third teaspoon of table salt for every quart (liter) of fluid is necessary to achieve this effect. Neither salt nor carbohydrate has been proven to be advantageous, except in very prolonged events with high fluid losses. For most activities, nothing beats water.

Digestion

The digestive tract—from lips to anus—is a tubelike structure inside the body. Whatever is inside the tube is not really inside the body. If a child swallows a penny, the coin gets passed from one section of the intestinal tract to another without ever being truly inside the child's tissues. Eventually, the penny emerges with neither the penny nor the child changed for the experience.

Most of what one swallows, however, is changed by the experience, and one is changed by what one chooses to swallow. In helping these changes along, the digestive system has several important tasks. The first task is to get food into the digestive system, or to ingest it. The next task is to move the food from place to place in the digestive tract and finally to eliminate whatever has not been taken into the body. During the trip, the food must be disassembled both mechanically and chemically into substances small enough to be absorbed by the cells lining the intestinal tract. It is instructive to trace the path from entrance to exit and note the changes that take place.

To start the process, the mouth has to open and bite off an appropriately sized piece of food. After the bite, tongue and jaw muscles work together with the teeth to chew the food. While the teeth do the actual grinding, the tongue and cheek muscles work to keep the food where it is supposed to be and to keep body parts out of the path of the teeth. This grinding process is aided by saliva, which not only wets the food but actually starts the chemical disassembly process.

Saliva allows the ground-up food to be moistened. When the food is chewed to a certain consistency, the tongue automatically flicks off a perfectly sized wad and flings it to the back of the throat, where it is swallowed. Meanwhile, enzymes in the saliva are breaking the complex carbohydrate chains into smaller chunks, and a different enzyme is peeling fatty acids off glycerol molecules. Chewing the food into small pieces means that more of the food makes contact with the saliva, so more of this initial chemical digestion can go on.

Once the food is swallowed, the muscular esophagus, which begins in the neck, propels the bolus (soft, chewed mass) of food to the stomach. The stomach is located under the lower part of the rib cage on the left side. The esophagus has a special structure at the stomach end that opens when food needs to get into the stomach, then closes to prevent food from returning from the stomach to the mouth. Malfunction of this structure allows stomach acid to flow back into the esophagus, resulting in heartburn.

The stomach is a muscular bag that serves as a holding tank; food can stay there for hours if necessary. People tend to shovel in food intermittently and in quantities that the intestines cannot handle. The stomach holds these large quantities, releasing only small amounts into the intestines. While in the stomach, the food is exposed to hydrochloric acid. This acid, which is made by some of the cells lining the stomach, kills most of the bacteria one swallows. Acid also unwinds the tangled, globular proteins. The stomach produces another substance called pepsin, which actually starts to break up the long amino acid chain of the proteins into smaller chunks. Carbohydrate and fat digestion, which began in the mouth, ceases in the stomach. The emphasis here is on breaking down proteins. Powerful stomach muscles slosh the liquid around, mixing it with the swallowed food bolus; the result is a substance called chyme. As the stom-

Mouth
Breaks up food.
Mixes food with saliva.

Salivary glands
Chemoreceptors and pressure receptors in the walls of the mouth and tongue trigger salivation to moisten food.

Pharynx
Swallows.

Esophagus
Transports food.

Liver
Produces bile that aids in digestion.
Stores many vitamins.
Destroys poisons.
Gets "first look" at most ingested nutrients.

Stomach
Stores and churns food.
Secretes mucus, hydrochloric acid, and the enzyme pepsin.
Mucus protects stomach walls.
Hydrochloric acid activates enzymes, which unwind proteins.
Pepsin breaks up protein molecules.
Kills germs.

Gallbladder
Stores bile.

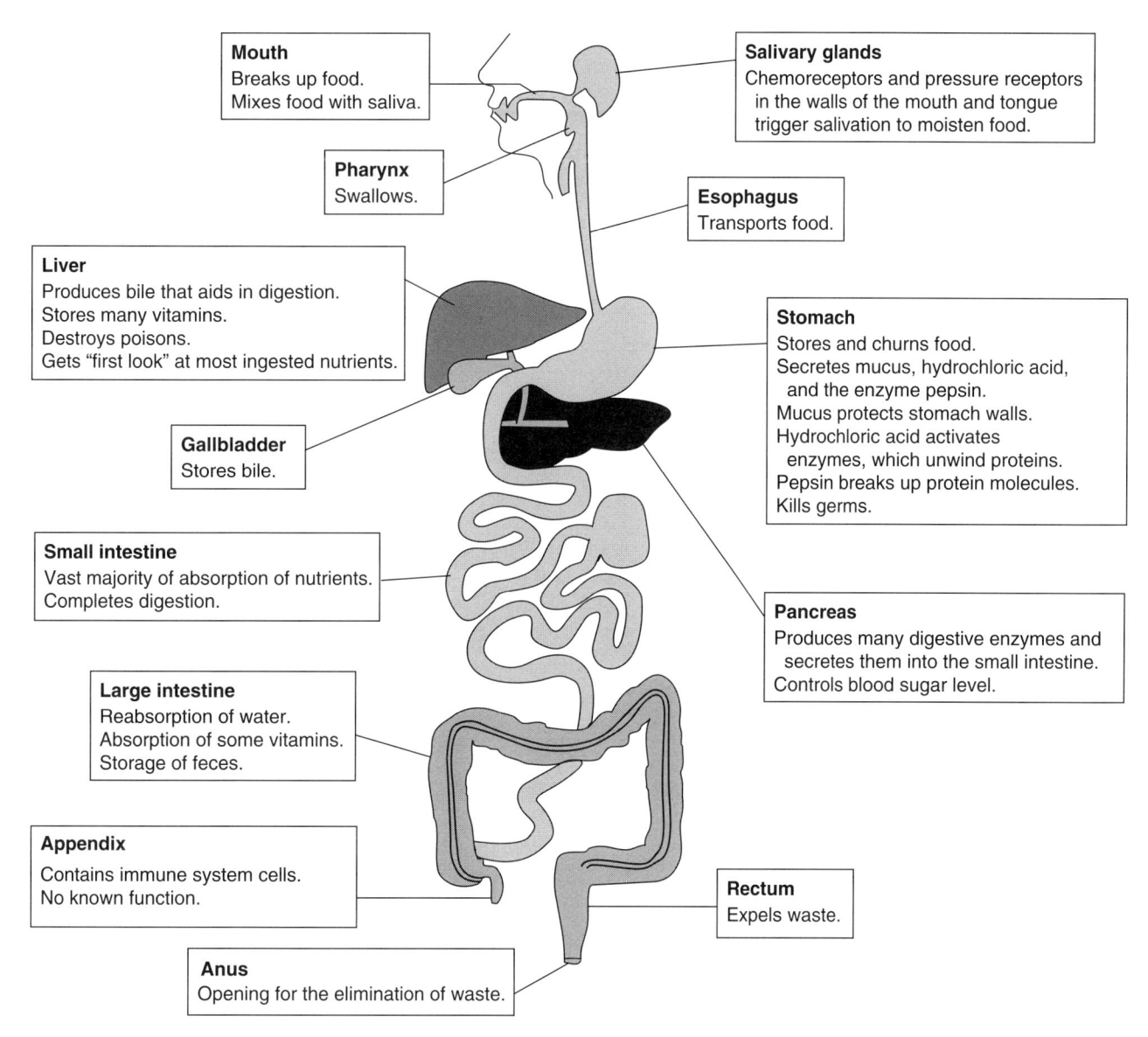

Small intestine
Vast majority of absorption of nutrients.
Completes digestion.

Pancreas
Produces many digestive enzymes and secretes them into the small intestine.
Controls blood sugar level.

Large intestine
Reabsorption of water.
Absorption of some vitamins.
Storage of feces.

Appendix
Contains immune system cells.
No known function.

Rectum
Expels waste.

Anus
Opening for the elimination of waste.

Figure 5. *The digestive system and how it functions.*

ach churns, a special muscle called the pyloric sphincter opens intermittently, allowing a small amount of chyme to leave the stomach with each contraction. The chyme enters the small intestine (which, for purposes of description, is divided here into three functional parts, although they are all continuous and there are no abrupt anatomical differences at the boundaries). The small intestine is called "small" because of its diameter. It is really a large organ, about 20 feet in length, and fills most of the abdominal cavity.

The first part of the small intestine is called the duodenum. Despite being only about 10 inches long, it is an extremely busy place. As chyme enters the duodenum, it consists of blobs of fat with some fatty acids removed from glycerol, chunks of glucose molecules strung together, and chunks of amino acids strung together, all floating in a wet, acid fluid. The duodenum is lined with specialized cells that "read" the contents of the chyme. These specialized cells then release hormones (chemicals produced by one cell that affect the activity of other cells) that regulate the activities of various parts of the intestinal tract and accessory digestive organs. About midway through the duodenum is a small hole through which the pancreas squirts a variety of chemicals and through which bile enters.

The pancreas is an accessory digestive organ, meaning that although no food passes through this organ, it is involved in digestion. As the special duodenal cells read the chyme, they respond with hormones, some of which act on the pancreas. Thus, if the duodenum is presented with acid, the pancreas squirts an antacid called sodium bicarbonate into the duodenum. If the chyme has an abundance of proteins, then the pancreas squirts enzymes that can take apart proteins. The same occurs for carbohydrates and triglycerides.

The liver also helps with fat digestion by producing a substance called bile. (Again, no food passes through the liver, but it is involved in digestion, so it is an accessory organ.) Bile is stored in the gall bladder. When one eats a fatty meal, the duodenal cells secrete a hormone (cholecystokinin) that causes the gallbladder to contract, Bile breaks the fat into smaller particles, making it easier for the fat-digesting enzymes to get at the chemical bonds they are supposed to break.

Now there is neutralized (no longer acidic) chyme in the duodenum, mixed with bile, and the pancreatic enzymes are disassembling chemical bonds. At this point, no nutrients have yet been taken into the body. It takes time for all of this disassembling to happen.

The remaining 19 feet of the small intestine consists of the jejunum and the ileum. The inside surface of these portions of the small intestine looks fuzzy, like very fine velvet. Each strand of fuzz in the small intestine is a tiny conelike projection called a villus (*see Figure 6*). Each tiny villus (barely visible to the unaided eye) is covered with specialized cells. One side of the cells comes in contact with the chyme. This side is covered with tiny hairlike projections (microvilli), so fine that they would have to be magnified 500 times to be visible. The villi and microvilli increase the surface area of the small intestine to a total area equal to the floor space of a two-story house. Inside each cone-shaped villus are blood-containing capillaries and a tiny lymphatic vessel.

Food sloshes around in the small intestine for hours after a large meal, as the absorbing process takes time and energy. The cells on the villi work to take in all of the nutrients. The intestinal cells make enzymes that finish off the process of disassembling the food molecules. In order to be absorbed, carbohydrates have to be in the form of monosaccharides, proteins have to be in the form of single amino acids or short chains of two or three amino acids, and triglycerides must be broken down to fatty acids and monoglycerides. Otherwise, most of the food molecules would be too large to be absorbed through the villi and into the blood and lymph. It is now the job of the intesti-

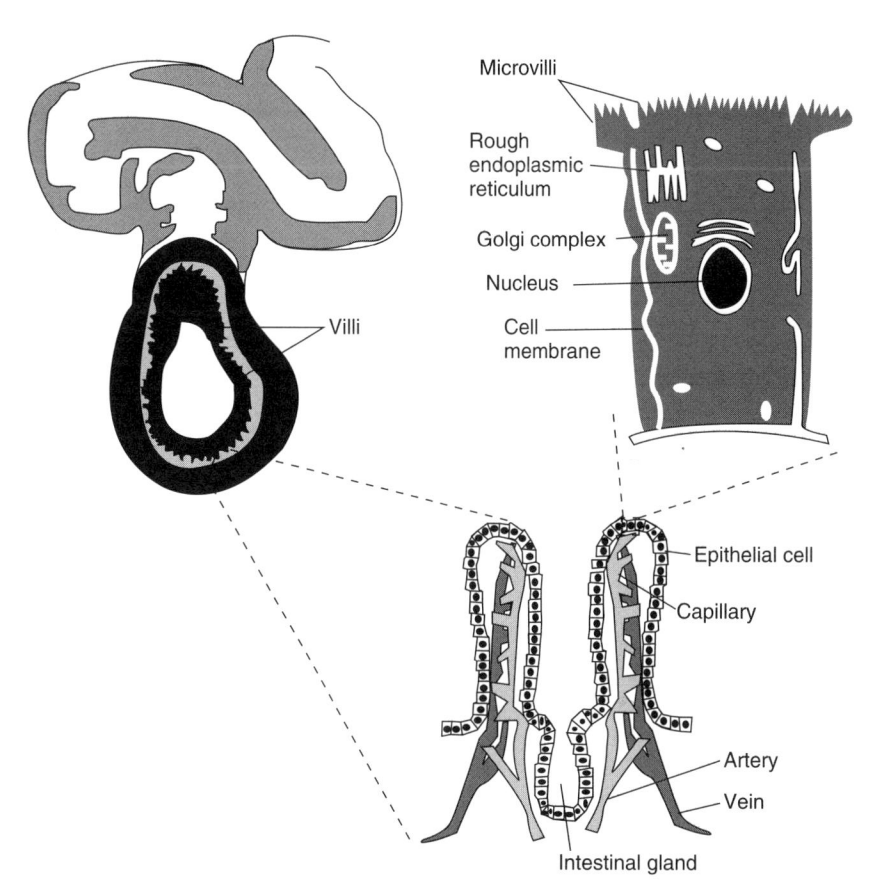

Figure 6. *Cross section of the small intestine.*

nal cells to absorb everything they can. The sugars, amino acids, and fatty acids are brought into the intestinal cells. The intestinal cells then transfer these small molecules into the blood and lymph. The resulting nutrient-rich blood collects into large veins, which carry it directly to the liver. There the veins break up into capillaries again and the nutrient-rich blood can slosh around the liver cells.

The liver is a remarkable organ that works to compensate for dietary indiscretions. The liver changes fructose and galactose into glucose, which can be used by all of the body's cells for energy. If one eats too much protein, the liver changes some of the amino acids to glucose. If one eats a few more calories than one needs, the liver can store glucose in the form of glycogen to a limited extent. If one has an even greater excess of calories, the liver converts what it can into fats. Most of the fatty acids that are absorbed are reconstituted into triglycerides by the intestinal cells and packaged into chylomicrons. These packages are too large to get into the capillaries, so they travel in the lymphatic system until they empty into a large vein close to the heart, where the contents are dumped into the general circulation.

An average meal spends about 5 hours in the small intestine. The chyme then leaves the small intestine and enters the large intestine through a valve that opens and shuts in response to food in the stomach. The chyme at this point contains fiber, as well as dead intestinal cells. Intestinal cells die, fall off, and are replaced rather quickly. If a cell falls off near the beginning of the jejunum, it gets digested and absorbed just like any other animal cell. If it falls off later, there is not enough time nor are there enzymes to digest it, so it passes into the large intestine. The chyme is also watery. The large intestine removes much of the water from chyme to form the firm feces. Bacteria in the large intestine digest fiber. These bacteria make the gases that cause flatulence. Intestinal bacteria also make some vitamins (the most important is vitamin K), which are absorbed from the large intestine into the bloodstream. The large intestine is also responsible for storing the feces until a socially acceptable moment and then eliminating them. The large intestine is muscle and, just like any other muscle, it needs to be exercised on a regular basis. Low-fiber diets contribute to a variety of large intestine disorders by not providing enough bulk for the large intestinal musculature. Fiber is material which we lack the enzymes to digest. Most people in the United States eat 4 to 6 grams of dietary fiber daily. While there is no RDA for fiber as yet, most experts agree that 20 to 25 grams would be ideal. Fiber is healthful in many ways. People who eat high-fiber diets tend to be leaner than those who do not. High-fiber diets protect against colon cancer and other intestinal disorders. High-fiber diets also protect against atherosclerosis by binding with bile, so that bile is not reabsorbed by the ileum. The cholesterol in the bile is then eliminated from the body. High-fiber diets regulate the levels of glucose in the blood, providing a steadier amount of this optimal fuel for exercise. Fiber is easily obtained from eating a wide variety of fruits and vegetables. Legumes and whole grains are also excellent fiber sources.

The digestive system is truly remarkable in its ability to ingest, take apart, and absorb the food one eats. It usually does its job so efficiently and quietly that one is scarcely aware it is happening. The vast majority of digestion and absorption happens in the small intestine with help from enzymes secreted by the pancreas. Fiber, intestinal cells, and bacteria, which are left over after this process, are eliminated from the large intestine. All of the work done by the intestines after a meal takes energy. To do this work, the cells of the digestive tract need oxygen and nutrients. Providing adequate blood flow to the intestines after a meal requires that blood be diverted from someplace else—primarily the skeletal muscles. When a person exercises, blood is diverted from the gastrointestinal system to the muscles. This is why one cannot digest and exercise at the same time: one cannot maximize one's blood flow to both places at once.

Weight Control

Never before has there been so much concern about weight, and never before has there been so much confusion, misinformation, and harmful practice in pursuit of the "ideal" body weight. A healthy body weight varies from individual to individual. If good health is defined as the ability to do work, then a good weight is one which allows a person to perform efficiently the work or exercise she chooses to do. Obviously, a healthy weight for a long-distance runner would be different from that for a power lifter. How, then, can a person determine what he should weigh?

Body mass is made primarily of three components: muscle, bone, and fat. It is the ratio of these components, or one's body composition, that determines if a person is overweight. For example, a professional football player who is 6 feet, 4 inches tall and weighs 255 pounds is clearly overweight by any height-weight table one might consult. If only 15 percent of that mass is fat, however, then this individual's excess weight is due to muscle, not fat—a desirable body composition for an offensive lineman.

Within the limitations imposed by each person's genetic makeup, an individual can change her muscle mass and fat mass. Building muscle shows up as weight gain on the scale. Losing fat will also be reflected on the scale. A person in training may be losing fat while gaining muscle and may therefore see no changes in actual weight. Clearly, then, weight is but a poor indicator of an athlete's health and ability to perform.

The best way to determine an "ideal" body mass is to determine body composition. This would tell the athlete and coach what percentage of total body weight is fat and what percentage is muscle. The individual could then be compared with top performers, and training adjustments could be made accordingly (*see also* BODY COMPOSITION).

The body needs some fat for good health. All nerves are wrapped in an essential layer of fat, and fat is a necessary part of the covering of various internal organs. There is fat in the bone marrow, and some fat under the skin is necessary for normal skin functioning. All these types of fat, which are necessary to well-being, are called essential fat. In men, essential fat accounts for 3 percent of body mass. For women, 14 percent body fat is considered essential.

Having less than the essential amount of body fat reduces the body's ability to withstand stress, including the stress of exercise. Such people get more infectious diseases and recover from them slowly, tire quickly, break bones more easily, and can actually suffer vital organ failure. Women with very low body fat appear to be especially prone to disorders of the reproductive system.

The ideal amount of body fat for athletes varies from sport to sport. Distance runners need to minimize fat while still maintaining good health, including normal reproductive function. Swimmers need not be as concerned about body fat, because fat improves buoyancy; being too lean can actually impede a swimmer's performance. Football linemen may want to have as much mass as possible without sacrificing speed and power. There are genetic limits that make a person more suited for one sport than another. Some women can tolerate 12 percent body fat with no ill effects, while others might find their lower limit to be 17 percent. Fat content is just one of the variables—which also include muscle fiber makeup and cardiovascular limitations—that affect performance. Trying to make a marathon runner out of someone genetically predisposed to higher than normal body fat could be frustrating, futile, and dangerous.

Changing one's body composition is an area in which there is much popular mythology but limited scientific information. Clearly, the amount of energy contained in ingested food must match the amount of energy expended, not only in voluntary activities but also in involuntary activities such as breathing, digestion, keeping warm, and so forth. If more calories are taken in than expended, the body converts the excess to fat and stores it. Some people tend to store the excess around the waist; others store the excess at the thighs and the buttocks. If energy expenditure exceeds caloric intake, the body uses these fat stores for fuel; thus, the simple solution to losing fat is to eat less than one expends.

Yet weight loss is not so simple. All people have a minimum energy expenditure for breathing, digestion, and all the other housekeeping functions. This energy expenditure is called the basal metabolic rate (BMR). BMR can vary from individual to individual, but it accounts for 60 percent of the total caloric expenditure by the average adult. For a moderately active woman in good health who eats about 2,000 calories a day, 1,200 of those calories are spent in cellular activities that would occur even if she were in a coma. The other 800 account for volitional activities, such as exercise. If this person exercised more, she would increase the 800-caloric expenditure. If she became sedentary, she would burn less than the 800-calorie allotment, although her basal metabolic rate would remain about the same. Some activities, such as body growth, actually increase BMR. Even a totally inactive child still grows, and growing takes energy. Another way to increase BMR is to increase muscle mass, as muscle tissue is active even at rest. All muscles have some degree of activity even when a person is not voluntarily using them. (This accounts for the difference in how a muscle looks and feels in a sleeping person as opposed to a paralyzed or dead person). Maintaining muscle tone takes energy. Fat cells are metabolically very inactive. A person with a high muscle-to-fat ratio will have a higher BMR than a person of the same gender and weight with a lower muscle-to-fat ratio. This means that the person with the greater muscle mass needs to eat more to keep his or her body composition the same. If the person with the smaller muscle mass ate the same diet, that person would gain weight, and the additional weight would be in the form of fat.

However, research suggests that each person has a regulatory center in the brain that determines how much body fat that individual needs. In experiments in which people grossly overeat in an attempt to increase their body fat, they do gain weight, but not as much as might be expected. Overeating may signal the body to speed up internal activities, increasing the BMR. When food intake returns to normal, these people quickly lose the additional pounds without needing to consciously diet. Their bodies diet for them by keeping the BMR higher than normal and regulating hunger until the original weight is restored. Similar events occur during starvation. Fat is lost, but at a much slower rate than one might expect mathematically. This slowdown occurs because under starvation conditions, the body reduces the BMR to conserve fat stores. This concept—that the body adjusts its BMR according to a perceived excess or scarcity of food—is called the set-point theory: the body has stored in the brain an idea of how fat it should be, and it adjusts appetite, hunger, and BMR accordingly. Though this theory is not yet proved, there is much evidence to support it. However, experts agree that this regulatory center is but one factor regulating body composition. Apparently the body's set point can be changed; aerobic activity done for 30 minutes three or more times a week without a change in diet influences body composition by reducing fat stores.

Suppose a 120-pound woman decides that she wants to lose 10 pounds. She starts her weight loss program with a body composition of 25 percent fat and has been maintaining this weight and body composition on a 1,800-calorie diet. She gives herself a month to lose the weight. To lose 10 pounds of fat, one needs to burn 35,000 calories more than one ingests. This dieter, then would have to reduce her caloric intake by 8,750 calories each week, or 1,250 each day, allowing her only 550 calories a day (for purposes of discussion, rounded to 600). If her BMR is 1,000 calories, her food will not provide her body with enough calories to perform housekeeping, let alone exercise. She will burn fat for fuel, but the body cannot run on fat alone. It must have some carbohydrate to initiate fat burning, and the brain cannot burn fat at all. If she does not get this carbohydrate from her diet, she will burn the glycogen stores in her muscles and liver. Each pound of glycogen contains only 1,700 calories.

During the first week, this woman maintaines a caloric deficit of 8,400 calories. Half of this she gets from her fat stores and half from glycogen. She loses 1.2 pounds of fat and 2.5 pounds of glycogen. Having lost almost 4 pounds in only one week, she sticks to the diet. Her body has now made some adjustments. Her BMR goes down, perhaps to 800 calories, and her caloric deficit drops to 7,000 calories per week. Again, she will compensate for half of those calories by burning body fat, yet her body will not allow her glycogen stores to be depleted further. She still needs glucose to burn the fat. Amino acids in her skeletal muscle will be converted to glucose, and she will now be losing muscle mass. In the second week, she loses 1 pound of fat and 2 pounds of muscle. She steps on the scale and sees that she has lost 3 pounds for the week. Again, she feels that the diet is working and she resolves to stick to it. In one more week she has lost a total of 9.7 pounds, but only 3.2 pounds in fat (plus 4 lb. in muscle and 2.5 lb. in glycogen). She now weighs 110 pounds. Before the diet, she carried 30 pounds (or 25% of her weight) as fat. Now 26.8 pounds (24%) of her new weight is fat. As soon as she resumes her regular diet, the weight returns. However, the lost muscle is not regained, the glycogen stores are restored, and the rest of the weight is restored as fat. Now she is 2 pounds fatter that she was before her diet, with a lower BMR (due to decreased muscle mass), making it harder for her to lose weight the next time. Repeated bouts of this leave her with too much fat, too little muscle, and lots of frustration.

A smarter and ultimately more successful regimen aims for reduced total body fat rather than for weight loss. Suppose that instead of trying to lose 10 pounds, the same 120-pound woman wants to change her body composition from 25 percent fat to a lean 18 percent fat. This would mean losing 9 pounds of fat. She decides wisely that this could be best accomplished over a 6- to 8-week period, with a modest fuel reduction of 400 calories per day. She eats plenty of vegetables and maintains her carbohydrate intake, while reducing the fat in her diet to 15 or 20 percent. The high-carbohydrate intake ensures the availability of glucose, so her body will not have to break down muscle in order to burn fat stores. She also embarks on an exercise program, exercising aerobically for 30 or 40 minutes four or five times per week, increasing her caloric expenditure by 300 calories a day. She also starts a modest weight-training program three times a week. At the end of 6 weeks, she has lost 9 pounds of fat and gained 4 pounds of muscle. She weighs 115 pounds but has reduced her body fat to 18 percent. Her BMR has increased, so now she has to eat 2,000 calories a day just to maintain this weight. She continues her exercise program to keep her set point adjusted to this new, higher level and to maintain her increased muscle mass. As long as she maintains her exercise regimen and a relatively low-fat diet (20 percent) she will maintain this body composition without "dieting."

For the person who feels the need to gain weight, there are two possibilities. Some people (young men especially) feel that they would like to be bigger, and some athletes need bulk to optimize performance in their sports. In both cases, mere overeating will not accomplish what is desired. The person who wishes to gain weight needs a high-quality diet that contains adequate protein and adequate nutrients so that the protein can be utilized properly. If the too-lean person is exercising, he or she needs to cut back on the aerobic work to perhaps 30 minutes three or four times a week and begin a resistance program to build muscle mass.

"Making weight" is a practice employed by athletes who must compete at or under a certain weight; it is common among jockeys and wrestlers (*see also* WRESTLING). Making weight is accomplished by fluid and food restriction in the few days prior to competition and may also be accompanied by techniques to enhance fluid losses, such as forced sweating without replacement of fluids. These are dangerous practices, especially for the athlete who has not completed growth. If an athlete is even mildly dehydrated, performance will suffer. Fluid shifts should never be used as a form of weight control. Instead, a preseason evaluation of body composition will allow a realistic assessment of lean body tissue. The athlete can then choose a strength program to increase lean body tissue while controlling diet and engaging in aerobic exercise to reduce body fat. A lower limit of 5 percent body fat should be established for high school wrestlers.

Jean Szilva, M.D.

References

Boyle, M., and G. Zyla. *Personal Nutrition*. St. Paul, Minnesota: West Educational, 1992.

Brown, J. *Nutrition Now*. St. Paul, Minnesota: West Educational, 1995.

Marieb, E. *Human Anatomy and Physiology*. Cambridge, Massachusetts: Benjamin Cummings, 1995.

Martini, F. *Fundamentals of Anatomy and Physiology*. Englewood, New Jersey: Prentice-Hall, 1995.

McArdle, W., et al. *Exercise Physiology*. Philadelphia: Lea and Febiger, 1991.

Merkin, M. *Physical Sciences with Modern Applications*. Philadelphia: Saunders, 1993.

Rhoades, R. *Medical Physiology*. Boston, Massachusetts: Little, Brown, 1995.

Tortora, G., and S. Grabowski. *Principles of Anatomy and Physiology*. New York: HarperCollins, 1996.

Pelvis, Hip, and Thigh

SOME ANTHROPOLOGISTS have spent their entire careers trying to understand why humans walk on two limbs while almost all other mammals walk on four. According to one school of thought, even the earliest members of the human family line were fully bipedal, much like modern humans. Another school of thought, however, holds that there was an extended period during which these hominids sometimes walked upright and sometimes went on all fours. In either case, however, the change from the quadrupedalism of hominoid species to the bipedalism of the human family (the hominids) entailed profound anatomical changes, particularly in the femur (thighbone) and pelvis (hips).

Modern humans—*Homo sapiens*—are much better able to stand erect (*see Figure 1*) than, for example, chimpanzees, which are mainly quadrupedal ("knuckle-walkers") but occasionally bipedal. This is because the center of gravity in a human lies at the pelvis, directly

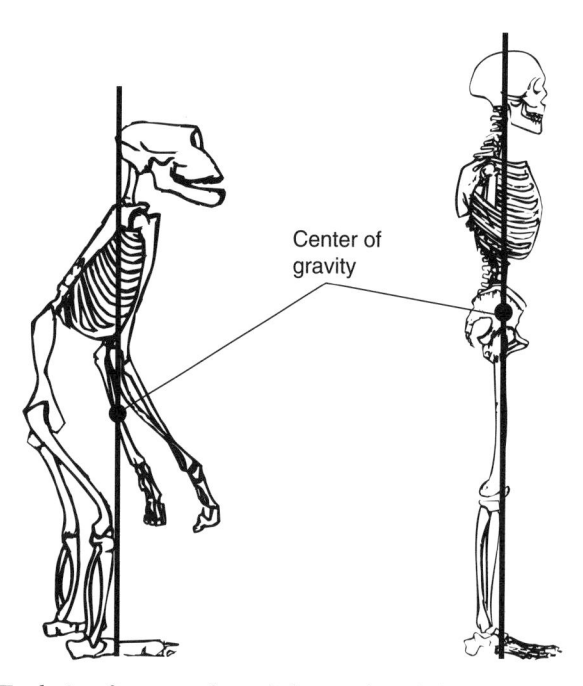

Figure 1. *Evolution from quadrupedalism to bipedalism had much to do with the evolution of the pelvis and femur (thighbone). A human can stand erect more easily than an ape because in the human body the center of gravity is at the pelvis and directly over the feet. (Adapted from Wilford, 1995)*

over the feet; in contrast, a chimpanzee's center of gravity lies away from the body. There are also significant differences between the human pelvis and the ape pelvis in shape, size, and structure. In comparing skeletons, scientists have identified a striking biomechanical difference: the unusually large joints that keep the human body upright (Jungers, 1988). The lumbosacral joint connecting the spine to the pelvis and the hip joint connecting the pelvis to the femur are much larger, relative to total body size, for humans than for apes. Because a larger joint surface area distributes the load more efficiently, some scientists believe that this evolutionary feature allows the human body to bear all its weight on two limbs rather than distributing the weight across four limbs. Human bipedal movement, then, is possible in part because of a more massive pelvis and larger hip joints, which combine to support the upper body.

In this regard, an interesting comparison can be made with the famous *Australopithecus* skeleton nicknamed "Lucy," an ancestral hominid more than 3 million years old: the size of these joints in Lucy lies much closer to those of modern humans than to apes (Jungers, 1988). Such evidence suggests that Lucy was fully bipedal, though other physiological features (such as the length of her arms) seem to indicate that she was also an agile climber; functionally, then, her bipedalism may have differed from that of modern humans. The comparative joint sizes support the theory that *Australopithecus* was an evolutionary phase combining a facility for climbing with proficient bipedalism. This combination may have persisted until the emergence of the genus *Homo* between 2 million and 2.5 million years ago, and the demise of the Australopithecines sometime between 1.2 million and 700,000 years ago.

Walking upright has inherent advantages: an upright creature can stand taller and reach higher in foraging for food; can see farther, spotting prey and predators more easily; and, of course, can use the forelimbs as arms and hands rather than for support and locomotion. However, the more massive pelvis required for bipedalism has certain drawbacks. It is believed that walking upright is related to women's difficulties with childbirth and to the general human susceptibility to back pain (*see also* SPINE). Humans are also much slower on foot—about 30 to 35 percent slower than quadrupedal chimpanzees and baboons, and about 50 percent slower than some of the larger mammalian carnivores (Haviland, 1985). Like many other evolutionary changes, the shift to bipedal movement came at some cost.

The Pelvis and Athletics

Pelvis is the collective name for the two hipbones and the sacrum—the five lower vertebrae fused together. The most important feature of the pelvis is its location. Within the pelvic cavity lies the body's center of gravity in the horizontal, vertical, and medial planes. Gravitational forces pull downward on each point of a body, and the distribution of these points determines the body's center of gravity. The center of gravity is the balancing point of the body in these three planes.

Most of the linear and angular motions that athletes perform take place around the body's center of gravity (*see Figure 2*). The pelvic girdle acts as the pivot and transfer point for all forces generated in the upper and lower extremities. Although movement of the pelvis itself is limited, it links the trunk with the lower extremities, coordinating the motion of each and providing the primary source of stability. It serves the important function of absorbing and redirecting some of the force of impact coming up through the legs before it reaches the spine.

Strong muscles in and around the pelvis are important to athletes for many activities. In running, jumping, swinging, or throwing, the large muscles of the upper legs and surrounding the hips initiate motion and provide most of the power. One study estimated that professional golfers deliver about 2 horsepower of energy when driving the ball, requiring at least 32 pounds of muscle mass to power the swing (Jorgensen, 1994). The study concluded that most of this 32 pounds of mass comes from the thigh muscles and the large muscles surrounding the pelvis. Because the pelvis is the major source of power for almost all sports, injuries in this area may significantly affect performance or sideline an athlete until they are fully healed.

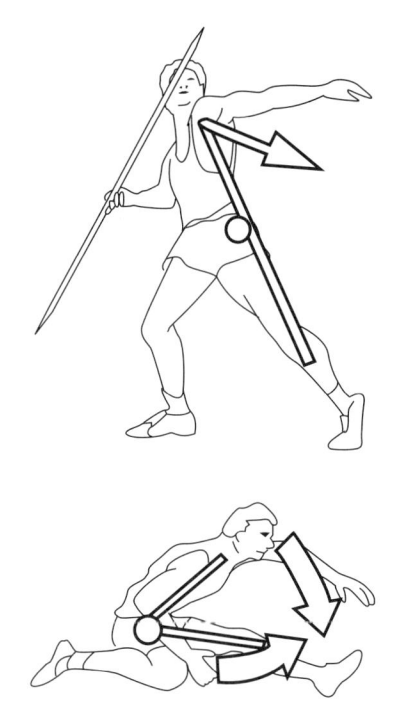

Figure 2. *Most athletic maneuvers require movement at or around the pelvis.*

Functional Anatomy

As noted above, the pelvis includes two hipbones. Each hipbone in turn consists of three bones: ilium, pubis, and ischium (*see Figure 3*). These three bones are separate during childhood but fuse together during adolescence. Anatomical differences between the male and female pelvis appear during puberty. Female bone structure is usually lighter, and bony protrusions for muscular attachments are less well-defined. The female pelvis is also smaller, shorter, and wider than the male pelvis. Moreover, the mean radius of the female femoral head is approximately 30 percent smaller than that of male (*see Figure 4 and Table 1*).

Some scientists believe that these anatomical differences give males certain athletic advantages over females. First, because a longer, narrower pelvis allows the surrounding muscles to transfer their energy in moving the legs more efficiently, males are able to run faster and jump higher. Second, the larger radius of the femoral head allows the male pelvis to withstand greater stress and compressive loads. The femur, the longest and strongest bone in the body, is connected to the pelvis at the acetabulum (hip joint). It is not in a vertical line with the axis of the individual standing erect. Instead, it slants inward at an angle. Because of the wider pelvis of the female body, the inward-slanting angle of the female femur is greater than that of the male. The larger angle formed also produces a greater imbalance of compressive forces on the knee joint.

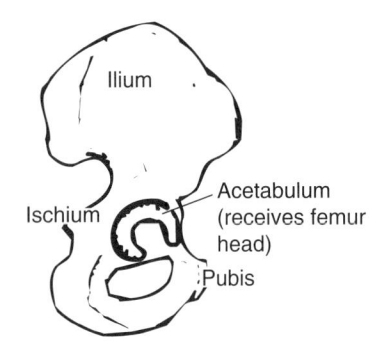

Figure 3. *The right hipbone viewed from the side. The hipbone consists of the ilium, pubis, and ischium.*

Figure 4. *There are significant anatomical differences between the male (left) and female (right) pelvic and femoral structure. These differences explain why congenital dislocation of the hip is six to seven times more common in females than in males. (Adapted from Albright, 1987)*

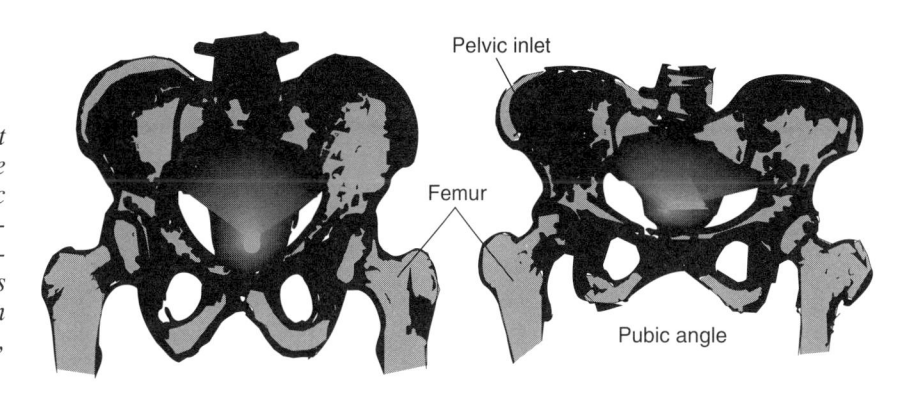

In both men and women, the gravitational force on the upper body during walking, running, and jumping bends the femoral neck. The structure of this part of the anatomy creates compression forces that are always greater than tension at the femoral neck. Hip fractures occur most often at the femoral neck because it is subject to these compressive and tensile stresses and is thinner than the rest of the femur.

The shape and slant of the femur also affect the weight-bearing force on the femoral neck. There are various angles between the femur neck and shaft angles, and extreme angles can cause vulnerability to injury (*see Figure 5*). For the coxa varus femur (angled at about 90°), the compressive force is less and the tension force greater. The femoral neck is subjected to greater compression and tension stresses, and a considerably greater shearing force. For the coxa valgus femur angle (an angle much greater than 90°), the compressive force is greater, making the resultant force greater on the femoral neck.

In addition to its weight-bearing function, the hip joint also functions as a ball-and-socket joint. In other words, it is able to move in all directions, providing the lower extremities with a substantial range of motion. The rounded head of the femur rests in the acetabulum, forming the hip joint. Along the posterior side of the femur's long shaft is a ridge called the linea aspera, which forms the attachment for several muscles of the hip and leg.

The hip joint is supported by a number of ligaments. The capsular ligament surrounds the joint, effectively deepening the cavity of the joint. These structures lend strength to the joint and prevent the leg from swinging outward and backward. Backward swinging is pre-

COMPARISON OF THE MALE AND FEMALE PELVIS

Pelvis	Male	Female
Type of bone	Heavy, rough	Slender
Structure	Deep but narrow, with less capacity	Shallow, wide, with great capacity
Shape of inlet	Heart-shaped	Oval, and larger than male
Pubic angle	Narrow, pointed; usually <90°	Wide, rounded; usually >90°
Direction	Tilted backward	Tilted forward
Femoral head	Larger radius	Smaller radius

Table 1.

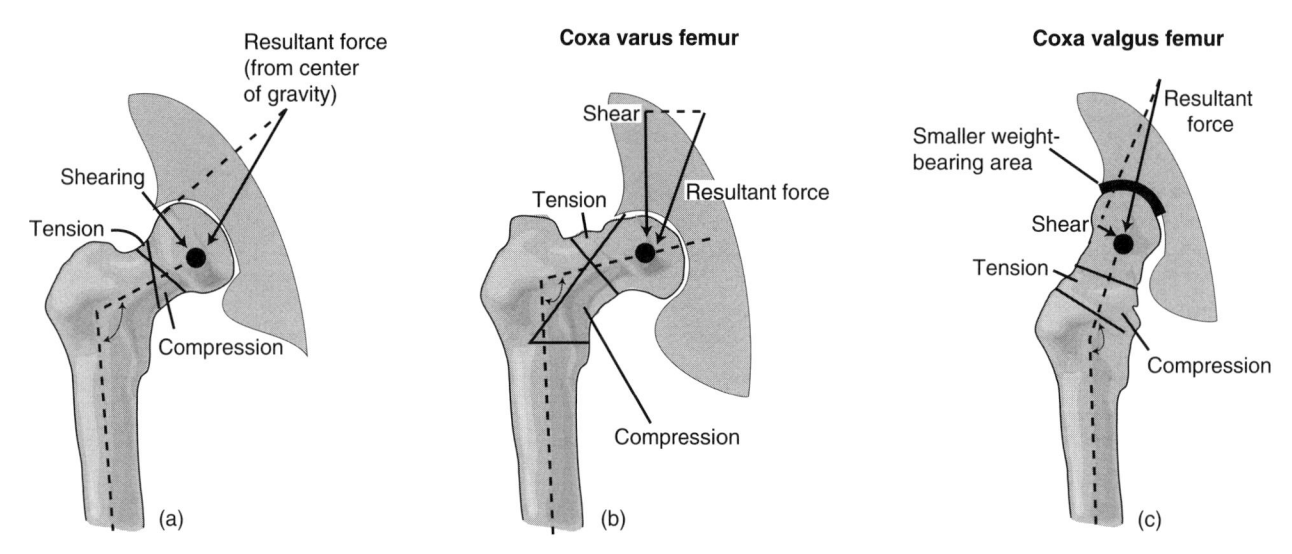

Figure 5. *(a) The stresses experienced by the femoral neck of a normal hip due to gravitational loads. (b) For the coxa varus hip, the compressive stresses are less but tensile stress is greater. This means that the hip must handle more bending stress than that of a normal hip. (c) For the coxa valgus hip, the compressive stress is greater, making the resultant force greater.*

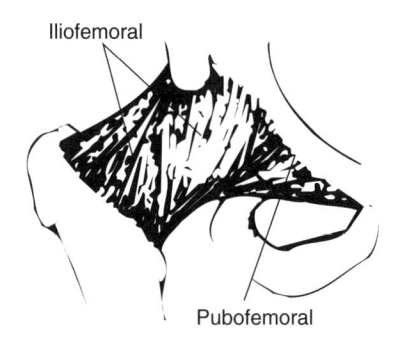

Figure 6. *The ligaments that support and stabilize the hip joint.*

vented by the iliofemoral ligament, which is attached to the ilium (a part of the hip) and reaches down to the thighbone. Outward swinging is restricted by the pubiofemoral ligament (*see Figure 6*). Both are extremely strong ligaments; in fact, the iliofemoral ligament, which is used to stand up, is the strongest ligament in the body.

The two hip joints and the joints of the lumbar spine are the basis of all pelvic girdle movement. Movements of the pelvic girdle include lateral twisting, or rotation, and tilting forward, backward, and laterally. Movements of the pelvis are often associated with motions of the spine and thighs and are often considered a secondary effect of spinal and thigh motion. But in some sports the motion is initiated by the pelvis itself, with the spine and thighs moving in reaction to a tilting of the pelvis.

Surrounding the pelvis lies the majority of the body's muscle mass. The gluteus maximus (large buttock muscle) is used to swing the leg backward and assists in keeping the knee straight; thus it is very important for sports requiring explosive power or acceleration. For example, in sprinting and football the hips are tilted forward so that the center of gravity lies directly over the accelerating feet. When the hips are tilted forward, the large buttock muscle works with greater force because the distance between its origin and insertion points becomes greater, which in turn increases potential power. The backward tilt of the male pelvis allows the gluteus maximus to generate more power than that of a female when the trunk tilts forward during sprinting.

The intermediate and small buttock muscles—the gluteus medius and gluteus minimus, respectively—are not important for power. However, they are vital for more precise movements and for stabilizing the hip joint. Their large area of origin makes it possible to move

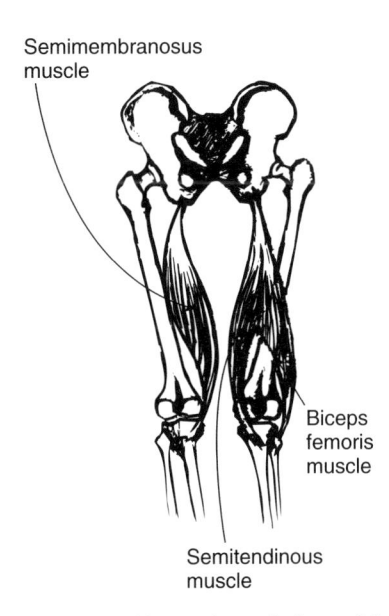

Figure 7. *Rear view of the pelvis and thigh. Because the tendons of the muscles shown all insert in close proximity—near the knee—they are referred to collectively as the hamstring muscles. They consist of the semimembranous, semitendonous, and biceps femoris.*

the thighbone in every direction, except inward toward the midline of the body. These muscles stabilize the hip joint when the body hits the ground during walking, running, and jumping. Without these outwardly stabilizing muscles, the upper body would fall across to the opposite side—fall inward—while running or walking.

The groin muscles are responsible for swinging the body toward its midline. Most of the groin muscles originate at the pubic bone of the pelvis and are attached to the posterior surface of the thighbone. In running, these muscles are used in the first part of the forward leg drive, as the foot leaves the ground and starts to move ahead of the body. These are also the critical muscles used by soccer players to accelerate the leg while kicking, and by figure skaters to initiate a twisting maneuver.

Hip flexor muscles are not as crucial to as many maneuvers as the buttock or groin muscles, but they are important in a number of sports. The hip flexor is able to contract in a variety of ways. It can bring the trunk toward the hips (in sit-ups and throwing) or bring the leg toward the hip (hurdling). Gymnasts depend on the contracting strength of the hip flexors to execute a number of maneuvers, and have shown a remarkable ability to increase their hip flexors' range of motion through stretching (*see also ACROBATICS*).

The hamstring muscle group, located on the posterior of the thigh, consists of the biceps femoris, semitendonous, and semimembranous muscles (*see Figure 7*). These bring the leg backward during the running stride. Athletes frequently pull a hamstring because these muscles are naturally tightly wound. Baseball players, whose hamstrings tighten up as they wait to play, are particularly susceptible to pulled hamstrings while sprinting to first base. This is, in fact, a perfect prescription for a hamstring injury: long periods of inactivity punctuated by an occasional all-out sprint about once every 40 minutes.

Pathophysiology and Treatment

Unlike the strong cortical long bones in the body, the pelvis consists of softer cancellous bone (*see SKELETAL SYSTEM*). However, the pelvis is protected by the significant amount of cushioning muscle mass around it. Further, the pelvis is in a position where it is less subject to the impacts and blows that the long bones regularly receive.

Direct blows to soft tissue cause contusions—subsurface bruising in which the skin is not broken. Contusions are the type of pelvic injury most frequently sustained by athletes. These direct blows can come from player-on-player collisions or from impacts with the playing surface (e.g., a volleyball player digging a spike, or a hockey player skating into the sideboards); impacts with equipment can also result in injury. Contusions may be superficial or deep within the large muscle mass that surrounds the pelvis. When severe muscular

Hip Replacement: Prospects for Young Athletes

At the peak of his popularity, the image of Bo Jackson, the professional football and baseball player, was ubiquitous. His image could be seen at playing fields, on billboards, and in many commercials. At the time of this writing, he was the only modern athlete to have become a superstar in both professional football and baseball. However, his career was cut short in 1991 by a routine tackle during a game between the Cleveland Browns and the Los Angeles Raiders. His awkward fall resulted in a severe hip injury, which required hip-replacement surgery in 1992, when he was 30.

The term *hip fracture* is a misnomer: what is commonly called a hip fracture is usually a break in the upper femur. This fracture is often difficult to heal because of a combination of stress—from bearing the weight of the upper body—and poor blood circulation.

For young, well-conditioned athletes like Jackson, the need for hip-replacement surgery is usually the result of one fall or collision, not the combined effect of hits taken over a 10- to 15-year career. If an athlete has a congenital condition, such as coxae vara or coxae valga, the risk of injury is greater. Weak or slow bone healing also is considered a contributing factor.

Hip-replacement surgery entails removing the patient's own joint and inserting an artificial ball-and-socket joint into the hip. A shaft, attached to the ball, is pushed down into the patient's thighbone (*see accompanying figure*). About 250,000 hip replacements are performed each year in the United States, and the procedure is considered very effective. In 1994, a panel formed by the National Institutes of Health to consider hip-replacement surgery concluded that it is associated with few complications. It has been performed since the early 1970s, mostly on the elderly. At the same time as a decline in bone mass with aging lowers the body's ability to withstand impacts, the body experiences a loss in motor control that increases the risk of falls. Older adults are more likely not only to fall but, when they fall, to suffer femur fractures.

Bo Jackson's case piqued the interest of doctors and sports fans because of his young age and his determination to continue to play professional baseball. It also focused attention on the effectiveness of the procedure. Hip replacement is considered very effective for the elderly, but would it be equally effective for a professional athlete? Specifically, would it hold up when Jackson (who weighed 240 lb.) started diving after fly balls and barreling into second base? After a hip replacement, doctors often recommend restricting athletics to low-impact activities such as walking, cycling, and swimming. (*see "Resumption of Activity"*). Thus many orthopedic surgeons did not think Jackson's replacement would last more than 2 years under the stress of competition. As it happened, however, Jackson's hip replacement held up well: he played major league baseball for two more seasons following the surgery (although he did not perform up to his pre-injury level and eventually retired, in 1995). Technology, of course, was a prime factor in this successful outcome.

Advances in the materials and procedures of implant surgery in general

Hip Replacement Surgery

Porous metal cup (to allow bone growth into material with polyethylene liner)

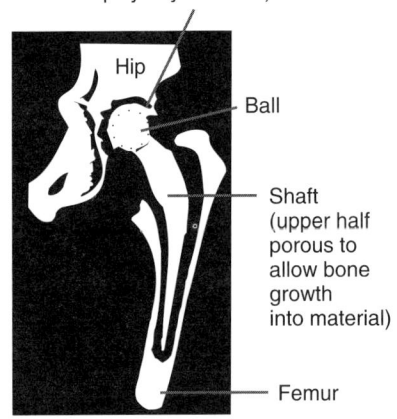

Hip

Ball

Shaft (upper half porous to allow bone growth into material)

Femur

hemorrhaging occurs, it may result in a long period of disability. But usually these injuries are mild and subside after a short period of rest (*see the box, "Pelvis and Thigh Injuries"*).

Athletes should not rush to resume activity, because muscle use must be restricted until healing is complete. Also, inactivity caused by injury results in a loss of strength and flexibility; therefore, if athletes begin playing again without first working to restore their pre-injury strength and flexibility, they are vulnerable to reinjury or prolonged disability.

have dramatically improved the results of hip-replacement surgery. Jackson's hip replacement consisted of a cobalt-chrome head in a cobalt-chrome cup with a polyethylene liner, and a titanium stem (shaft) implanted into the femoral canal. Tiny beads and pores on the upper end of the stem allow bone to grow into the pores and between the beads. This melding of bone with implant material is called osseointegration and is a vital aspect of hip-replacement surgery.

Surgeons need to create a strong bond between the implant and bone without triggering a response from the immune system. Until the mid-1980s, most hip implants used cement prepared in a vacuum and injected into the joint. Cement is adequate for elderly patients, but for the sprinting and diving that Bo Jackson would do on the baseball diamond, it would never have held up; in a case like his, osseointegration is essential. To aid osseointegration, some doctors use a chemical coating of hydroxylapalar over the stem so that new bone tissue bonds more quickly to the coating. Integrating growth hormones into the coating may also aid osseointegration; growth hormones stimulate the cells that form bone and may assist in the release of the body's own hormones that indirectly stimulate bone growth.

There are some problems with hip replacement. One problem has to do with the hydroxylapalar coating over the stem, applied to promote osseointegration: some experts are concerned about the strength of this substance and the possibility that it will flake off into the body, causing a rejection response from the immune system.

A second problem is that although the cobalt and ceramic material of the ball is extremely resilient and strong, the polyethylene socket is not. It has a tendency to wear and flake off, releasing particles into the femoral canal. This often triggers a response from the immune system, which attacks these invaders. In time, that may necessitate follow-up surgery to replace the joint again. To reduce the chance of socket deterioration, some manufacturers use particle accelerators to blast nitrogen-charged atoms into the ball, hardening and smoothing its surface; some have improved the smoothness of the finish; and some have used different materials as bearing surfaces, such as ceramics. These measures reduce friction when the ball rotates in the socket.

A third problem has to do with the hardness of the ball. Many people assume that the harder the ball, the better. This seems logical, but in fact a ball can be too hard, and such a ball may be detrimental, especially for young athletes.

A fourth problem is that bone (which is more elastic) ends up bending around the stiffer implant, loosening the bond between the two. For this reason, a titanium composite, because of its elasticity, may prove to be a better stem material. In other words, its material properties are more like those of bone (see EQUIPMENT MATERIALS).

A major concern of doctors performing hip replacements on young professional athletes is whether the replacement can withstand the impact forces created in sports. In climbing stairs or running, a force equivalent to five to six times body weight can be exerted on the hip joint; in landing from a jump, a force perhaps ten times body weight can exist (Maquet, 1985). Athletes are subject to even greater impact forces, and of course such forces are highest for very big men like Bo Jackson. Future advances, such as nondeteriorating composites, may result in more durable hip replacements, even for the very young and the very athletic. Such materials would more closely resemble the strength and flexibility of the pelvis and femur, and the strength of the weight-bearing surfaces.

RESUMPTION OF ACTIVITY
After hip-replacement surgery, orthopedic surgeons recommend avoiding high-impact sports and activities in which there is a high risk of falling or twisting the leg.

Recommended: Golfing, swimming, cycling, bowling, scuba diving, sailing, hiking

Questionable: Cross-country skiing, speed walking, ice skating, tennis, aerobics, volleyball, softball

Dangerous: Raquetball, running, hockey, baseball, water skiing, alpine skiing, basketball, soccer, football

Prevention of Injuries

Preventive measures can significantly lower the incidence of injury to the pelvis, hips, and thighs. Flexibility training (stretching) to increase range of motion, strength training to improve the working of muscles in the region, and wearing the proper equipment are among the most effective ways to prevent injuries.

Stretching. Because the majority of muscle mass is located in the

Pelvis and Thigh Injuries

Although the pelvis and thigh are less common sites of injuries than the knee or ankle, blows and falls can lead to chronic injuries.

Hip pointer. This is a contusion or a sharp tearing of the muscle attached to the iliac crest of the hip. In severe cases, the muscle tears away a small fragment of bone (avulsion fracture). Volleyball players frequently incur a contusion hip pointer injury when diving to the floor to "dig" a spike. Football players experience this injury from collisions and from sudden stretching of the muscles while making a quick turn to block. Minor injuries heal in a few days, but the severe cases, including avulsion fractures, can take 8 to 10 weeks.

Groin pull. This is a muscle tear from the groin. Groin pulls can be avoided by improving flexibility and muscular strength in the groin muscles. A mild pull takes a few days to heal; a more severe tear may take as long as 8 to 10 weeks to heal fully.

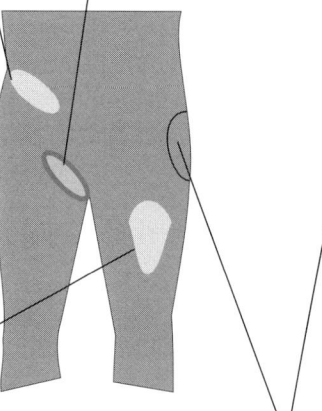

Hamstring tear. The bane of sprinters, jumpers, and hurdlers, hamstring tears make training impossible. The injured muscle fibers are replaced by scar tissue that is not elastic and does not contribute to the functioning of the muscle. It is necessary to increase the bulk and power of the remaining muscles before returning to action. People who suffer extreme hamstring pulls can never perform quite as well as before the injury.

Myositis ossification. This condition is caused by a blow to the thigh. After massive bleeding in the thigh muscle, "bone in the muscle" results, triggering new bone growth (ossification) into the hematoma. The quadriceps muscle is the large muscle located at the front of the thigh, a common target for blows in sports such as football, hockey, and rugby. When a blow is severe, this muscle may take as long as 3 to 6 weeks to regain strength and enough flexibility to bend and straighten the leg completely.

Trochanteric bursitis. This inflammation injury is common among women runners because of their wider hip structure, and among all athletes with a discrepancy in length of the legs. It can be easily treated by correcting running form, by running only on flat surfaces, or—in severe cases—by ceasing running altogether.

pelvis and thigh region, and because that region is near the body's center of gravity, it is important to stretch and increase the range of motion in this region. Muscles should be stretched gently and slowly both before and after exercise—before exercise to improve performance and avoid injury, and after exercise to increase range of motion. Following exercise, the muscles are still warm, so they are less likely to be injured by efforts to increase range of motion.

Inadequate stretching may have several consequences. For example, a lack of flexibility around the hips necessitates compensation by other body parts. This is especially true for hurdlers. Hurdlers use a powerful hip flexor (bending) action to bring the lead leg up to clear a hurdle. If a tight hamstring muscle restricts this action, either the hurdler's lead foot will topple the hurdle or the hurdler will have to jump higher to clear it. A tight iliopsoas—the hip flexor muscle that runs from the lumbar vertebrae to the femur—can lead to poor posture and eventually to back pain. When the iliopsoas is too tight, it tends to sway the spine slightly, which in turn increases the stress between the vertebrae. Thus, the more flexible the iliopsoas, the less countering action is needed by the abdominal muscles to hold the spine in place.

Strength training. Although strength training for this region of the body is important, it is not as critical as for other regions; the reason is that the pelvis, hip, and thigh are exercised by everyday activities, such as walking, running, and climbing stairs. Specific strength exercises for this region should include the abdominal muscles as well as the hip flexors and the hamstrings.

Protective equipment. In sports like football, in which the hip and thigh region is subjected to impact collisions from other players, protective equipment is necessary. To prevent muscle bruising and protect the hips, football pants come with pads over the hips and thighs to distribute the impact from collisions. These pads are quite effective at limiting injuries. Some volleyball players also wear hip-padded shorts to prevent hip injuries from dives across the floor.

Many athletes wear neoprene shorts or thigh sleeves that extend to the knee. There is little conclusive evidence that these sleeves prevent injuries by providing support, but they do help muscles warm up faster. Because warm muscles have a greater range of motion, such equipment may indirectly reduce the number of pulled hamstrings.

John Zumerchik and Robert J. Daley, M.D.

References

Albright, J., and R. Brand. *The Scientific Basis of Orthopaedics*. New York: Appleton and Lange, 1987.

Appenzeller, O. *Sports Medicine: Fitness, Training, Injuries*. 3rd ed. Baltimore: Urban and Schwarzenberg, 1988.

Arnheim, D. *Modern Principles of Athletic Training*. St. Louis, Missouri: Times Mirror Mosby, 1989.

Bloomfield, J., et al. *Textbook of Science and Medicine in Sports*. Champaign, Illinois: Human Kinetics, 1992.

Brinckmann, P., et al. "Sex Differences in the Skeletal Geometry of the Human Pelvis and Hip Joint." *Journal of Biomechanics* 14, no. 6 (1981): 427–430.

Jacob, S., et al. *Structure and Function in Man*. Philadelphia, Pennsylvania: Saunders, 1982.

Jefferson, J. "The Thighbones Connected to the . . . Artificial Hipbones." *New York Times*, 29 November 1992, sec. III, p.7.

Jorgensen, T. *The Physics of Golf*. Woodbury, New York: American Institute of Physics, 1994.

Jungers, W. "Relative Joint Size and Hominoid Locomotor Adaptations." *Journal of Human Evolution* 17 (1988): 247ff.

Haviland, W. *Anthropology*. 4th ed. New York: Holt, Rinehart and Winston, 1985.

Frankel, V. *Basic Biomechanics of the Skeletal System*. Malvern, Pennsylvania: Lea and Febiger, 1980.

Gamble, J.G. *The Musculoskeletal System: Physiological Basics*. New York: Raven, 1988.

Helminen, J. *Joint Loading: Biology and Health of Articular Structures*. Bristol, England: Wright, 1987.

Maquet, P. *Biomechanics of the Hip: As Applied to Osteoarthritis and Related Conditions*. New York: Springer-Verlag, 1985.

Saul, H. "Hip Bone Connected to the Titanium Implant." *New Scientist* 143, no. 1934 (16 July 1994): 34–38.

Tietz, C. *Scientific Foundations of Sports Medicine*. St. Louis, Missouri: Mosby, 1989.

"Total Hip Replacement." *National Institutes of Health Consensus Statement* 12, no. 5 (12–14 September 1994): 1–31.

Wilford, J. "The Transforming Leap: From Four Legs to Two." *New York Times*, 5 September 1995, sec. see C, p 1.

Wirhed, R. *Athletic Ability and the Anatomy of Motion* (trans.). New York: Wolf Medical, 1984.

Rehabilitation

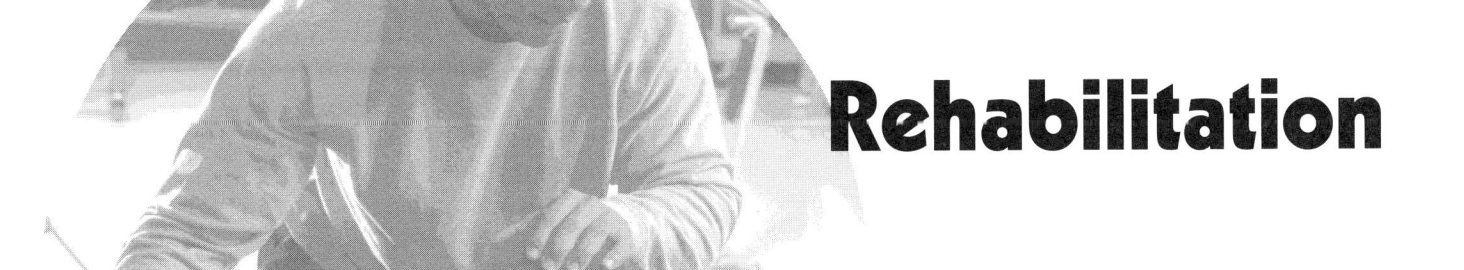

INJURIES TO THE MUSCULOSKELETAL system have been experienced by many—perhaps nearly all—athletes. The type and severity of these injuries, however, vary greatly. Amateurs and casual participants typically suffer overuse injuries after increasing the duration or intensity of exercise too quickly. Without adequate warm-up, the muscles, tendons, and bones are insufficiently prepared for vigorous workouts. Professional athletes, on the other hand, are not very susceptible to overuse injuries, partly because they are not prone to common musculoskeletal problems (if they were, they would never have reached the elite level), and partly because of their superior degree of athleticism. Thus professionals face different kinds of risks: their injuries usually come from more serious trauma. While a weekend jogger might suffer from tendinitis or a pulled muscle (strain), an ultramarathoner would be more likely to rupture a tendon or a muscle.

Rehabilitation is the process of recovery after injury; it involves not only healing but also becoming skillful and dexterous again. This process has come a long way in recent years.

In the past, an athlete with a moderate to severe injury would simply be told to rest until the injury was completely healed. Immobilization with a cast, a splint, or athletic tape was common, and it was maintained almost up to the actual day the athlete returned to play. Cold therapy, usually in the form of ice, was prescribed for only the first 24 to 48 hours after an injury; this was followed by heat applications until full healing had occurred. Along with some gentle stretching and strengthening, that was all that was done, and it was considered adequate rehabilitation.

Advances in exercise physiology and physical medicine have led to a different, and more scientific, approach to treating and preventing injuries. Except for serious injuries such as bone fractures, immobilization is limited to the minimum duration needed to prevent further damage. For many common sports-related injuries, like tendinitis, immobilization is not recommended at all. Instead, "range of motion" (ROM) exercises and gentle stretches are started immediately, as a precursor to more active exercises. Cold therapy, or cryotherapy, is no longer restricted to the first day or two but lasts as long as there is active inflammation or irritation around the injury—

though typically it still takes the form of application of ice. Heat therapy has become much less important, since research studies have found that superficial heat, such as a hot pack or an over-the-counter ointment, has little effect on deep tissues. Deep heating is available—for instance, from the ultrasound machines in physical therapy clinics—but even that is used only for specific reasons. (One prevalent use is for pitchers and quarterbacks: heat is directed to an inflamed rotator cuff tendon in the throwing shoulder.) For most sports injuries, ice is used as long as the area is irritated, usually until the inflammation subsides.

If there are no contraindications—that is, no medical reasons not to proceed—active exercise is recommended as soon as pain has subsided enough to allow it. This exercise typically takes the form of stretching and strengthening. The same advice that applies to so many other things in life applies to rehabilitation as well: "Crawl, walk, then run." That is, exercise starts at a low level so as not to aggravate the injury, and then becomes more challenging as time passes and healing progresses.

This article will discuss reactions to injury and phases of rehabilitation after injury.

Responses to Tissue Injury

All soft-tissue injuries have some elements in common. Because a great deal is known from research studies about injuries to tendons and about how the tendons respond to injury, they will serve as a useful model here. Tendon injuries are common, and what is known of the physiology of these injuries can be extrapolated to other soft tissues, including ligament, muscle, and cartilage.

Injuries can be roughly divided into acute and chronic. The terms *acute* and *chronic* refer only to time, not to severity: an acute injury is one that started within the last few minutes or hours; a chronic injury is one that has been present for weeks, months, or even longer. Although degree of severity is not a direct part of the definition of *acute* or *chronic*, severity is another useful way to categorize injuries—for one reason, because an athlete often cannot pinpoint the exact time a problem started. In fact, acute injuries do tend to be more severe and more dramatic; a good example is an out-of-condition softball player who ruptures a hamstring muscle. Chronic soft-tissue disorders, on the other hand, are often "overuse" injuries: minor repetitive stresses to the structure have accumulated over time and have eventually resulted in pain and dysfunction. Typically, with a chronic injury, an athlete has not allowed enough time for soft tissues to adapt to the increasing duration or intensity of exercise; good examples are tennis elbow and most cases of tendinitis.

At the microscopic level, sports trauma results in a loss of cells or cellular material (matrix). This occurs with a sudden overwhelming of the tissue (acute injury with abrupt onset) or an accumulated over-

GENERAL GUIDELINES IN CATEGORIZING INJURIES

Type of Injury	Usual cause	Location	Examples
Acute	Traumatic accident	Easy to identify	Ruptured hamstring muscle
Chronic	Minor repetitive stress	Difficult to pinpoint	Tennis elbow; shoulder stiffness (problem with rotator cuff)

Table 1.

load (chronic injury with gradual onset). With tendons, acute sudden trauma often leads to rupture, frequently at the point where the substance of the tendon blends into the muscle fibers: the musculotendinous junction, which is a mechanical weak point. This sets off a predictable tissue response, lasting at least several months.

The first step in this response process is inflammation (from the Latin *inflammare*, "to set on fire"), which is initiated when blood vessels are injured. This is called a "vascular" event—a term that indicates the integral role of blood vessels—but certain well-defined chemical events are also involved. These chemical events lead to the classic signs of inflammation: redness, swelling, heat, and pain. Pain is perhaps the most familiar indicator of inflammation. Some pain receptors are set off by mechanical stresses, such as the pressure from swelling. Other receptors are sensitive to the release of chemicals like bradykinin and "substance P." (One medical puzzle yet to be solved is why some people experience pain long after stimulation of the pain receptors has apparently ended. This can lead to a "chronic pain syndrome" that is difficult to treat.) For a one-time injury, without ongoing damage to the involved tissues, the acute changes of inflammation start within minutes of injury and last 3 to 5 days.

Once a sports injury has resulted in inflammation within or around a tendon, the second step in the tissue response is healing. Platelets, cells involved in the clotting response, are the first to appear after an acute injury. Other cellular building blocks follow, and formation of new blood vessels (neoangiogenesis) soon begins. Thereafter, healing proceeds along one of several pathways.

The most common pathway of healing is repair: replacement of cells that were injured—lost or damaged—during the initial trauma. One type of repair is regeneration, which results in tissue that is identical to the injured part. Except in a fetus, however, repair is virtually always of a second type: scar formation. In this type of repair, the new tissue—scar tissue—is less than optimal, compared with the original tissue, in terms of its functional characteristics: strength, flexibility, and endurance.

This second step of tissue response, repair, starts 24 hours after an injury and lasts up to 2 months. White blood cells called macrophages coordinate the process. Immature replacement cells for injured tendinous structure (tenocytes) are also seen during the repair stage.

When repair fails to proceed, there is usually a third step: degen-

Bodily Responses to Injury

Inflammation

Repair
- Regeneration
- Scar formation

Degeneration
- Chronic inflammation

eration: a progressive decrease in the functional status of the tissue; that is, the tissue becomes weaker. Atrophy, the shrinkage of cells, causes much of the degeneration, especially if the injured part is immobilized in a cast or splint. Degeneration makes a tendon more susceptible to future injury. It is important for the physician, therapist, or trainer to alert the athlete to this potential problem, so that rehabilitation efforts can be directed at prevention of future injuries as well as initial healing.

In cases of degeneration, chronic inflammation may occur in certain susceptible soft tissues, particularly when ongoing overuse never allows the structures to fully adapt to repetitive stresses. Microscopically, this occurs in regions of the body with an abundance of blood vessels. The rotator cuff tendons and the forearm muscles involved in tennis elbow are two of the most common examples.

It is worth noting that not all chronic conditions—that is, not all long-term conditions—are characterized by chronic inflammation. The processes of inflammation, repair, and degeneration form a spectrum of responses to an injury. Which, if any, of them will predominate at a given time depends on the mechanism of the initial injury, and on the efficacy of treatment and rehabilitation.

The following discussion will consider the four phases of rehabilitation after athletic injuries. Phase 1 (acute) encompasses diagnosis and immediate treatment; phase 2 is the subacute phase of treatment; phase 3 involves resumption of normal activity; phase 4—the crucial final phase—involves education for maintenance and prevention. It should be noted, though, that there are no clear demarcations between the four phases of rehabilitation after a sports-related injury. Some aspects of all four may be occurring throughout recovery, and even after return to play.

Phase 1 of Rehabilitation: Acute

The overriding goals of the first, acute, phase of treatment are prevention of further tissue damage and control of pain. Considerations of importance during phase 1 are diagnosis, rest, heat and cold therapy, compression, elevation, and anti-inflammatory drugs.

Diagnosis. Before an athletic injury can be successfully treated, the mandatory first step of phase 1 is an accurate and specific anatomic diagnosis. It is not adequate to label an injury "knee strain" or "foot sprain"; such a label merely describes the location of pain or dysfunction. The practitioner must be sufficiently skilled to pinpoint the cause, including any underlying biomechanical abnormalities.

Rest. Many physicians tell athletes to rest after an injury. It is true that some serious injuries, including most fractures, may require temporary total rest, but most overuse injuries and even many acute problems do not. Moreover, very competitive athletes may not follow the advice to rest if they think they can continue to play through the pain. Thus sports medicine practitioners who always prescribe complete rest after all injuries lose credibility, and rightly so. In many cases no further harm will be done to the affected tissues by "relative rest," which means cutting down to about 80 percent of the previous pain-free level of physical activity. The athlete can then gradually increase activity until it is back to 100 percent.

Relative rest may be prescribed, for instance, for a runner who has developed shinsplints (medial tibial stress syndrome) from increasing mileage or speed too quickly. In this case, relative rest allows the muscular attachments to the tibia, the fibula, and the membrane between the bones adequate time to adapt and accommodate to the stresses of activity—a necessary condition for healing. Consider a runner who usually logs 30 miles (48 km) a week at a pace of 8 minutes per mile (1.6 km), but then begins to train rigorously for a half marathon by doubling the distance to 60 miles (96 km) a week and increasing the pace to 6:45 per mile. Such an abrupt change in training often causes shinsplints that need to be treated with relative rest. Here, training might be adjusted to a 6-mile (10-km) run four times a week at a moderate pace of 8 minutes or 8:15 per mile. Mileage and speed can then be slowly increased, as long as the runner can do so with little or no pain.

Cold and heat therapy. Rest, properly prescribed, is perhaps the most effective treatment. The issue of heat versus cold therapy is a bit more tricky. However, in cases where soft tissue is inflamed or irritated, several factors make cold preferable to heat. First, cold therapy (cryotherapy) slows down the nerve fibers that carry pain signals; thus ice acts as an anesthetic. Second, blood vessels constrict when cold is applied (this effect is called vasoconstriction), so the swelling that accompanies many injuries is at least somewhat controlled. Third, vasoconstriction also means that warm blood is kept away from the area, allowing the beneficial effects of the ice to continue after it is removed from the skin. Fourth, cold limits internal bleeding and inflammation, both of which can cause further damage to tissues.

For these reasons, cold therapy, typically in the form of ice packs, is prescribed as soon as it is feasible for most acute injuries. A familiar example is an acute ankle sprain, in which swelling from ruptured blood vessels is often rapid and dramatic. The components of such swelling, particularly breakdown products of blood, can themselves irritate the surrounding tissues. Twenty minutes of ice application several times daily can limit the swelling and its secondary effects—irritation and immobility. Periodic, not continuous, icing is recommended because a 20-minute application of an ice pack to the injured ankle produces up to 1 hour of decreased temperature deep in the joint; also, prolonged application of cold may injure the skin or nerves lying just under the skin.

Cold is preferred to heat as long as inflammation, irritation, or swelling persists in or around an injured area. There is no preset time, such as 24 or 48 hours, for switching from ice to heat; the guide should be cessation of inflammation, irritation, and swelling.

As noted earlier, heat applied to the skin—in the form of hot packs or warm water, for example—penetrates only a short distance under the surface. (For example, only a minimal amount of heat can penetrate very far into the ankle.) Although some mild heating of deeper-lying tissues does occur as a reflex effect of superficial heat, this results in no more than a slight increase in temperature. Also, heat (unlike cold) causes blood vessels to dilate (vasodilation), and this effect counteracts its warming effect, because increased amounts of blood at body temperature are brought to the injured area. On the other hand, this last point means that whenever temperature does increase in soft tissues, the primary effect is to increase the blood flow locally. In the late stages of the healing process, that might be beneficial, because all substances required for tissue repair are blood-borne.

Generalized heating, as in a hot tub, is rarely useful in the acute phase of treating athletic injuries. If superficial heat is applied to a large area of the body, the major (and well-known) physiologic effect is relaxation, sometimes to the point of sedation. Most of us have experienced this in a warm bath, a hot tub, or a sauna. It is a "central" effect, however—meaning that it arises in the brain, not in the injured area.

There are (as noted above) forms of heat application that can reach deep-lying structures unaffected by superficial heat. The most common is ultrasound, which requires the special machinery provided by physical therapy clinics and athletic training facilities. Ultrasound treatment uses high-frequency sound waves; this acoustical energy causes molecules in soft tissue to vibrate, producing mechanical and heat energy. Ultrasound has raised the temperature of joint capsules to well over 115 degrees F (46° C; Arnheim, 1985). The most important effect of ultrasound is "deep heating" near the interface between two structures of different densities, as where muscle or tendon attaches to bone. Ultrasound treatment is particularly effective for the rotator cuff in the shoulder, the hip, the knee joints, and certain other deep structures.

Compression. Compression of an injured area with a elastic bandage or athletic tape may be prescribed for several reasons. Swelling can be controlled by the proper application of a bandage or tape. Also, the injured area can be somewhat immobilized in this way, preventing the damage from worsening.

However, compression treatment involves other considerations. For one thing, the sensation of a compressive wrap on the skin and deep-lying tissue may minimize or cover up sensations of pain in the same tissues—that is, these tissues may be sending pain signals that are being delivered but not fully perceived. Second, taping can necessitate a trade-off, a balance between support and mobility. Too tight

> ## Why Cold Is Preferable to Heat in Phase 1
>
> 1. Cold slows down pain-carrying nerves.
> 2. Cold constricts blood vessels, so that swelling is controlled.
> 3. Constriction of blood vessels also keeps warm blood away from the injured area.
> 4. Cold limits the internal bleeding and inflammation that cause further tissue damage.

The Taping Problem

It is important to have professional assistance in deciding how tightly to tape an injury because:

1. Too tight a wrap reduces the risk of further injury by giving added support, but it limits mobility and therefore impairs performance.

2. Too loose a wrap allows better mobility but does not reduce the risk of further injury as much as wrapping tightly does.

a wrap gives support but limits mobility and therefore is detrimental to performance; too loose a wrap allows more mobility but (obviously) does not give as much support and therefore does not reduce the risk of injury as much. Thus an appropriate balance must often be found. At one extreme is a bone fracture, in which preventing motion is more important than avoiding any negative effects of immobilization. With most sports-related injuries, however, recovery is promoted by an early resumption of activity, and so immobilization is used, if at all, only as long as it is absolutely needed medically.

Elevation. If the acute management of an injury calls for immobilization or compression, the treatment will usually also include elevating the body part. Again, perhaps the most common example is a sprained ankle: elevating the ankle on a footstool allows gravity to limit blood flow to the injured area and thus helps reduce swelling. Elevation of the injured part is likely to be helpful for up to 3 days after the injury.

Anti-inflammatory drugs. The physician will often prescribe a nonsteroidal anti-inflammatory (NSAI) medication, not only to inhibit the local inflammatory process but also to relieve pain. After a few days, these drugs should be taken only "as needed," much as an analgesic is taken for a headache.

Phase 2 of Rehabilitation: Subacute

During the second, subacute, phase of treating athletic injuries, the focus changes: the major goal in phase 2 is to promote the healing of soft tissue. However, many of the same therapeutic measures used in phase 1 should be continued, although perhaps with slightly different objectives.

Cold and heat therapy in phase 2. There is no universally applicable endpoint for cold therapy (cryotherapy); it is recommended as

Rest, Ice, Compression, and Elevation (RICE)

When a muscle, tendon, or ligament is injured, recuperation can take a few days or a few weeks—depending on what treatments are applied, and in what order.

REST the injured area until pain and swelling subside, usually around 24 to 72 hours.

ELEVATING the injury—allowing gravity to help limit blood flow to the area—limits the amount of swelling.

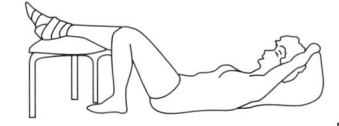

24 hours	48 hours	72 hours	Beyond

ICE the injury immediately, then for 20 minute intervals several times a day. Depending on the severity of injury, icing usually is continued for 24 to 72 hours.

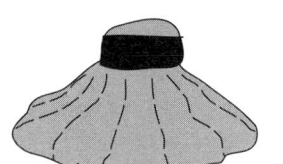

HEAT treatment should not begin until inflammation, irritation, and swelling stop, usually after two or three days; sometimes, however, heat should be avoided for several weeks. Resist the urge to begin training again too soon.

EXERCISE. "Relative rest" (e.g., training at 80% of pre-injury level) often is the best course of action. However, stretching and strengthening exercises should begin much sooner than that: as soon as pain and swelling subside.

long as irritation or inflammation of soft tissue persists. Applications of cold may be less frequent, though; for example, they might be tied to a twice-daily or three-times-daily exercise program. Some athletes find it easier to do the prescribed ROM or stretching if ice is applied first; others find icing helpful after exercising, to minimize the pain and irritation the activity produces. Once swelling subsides and exercise is no longer painful, there is usually no need for further cold therapy. However, exceptions do exist: many patients find long-term icing helpful as an accompaniment to an ongoing exercise program.

During the subacute phase of treatment—that is, once inflammation has subsided—generalized heating (whirlpool, hot packs over a broad area of skin, etc.) might prove useful for relaxing the muscles as a prelude to exercise, especially stretching. About 20 minutes of heating is required before this effect is noticeable.

Many athletes find it helpful to take a warm bath before exercise, in conjunction with whirlpool stretching and ROM exercises. Tanks for this purpose are made in various sizes to accommodate the leg or the arm and shoulder. A therapy pool large enough to stand in chest-high—available in many modern physical therapy clinics—is useful not only for specific exercises but also for aerobic training (running in place) during rehabilitation (*see SWIMMING*).

Deep heating in the form of ultrasound therapy, as described earlier, is most commonly used at this stage. Such heating can reach the joints at the knee, hip, and shoulder or can concentrate heat in a localized area, such as the outside of the elbow (in a case of tennis elbow). The main disadvantage of ultrasound therapy (and the main reason why its use is not more widespread) is that it can be given only in a therapy clinic or a doctor's office.

Anti-inflammatory drugs in phase 2. To prevent further damage, the physician may prescribe NSAI medication. Aspirin is effective and usually well tolerated. For patients who experience gastrointestinal irritation with aspirin, one of numerous other NSAIs is prescribed, such as ibuprofen or naproxen. (It is very rare for a patient to be unable to tolerate any NSAI medication.) When taken at the full prescribed dosage, these drugs work as both pain relievers (analgesics) and anti-inflammatory agents. If taken at a lower dosage, they act only on pain.

Another method of reducing inflammation, and thereby promoting healing, is for the physician to introduce anti-inflammatory medication directly around the injured tissue, typically by injection. A small amount of a potent cortisone-related compound (that is, a steroid, although not the same type used by some athletes for muscle building) is deposited by needle and syringe. The patient is instructed to avoid heavy exercise of the affected area for about 48 hours. Steroid injections are not used routinely. Generally, a steroid injection should not be repeated more than three times in a given region. Note that *no* material—particularly a corticosteroid—is ever injected directly into the substance of a tendon. Such an injection could weaken the tendon and contribute to a subsequent rupture; also, a poorly placed injection to treat ankle tendinitis could contribute to the rupture of the achilles tendon.

GENERAL GUIDELINES FOR REHABILITATION AFTER SPORTS INJURIES

Time Frame	Goal	Treatment
Immediate (minor; playing)	Control further damage without adversely affecting performance.	Ice. Continue play by using tape and protective padding and braces.
Short-term (minor; playing)	Speed healing process and minimize risk of further injury.	Rest the injured area as much as possible. Use heat after swelling subsides, and tape injured joint before play.
Immediate (major; sidelined)	Control and minimize pain and swelling.	Rest, ice, and elevate the injured area.
Short-term (major; sidelined)	Speed healing of injured area and maintain normal function of uninjured body parts.	Continue to ice at 20-minute intervals until swelling subsides. Start strength and flexibility training of uninjured body parts.
Long-term (major; sidelined)	Regain as much preinjury strength, flexibility, balance, timing, and coordination as possible.	Aqua training for cardiovascular training and muscle toning. Continue strength and flexibility training.

Table 2.

Phase 3 of Rehabilitation: Resuming Full Activity

The goal of the third phase of treatment is to return to full activity—ideally, free of pain and functioning at least at the level that existed before the injury. It might seem as if this would simply be a matter of advising the patient to increase activity as tolerated until that goal is achieved. In fact, though, this is the most complex phase of rehabilitation. It requires careful monitoring and a genuine "feel" for sports medicine as a science and an art.

By the time phase 3 of rehabilitation gets under way, the physician and the athlete should have determined the following; answers to these questions are necessary before an appropriate exercise program can be designed and begun:

• Why did the injury occur? Was it because of poor technique, improper conditioning, or just happenstance?

• Did an inherent or acquired biomechanical problem contribute to the injury? (Common inherent problems include flat feet and legs of different lengths; common acquired problems include imbalance of muscle strength or flexibility.)

• What steps can be taken to prevent a recurrence?

There are at least five areas to address and monitor during phase 3: (1) flexibility, (2) strength, (3) aerobic training, (4) coordination, and (5) graduated return to activity. For optimum progress, active exercise is designed to improve the patient's physical status through an individual program that can be closely monitored by a therapist, an athletic trainer, or an exercise physiologist.

Flexibility. The term *flexibility* refers to the "stretchiness" of a structure. Inflexibility, usually of muscles, may be a predisposing factor in injuries. In a sprinter, for example, tight hamstring muscles could result in a strain or even a rupture of that group. By the same token, if a muscle group is injured for other reasons, it can become inflexible because of immobility, weakness, inhibition of motion by pain, and other factors. It is therefore important to assess flexibility early in the course of treatment, and for the therapist and the patient to devote part of each exercise session to stretching. During phase 3 of rehabilitation, stretching should be done both before and after the remainder of the exercise program. Stretching before a workout is useful for avoiding further injury (e.g., muscle fiber tear); stretching afterward, when the muscles are warm and more extensible, helps increase baseline flexibility.

Stretching before athletic activity may reduce the risk that muscle fiber will tear away from the bone or tendon to which it is attached.

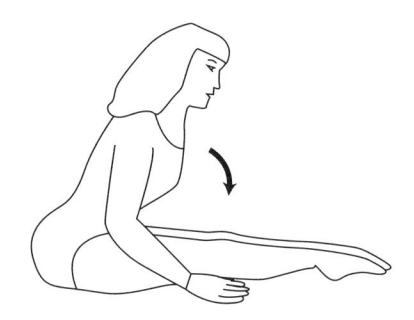

Figure 1. *Hamstring muscle stretch. Stretching and warming up should never be rushed by bouncing (using momentum from motion). The position that stretches the muscle should be held for at least a minute.*

When the temperature of muscle cells increases even slightly, as it does during a minor warm-up, metabolism speeds up. Also, oxygen dissociates from blood, an effect that in turn increases blood flow. These factors combine to reduce muscle viscosity (force resisting fluid flow), with the beneficial effect of reducing injuries. In addition, oxygen is in more plentiful supply during muscular work, and nerve impulses speed up. This heightened metabolic state of muscle improves an athlete's quickness and maximum capacity for work.

Stretching or warming up should never be rushed by "bouncing"; bouncing is never appropriate as a means of stretching. Rather, the position that stretches a muscle should be held for at least 1 minute, leading to the familiar pulling sensation—not to pain.

Strength. As with flexibility, a deficiency or an imbalance in strength may be a preexisting condition that contributes to a sports injury, or it may itself be a primary or secondary effect of an injury. The physician must not only examine the strength of each muscle in the injured area but also judge whether there is any imbalance in the major muscle groups locally.

In this regard, perhaps the most common example—although it is not well recognized—has to do with the shoulder. A quarterback might have a typical rotator cuff injury, leading to inflammation and pain in the throwing shoulder. By the time phase 3 of rehabilitation is reached, the relative strength of the muscles in front and in back of the shoulder should have been studied. Typically, the muscles in back, those responsible for stabilizing the shoulder blade against the rib cage, are weaker than those in the front of the shoulder and chest. This is an underlying condition that allows the ball-and-socket joint of the shoulder too much slippage, leading to irritation of the cuff. If only the cuff muscles are treated, without a program to balance the strength, the problem will recur after the athlete returns to throwing.

Finally, other muscles in the kinetic chain must be strengthened or stretched as necessary. The term *kinetic chain* refers to all portions of the musculoskeletal system that link together to perform a given motion. For a pitcher or a quarterback, this includes the abdominal, lumbar, and leg muscle groups. This type of "big picture" analysis is mandatory for the successful treatment of any musculoskeletal athletic injury, regardless of its location.

The athlete should not feel discouraged if there are no immediately noticeable gains from a strengthening program. At least 6 to 8 weeks will be needed before improvements in strength can be felt, although computerized machinery will be able measure gains well before that.

Aerobic training. Any athlete must reach a certain level of general endurance and fitness to optimize performance in a given sport. But certain sports—like rowing, cross-country skiing, cycling, and marathon running—primarily involve aerobic training. These sports push athletes up to, or close to, the body's maximum capacity for oxygen utilization. They require the ultimate level of cardiovascular training.

A period of inactivity, or a drop-off in activity, leads to a decline in aerobic conditioning. Whether this decline is significant depends on the sport. For example, aerobic fitness is of secondary concern for baseball players, important for hockey and soccer players, and critical for long-distance runners. (Despite this, however, long-distance runners should not return too soon after an injury, because reinjury is probable and could set them back even further.)

Following a sports-related injury, a primary objective of rehabilitation, during all phases of recovery, is to prevent a decline in the athlete's previous level of aerobic conditioning. But for many athletes, running is the primary means of maintaining fitness, and many injuries preclude running. In these cases, an alternative exercise is needed, one that will keep the heart, lungs, and musculoskeletal system in top shape while the injured area heals. There are several options: exercise bicycle, stair climber, rowing machine, and (if a pool is available) swimming. Pool exercise is particularly effective as a substitute for running, because the buoyancy of the water minimizes impact forces on the lower leg (*see also SWIMMING*). Cross-training—in which several different aerobic activities are done at different times throughout a typical week—is strongly encouraged. By these means, all areas can be kept in top condition for the return to the particular sport.

Coordination. If an injury causes only a brief time away from the primary sport, coordination will probably not suffer. There are two general instances, however, in which attention to coordination as part of the rehabilitation program is essential: first, when more than a few weeks have elapsed since playing; second, when the injured area plays a primary role in coordination.

Coordination and timing drop off whenever an athlete stops training for any period of time, whether the time away is due to injury or simply to disuse during an off-season. In fact, this phenomenon is the reason why every major sport schedules preseason training and exhibition games. Returning to action after injury and returning after an off-season both require the athlete to start out slowly and to use progressively more difficult exercises that simulate the skills required. Depending on the sport, higher-level skills such as bounding and leaping are simulated with "plyometric" exercises (*see the boxes on plyometrics in VOLLEYBALL and MOTOR CONTROL*). Of course, the maximum level of coordination is reached only when an athlete, now fully recovered from injury, has been back in play for several weeks, fine-tuning these skills in the competitive arena.

Returning to play. For most sports-related injuries, there is no universally applicable "definitely safe" time for an athlete to return to play; injuries vary in severity, and individuals heal at different speeds. Given this fact, and the fact that reinjury is likely if sports activity is

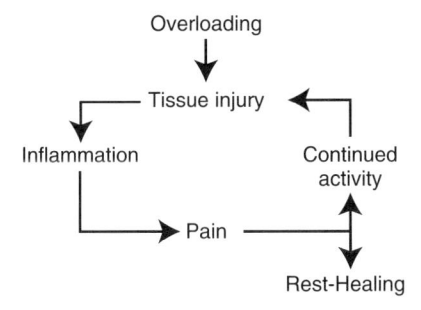

Figure 2. *When pain is experienced, stop. See a doctor. Continued activity can lead to more tissue damage, further delaying the return to play. Resuming play too early after an injury can result in a never-ending cycle of injury and reinjury. Rest is often the only way to break out of that cycle.*

resumed too soon, especially at full intensity, the best course of action is a gradual return under the supervision of a trainer, a therapist, or a coach. Also, periodic reevaluation by a physician is needed to ensure that no further damage is occurring.

All athletes need to use some common sense, too: if pain persists or seems to be increasing, they should stop. Unfortunately, however, pain is not always a clear-cut guideline. The initial return to play typically increases pain in the area of injury. The athlete and the physician must therefore distinguish between the usual soreness after a layoff and a reaggravation of the underlying problem.

A competitive tennis player, returning to action after experiencing a shoulder injury, might take the following steps: First, on-court activity might begin with hitting against a backboard, using only routine forehand and backhand strokes. Alternating between backhand and forehand ground strokes works on the needed lateral movements. Simple half-speed serves can be added next, progressing to topspin and three-quarter-speed serves. This can be followed by work with a skilled hitting partner who alternates baseline and short shots, encouraging movement forward and back. These controlled drills eventually progress to match-level play, but not yet at a highly competitive level. If all goes well, return to unlimited play soon follows.

Phase 4 of Rehabilitation: Maintenance and Prevention

Advances in rehabilitative sports medicine now allow injured athletes to return to their sports not only free of pain but perhaps in better physical shape than they were before being injured. Too often, though, sports medicine practitioners ignore the crucial fourth phase of rehabilitation: education for maintenance and prevention. This final phase is essential to preserve and improve on the achievements made during treatment, so that athletes can not only optimize their performance but also prevent future injuries.

As noted earlier, there are no sharp boundaries between the four phases of rehabilitation, and phase 4 is a good example: aspects of this phase appear in earlier phases as well. Thus the principles of prevention are introduced early on, when the underlying biomechanical problems that may have predisposed the athlete to injury in the first place are identified. These problems are discovered by analyzing movement patterns and predicting forces acting on the joints. Designing an individual exercise program, along with properly fitted aids (shoe inserts, bracing, taping, or splinting), will help ensure that an athlete can safely return to action.

Training errors should of course be avoided—especially the common mistake of increasing the duration or intensity of exercise too quickly. The athlete must be educated at the beginning of self-training about the importance of avoiding such errors.

Cross-training techniques (as mentioned above, these involve varying the exercise routine throughout each week) are very important in preventing injury. Cross-training gives any particular bone or soft tissue time to recover from the preceding workout. Athletes, especially those who are highly committed to a single sport, often have not considered the idea that this kind of variety can also help improve performance in their primary activity. Middle- and long-distance runners, for instance, routinely include interval training—wind sprints—in their usual routine. (This needs to be supervised, though, to achieve the desired effect: improving the "kick" at the end of a race without diminishing overall endurance.) Basketball players also add some middle-distance running for cross-training, even though most of the game itself is spent doing interval sprints.

Selecting equipment and making adjustments to it are also important. Regularly replacing running shoes to prevent shinsplints and stress fractures, lowering a tennis racket's string tension to prevent tennis elbow, and adjusting a bike seat to prevent knee problems are just three of the many steps athletes can take to avoid disabling injuries.

For fitness "fanatics," such as obsessive-compulsive runners, prevention of injury might require insight into psychological issues that underlie habitual overexertion. Obsessive-compulsive athletes often repeat the same activity that has already resulted in a disability.

If the principles of phases 1 through 4 are followed, successful rehabilitation is usually achievable. To recapitulate: Successful rehabilitation must begin, in phase 1, with an accurate, specific, anatomic diagnosis rather than simply a description of symptoms. Initial treatment in phase 1 is critical in preventing the spread of damage, often by controlling inflammation. Shortly thereafter, in phase 2, healing is promoted using the various techniques at the disposal of a physician or another sports medicine practitioner. In phase 3, return to active exercise, and eventually to actual play, is often a gradual process. Generally, it should start only when it will cause no further tissue injury. The timing of return to unlimited participation in sports must be geared to the individual athlete, with an awareness of the demands of the sport and of how well the athlete has responded to treatment. Phase 4, the critical final phase of treatment, encompasses prevention, which completes the full circle of rehabilitation for any sports-related injury.

Steve R. Geiringer, M.D.

References

Arnheim, D. *Modern Principles of Athletic Training*. 7th ed. St. Louis, Missouri: Times Mirror Mosby, 1985.

Halvorson, G. "Principles of Rehabilitating Sports Injuries." In C. Tietz (ed.), *Scientific Foundations of Sports Medicine*. Philadelphia, Pennsylvania: Decker, 1989.

Respiration

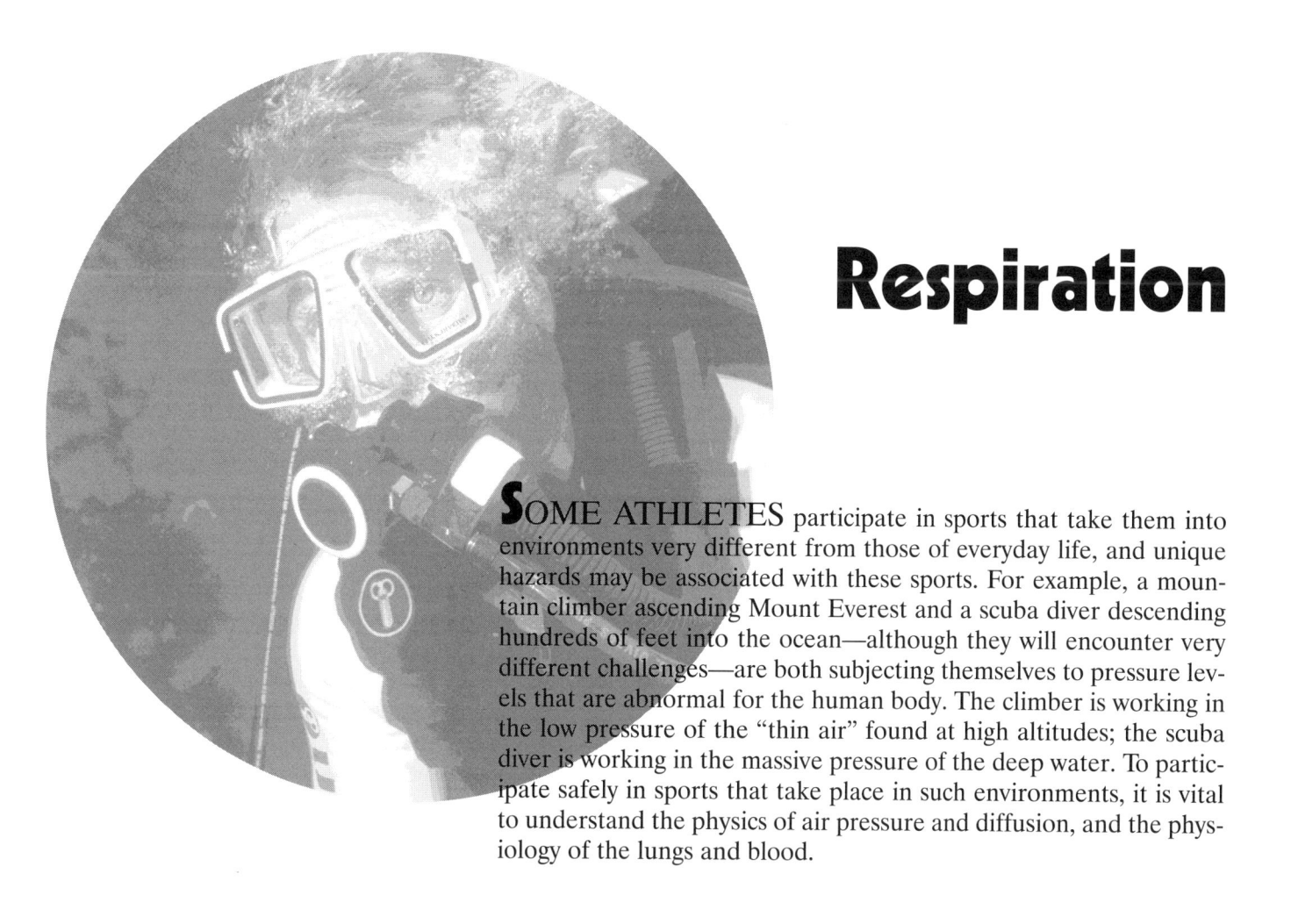

SOME ATHLETES participate in sports that take them into environments very different from those of everyday life, and unique hazards may be associated with these sports. For example, a mountain climber ascending Mount Everest and a scuba diver descending hundreds of feet into the ocean—although they will encounter very different challenges—are both subjecting themselves to pressure levels that are abnormal for the human body. The climber is working in the low pressure of the "thin air" found at high altitudes; the scuba diver is working in the massive pressure of the deep water. To participate safely in sports that take place in such environments, it is vital to understand the physics of air pressure and diffusion, and the physiology of the lungs and blood.

Physics of Respiratory Gases

Studying the physics of gases will allow us to understand how gases exert pressure, dissolve in liquids, and diffuse from one location to another.

Air Pressure

We live at the bottom of an "ocean" of air many miles in thickness, called the atmosphere. The atmosphere exerts pressure on the body.

Atmospheric pressure is expressed in mm Hg. (Hg is the chemical symbol for mercury and mm is the abbreviation for millimeters.) The atmospheric pressure (in mm Hg) is the height of a column of mercury that the air pressure will support. At sea level, air pressure will support a column of mercury 760 millimeters high; thus at sea level, air pressure = 760 mm Hg, or 1 atmosphere (atm).

As we ascend in altitude, the thickness of the atmosphere above decreases. This reduces the air pressure on the body. A skier in the Rocky Mountains at an altitude of 10,000 feet (3,030 m) experiences air pressure of only 523 mm Hg (0.69 atm). A climber near the summit of Alaska's highest mountain, Denali (previously called Mount McKinley), is at an altitude of 20,000 feet (6,060 m) and experiences air pressure of only 349 mm Hg (0.46 atm). A climber at the summit of Mount Everest, the world's highest peak, is at an altitude of 28,000 feet (8,484 m) and experiences even lower air pressure: 250 mm Hg (0.33 atm).

The air we breathe is 21 percent oxygen (whose chemical symbol is O_2) and 79 percent nitrogen (N_2). (There are small amounts of several "trace" gases, but these are not of great physiologic importance and can be ignored for the purposes of this discussion.) Just as (disregarding the trace gases) oxygen and nitrogen together make up the atmosphere, the pressures produced by oxygen alone and nitrogen alone combine to make up atmospheric pressure. The pressure exerted by any one gas is known as partial pressure and is determined by two factors: (1) total atmospheric pressure and (2) the fraction of the atmosphere made up by the given gas. Thus at sea level, the pressure exerted on the body by the oxygen in the air is 760 mm Hg × 0.21 = 160 mm Hg. This pressure is called the partial pressure of oxygen, or PO_2.

The proportions of oxygen and nitrogen in the air do not change at higher altitudes. But because the total air pressure is reduced at a higher altitude, the partial pressure of oxygen in the air also falls. At 10,000 feet, the atmosphere has a PO_2 of 110 mm Hg (523 × 0.21 = 110 mm Hg). At the summit of Mount Everest, PO_2 is only 52.5 mm Hg (250 × 0.21 = 52.5 mm Hg). The atmosphere at higher and higher altitudes, then, provides less and less oxygen. We gasp for breath on a mountaintop because PO_2 is greatly reduced. Thus ascending to high altitude presents a challenge because the air at a high altitude has a far lower partial pressure of oxygen than would be the case at sea level.

When we go underwater, by contrast, we are subject to increased pressure. Because water is far denser than air, 1 atm (760 mm Hg) of pressure is exerted by a mere 33 feet (10 m) of seawater. Thus, at a depth of 33 feet the body is subjected to 2 atm of pressure (1,520 mm Hg): 1 atm from the water plus 1 atm from the air above the water. At a depth of 66 feet (20 m), the body is subjected to 3 atm (2,280 mm Hg) of pressure: 2 atm from the water plus 1 atm from the air.

Underwater, the combined pressure of the atmosphere and the water is exerted on all parts of the body, including the chest. For this reason, in order to breathe comfortably it is necessary breathe air that has the same pressure as the pressure being exerted on the outside of the body. This means that at a depth of 33 feet a scuba tank must supply air at a pressure of 2 atm. If the tank has been filled with air that has the same proportions of oxygen and nitrogen as the atmosphere, at a 33-foot depth it will supply air with a PO_2 of 320 mm Hg (1,520 × 0.21 = 320 mm Hg). At a 66-foot depth it must supply air at 3 atm of pressure, with a PO_2 of nearly 480 mm Hg.

Dissolved Gas

Virtually all gases dissolve to some extent in water. Because the blood plasma is made up primarily of water, all gases dissolve to some extent in blood plasma as well. The amount of a gas dissolved in a fixed volume of water is determined by the product of two factors: (1)

the solubility of the gas in water and (2) the partial pressure of the gas over the water.

Factor 1, the solubility of a gas in water, is a physical property of each gas. Because of their chemical makeup, some gases are more soluble in water than others. For instance, at a temperature of 15° C (59° F), when oxygen has a partial pressure of 1 atm over water, 34 milliliters (ml) of oxygen dissolve in 1 liter of water. However, when carbon dioxide has a partial pressure of 1 atm over water, 1,019 ml of carbon dioxide dissolve in 1 liter of water. Thus the solubility of carbon dioxide in water is almost 30 times that of oxygen. Nitrogen, by contrast, has a solubility in water about half that of oxygen. When the partial pressure of nitrogen over water is 1 atm, 17 ml of nitrogen dissolves in each liter of water.

Factor 2 is the partial pressure of the gas over the water. The amount of a gas dissolved in a fixed volume of water is directly proportional to the partial pressure of the gas above the water. This means that if the partial pressure of a gas above a liquid is doubled, the amount of the gas dissolved in that liquid is also doubled.

Because there is direct link between the partial pressure of a gas over a liquid and the amount of that gas dissolved in the liquid, it is possible to refer to the partial pressure of a gas in a liquid. For instance, if water is exposed to air at a pressure of 1 atm and allowed to dissolve as much oxygen as it can, the partial pressure of oxygen in the water is said to be 160 mm Hg, just as the partial pressure of the oxygen in the air above the water is 160 mm Hg.

Since the amount of a gas dissolved in water is highly dependent on the partial pressure of the gas over the water, the relative solubility of gases can be compared only under the same pressure conditions. Therefore, in the examples above, the solubility of nitrogen, oxygen, and carbon dioxide in water was compared under conditions where each gas had a partial pressure of 1 atm over the water. Another way to compare the solubility of different gases in water is to measure the volume of the gas that dissolves in 1 liter of water for each 1 mm Hg partial pressure. Expressed in these terms, the solubility of oxygen in 1 liter of water is 0.045 ml O_2 / mm Hg partial pressure (34/760 = 0.045); the solubility of nitrogen in 1 liter of water is 0.022 ml N_2 / mm Hg partial pressure (17/760 = 0.022).

To clarify the concepts of partial pressure and gas solubility, it is helpful to consider the following problem: Given a mixture of gases with the same proportions of oxygen and nitrogen found in the atmosphere, how much of each of these gases can dissolve in 1 liter of water at the pressure found at sea level? This problem can be approached in two steps. First, the partial pressures of both oxygen and nitrogen at 1 atm total pressure (sea level) are determined by multiplying total pressure times the fraction of the atmosphere made up by each gas. Second, the amount of each gas dissolved in the water is determined by multiplying the partial pressure of the gas times the solubility of the gas.

Step 1 is straightforward. Indeed, some of the required calculations have already been done, when PO_2 at different air pressures was determined. The partial pressures of oxygen and nitrogen at sea level are $PO_2 = 160$ mm Hg and $PN_2 = 600$ mm Hg ($760 \times 0.79 = 600$). In step 2, each partial pressure is multiplied by the solubility of the gas to determine the amount of the gas dissolved in 1 liter of water. At sea level, 7.2 ml oxygen ($160 \times 0.045 = 7.2$) and 13.2 ml nitrogen ($600 \times 0.022 = 13.2$) are dissolved in each 1 liter of water. Note that the amount of nitrogen dissolved in the water is greater than the amount of oxygen, even though the solubility of oxygen is twice that of nitrogen. This occurs because the partial pressure of the nitrogen is nearly four times that of oxygen.

Pressure and Gas Volume

One way to understand how gases behave is to visualize a gas as a collection of moving, colliding particles. As the molecules that make up a gas move randomly through space, they bump into each other and into the walls of the container they are in. The pressure of a gas is really the force of these individual collisions between the gas molecules and the wall of the container added together. When a football or a bicycle tire is blown up with a hand pump, or a balloon is blown up by mouth, it is apparent that the more air is put into the container, the higher the pressure in the container becomes. The reason is that if more air molecules are crowded into a given space, the chance increases that air molecules will collide with the walls of the container.

In fact, if a fixed amount of gas is sealed in a container that can change volume, like the cylinder of an automobile engine, there is an inverse relationship between the volume of the container and the pressure of the gas on the walls of the container (*see Figure 1*). If the piston is pulled out, expanding the volume of the cylinder, the pres-

Figure 1. *A piston pump works as follows. During the suction stroke (piston pulled up), decreased pressure causes the inlet valve to open and fluid to flow into the cylinder. When the piston is pushed down, increased pressure causes the inlet valve to close and fluid to be forced out of the opened outlet valve. Whenever a fixed amount of gas is sealed in a container that can change volume (no valves), there is an inverse relationship between container volume and gas pressure on the walls of the container. Greater volume means less pressure; less volume means greater pressure.*

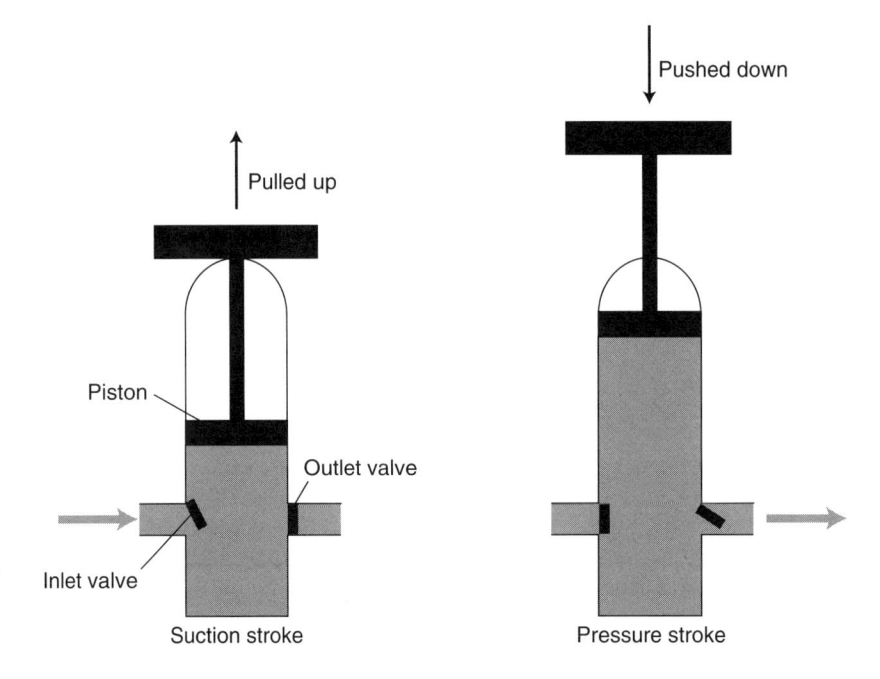

sure on the gas inside drops proportionately. If the piston is pushed in, the pressure increases. This inverse relationship can be expressed as an equation: $P \times V = K$, where P is the pressure of the gas, V is the volume occupied by the gas, and K is a constant. Another way to describe the inverse relationship between pressure and volume is $P_1 \times V_1 = P_2 \times V_2$. That is, given a fixed amount of gas in a container at an initial pressure P_1 and volume V_1, if the pressure is increased to P_2, the new volume V_2 will be proportionally lower.

The practical consequences of this inverse relationship between volume and pressure are striking. For example, consider a diver swimming toward the surface. Let us begin with the diver at a depth of 66 feet (20 m; 3 atm pressure), filling the lungs to a volume of 5 liters. If the diver then swims to the surface (1 atm pressure) while holding his or her breath, the volume of the lungs will expand to 15 liters ($5 \times 3 = 15 \times 1$). This will almost certainly cause the lungs to burst; that is why scuba divers are to taught breathe continuously, particularly as they ascend.

Diffusion of Gases

Diffusion is a passive process whereby gases can move from areas of higher partial pressure to areas of lower partial pressure. To understand how diffusion of gases works in the body, it is helpful to imagine the following experiment.

An airtight box is divided in half with a membrane through which both oxygen and carbon dioxide can pass. Then the right side of the box is filled with oxygen at 1 atm pressure and the left side with carbon dioxide at 1 atm pressure. The oxygen has a higher partial pressure on the right side of the box than on the left. Thus the oxygen diffuses from the right side to the left. The carbon dioxide has a higher partial pressure on the left side of the box than on the right. This causes the carbon dioxide to diffuse from the left side to the right. When the partial pressures of the gases in the box finally stop changing, there will be 0.5 atm partial pressure of oxygen and 0.5 atm partial pressure of carbon dioxide on each side of the membrane. No further net diffusion of gas can occur, because the partial pressures of each gas are the same on both sides of the membrane. Under these conditions, for every oxygen molecule that moves from the right side of the box to the left, another molecule moves from the left to the right. The gas is said to have reached equilibrium.

Likewise, gases that are dissolved in liquids diffuse from areas of higher partial pressure to areas of lower partial pressure. This phenomenon is vital to the ability of the human body to deliver oxygen to its interior. Oxygen diffuses from the lungs into the blood and from the blood out to the tissues. In both cases, the oxygen is moving from an area of higher to an area of lower partial pressure.

Several physical factors affect the rate at which a gas diffuses across a membrane. Three of these are particularly important to this discussion. First, the larger the difference between the partial pressures of the gas on the two sides of the membrane, the faster the net rate of diffusion will be. In the simple example of the airtight box, at the beginning of the experiment oxygen has a high net diffusion rate because the difference in partial pressure between the two sides of the membrane is large. However, as the oxygen approaches equilibrium, the net rate of diffusion slows because the difference in partial pressure between the two sides of the box decreases. Net diffusion stops completely when equilibrium is reached because at equilibrium there is no difference in partial pressure between the two sides of the box.

Second, the larger the surface area of the membrane, the more rapid the diffusion. The membrane across which oxygen diffuses as it travels from the lungs to the blood (the respiratory membrane) is a delicate structure with a huge surface area. Diseases such as emphysema, which can be caused by smoking, destroy parts of this membrane and reduce its surface area. This slows the diffusion of oxygen into the blood and therefore has a serious impact on health.

Third, some membranes allow gases to pass more readily than others. When a membrane allows a gas to pass easily, it is said to be very permeable to the gas. Thin membranes are generally more permeable than thicker ones. Thus, gases generally diffuse more rapidly across thin membranes than thicker ones. Exposure to the low PO_2 of high altitudes can cause water to leak into the respiratory membrane and thicken this usually thin structure. The extra thickness of the respiratory membrane slows the diffusion of oxygen into the blood, and this can be a serious problem for mountain climbers.

Physiology of Respiration

Every body cell needs to break down sugars and fats for energy (*see also ENERGY AND METABOLISM*). When they burn these fuels, body tissues use oxygen and produce carbon dioxide. The two primary functions of the lungs are to move oxygen from the atmosphere to the blood, and to remove carbon dioxide from the blood and send it into the atmosphere. Once the blood has picked up oxygen at the lungs, it is pumped by the heart to the body tissues. Carbon dioxide, which is produced by body tissues, enters the blood as it flows through the tissues. This carbon dioxide–rich blood circulates through the veins to the lungs, where it is removed from the body (*see also HEART AND CIRCULATORY SYSTEM*). Thus to understand the function of the lungs, it is necessary to consider three processes:

1. *Ventilation*—the process by which air is moved in and out of the lung

2. *Gas exchange*—the process by which oxygen leaves the air in the lung and enters the blood, while carbon dioxide moves in the opposite direction

3. *Gas transport*—the process by which oxygen and carbon dioxide are carried in the blood

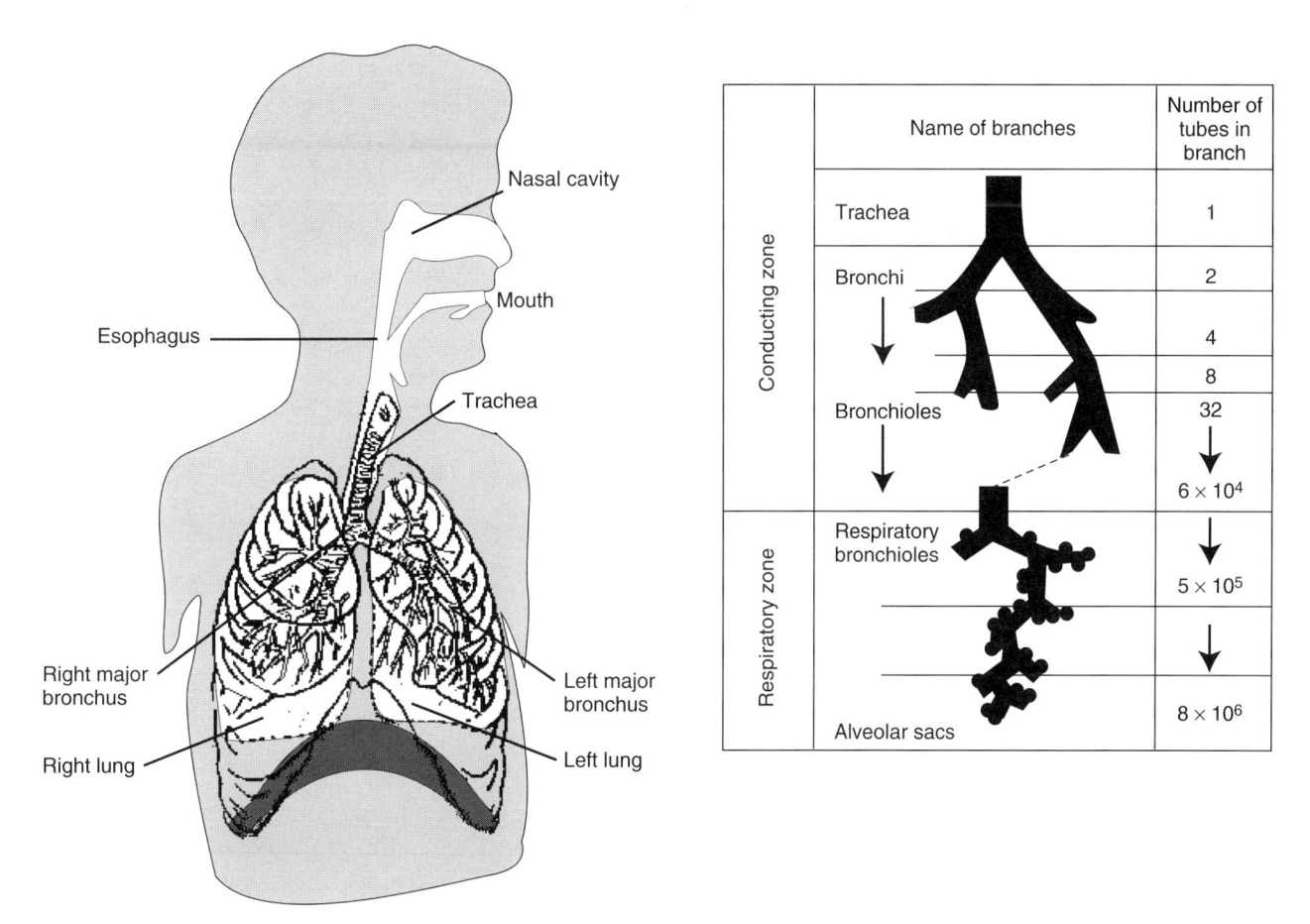

	Name of branches		Number of tubes in branch
Conducting zone	Trachea		1
	Bronchi		2
	↓		4
			8
	Bronchioles		32
	↓		6×10^4
Respiratory zone	Respiratory bronchioles		5×10^5
			↓
	Alveolar sacs		8×10^6

Figure 2. *Shown here are (left) the organization of the respiratory system, and (right) the airway branching pattern, from the single trachea to the millions of alveolar sacs.*

Ventilation

The lungs are located in the thoracic (chest) cavity and are connected to the outside atmosphere by a series of branching tubes. Starting at the mouth, the initial part of the passage, known as the pharynx, is a common pathway for the respiratory system and the digestive system. From the pharynx, air passes through the larynx, or voice box, into the trachea in the throat. The trachea branches into bronchi, which branch further into smaller tubes called bronchioles. The bronchioles end in blind sacs called alveoli (*see Figure 2*). As will be discussed later, gas exchange between the air in the lungs and the blood occurs in the alveoli.

Ventilation of the lungs works very much like a bellows. During inspiration (breathing in), the diaphragm—a dome-shaped muscle that makes up the floor of the thoracic cavity—contracts (*see Figure 3*). This causes the diaphragm to fall and flatten. At the same time, other muscles attached to the ribs lift the rib cage up and out. The combined effect of these actions is that the volume of the thoracic cavity is increased during inspiration. As the volume of the thoracic cavity increases, the lungs are stretched to an expanded volume. This increase in volume causes the air pressure in the lungs to drop below

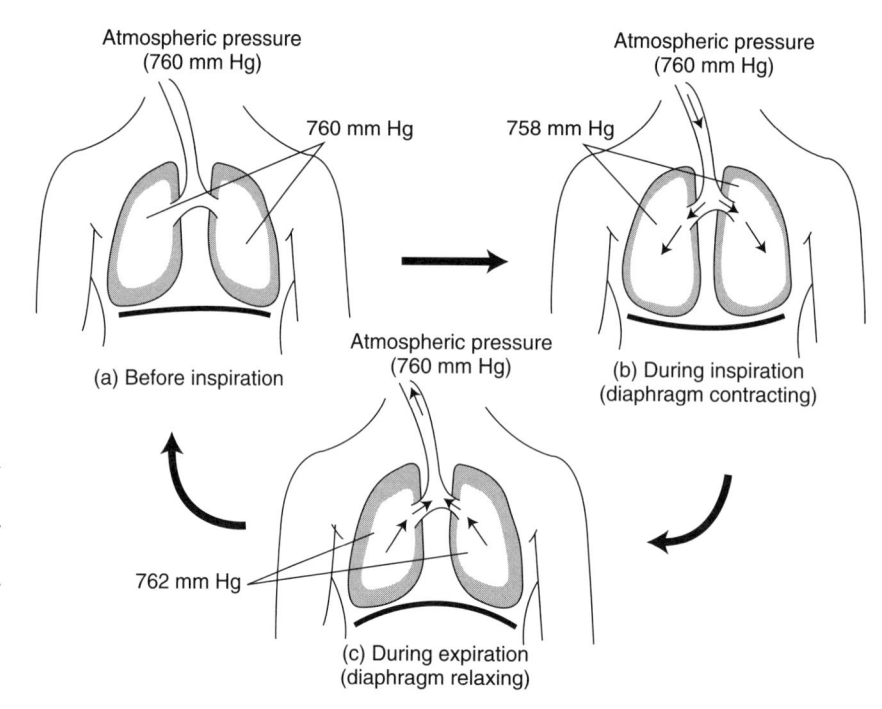

Figure 3. *Pressure changes during breathing. (a) Pressure before inspiration. (b) During inspiration, alveolar pressure decreases. (c) During expiration, alveolar pressure increases. Air pressure seeks a state of equilibrium so that alveolar pressure = atmospheric pressure.*

the pressure of the atmosphere outside the lungs. As a result of this difference in pressure, air flows into the lungs. Because inspiration occurs when the lung pressure falls below atmospheric pressure, this type of ventilation is called negative pressure ventilation.

Expiration (breathing out) is the opposite of inspiration. The diaphragm relaxes and returns to its higher position and its dome shape. The chest muscles relax, and the rib cage falls. The volume of the thoracic cavity is reduced, and the lungs are compressed. This causes the air pressure in the lungs to rise above atmospheric pressure, and air is forced out of the lungs.

At the end of a quiet inspiration, an adult male has about 3,000 ml of air in his lungs. When he exhales, he breathes out about 500 ml. Thus, there is still about 2,500 ml of "old" air left in the lungs at the end of a quiet expiration. The volume of air breathed in and out with a breath (in this example, 500 ml) is known as the tidal volume. At rest, a person may breathe in and out about 12 times per minute. This value is known as the respiratory rate. The total amount of air breathed in and out of the body every minute, known as the minute ventilation, is found by multiplying respiratory rate times tidal volume. The minute ventilation of an adult male at rest is thus 500 ml/breath × 12 breaths/minute = 6,000 ml/minute. Note that 6,000 ml = 6 liters.

During exercise, the need for energy is increased, and to meet this need the body requires far more oxygen. During extreme exertion, the lungs expand to 6,000 ml volume at the peak of inspiration and empty nearly to 1,000 ml on expiration. This achieves a tidal volume of almost 5,000 ml, a tenfold increase over resting tidal volume. The respiratory rate also increases during exercise. An adult who takes 12 breaths per minute at rest may take 20 or more breaths every minute during heavy exercise. Thus the minute ventilation during extreme exercise may be as much as 100,000 ml/minute, a fifteenfold increase over the resting value. This amount of respiratory activity is necessary to deliver to the body the amount of oxygen that is needed during very intense exercise, which is 15 times more than the amount needed at rest.

The rate and depth of ventilation are controlled by respiratory centers in an area of the lower brain called the brain stem, located just above the spinal cord. The brain stem contains groups of cells capable of responding to changes in the levels of carbon dioxide and oxygen in the arterial blood. When the carbon dioxide level rises too high or the oxygen level falls too low, the brain stem signals the muscles of respiration to increase the rate and depth of ventilation. This brings extra oxygen to the blood and removes the excess carbon dioxide, thus returning the oxygen and carbon dioxide levels to their proper values. Under normal conditions the oxygen level in the arterial blood remains quite constant and the respiratory centers of the brain stem respond predominantly to changes in blood carbon dioxide. However, if the level of arterial oxygen falls, either as a result of lung disease or when a person enters a low-oxygen environment (as at a high altitude, for example), the low level of arterial oxygen will act as a stimulant to respiration.

How ventilation is regulated during exercise is not as straightforward as might be expected. Certainly, the demand for oxygen and the production of carbon dioxide both increase during exercise, and it might be predicted that these changes would produce a fall in arterial oxygen and a rise in carbon dioxide, which in turn would stimulate ventilation. However, careful measurements show that the levels of blood oxygen and carbon dioxide actually change very little during exercise, in part because when a person anticipates strenuous exercise, ventilation increases before the exercise even begins. It appears that higher brain centers stimulate the muscles of respiration to increase ventilation in preparation for exercise. Once exercise begins, the strenuous activity of the skeletal muscles itself can maintain this stimulation.

A note on artificial ventilation. People who cannot breathe (a condition known as respiratory arrest), can be connected to a machine, called a ventilator, that will breathe for them.

In the polio epidemics of the 1940s and 1950s, some people who contracted polio became paralyzed, lost the use of the diaphragm, and therefore were unable to breathe and had to connected to ventilators. At that time, the only type of ventilator available was the "iron lung." This primitive piece of equipment is a metal shell that surrounds the entire patient except for the head. A leather or rubber gasket around the patient's neck seals off the inside of the box from the atmosphere, and a vacuum pump is connected to the inside of the box. When the pump is turned on, the pressure in the box drops below atmospheric pressure and the patient's chest is sucked outward toward the wall of the box. The patient inhales even without being able to move the diaphragm. When the pump is turned off, the pressure in the box returns to atmospheric pressure, the patient's chest falls passively, and the patient exhales. The iron lung repeats this process for every breath. Iron lungs are negative-pressure ventilators: that is, the patient inhales when the pressure in the lungs drops below atmospheric pressure.

Beginning in the 1960s, a more sophisticated ventilator—a positive-pressure ventilator—came into use. One end of a tube is inserted down the throat of a patient in respiratory arrest, past the larynx, and into the trachea. The other end of the tube protrudes through the patient's mouth or nose. This tube, called an endotracheal tube, is about 10 millimeters (1/4 in.) in diameter and has an inflatable cuff around its lower end. When the cuff is blown up, it makes a seal between the outside of the tube and the wall of the trachea so that air can enter the patient's lungs only through the tube. The mouth end of the tube is connected to the positive-pressure ventilator, a machine capable of pumping air (or any desired mixture of gases) directly into the patient's lungs.

For a patient connected to a positive-pressure ventilator, the ventilation cycle is as follows. First, the ventilator pump turns on, pumping air into the patient's lungs at a pressure greater than atmospheric pressure (inspiration). Then the pump turns off, and the air in the patient's lungs escapes passively (expiration). The ventilator repeats this process 10 to 20 times every minute. Positive-pressure ventilators are so called because they deliver air to the patient's lungs at a pressure above atmospheric pressure.

Positive-pressure ventilators are extremely useful for patients having surgery under general anesthesia. During some surgical procedures, such as the removal of the appendix or part of the lung, the surgeon must open the patient's abdominal or thoracic cavity. To do this, the surgeon must cut through several layers of muscles and spread the cut edges of the muscles apart. It will obviously be much easier for the surgeon to do this if the patient's muscles are relaxed (and what is easier for the surgeon is usually what is best for the patient). One approach to the problem of relaxing the muscles for surgery is to administer general anesthesia and muscle relaxants. The anesthetist places the patient under general anesthesia (usually with sodium pentothal or a similar drug administered through an intravenous line) and then administers a muscle relaxant (also through the intravenous line) that paralyzes all skeletal muscles, including the diaphragm. (The muscle relaxant is usually a chemical relative of curare, the arrow tip poison used by native peoples of South America.) An endotracheal tube is then inserted into the patient's trachea, and the patient is placed on a positive-pressure ventilator. The anesthetist usually maintains the patient under general anesthesia with a gas anesthetic agent and administers additional doses of muscle relaxant if necessary. When the surgery is over, the anesthetist turns off the anesthetic gas and administers an intravenous medication that reverses the effects of the muscle relaxants. The patient wakes up and begins to breathe independently. Then the anesthetist removes the patient's endotracheal tube.

Positive-pressure ventilators have several advantages over negative-pressure ventilators. They allow a health care worker to adjust the volume of air the patient receives with each breath. They also allow the health care worker to change the composition of the gas administered to the patient. For instance, a patient in respiratory arrest may need more than 21 percent oxygen. A patient on positive-pressure ventilation can easily be given an oxygen-enriched gas mixture to meet this need.

However, positive-pressure ventilation also has some disadvantages. A person can be connected to a positive-pressure ventilator only by a tube that seals against the tracheal wall. Thus a patient on a positive-pressure ventilator must have either an endotracheal tube (inserted through the mouth or nose) or a tracheostomy tube inserted directly through an incision in the throat (-*ostomy* means "opening into"). Neither option is particularly comfortable for a conscious patient. Also, with an endotracheal tube or tracheostomy tube in place, complications can arise. The inner surface of the trachea is covered with sticky mucus that traps bacteria and viruses. Small, hairlike projections called cilia on the tracheal cell surface beat rhythmically and push the mucus—with the bacteria entrapped in it—out of the larynx and into the pharynx, where it can be swallowed. A patient with an endotracheal tube or tracheostomy has a huge pathway through which bacteria can enter the trachea. However, because the inside of the tube does not have cilia, the patient cannot eliminate the bacteria from the respiratory system. This creates a risk of respiratory infections such as pneumonia.

Gas Exchange

As discussed earlier, air at sea level has a PO_2 (partial pressure of oxygen) of 160 mm Hg. When this air is inhaled into the alveoli—the tiny air sacs that fill the lung—it mixes with the "old" air still present from the last breath. The old air has a more carbon dioxide and less oxygen than the atmosphere. This mixing, along with the fact that water vapor is added to the air as it moves through the bronchi, reduces the PO_2 of the gas in the alveoli to about 105 mm Hg.

The alveoli are small sacs about 0.25 mm (0.009 in.) in diameter. The lungs of a heathy adult have some 300 million alveoli. Thus, the total surface area of all alveoli combined is 70 to 80 m^2, an area approximately equal to one side of a tennis court. This large surface area is vital to survival because oxygen must diffuse from the alveoli into the blood. Diseases such as emphysema, which can be caused by smoking cigarettes, reduce this surface area and limit the ability of the body to move oxygen from the alveoli to the blood.

The walls of the alveoli are very delicate structures made up of a single layer of cells and a thin membrane (*see Figure 4*). The pulmonary capillaries (capillaries of the lung), located immediately out-

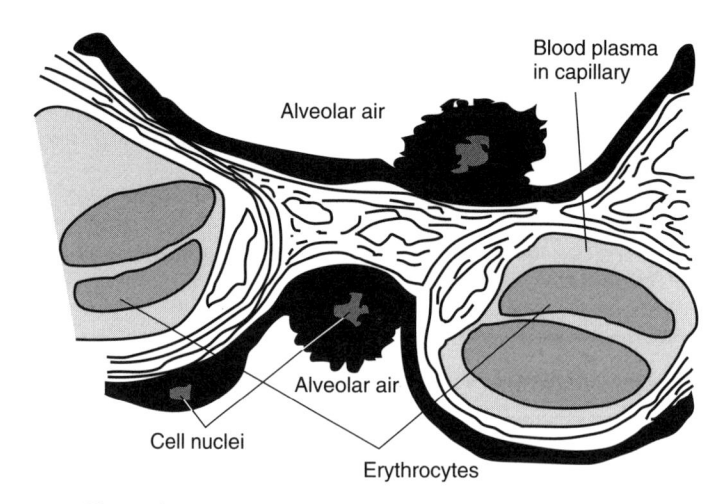

Figure 4. *Shown here is a magnified view of a portion of the alveolar wall.*

side the alveoli, also have very delicate walls made up of a single cell layer and a thin layer of membrane. There is only a very narrow space—known as the interstitial space—between the alveolar and pulmonary capillary walls. Thus, only two cell layers, two thin membranes, and a very narrow space separate the gas in the alveoli from the blood. The structures that separate the alveolar gas from the blood are called the respiratory membrane.

At the respiratory membrane, oxygen must diffuse from the alveolar gas to the blood, and carbon dioxide must diffuse from the blood to the alveolar gas. The total distance between the blood in the pulmonary capillaries and the gas in the alveoli (thickness of the respiratory membrane) may be as little as 0.2 micrometer (μm). For the lungs to function properly, the distance between the blood and the air must be very short, so that gas exchange can proceed efficiently.

As discussed above, diffusion can occur quickly and efficiently only over very short distances. The diffusion of oxygen across the normal respiratory membrane is so efficient that PO_2 drops only from 105 mm Hg in the alveolar gas to 100 mm Hg in the blood leaving the pulmonary capillaries. When the oxygenated blood reaches the tissue capillaries throughout the body, the oxygen diffuses out of the blood and enters the cells of the tissues, where it is used in the breakdown of sugars and fats for energy. As the oxygen diffuses out of the blood and into the cells, the blood PO_2 falls from 100 mm Hg to 40 mm Hg by the time the blood reaches the veins (*see Figure 5*).

Gas Transport

Blood is made up of a clear liquid known as blood plasma, with blood cells suspended in it. There are several types of blood cells, the most common of which is the red blood cell, or erythrocyte. A small amount of the oxygen that diffuses from the alveolar gas into the blood simply remains dissolved in the blood plasma and thus creates a partial pressure of oxygen in the blood. Most (98 percent) of the oxygen in the blood enters the erythrocytes and combines with the protein

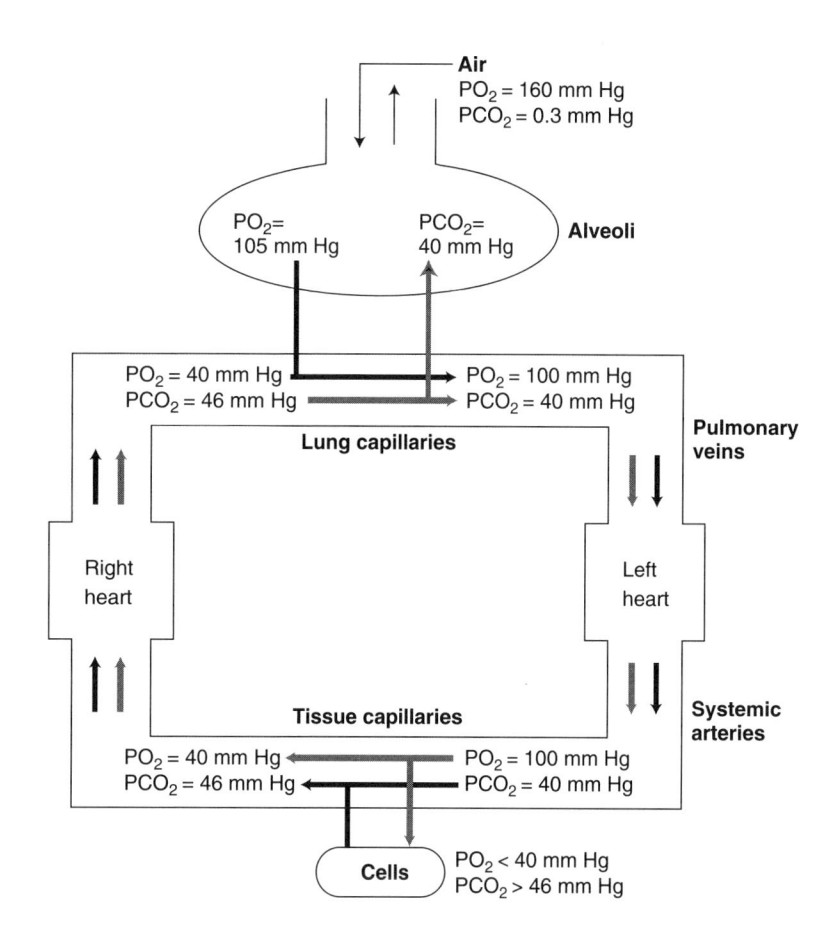

Figure 5. *Shown here is partial pressure of oxygen and carbon dioxide in the air, lungs, blood, and body cells. (Adapted from Vander, 1994)*

hemoglobin in those cells. Because a molecule of oxygen must first dissolve in the blood plasma before it can enter an erythrocyte, the higher the partial pressure of oxygen in the blood plasma, the more oxygen will be bound to hemoglobin. Each molecule of hemoglobin can carry only four molecules of oxygen. Thus when all the hemoglobin molecules in the erythrocytes of a given blood sample are carrying four oxygen molecules, the hemoglobin is 100 percent saturated.

The relationship between the partial pressure of oxygen in the blood plasma and the percent saturation of hemoglobin in the erythrocytes of that blood (*see Figure 6*) is complex. As the PO_2 increases from low levels, the hemoglobin saturation increases too, steeply at first and then more gradually. At a PO_2 of about 100 mm Hg, the hemoglobin is virtually 100 percent saturated. Even if the PO_2 is increased above 100 mm Hg, no more oxygen can be carried on the hemoglobin. Because virtually all of the oxygen in the blood is carried on the hemoglobin, this means that above 100 mm Hg, further increases in the PO_2 add very little to the amount of oxygen in the blood.

It can be seen, then, that evolution has produced a hemoglobin molecule very well adapted to environmental conditions. Under normal circumstances, the PO_2 delivered from the alveolar gas to the blood of the pulmonary capillaries is 100 mm Hg, exactly sufficient to produce a nearly maximum amount of oxygen in that blood. It can also be seen that the common practice of having players breathe from an oxygen tank at the sidelines during a sporting event probably has more psychological than physiological effect—this can add very little extra oxygen to a player's blood. There is one exception to this statement, however: a player who comes from sea level (New York or San Francisco, for example) to compete in a high-altitude location (say, Denver, at an altitude of 5,300 ft., or 1,606 m), might find it more difficult to exercise strenuously, because of the low PO_2 in the atmosphere at this altitude. This player might indeed benefit from breathing 100 percent oxygen from a tank at the sidelines, although the effect will last only a few minutes once play is resumed (*see the section below, "Sports at High and Low Air Pressure"*).

Oxygen is not the only important gas carried in the blood. Carbon dioxide, produced in the tissues as a waste product when sugars and fats are broken down for energy, enters the blood as it passes through the tissue capillaries. Like oxygen, carbon dioxide is carried both in chemical solution in the blood plasma and bound to hemoglobin in the red blood cells, although a smaller fraction of carbon dioxide is bound to hemoglobin than is the case for oxygen. In the capillaries of the lung, carbon dioxide leaves the blood, diffuses across the respiratory membrane, and enters the alveoli. It is then exhaled. Because carbon dioxide leaves the blood at the lungs, the partial pressure of carbon dioxide (PCO_2) is higher in the blood flowing toward the lungs than it is in the blood flowing away from the lungs. The PCO_2 of the arterial blood pumped by the heart to the body tissues is normally 40 mm Hg, while the PCO_2 of the venous blood that returns from the tissues to the heart is normally about 46 mm Hg.

Carbon dioxide has a very important effect on the acidity of blood. When carbon dioxide dissolves in the blood, it combines with water to form carbonic acid (H_2CO_3). The carbonic acid then under-

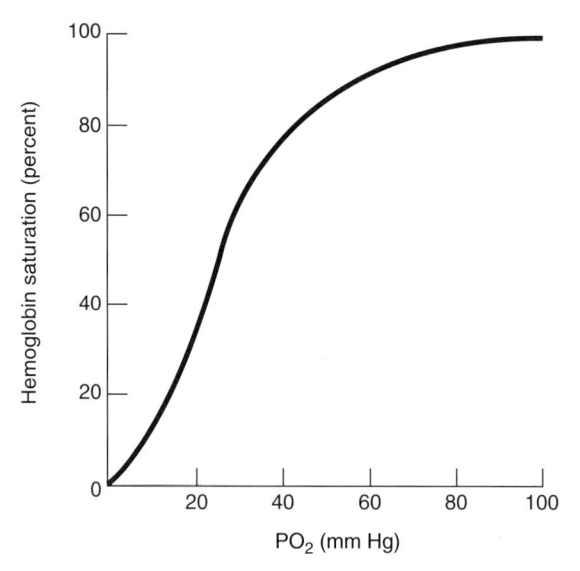

Figure 6. *This graph shows the relationship between the partial pressure of oxygen in the blood plasma and the percent saturation of the hemoglobin in the erythrocytes of that blood.*

goes a chemical splitting to produce bicarbonate ions (HCO_3^-) and hydrogen ions (H^+): $CO_2 + H_2O \rightarrow H_2CO_3 \rightarrow HCO_3^- + H^+$. The concentration of hydrogen ions in the blood is important because it directly determines the acidity of the blood. Acidity is measured with a pH scale that runs from 0 to 14. Because pH is an inverse scale, lower pH values indicate a higher concentration of hydrogen ions and more acidity; higher pH values indicate a lower concentration of hydrogen ions and less acidity. Thus the greater the partial pressure of carbon dioxide in the blood, the greater the concentration of hydrogen ions, and the more acidic the blood will be (lower pH). Conversely, the lower the carbon dioxide level in the blood, the lower the concentration of hydrogen ions in the blood and the less acidic (more alkaline, higher pH) the blood will be.

Because nitrogen is the most abundant gas in the atmosphere, it too might be expected to cross the respiratory membrane from the alveoli into the blood. Nitrogen certainly does enter the blood; however, it dissolves in the blood plasma only in small amounts and is not carried on hemoglobin. Because nitrogen gas is neither used nor created in metabolism, it is described as metabolically inert and is usually ignored in discussions of physiology. Still, in some situations such as scuba diving, where the environmental pressure is unusual, even the relatively small amount of nitrogen dissolved in the blood can have serious consequences.

Respiratory Diseases

Respiratory diseases are major killers in the United States and, as a result, society puts a great deal of effort into education about the dangers some behaviors pose to our lungs. The image of patients with emphysema holding a cigarette up to their tracheostomy opening is familiar to most of us; and virtually everyone who smokes has seen the warnings printed on every cigarette pack—but many smokers ignore all this. Some younger people, including some athletes, may trivialize the threat of respiratory disease because they believe that respiratory diseases strikes only older people. Unfortunately, this is not the case.

This section focuses on two respiratory diseases: first, asthma, a disease that often strikes young people; second, emphysema, a disease that also begins when a person is young, though it does not show itself until later in life.

Asthma

Asthma is a very common disease. In the industrialized countries, about 1 person in 20 suffers from asthma. People with asthma usually feel perfectly normal most of the time but suffer periodic attacks during which they have great trouble breathing and may require medication or even hospitalization. An asthma attack can be triggered by a variety of stimuli: emotional upsets, respiratory infections, or inhalation of an allergen (pollen, for example). In some people, exercise can trigger asthma attacks.

Whatever the cause, an asthma attack usually involves several responses. The muscle surrounding the bronchi contracts (bronchospasm). The bronchi also produce excess mucus, and the inside of the bronchi becomes inflamed and swollen. These responses combine to narrow the bronchi, making it difficult to breathe out (exhale). The air moving through the narrowed bronchi produces the characteristic wheezing sound made by a person who is having an asthma attack.

Once an attack begins, it must be treated and terminated as soon as possible. The struggle to breathe during an attack expends a huge amount of energy, and if the attack continues, the person may tire. Blood oxygen can fall and blood carbon dioxide can rise because the lungs are not being ventilated enough to meet the metabolic needs of the tissues. If a severe asthma attack goes on for a long time, the patient can stop breathing (go into respiratory arrest) and require mechanical ventilation.

Severe asthma attacks can also damage the lungs. Because the patient is unable to breathe out well, air becomes trapped in some parts of the lungs, and the alveoli in these areas become overinflated. This can damage the delicate walls of the alveoli and lead to emphysema later in life.

Asthma attacks can often be controlled with a variety of medications. Steroids, which block the inflammatory response; and bronchodilator medications, which cause the muscle surrounding the bronchi to relax, are particularly helpful for people with asthma. Some of the most useful medications for people with asthma are administered through an inhaler—a small handheld device that allows the patient to stop an attack by delivering medication directly into the lungs.

People with severe asthma may have to limit sports-related activity, particularly during certain times of the year, such as pollen season, when they are very prone to attacks. However, many young athletes with asthma find that they can participate in sports if they follow some very simple rules:

1. *Seek advice, and keep others informed.* Consult a physician about plans to participate in sports. Work with a doctor to develop a plan for specific athletic goals and the specific medical problem. Also, players should inform their coaches about any medical conditions, so that a coach will be prepared to react quickly to any emergency that does occur.

2. *Listen to the body.* Learn what situations and stresses are most likely to trigger attacks, and avoid these situations. Learn to recognize the early signs of an asthma attack. When an asthma attack begins, stop exercising and treat the asthma promptly.

3. *Keep appropriate medications available.* Anyone who uses an inhaler to treat asthma attacks should always have the inhaler on hand, par-

ticularly during exercise. As already mentioned, exercise itself can trigger asthma attacks in some people, and it is very important to terminate an asthma attack as quickly as possible.

Emphysema

Emphysema is an insidious, debilitating, and deadly respiratory disease caused by the destruction of the delicate walls of the alveoli. As the walls of the alveoli deteriorate, the boundaries between these small, individual sacs break down, and the patient is left with a reduced number of larger sacs with scarred walls. One large sac has less surface area than many small ones. Furthermore, alveolar walls thickened by scarring block the diffusion of respiratory gases. For these reasons a person with emphysema will have a low level of blood oxygen and a high level of blood carbon dioxide.

Emphysema develops for a variety of reasons. No one event damages the lungs enough to cause emphysema; it takes many separate injuries, over many years. Smoking, air pollution, and chronic lung infections can put a person at risk.

Smoking is a particularly potent, and totally avoidable, cause of emphysema. A person who smokes a pack of cigarettes a day is 15 times more likely to develop emphysema than a nonsmoker. Cigarette smoke irritates the lungs; in response, the airways produce extra mucus. This mucus would ordinarily be swept out of the airways by the beating action of the cilia. However, cigarette smoke also paralyzes the cilia, so that the extra mucus remains in the lungs until it is coughed up. The need to cough up this extra mucus produces the characteristic "smoker's cough." Because mucus builds up overnight, smokers usually cough most just after getting up in the morning. This buildup of mucus is more than just a minor nuisance that causes coughing. Because the cilia cannot remove the mucus from the lungs, bacteria and viruses build up in the respiratory system. This is the reason that smokers get more colds and other respiratory infections than nonsmokers. The extra mucus clogs the airways and blocks the passages to groups of alveoli. When the smoker coughs, the pressure in these blocked alveoli shoots up to very high levels because the air in the alveoli cannot escape. This high pressure damages the alveolar walls. The smoker is then on the way to developing emphysema.

Of course, emphysema is not the only risk entailed by cigarette smoking. Smoke is a combination of gases and small solid particles. When a smoker draws this deadly mixture into the lungs, the particles can stick to the walls of the airways, particularly at places where the airways branch. Under normal circumstances, the cilia might sweep these particles away, but because (as noted above) cigarette smoke paralyzes the cilia, the particles are more likely to remain in the lungs. These particles can cause lung cancer. Indeed, smoking is the major cause of lung cancer in the United States. Four out of five cases of lung cancer are caused by smoking. Furthermore, lung cancer is a particularly deadly form of cancer. Among patients diagnosed with lung cancer, only 1 in 8 will be alive 5 years after diagnosis.

Perhaps one reason why some young people disregard the dangers of smoking is that damage from smoking often cannot be recognized until later in life, when it has already progressed to a dangerous level. Most organs of the body are constructed with some level of redundancy: they can perform their normal resting functions even when working at less than 100 percent efficiency. Redundancy allows the organs to perform at above-normal levels during times of need. For instance, the heart can pump more blood and the lungs can ventilate more air than is necessary to maintain the body at rest; that, of course, is what makes work and exercise possible. Redundancy also means that an organ can often maintain its functions, at rest, even after it has been damaged, if activity is limited so that the damaged organ is not subjected to stress.

However, when a person with emphysema continues to expose the lungs to cigarette smoke, lung damage is progressive. Sedentary people may not even realize that they have emphysema until lung damage is so severe that it prevents them from performing normal activities such as climbing stairs. At that advanced stage of the disease, so many alveoli have been destroyed that the normal physiological redundancy of the lungs is gone. Any more damage will leave a person a respiratory cripple, gasping for breath and permanently connected to an oxygen tank. Such a person may eventually die from inadequate oxygen delivery to the brain and heart.

Fortunately, quitting smoking can help stop the progression of emphysema at almost any stage. Alveolar walls that have already been destroyed cannot repair themselves: this damage is permanent. However, once a smoker quits, the lungs are less irritated and produce less mucus. This reduces coughing. Also, the cilia regenerate and begin to clear out the accumulated mucus, reducing the risk of airway obstruction and further lung damage. Thus, even though cigarette smoking is notoriously addictive, it makes sense for anyone who smokes to try to quit immediately.

Sports at Low and High Air Pressure: Mountaineering and Scuba Diving

High-altitude mountain climbing and scuba diving are exhilarating and rewarding sports that bring tremendous personal satisfaction. However, both sports also entail risks, because participants are exposed to potentially hazardous environments. Although the hazards associated with climbing and scuba diving are very different, they have one thing in common: the athlete must deal with the effects of altered air pressure. An understanding of the physics of the atmosphere and the physiology of respiration will help athletes avoid potentially lethal mistakes underwater and in the mountains.

Climbing: Low-Pressure Exercise

Respiratory physiology at high altitudes. As discussed earlier, the atmosphere has a lower total pressure and a lower partial pressure of oxygen (PO_2) at high altitudes than at sea level. Thus, when climbers ascend to a high altitude, they are exposed to an atmosphere containing less oxygen than the atmosphere at sea level. When this "thin" air is breathed into the lungs, it is diluted with "old" air from the previous breath and with water vapor supplied by the lungs. This further reduces PO_2. Moreover, because oxygen moves from the lungs to the blood by diffusion, the PO_2 of the arterial blood must be even less than that found in the alveoli of the lungs.

Some "hard numbers" will demonstrate the importance of this reduction in oxygen level. At sea level, the atmospheric pressure is 760 mm Hg and the PO_2 in the atmosphere is 160 mm Hg. If the lungs are functioning normally, this means that the PO_2 in arterial blood will be 100 mm Hg and that hemoglobin, the protein that carries oxygen, will be 100 percent saturated with oxygen. At the summit of Denali in Alaska (the highest peak in the United States), an altitude of 20,000 feet, the atmospheric pressure is 349 mm Hg and the atmospheric PO_2 is 110 mm Hg. For a person standing there, the PO_2 in the alveoli will be 40 mm Hg, and the PO_2 of the arterial blood will be in the mid-30s, depending on how well the person's lungs are functioning. The oxyhemoglobin dissociation curve (*refer back to Figure 6*) shows that when arterial PO_2 is this low, the hemoglobin in the red blood cells is less than 70 percent saturated. This means that the blood is carrying less than three-fourths of the normal amount of oxygen.

Low arterial oxygen is called hypoxia (*hypo*, "low"; *oxia*, "oxygen level"). The effects of hypoxia are dramatic. Respiratory centers in the brain stem sense the low arterial oxygen level and respond by signaling the respiratory muscles to increase the rate and depth of lung ventilation. This response is helpful because it brings more air into the lungs, though because the air breathed in at high altitude is low in oxygen, it cannot completely correct the problem of low arterial oxygen.

However, the increase in ventilation also has an undesired effect: it removes too much carbon dioxide from the blood. This is a problem because the level of carbon dioxide is closely tied to blood acidity. When too much carbon dioxide is removed from the blood, the blood becomes too alkaline. Alkaline blood depresses the respiratory centers in the brain stem and tends to reduce lung ventilation. The conflicting messages sent by low oxygen and low carbon dioxide to the respiratory centers of the brain stem can produce very uneven respiratory patterns. As a result, climbers at high altitude sometimes fluctuate between fast and slow respiration, particularly when asleep.

Hypoxia produced by high altitude has a variety of other effects. Arteries to the brain and eyes dilate, so that blood flow to these organs increases. Small pulmonary (lung) arteries (vessels) constrict, raising the pressure in the pulmonary artery. This constriction also stretches the delicate lung capillaries, making it easier for water and fluid to leak out into the lung tissue. In addition, the kidneys are stimulated to release erythropoietin, a hormone that increases the production of erythrocytes (red blood cells). Because the erythrocytes carry most of the oxygen in the blood, this adaptation to hypoxia increases the oxygen-carrying capacity of the blood.

Acute mountain sickness. As many as 25 percent of people who ascend rapidly from sea level to 10,000 feet experience unpleasant symptoms associated with altitude. The exact nature and the severity of these symptoms vary from person to person, but in general they may include headache, nausea, malaise, and sleep disturbances. Some people also experience a decrease in visual acuity, particularly in dim light, probably as a result of a decrease in the delivery of oxygen to the photoreceptors of the eye (*see also VISION*). Together, these symptoms are referred to as acute mountain sickness.

Headache is the most common symptom of acute mountain sickness, but its cause is not fully understood. One possible explanation is that the increase in blood flow to the brain caused by hypoxia may put pressure on the sensitive membranes that surround the brain, producing pain.

Most people who experience early symptoms of acute mountain sickness recover in a few days with no treatment other than rest. However, a few develop serious and even life-threatening complications. The constriction of the smallest branches of the pulmonary artery and the increase in fluid and protein leaking from the pulmonary capillaries combine to allow fluid to accumulate in the interstitial space between the alveoli and the pulmonary capillaries. Fluid accumulation in this vital space is known as pulmonary edema. Pulmonary edema thickens the pulmonary membrane and slows the diffusion of oxygen from the alveoli to the blood. This exacerbates high-altitude hypoxia. At its worst, pulmonary edema may allow fluid to leak into the alveoli themselves. Once this occurs, air can no longer enter the alveoli, and people may drown in their own bodily fluids. Symptoms of pulmonary edema include a cough—particularly a cough that brings up pink-tinged fluid—and moist, crackling sounds known as rales which can be heard, sometimes even without a stethoscope, when the patient inhales.

An extremely grave complication of acute mountain sickness occurs when fluid leaks from the brain capillaries into the brain tissue and produces cerebral edema. This may result from the increase in blood flow to the brain that occurs with hypoxia. However, autopsies on the brains of people who have died from high-altitude cerebral edema suggest that bleeding from both small and large brain arteries also may play a role. Whatever its exact cause, cerebral edema produces a loss of coordination, often first seen when the climber develops a staggering gait as if intoxicated (ataxia), or problems with fine motor skills. Unfortunately, cerebral edema also makes it difficult or impossible for a climber to think logically. Losing both motor skills and logical thought high on a dangerous mountain can be a virtual death sentence for even the most skilled and experienced mountaineer.

Acute mountain sickness can also lead to retinal hemorrhage: bleeding from the small arteries in the eye. The retina is the part of the eye that acts like the film of a camera. Just as film receives light and changes this light into something interpretable as a visual image, the retina receives light and changes it into an electric signal, which is then sent to the brain, where it is interpreted as a visual image. Retinal hemorrhage may result from the increase in retinal blood flow that occurs with hypoxia. The hemorrhage can destroy parts of the retina, producing small blind spots that can no longer respond to incoming light. Because there are two eyes to gather visual information, a climber may not notice a small blind spot in one eye, although an optometrist would be able to see it during an eye exam. However, if retinal hemorrhage occurs in the part of the retina necessary for very acute vision, a permanent decrease in visual ability will result.

Preventing acute mountain sickness. As is so often the case in medicine, preventing acute mountain sickness is far preferable to treating it. Each person reacts differently to altitude, and some people can ascend to moderate altitudes quite quickly with no ill effects. However, for most people a slow ascent is the best way to avoid acute mountain sickness. On high mountains, which take many days to climb, most experts recommend that climbers ascend no more than 2,000 vertical feet (606 m) per day. This gives the body time to adjust to the effects of decreased pressure.

It isn't always easy to abide by this strict limit on ascent rate. A variety of factors—including short periods of good weather and limited vacation time—may tempt climbers to ascend more rapidly. However, it is vital to resist the impulse too climb too high too fast. In the words of Charles Houston, a world-renowned expert on acute mountain sickness who was (in 1960) the first physician to correctly diagnose high-altitude pulmonary edema, "It is the impatient who are likely to become patients" (Houston, 1993).

Getting enough rest and maintaining a good diet are also crucial in avoiding acute mountain sickness. Again, though, the situation makes this advice difficult to follow: a person experiencing nausea and sleep disturbances from high altitude is unlikely to get enough rest or food. Thus when the first symptoms of acute mountain sickness begin, climbers should, if possible, descend to a lower camp where they feel better and rest there for a day or two before starting up again.

A diet rich in carbohydrates offers at least a theoretical advantage at high altitudes over a diet rich in fats or protein. This is because when carbohydrates are used for energy, they produce one molecule of carbon dioxide for every molecule of oxygen consumed, whereas burning fats and proteins produces only 0.8 molecule of carbon dioxide for every molecule of oxygen used. The extra carbon dioxide produced when the body uses carbohydrates should keep the blood pH closer to normal during the respiratory stimulation produced by high-altitude hypoxia.

In practice, however, the advantage of a high-carbohydrate diet may be very small; and in fact an all-carbohydrate diet would probably be a poor choice. The body needs both fats and proteins at high altitudes, just as it does at sea level; fats are particularly important in helping withstand the cold weather so often encountered. Also, in addition to the nausea noted above, loss of appetite and monotonous meals make it difficult for a climber at high altitude to consume enough food of any type. Therefore, a climber's primary concern should be adequate food intake. Probably the best way to ensure adequate food intake at high altitude is to arrange for a diet that tastes good. Every climber will have different dietary preferences, but for most of us tastiness indicates the presence of at least some fat.

It is also vital to stay well-hydrated. Increased production of erythrocytes (red blood cells) and loss of fluid from capillary beds can occur at a high altitude. Also, more body water is lost in exhaled breath because the air tends to be cold and dry. These problems combine to produce very thick, viscous, slow-moving blood which is susceptible to abnormal clotting. Once clots form, usually in the veins of the arms or legs, they can break off and move to other locations. A moving clot is called an embolus (plural, *emboli*). Emboli that originate in the extremities can move with the blood through the right side of the heart and lodge in the pulmonary artery. These pulmonary emboli are life-threatening because they limit the blood flow to the lungs. Staying well-hydrated does not infallibly prevent pulmonary emboli, but climbers who allow themselves to become dehydrated are definitely asking for trouble.

Someone who has never been at a high altitude may think that staying well hydrated is just a matter of common sense and easily accomplished. Unfortunately, this is not the case. Because of the low temperatures encountered at high altitude, no water will be found in liquid form. This means that the climber must either carry water up or bring a stove and fuel to melt snow. Both of these solutions require the climber to carry substantial weight, and melting snow for drinking water takes a great deal of time and effort, particularly in bad weather. Nevertheless, staying well hydrated at high altitude is literally a matter of life and death.

One medication that may help some people avoid acute mountain sickness is Diamox. Diamox acidifies the blood slightly, balancing the decreased acidity that usually accompanies the respiratory stimulation of hypoxia. This allows deep breathing, which delivers more oxygen to the body, while still maintaining a near-normal blood pH.

Treating acute mountain sickness. Once acute mountain sickness has developed, the definitive treatment is descent. Descent almost always cures acute mountain sickness.

However, there are rare exceptions to this reassuring rule: a few people who become very ill at high altitudes die, usually of pulmonary or cerebral edema, despite being evacuated to a lower elevation. Also, it is not always possible to descend quickly from a high altitude. Bad weather and difficult terrain may keep even expert mountaineers from descending. Further, serious acute mountain sickness may make a person incapable of descending without assistance; in the worst-case scenario, climbers may be so incapacitated by acute mountain sickness that they cannot assist in their own rescue. And as anyone who has helped evacuate a sick or injured climbing partner knows, descending from a high peak while carrying or dragging a partner is difficult, dangerous, and very slow.

Some inexperienced climbers believe that if disaster strikes, they can rely on help from outside to evacuate them. Although outside help is sometimes available, and is certainly welcome in any emergency, climbers should have their own contingency plans in place rather than relying on outside help. Rapid evacuation from a high altitude usually implies an airlift, but fixed-wing aircraft require a large flat area with a firm, even surface for takeoff and landing, and such natural airports are seldom available in the mountains. Because helicopters have very strict altitude limitations, sick climbers must often be brought down a long distance on the ground before they can be picked up by a helicopter. In addition, climbing emergencies seldom occur under perfect weather conditions. The extreme cold and bad weather that lead to trouble in the first place can make an emergency air evacuation difficult or impossible.

For these reasons, it is important for every climber to understand the emergency treatment of acute mountain sickness. If an oxygen tank is available, a person suffering from a severe case of acute mountain sickness should be given 100 percent oxygen to breathe. Even though a sick person is in an environment with a low total atmospheric pressure at high altitude, administering pure oxygen will increase the partial pressure of oxygen breathed. This will increase the PO_2 in the alveoli and arterial blood, reducing hypoxia. A reduction in hypoxia will help decrease the severity of high-altitude pulmonary and cerebral edema.

It is also helpful to artificially raise the atmospheric pressure around a person suffering from acute mountain sickness. This can be accomplished by placing the person in a bag known as a Gamow tent, which can be pressurized. Exposing a person to a pressure greater than that of the surrounding atmosphere is equivalent to descending to a lower altitude. The pressurized tent increases the partial pressure of oxygen in the air and the PO_2 in the arterial blood. As they become lighter and less expensive, Gamow tents, or similar devices, are becoming increasingly popular as safety equipment for high-altitude expeditions.

Diamox, the medication sometimes used to prevent acute mountain sickness, can also be used to treat it. In addition to its action on blood pH, Diamox is a mild diuretic—that is, it increases urine output—and thus it can remove excess fluid from the lungs. A number of other drugs, including the steroid dexamethasone and the antihypertensive nifedipine, may be very helpful treatments. However, these medications are best administered by a physician.

In the past, a variety of very powerful diuretics were used to treat severe acute mountain sickness. The rationale for using these drugs stemmed from the fact that they are helpful in reducing the symptoms of acute pulmonary edema. Unfortunately, these drugs also produce dehydration by reducing blood volume. This effect can make acute mountain sickness worse by favoring the production of blood clots (thrombi). For this reason, powerful diuretics are now seldom used to treat acute mountain sickness.

Acclimatization to high altitudes. Imagine skiers who ascend quickly from sea level to a ski resort in Colorado at 8,500 feet (2,575 m) and then ski in the nearby Rocky Mountains at 10,000 feet (3,030 m). For the first few days, they may experience minor symptoms of acute mountain sickness, often including headache and a reduced ability to perform strenuous exercise. However, if they remain at these altitudes for several days or weeks, they will find that the body acclimatizes to the higher altitude. They may first notice this acclimatization process when they discover that they can ascend to higher altitudes without symptoms of acute mountain sickness (such as headache) and that they can exert themselves more than when they first arrived.

Several factors are involved in this acclimatization process. Throughout a climber's stay at a high altitude, hypoxia continues to stimulate an increased rate and depth of ventilation. This keeps the climber's blood carbon dioxide low and initially tends to increase blood pH. However, over the course of a week or more, the climber's kidneys compensate for this excess of base in the blood by excreting more base in the urine. This returns the blood pH toward normal. Hypoxia also stimulates the climber's kidneys to produce erythropoietin, the hormone that stimulates the formation of more red blood cells (erythrocytes). More red blood cells allow the lungs and circulation to supply oxygen more efficiently to body tissues to compensate for the low atmospheric oxygen levels found at the high altitude. The changes that occur during acclimatization extend to the tissues and individual cells of the body. After days or weeks at a high altitude, the capillaries—the smallest blood vessels that are directly responsible for supplying oxygen to the tissues (*see* HEART AND CIRCULATORY SYSTEM)—dilate to allow more blood flow. The cells themselves produce more mitochondria—the subcellular organelles where carbohydrate metabolism occurs (*see* ENERGY AND METABOLISM)—so that oxygen can be used more efficiently. These changes allow an acclimatized climber to perform more work than, say, a newly arrived partner.

Unfortunately, however, no amount of acclimatization will make climbers at high altitudes capable of matching the extreme levels of exertion they could achieve at sea level. Also, there is a limit to the

HAZARDS OF ALTITUDE

Feet above sea level	Atmospheric pressure (atm)	Comments
28,000	0.33	Highest peak in world (Mount Everest, Nepal: 28,000+)
20,000	0.46	Highest peak in North America (Denali, Alaska: 20,320)
18,000		Most climbers deteriorate faster than they acclimate
17,000		Highest permanent human settlements
10,000	0.69	25% of people experience acute mountain sickness

Table 1.

benefits of acclimatization. Above 18,000 feet (5,454 m), most climbers find that they deteriorate faster than they acclimatize. Over the course of weeks, a climber who remains at these extreme altitudes will lose weight and eventually become weaker rather than stronger. Extreme altitudes adversely affect the entire range of human functions, from work to reproductive capacity. In fact, the destructive effect of extremely high altitudes on human physiology is probably the reason that there are no known examples of permanent human settlements at altitudes above 17,000 feet (5,151 m).

Furthermore, the process of acclimatization is temporary. This is particularly unfortunate for climbers who live at low altitudes but make periodic trips to high altitudes. When acclimatized climbers descend to sea level, they will lose their acclimatization over the course of several weeks, about as quickly as they acquired it. People who live permanently at high altitudes become very well acclimatized, but even they can experience mountain sickness if they descend to sea level, spend several weeks there, and then return home.

Scuba Diving: High-Pressure Exercise

Scuba diving is a popular recreation for people with a wide range of physical abilities. Diving appeals to the sense of adventure because it allows exploration of a watery world that is otherwise hidden from view. This underwater world, however, poses physical challenges for a number of reasons. In contrast to mountaineering, a sport which involves coping with low air pressure, many of the challenges of scuba

THE HAZARDS OF DEPTH

Feet below sea level	Atmospheric pressure (atm)	Comments
21	1.63	Depth where bends becomes a danger
60	2.8	Maximum depth for beginners
100	4.0	Depth where nitrogen narcosis begins
130	4.9	Maximum depth for recreational divers
200	7.0	Severe nitrogen narcosis
250	8.5	Extremely dangerous depth

Table 2.

diving result from the extremely high pressures to which the body is subjected underwater.

The underwater world is inhospitable to humans—unlike fish—because their bodies are not designed to obtain oxygen from water. Scuba divers solve the problem of acquiring the air necessary for cellular metabolism by carrying an artificial air supply on trips beneath the surface. The word *scuba* is an acronym for "*s*elf-*c*ontained *u*nderwater *b*reathing *a*pparatus." The equipment needed for underwater respiration includes the scuba tank or cylinder, which stores a large amount of highly compressed air in a relatively small space; a valve, which controls the flow of air; and a regulator, which is the mechanism through which the diver breathes. The regulator is the device that reduces the pressure of the air in the scuba tank, and delivers that air to the diver at the same pressure as the surrounding water. The pressure of the water around the diver is known as the "ambient pressure." Because ambient pressure pushes in on the diver's chest at all times, a diver can breathe comfortably only by inhaling air at the same pressure as the ambient pressure—the pressure outside the body.

Scuba equipment is remarkably effective at solving the basic problem of air delivery to humans underwater. Leaving aside any concern about equipment failure, one might assume that a diver could stay underwater for periods of time limited only by the supply of air. However, as discussed below, the high ambient pressures underwater have significant effects on the human body that greatly limit the length of time for diving and the depths that can be explored. To date, no one has completely solved the problems posed by increased pressure on divers. One of the best ways divers can improve their safety is by learning how pressure affects physiology.

Physiology underwater. The human body is affected in many ways by the high pressures encountered under water. For example, there is direct compression of the gas in the body's air spaces. Natural air spaces are found in the middle ear (the space behind the eardrum), the sinuses (spaces within the bones of the skull), and the lungs. There is also an artificial air space between the diver's mask and face. As pressure increases, the volume of a fixed amount of gas in these spaces decreases. Bodily air spaces are the most sensitive to pressure, because gases are compressible whereas the rest of the body is made up of liquids and solids, which are essentially incompressible.

To function properly, air sacs in the body must contain air that has the same pressure as that of the surrounding environment. On land, the body automatically adjusts or "equalizes" pressure, because the air sacs are open to the surrounding atmosphere. The lungs, of course, are connected to the atmosphere by the pharynx and trachea. The middle ear is connected to the back of the throat by a passage called the eustachian tube. The sinuses are connected to the nasal airway by thin passages. Because air travels through these passages during breathing, pressure equalization is usually unnoticeable. For example, in hiking up a mountain, as the atmospheric pressure drops, the air pressure is equalized in the lungs, middle ear, and sinuses with every breath taken. By contrast, when changes in air pressure happen suddenly—for example, on takeoff or landing in an airplane—the ears may "pop" or the sinuses may ache.

The air sacs are compressed by ever-increasing ambient pressure as a person dives underwater. On descent in seawater, the ambient pressure increases at a rate of 0.03 atm (23 mm Hg) per 1 foot (0.3 m) of depth. Thus (as discussed earlier), at a depth of 33 feet (10 m) the ambient pressure is equal to 2 atm: 1 atm from the water plus 1 atm from the air above it. If the air pressure in the air sacs is not equalized to that in the surrounding water, the ambient pressures are great enough to collapse the lungs, rupture the eardrum covering the middle ear, force tissues into the sinus cavities, and push the mask tightly against the diver's face.

With scuba gear and proper training, these so-called "squeeze" injuries can be avoided. A diver equalizes the pressure in the lungs to ambient pressure by breathing compressed air. The sinuses usually equalize as the diver breathes, unless they are congested from a cold or an allergy. The diver equalizes the pressure in the mask (which covers the nose as well as the eyes) by breathing a little compressed air into it as needed. Divers are constantly alert for a telltale feeling of pressure in the ear, which signals an imbalance between the ambient pressure and the air pressure in the middle ear. Swallowing can open the eustachian tubes and equalize the pressure in the middle ear to ambient pressure.

Problems also can occur as a diver ascends. During ascent, the ambient pressure falls. Unless equalization occurs, the pressure in the air spaces will become greater than ambient pressure. This difference in pressure can allow the gases in the air sacs to expand and produce an ascent injury. An ascent injury to the ears or sinuses is known as a "reverse block."

Ascent injuries to the lungs are particularly dangerous. Therefore, divers must understand how they occur and how they can be avoided. If a swimmer takes a breath of air at the surface, dives 33 feet down to the sea bottom, and ascends, there will be no adverse effects on the lungs. The air-filled lungs will be compressed to half their original volume on descent, and will return to the original volume as the diver surfaces. However, a diver who takes a breath of compressed air while submerged and then surfaces while holding the breath is at serious risk of an ascent injury.

One might imagine that a diver breathing from a scuba tank would never be so foolish as to surface while holding the breath. Unfortunately, though, divers sometimes do this. An inexperienced scuba diver can panic in an "out of air" emergency and lose control of the ascent. A snorkeler might locate a cave underwater and take a breath of air trapped inside. Or a snorkeler might swim down, encounter a scuba diver, and take a breath of compressed air from the scuba diver's regulator. In any of these situations, if the lungs are filled with compressed air 33 feet below the surface and the diver then ascends without exhaling, the air in the lungs will double in volume, and the expanded air volume can cause a serious lung-expansion injury.

A lung-expansion injury begins when the alveoli inflate to full volume and then rupture. This may happen without the diver's knowledge, as it causes no discomfort. Rupture of the alveoli causes the lungs to collapse (pneumothorax). Air from the lungs may escape into the space surrounding the heart (mediastinal emphysema) or become trapped underneath the skin (subcutaneous emphysema). The most serious result of a lung-expansion injury is a life-threatening condition known as an air embolism, in which air enters the bloodstream and blocks the flow of blood to the brain and other vital organs. This can cause paralysis and permanent brain damage and can even be fatal. Diving is not a sport to be taken lightly.

The bends. Most recreational divers fill their tanks with air that is composed of the mix of gases found in the atmosphere: 79 percent nitrogen and 21 percent oxygen. At sea level, nitrogen has no physiologic impact on the human body; it is carried in the blood and enters the tissues, but it is neither produced nor broken down by the body. However, in the high pressures underwater, nitrogen interacts very differently with the body. In order to minimize their risk of decompression sickness—"the bends"—divers need to be aware of these effects and plan their dives accordingly.

In breathing air at sea level, the partial pressure of nitrogen in the lungs is the same as the partial pressure of nitrogen in the blood. Because of this equilibrium, nitrogen enters and leaves the bloodstream at a 1-to-1 rate of exchange: that is, 1 molecule of nitrogen enters the blood from the lungs for every 1 molecule of nitrogen that leaves the blood and enters the lungs.

As the ambient pressure on a diver increases, total air pressure and partial pressure of nitrogen in the lungs increase as well. Under these conditions, the partial pressure of nitrogen in the lungs exceeds the partial pressure of nitrogen in the bloodstream, and more nitrogen enters the blood from the lungs than leaves the blood for the lungs. The amount of nitrogen in the blood increases.

Nitrogen dissolved in blood plasma is carried throughout the body. (Blood plasma is all the blood except for the blood cells.) Because the partial pressure of nitrogen in the blood reaching the tissues is now greater than the partial pressure of nitrogen in the tissues themselves, nitrogen leaves the blood and enters all body tissues. The rate at which nitrogen is absorbed by the tissues of a particular part of the body depends on the tissue's blood supply. Some tissues—including the brain, spinal cord, muscles, lungs, and heart—have high blood flow and quickly become saturated with nitrogen. These tissues are called "fast tissues." Other tissues, such as bone and fat, have lower blood flow, so they become saturated with nitrogen more slowly. These tissues are called "slow tissues." However, the greater the depth and the longer the dive, the more nitrogen is absorbed by all body tissues.

As a diver swims to the surface, the ambient pressure and the partial pressure of nitrogen in the lungs both decrease. The process of nitrogen uptake by the body tissues is now reversed. Nitrogen, which has been dissolved in the tissues, moves back to the blood but is still in dissolved form. At the lungs, this nitrogen once again becomes a gas and is then eliminated from the body at the lungs when the diver exhales. Problems can occur if a diver surfaces too quickly, that is, before the excess nitrogen has been eliminated. When that happens, excess nitrogen may form bubbles inside the blood and tissues of the body. The resulting condition is called decompression sickness or "the bends."

The bends can be serious or even fatal. This is the case because bubbles of nitrogen are particularly likely to form in very sensitive tissues such as the brain, spinal cord, and joints. Nitrogen bubbles can impair circulation of the blood and distort various tissues. Symptoms of the bends may be as benign as fatigue, skin rash, and painful joints. However, the bends can also produce more serious symptoms, including difficulty speaking, personality changes, convulsions, leg weakness, loss of sensation, impaired bowel and bladder control, paralysis, and unconsciousness.

Researchers have found that 50 percent of divers with serious decompression sickness have patent foramen ovale, a heart defect in which there is a small opening between the right and left atria. This opening allows some blood to flow directly from the right atrium to the left atrium, bypassing the lungs. If a diver with patent foramen ovale ascends too quickly and nitrogen bubbles form in the blood, these bubbles can reach the left side of the heart and be pumped directly to the brain and spinal cord, where they may block small arteries. Blocking the blood flow to these vital organs produces some of the most serious complications of the bends, such as paralysis and unconsciousness.

The U.S. Navy, the Divers Alert Network (DAN), and private professional diving associations have done research on the physiology of nitrogen absorption and its effect on diving. Their studies have shown that by planning ahead, a diver can minimize the risk of the bends. Using tables or computers, divers calculate the amount of nitrogen that will be present in their bodies after one or more dives, depending on the depth and duration of each dive. If too much nitrogen has accumulated in the tissues during a dive, the diver must plan to delay the final ascent to the surface during a "decompression stop" that allows excess nitrogen to be breathed off underwater. Cautious divers ascend slowly, or take a temporary stop during the ascent. It has been shown that 50 percent of nitrogen bubbles in venous blood are reduced during a 3-minute stop at a depth of 6 meters (about 20 ft.). A "safety stop" might not be very exciting, but it's a good idea nonetheless.

Treating decompression sickness. A recent report described the following treatment for decompression sickness. A man vacationing on the North Carolina coast felt fine after surfacing from his second dive of the day. Forty-five minutes later, he developed a headache, became dizzy, had trouble walking, and felt a tingling sensation on his abdomen. Next he developed vision problems and nausea, lost his way while driving back to his hotel, and didn't recognize a friend who was waiting for him there. It was clear that these symptoms were caused by nitrogen bubbles that had formed in the brain.

Fortunately, this diver received rapid, expert medical attention. Specially trained medical personnel placed him in a sealed recompression ("hyperbaric") chamber and raised the pressure inside the box to 2.8 atm. This high pressure forced the nitrogen bubbles inside the brain from a gas back into dissolved form. Over a period of 6 hours, the pressure was reduced in stages to 1 atm while the patient breathed pure oxygen. The man recovered fully.

Preventing the bends: Nitrox. Adverse physiologic effects of nitrogen are a crucial reason to limit the depth and duration of dives. To counter these effects, divers sometimes breathe a mixture of gases containing a reduced fraction of nitrogen, thus reducing the partial pressure of nitrogen at any depth in comparison with air at the same depth.

Nitrox is a mixture of oxygen and nitrogen. Among divers, Nitrox, Enriched Air, and EANx are terms used for oxygen-nitrogen mixtures that contain less nitrogen than air. There are two standard Nitrox mixtures, Nitrox I with 68 percent nitrogen and 32 percent oxygen, and Nitrox II with 64 percent nitrogen and 36 percent oxygen. (By comparison, air is 79 percent nitrogen and 21 percent oxygen.) The principal reason divers use Nitrox is to reduce the risk of developing the bends. The higher the partial pressure of nitrogen in the lungs, the greater the amount of nitrogen that can dissolve in the body tissues. Thus, if a diver breathes a Nitrox mixture with a smaller fraction of nitrogen than air, this will reduce the partial pressure of nitrogen in the lungs and the amount of nitrogen dissolved in the tissues. When the diver surfaces, less nitrogen will be dissolved in the tissues. This reduces the risk of nitrogen bubbles in the blood and thus lowers the risk of the bends.

By using Nitrox, a diver may reduce the risk of the bends while following a standard dive plan. Divers can also use Nitrox to extend the length and depth of dives and to increase the number of dives they can safely make in a single day.

Nitrogen narcosis. The bends are not the only risk divers face from nitrogen. At sea level, the amount of nitrogen dissolved in the body tissues is too small to have an important effect. However, as a diver descends to greater depth and the ambient pressure increases, the amount of nitrogen dissolved in the body tissues increases as well. In the brain, the nitrogen dissolves in the membranes surrounding individual brain cells and produces a narcotic effect, just as anesthetic agents such as nitrous oxide do. This phenomenon is known as nitrogen narcosis or "rapture of the deep."

While it may sound amusing or mildly enjoyable, nitrogen narcosis is extremely dangerous to scuba divers. Nitrogen narcosis can start at depths of about 80 feet (24 m), where the ambient pressure is 3.4 atm. The diver begins to feel dizzy or intoxicated and soon becomes unable to communicate or perform motor or mental tasks. In addition to greatly endangering the diver's own safety, this also puts the diving buddy at risk. Fortunately, it is very easy to treat nitrogen narcosis: the symptoms quickly end if the affected diver ascends to a shallower depth.

Oxygen toxicity. Oxygen toxicity is oxygen poisoning of the human body. There are two types of oxygen toxicity: (1) central nervous system (CNS) oxygen toxicity, which affects the brain and spinal cord; and (2) pulmonary oxygen toxicity, which affects the lungs.

Type 1, CNS oxygen toxicity, is caused by short-term exposure to high oxygen partial pressures. These can be encountered during very deep dives—that is, to depths of more than 150 feet (about 45 m). CNS oxygen toxicity begins with symptoms that are very similar to the bends and may include muscle twitching, nausea, hearing problems, tunnel vision, light-headedness, and breathing problems. As the poisoning progresses, the diver loses consciousness, becomes completely rigid, stops breathing, and goes into convulsions. A diver in this condition usually drowns. Because these convulsions often cause divers to lose the regulator, they will still drown even if they start breathing again while unconscious. The cause of CNS oxygen toxicity is not known. However two possible factors are disruptions in the machinery that the brain uses to extract energy from glucose, and a reduction in blood flow to the brain.

Type 2 of oxygen toxicity, pulmonary toxicity, is caused by longer exposure to more moderate oxygen partial pressures. Oxygen at these partial pressure directly irritates the lungs. The resulting symptoms are like the flu or pneumonia and include coughing, breathing difficulties, lack of coordination, and sore throat and chest. The onset of symptoms usually occurs after the dive (*see also SWIMMING*).

David E. Harris and Barbara Lelli

References

Guyton, A., and J. Hall. *Textbook of Medical Physiology*. Philadelphia, Pennsylvania: Saunders, 1994.

Houston, C. *High Altitude: Illness and Wellness*. Merrillville, Indiana: ICS, 1993.

McArdle, W., et al. *Exercise Physiology: Energy, Nutrition, and Human Performance*. Philadephia, Pennsylvania: Lea and Febiger, 1986.

Moon, R., et al. "The Physiology of Decompression Illness." *Scientific American* 273, no. 70 (1995).

Schmidt-Nielson, K. *Animal Physiology: Adaptation and Environment*. New York: Cambridge University Press, 1994.

Vander, J., et al. *Human Physiology*. 6th ed. New York: McGraw-Hill, 1994.

Wilmore, J., and D. Costill. *Physiology of Sport and Exercise*. Champaign, Illinois: Human Kinetics, 1994.

Shoulder, Elbow, and Wrist

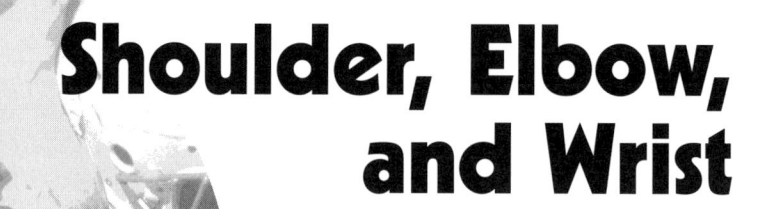

THE BODY'S UPPER EXTREMITIES often bear the brunt of injuries suffered in sports. The arm and shoulder usually are the first parts of the body extended to brace falls, lead the way during collisions, and perform the repetitive throwing motions that many sports require.

Of all upper extremity actions in sports, the ability to throw and strike are among the most vital skills. For the shot put, discus, bowling, and baseball pitching, for example, throwing is the central skill. These activities require little, if any, running but extensive throwing. On the other hand, the striking sports—such as tennis, badminton, racquetball, and field hockey—equally emphasize running and throwing or striking movements.

Most sports require an overarm throwing or swinging motion, but several, such as softball, bowling, curling, and hammer throwing, use a sidearm or underarm motion. However, not all overarm and underarm throwing motions are the same. Some sports use very similar throwing motions (e.g., the stepping approach and underarm release of curling and bowling); other sports require considerably different throwing techniques (e.g., the overarm football pass, baseball pitch, and shot put).

Although sidearm and underarm motions may be necessary for a variety of reasons (some based on rules, others on mechanics), an overarm motion remains the most common way to throw. Sometimes, the preference for overarm throwing reflects negative stereotypes connected to underarm throwing. Despite some popular beliefs to the contrary, underarm throwing is not inherently inferior to overarm. In fact, one of the highest career free-throw percentages in the history of the National Basketball Association belongs to Rick Barry, who threw underhand. Furthermore, the fast ball of Joan Joyce, an underhand softball pitcher, was clocked at 193 kilometers per hour (120 mph)—approximately 25 percent faster than many top major league baseball pitchers.

Mechanics of Throwing and Swinging

To understand the nature of upper extremity injuries, the entire body must be considered. Since the arms and shoulders are anchored to the trunk, back injuries can cause arm injuries, and likewise, arm injuries can cause back injuries. Throwing and striking entail an acceleration starting from the lower body, through the trunk, and finishing through the arm segments. For a right-hander's tennis serve, the bent knees extend as the tilted pelvis and trunk straighten and rotate, and the arched back begins to flex forward. This gets the whole body "springing" forward before the shoulder and arm motion ever begins. If the motion is smooth, an efficient transfer of momentum (mass × velocity) occurs. Well executed throwing and swing motions entail a summation of body part velocities so that there is a complete transfer of momentum from the trunk to the arm. A lower back injury often forces an athlete to adjust his or her normal motion to alleviate lower back stress. Even the slightest adjustment may trigger a greater reliance and stress on the shoulder and elbow to compensate for the reduction in force provided by the lower back.

Most of the energy produced by the slower, more massive muscles in the legs and lower body gets transferred to the muscles surrounding the shoulder, elbow, and wrist joints. Because the upper extremities are farther from the body's center of gravity and axis of rotation, they experience far more torque (force that gives rise to rotational movement) than the trunk and lower body. This transfer of energy makes the upper extremities more prone to serious injuries.

For baseball pitchers, angular momentum of the arm developed during the acceleration phase must somehow be stopped by a deceleration torque applied by the shoulder's rotator cuff. An excessive deceleration torque would result in injury. Even so, there is torque of about 300 inch-pounds (1335 newtons, N) at the beginning of this phase (McLeod, 1985). This would be the equivalent force of holding a 4.5-kilogram (12-lb.) weight (three 1,000-page encyclopedia volumes) parallel to the ground at arm's length.

Another important factor is anatomical variation among individuals. The differences in lengths of bones, which act as levers, affect the strength, velocity, and range of motion, resulting in different mechanics and torque (*see Figure 1*). For example, if two individuals can move the forearm at the same angular velocity, the hand of the person with a longer forearm moves at a greater linear velocity than the hand of a shorter-limbed individual. Of equal importance is muscular anatomy. Because the distance of the muscular attachment from the joint differs among individuals, everyone has different capacities for strength and limb velocity. Muscle structure also affects mobility. For example, a bulky bodybuilder would have less shoulder mobility than a gymnast.

Equipment is an important factor, too. For example, it may seem odd that professional baseball pitchers suffer far more arm injuries than tennis players, despite the fact that a pitcher throws far less in a typical game than a tennis player serves in a typical match. The difference is the equipment. Major league starting pitchers throw, on average, 100 pitches in a game at an average velocity of 137 to 145 kilometers per hour (85 to 90 MPH), and then take 4 days off to rest. Professional tennis players may hit 500 serves, at an average speed of 161 kilometer per hour (100 MPH), during one match. They then

Figure 1. *The arm and body motion used to throw and strike balls varies by sport, as seen in the football pass (a), softball pitch (b), shot put (c), baseball pitch (d), and tennis serve (e). The solid line shows the arm lever, and the dashed line shows the hip lever. These different dynamics account for the variety of upper extremity injuries in different sports.*

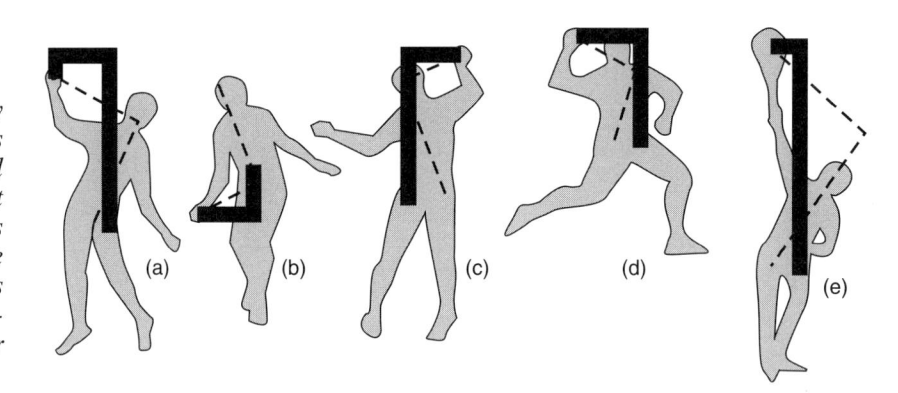

return to the court the following day to play another match of 500 serves. Tennis players can play full matches day after day because lengthening the lever of the body (racket + arm) greatly increases the speed of the racket head imparting the force. Because the weight of the racket is far from the axes of rotation (e.g., elbow and shoulder), a relatively small difference in the weight of a racket makes a considerable difference in demands on the muscles involved in moving the racket (Adrian and Cooper, 1989).

Ball velocity depends on the momentum imparted up through the point of ball release (in throwing) or the point of contact between ball and racket (in striking). In the case of the baseball pitcher, the arm must accelerate at a faster rate, achieving a greater velocity, because the pitcher does not have the luxury of the extended lever—the racket. It is useful to think of the arm, or the arm and racket, as similar to a whip. The pitcher's arm velocity is analogous to the sound-breaking velocity reached at the tip of a whip when it cracks, whereas the tennis player's arm needs to achieve only a fraction of that velocity. Only the racket reaches extreme velocities. The pitcher can release the ball only at the same velocity that the hand has accumulated. The tennis player, by contrast, not only sends the ball off at a much faster velocity, but also does so using far less hand velocity. And as soon as a pitcher reaches his top arm speed at release, he quickly must exert a much more forceful muscle and tendon action to put the brakes on the much greater internal rotation.

A tennis player has another advantage: momentum is accumulated in the racket during the swing and is transferred to the ball quickly in the moment of collision, rather than being transferred gradually, as in the case of throwing a baseball. For a perfectly elastic collision (no loss of kinetic energy) a tennis ball would travel at nearly twice the speed of the racket. In reality, the collision is not perfectly elastic, but there is still a considerable "velocity bonus" from the dynamics of the collision.

A hitter has a further advantage over the thrower in that a struck ball must travel faster than the object that hit it. A large moving object colliding with a small stationary object will knock the small object away at twice its speed. For example, a tennis ball hit with a racket and a golf ball driven with a club travel at a much greater velocity than a baseball thrown by a pitcher. Consider the dynamics in reverse: a tennis player can use half the force, and experience half the stress, to generate the same ball velocity as a pitcher.

Functional Anatomy

Physicians categorize arm injuries as either acute or chronic (overuse). Acute trauma is the result of a singular event, such as a collision or a fall on the shoulder. Overuse injuries are caused by repetitive motions like those of a baseball pitcher who throws 4,000 pitches a season, or swimmers whose daily workout might entail 10,000 arm strokes. Some injuries can have both acute and overuse causes. For instance, by slipping during delivery, baseball pitchers can experience an acute arm injury, such as a tendon tear or contusion, superimposed on a shoulder that has an ongoing overuse injury.

Because acute injuries occur from a singular incident, a definite causal relationship exists. An athlete knows exactly what action caused the injury. The same does not hold for overuse injuries. They are more difficult to detect and often subside with rest but then recur with a resumption of activity. While it is difficult to pinpoint the specific population suffering from overuse injuries, many experts believe they are far more prevalent than acute injuries.

Shoulder

Shoulder rotation is most common in sports requiring overhead throwing and swinging. Despite differences in equipment and mechanics, from the point of view of rotational mechanics, such sports are very similar.

Although the motions used in other sports—such as the various swimming strokes—seem very different, they also depend upon a motion remarkably similar to overhead throwing. This similarity is true despite differences in body motion, shoulder action, equipment used, and forces involved in the action. The biomechanical function of the rotator cuff is the same in all these activities, and this makes the swimmer susceptible to the same shoulder dysfunction as the baseball pitcher.

The shoulder possesses both great power and great mobility. Its primary purpose is to put the hand in position to perform tasks. One of the most mobile joints in the body, the shoulder can move up, down, out, and around, and it is the only joint that allows 360-degree rotation (*see Figure 2*). Using the power of the shoulder, athletes can throw or strike objects not only at great speed but also from several angles: overhand, three-quarters, sidearm, and underhand.

Unfortunately, the shoulder's tremendous range of motion comes at the expense of stability. A large number of muscles and bones in the arm-shoulder complex are involved in shoulder motion. The bony

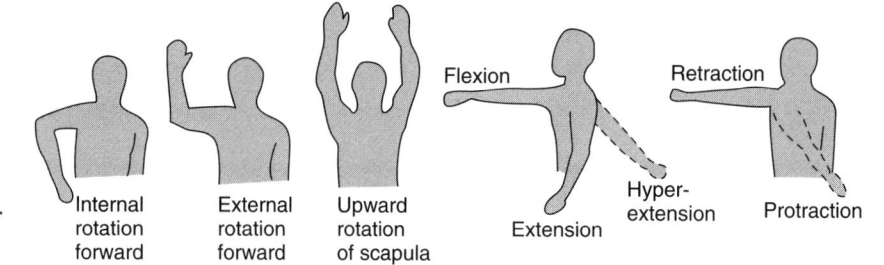

Figure 2. *The shoulder's range of motion.*

anatomy of the shoulder consists of the scapula, humerus, and clavicle (*see Figure 3*). These three bones share two joints: glenohumeral and acromioclavicular. By itself, the glenohumeral is relatively unstable because a proportionately large humeral head moves about a shallow glenoid socket—similar to the way a golf ball sits on a tee.

The muscles and tendons surrounding the joint—vital stabilizers

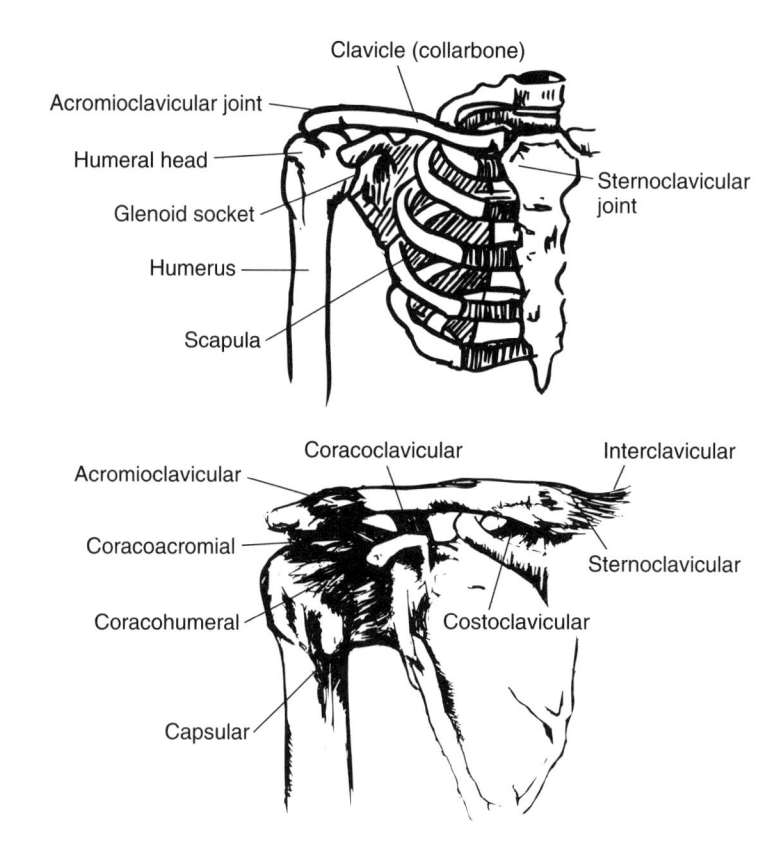

Figure 3. *The bony anatomy (above) and ligaments (below) of the shoulder girdle. The size and range of movement of the scapula are two of the best measures of the body's ability to generate arm velocity. During the throwing motion, the scapula moves forward over the back (torso) by as much as 15 centimeters (6 in.) or more. A large scapula, with a large range of motion, seems a key to high-velocity throwing and swinging. The longer the scapula, the farther down are the muscles attached to it. This creates the potential for greater force production. In part, this may explain why most of the hardest-throwing pitchers in major league baseball are much taller than average.*

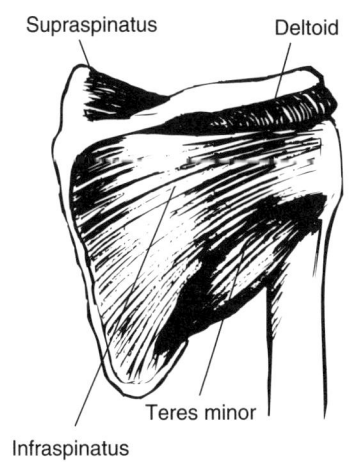

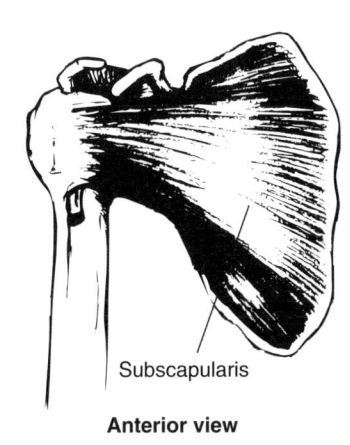

Figure 4. *The posterior and anterior view of the rotator cuff muscles and their insertion points. The primary function of the supraspinatus muscle is to stabilize the shoulder (glenohumeral joint).*

of the glenohumeral joint—are collectively called the rotator cuff. Tendons from four muscles—the subscapularis, the supraspinatus, the infraspinatus, and the teres minor—blend together and are inserted into the humerus (*see Figure 4*). These soft tissues are tremendously elastic, but when they are strained or torn, they can cause considerable pain.

The joint capsule, which is also composed of soft tissue, is relatively weak and has considerable leeway, or "slack," to assist in the joint's mobility. This slack improves mobility but also makes the joint one of the easiest to dislocate. Consciously and unconsciously, the brain can play a significant role in preventing dislocation. By anticipating a forthcoming dislocating force, the muscles *pre*stress the joint, working in the opposite direction. When an athlete expects the shoulder to be yanked in a way that may dislocate the joint, the brain sends a signal to the rotator cuff muscles to contract (pull) the humerus and scapula more tightly together. This *pre*stress phenomenon means that even before the thrown object nears the release point, a countering decelerating recoil has already begun. In other words, the rotator cuff muscles get an early start, "bracing" against the forthcoming force to maintain shoulder stability (*see also SKELETAL SYSTEM*).

The effectiveness of the rotator cuff depends on its force of action, which in turn is determined by the size of the cuff, the type of contraction, and the speed of contraction. It also depends on arm length, leverage, and angle of pull. Studies have found that the supraspinatus muscle functions primarily as a stabilizer of the glenohumeral joint (*again, see Figure 4*). The 75-degree angle of insertion of the supraspinatus with respect to the glenoid provides the countering compressive forces that allow the powerful deltoid muscle to function efficiently. The deltoid maintains its fulcrum of action (pivot point) at the glenohumeral interface. Complementary action between the deltoid and supraspinatus keeps the fulcrum in place during rotation and avoids impingement (pinching) of the humeral head and rotator cuff into the acromion. (The acromion acts like a roof over the cuff and shoulder joint.)

The infraspinatus and teres minor work primarily as external rotators of the shoulder, effecting a motion such as the external rotation used by a tennis player hitting a backhand. They also help stabilize the humeral head against the internal rotation force created during overarm throwing.

The subscapularis is an internal rotator that also acts as a humeral head stabilizer against anterior and forward movement away from the joint capsule. Working in tandem, the infraspinatus and subscapularis are important stabilizers, especially during stabilizing (eccentric) contractions, such as those that occur when the pitcher's arm decelerates after releasing the ball.

The more exterior large superficial muscles—the deltoid, trapezius, latissimus dorsi, and pectoralis—provide power for movements of the shoulder (*see Figure 5*). The rotator cuff muscles pro-

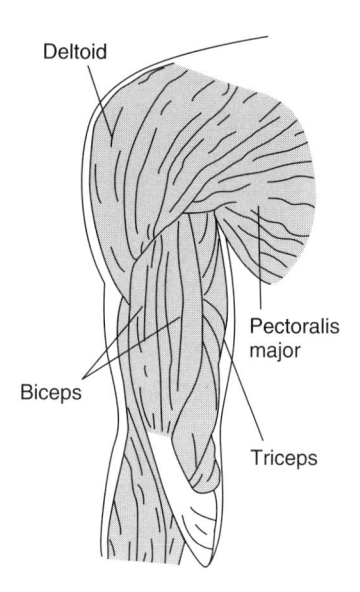

Figure 5. *The primary shoulder muscles. They function primarily as the "power" muscles but also assist in rotation.*

vide the fine-tuning, critical for "soft touch" actions like drop shots in tennis and hook shots in basketball. Not all muscle action is the same.

Because these larger muscles are stronger than the rotator muscles (particularly the supraspinatus), the rotators are much more susceptible to injury. As these larger muscles jerk the arm out of the glenohumeral joint, the body uses the relatively much weaker supraspinatus to hold everything together. Repetitive motions strain and fatigue these stabilizers, loosening the rotators' "grip" on the joint. This often leads to impingement of the stretched out supraspinatus muscle against the shoulder bones. Every time the arm is lifted or lowered, it creates a sharp pain at the point of muscle pinching against bone.

Probably the biggest muscle attached to the shoulder is the biceps. Although it acts mainly as a humeral head depressor or stabilizer, the long head of the biceps is also a passive participant in shoulder motion. Ironically, athletes who spend hours in the weight room building up their "beach biceps" do little to improve shoulder strength and speed. Nevertheless, the bicipital tendon can play an important stabilizing role. When a tear occurs in the rotator cuff, the bicipital tendon may enlarge as it compensates for the impaired rotator cuff muscles. This is particularly prevalent among more active older athletes. Although a minor, secondary contributor in shoulder rotation in younger athletes, the biceps muscles play a much greater role during combined shoulder and elbow functions, such as in the deceleration phase of the throwing motion.

Shoulder injuries. An overhead throwing motion, whether it takes the form of pitching, passing a football, or serving in tennis, consists of three phases: cocking, acceleration, and deceleration.

The windup or cocking phase involves moving the arm away from the body, straightening, and external rotation, primarily involving the deltoid muscle. Arm impingement problems usually show up in the cocking phase, and joint stress in a forward direction is common, particularly when the infraspinatus and teres minor fail to keep the humeral head in place.

The acceleration phase of the throw begins an almost instantaneous and complete reversal of muscle action and arm motion. The internal rotators—subscapularis and pectoralis major—provide the force for this motion, made possible by the synergistic relaxation of the posterior rotator cuff muscles. The latissimus dorsi, the serratus anterior, and the triceps also provide additional force.

The final phase, the deceleration or follow-through, involves the entire rotator cuff. The subscapularis continues to rotate internally. The posterior cuff works to decelerate the arm and to maintain the humeral head within the glenoid. The supraspinatus, active through all phases of the throwing motion, subsides during the deceleration phase (*again, see Figure 4*).

Many injuries in throwing and racket sports occur because the shoulder joint experiences tremendous torque during the acceleration phase as the body moves forward ahead of the shoulder and arm. These forces require the muscles and tendons around the shoulder to keep the pivotal shoulder joint in place as the arm moves forward. If the muscles and tendons around the shoulder are out of condition, become fatigued, or move suddenly, the shoulder can slip anteriorly (toward the front of the body) or posteriorly (toward the back of the body) away from the shoulder socket during the acceleration phase or, more likely, during the deceleration phase. Extreme acceleration and deceleration forces combine with extreme external and internal rotational velocities of the humerus. These "pulling" and "pushing" velocities can create a "grinding" of the rotator cuff.

For baseball pitchers, the type of pitch plays a major part in determining the magnitude of stress to the shoulder. The fastball tends to be less traumatic to the shoulder than the curveball or the slider. The latter two pitches require the pitcher to move the wrist and elbow in order to impart a high rate of spin. And because the thrower releases the ball slightly later for the curve or slider than for the fast ball, the pitcher has less distance and time to decelerate the shoulder, producing greater deceleration torque. Thus, it is vital that young pitchers develop correct deceleration mechanics to safely absorb the deceleration energy. Tennis players can also develop shoulder injuries during the follow-through. But for tennis players, unlike baseball pitchers, many shoulder problems result from poor mechanics, particularly overextension, such as an exaggerated reach necessary to reach an errant ball toss (serving).

Water polo players are among the most prone to shoulder injuries. Despite the fact that water polo players' peak shoulder angular velocity is nearly half that of baseball pitchers (about 1,200° per second, compared with 2,200° per second for baseball pitchers), one study found that 36 percent of the U.S. national water polo team experienced rotator cuff tendinitis (Adrian and Cooper, 1989). This extremely high incidence of rotator cuff tendinitis seems plausible because in all throwing, the greatest risk of injury occurs during deceleration. When a water polo player tries to throw the ball, usually two-thirds of his or her trunk remains above water, while the rest of the body remains submerged. Water density is 832 times that of air. This density difference means that the upper body is moving through the air at great speed, but the lower body cannot assist in deceleration because the denser water prevents the lower body from following through at the same velocity as the upper body. A water polo thrower must absorb the additional torque of the shoulder at the shoulder because of the hip's inability to rotate forward. As a result, most of the deceleration of the arm occurs in the shoulder complex and is not distributed throughout the body.

Elbow

Three bones come together to form the elbow joint: the humerus (upper arm bone), radius, and ulna (two forearm bones). The longer

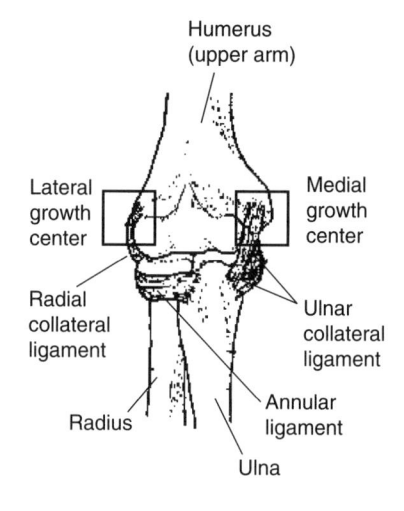

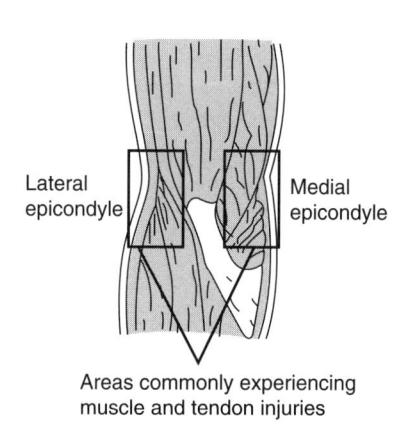

Figure 6. *The lateral epicondyle is the "outside" growth center, and the medial epicondyle is the "inside" growth center. Most elbow injuries are caused by a tearing of the lateral and medial epicondyle tendons. Little League elbow is an injury to the medial epicondyle; tennis elbow is an injury to the lateral epicondyle.*

forearm bone, the ulna, hooks around the joint and attaches to the humerus. It allows the hingelike motion that bends and straightens the elbow. The shorter forearm bone, the radius, has a rounded shape that allows for the turning motion of the forearm, either upward (supinate) or downward (pronate). Powering forearm movement are the upper arm muscles—the biceps and triceps—that join at the elbow. The biceps muscles (front of upper arm) allow the arm to bend with power and the wrist to rotate inward; the triceps muscles (back of upper arm) attach to the ulna and allow the elbow to straighten with power and rotate outward.

The two groups of forearm muscles and tendons originating at the lateral (outside) and medial (inside) humeral epicondyles stabilize the elbow joint and power the wrist (*see Figure 6*). The lateral humeral epicondyle (outside growth center) and its associated musculature are located on the top portion of the elbow (if palm and arm lie flat on a table) and permit the wrist to straighten or extend. The medial humeral epicondyle (inside growth center) and its associated musculature are located on the opposite side of the elbow and give the wrist the power to snap downward or flex. Most elbow injuries occur to the accompanying tendons: the lateral and medial epicondyle.

Elbow injuries. The types of elbow injuries experienced in throwing sports differ from those experienced in racket sports. Baseball pitchers suffer an inordinate number of injuries to the elbow. Contrary to common belief, and even though the curveball places more torque on the shoulder than the fastball, the fastball creates more torque on the elbow than does the curveball. The pitcher is more likely to overextend the elbow when throwing the fastball, increasing the chance of hyperextending the elbow.

Whatever the type of pitch, it is important to pitch with a slightly bent elbow so that as the elbow fully extends, it absorbs the torque that pulls the forearm from the elbow during deceleration. Releasing the ball with a fully extended elbow creates a tremendous amount of torque on the elbow joint. This strains the tendons around the elbow and can eventually lead to serious injury. The tremendous torque caused by this arm velocity is linked to a high incidence of elbow injuries among baseball pitchers. Adverse conditions add to this natural stress on the elbow. When a pitcher loses footing and slips off a damp pitcher's mound, the chances of injury increase tremendously.

Although there is a potential for injury from throwing a fastball, the curveball is more likely to create the strong rotational forces on the elbow that can, through improper technique, lead to injury. For example, when throwing a curve, a pitcher may try to add spin by turning the elbow and wrist over with a twisting motion (eversion or supination). This twisting causes the elbow to work against its natural motion, resulting in constant joint irritation. Rather than twisting the throwing arm at ball release, pitchers can create spin by varying ball grips and finger pressure points. A pitcher can greatly reduce the risk of elbow injury by avoiding the tendency to fully extend the elbow and twist the arm.

These types of acute elbow injuries are less common among tennis players. However, tennis players are susceptible to tennis elbow, which physicians call lateral epicondylitis, because of the tremendous angular velocities required of the elbow for tennis ground strokes. Along with rotator cuff tendinitis, lateral epicondylitis is the most common upper extremity injury suffered by tennis players. However, the incidence of tennis elbow has been dropping over the last decade because rackets made of composite material dampen vibrational energy more effectively.

This dampening of vibrational energy was made possible by advances in materials, as players traded their wooden rackets for lighter composite rackets. The new rackets have resulted in a causal shift: the majority of injuries now stem more from improper technique than from a too heavy racket. In particular, tennis players who extend the elbow forward during the backhand, pointing in the direction where they plan to hit the ball, are much more likely to experience elbow injuries. The grip size of the racket also can be a factor in tendinitis symptoms. If symptoms occur, leading to grip weakness and restricted wrist extension due to pain, it is possible to play with the pain because the motion of the elbow usually remains stable and normal.

Wrist

The wrist forms the junction between the radius and ulna and the eight wrist or carpal bones. Eight small semiround bones arranged in two rows of four make up the bony complex, which is held together by many small flexible ligaments. These small semiround bones easily move about each other like ball bearings, giving the wrist joint its tremendous flexibility and mobility.

Four large tendons attached to the forearm muscles power wrist movement—up, down, left, and right. While it is possible to continue competing fairly effectively after the onset of tennis elbow, tendon injuries to the wrist usually halt activity. These tendons are delicate, so injuries to them make using a bat or racket impossible. The tendons are too delicate to withstand the torque applied to the wrist.

The wrist torque is the last torque throwers exert on the ball before release. As the wrist snaps forward, it gives the ball speed and spin. Finger pressure points and the speed of the wrist snapping forward determine the degree of spin on the ball but also create additional torque to the elbow. Without a strong wrist snap to maximize rotation, the amount of ball movement would be limited.

Wrist injuries. Because of the short extension from the wrist to the fingertips, and the simple back-to-front snap, wrist injuries among baseball pitchers are much less common than are injuries to the shoulder and elbow. As the prevalence of elbow injuries has declined among tennis players, the number of wrist injuries may be increasing. The same large-head high-tech rackets that reduce vibrations also have changed the way players hit the ball. Until the early 1990s, most tennis professionals advised striking the ball with a firm, locked wrist.

Common Shoulder, Elbow, and Wrist Injuries

The participants in most throwing and swinging sports are recreational athletes, not professionals. These athletes play tennis, golf, and softball for fun and exercise. Of course, a significant group of recreational athletes play as aggressively as professional athletes, putting themselves at risk for injury. Thus, understanding of the potential long-term effects of upper extremity injuries is useful for all athletes. Often, the all-star high

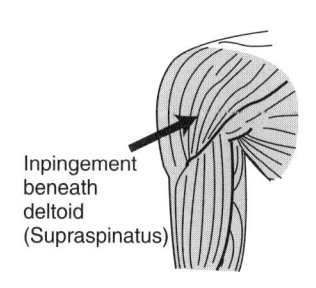

Inpingement beneath deltoid (Supraspinatus)

Rotator cuff. Rarely seen in youth and high school sports, this arm injury is more likely to trouble an athlete later in life because it is a repetitive or overuse problem. There is an angle of the arm at which the ball of the upper end of the humerus hinges in the shoulder, and the attached tendon begins to experience wear. Over time, the movement of the bone can impinge on and damage the rotator cuff tendon that provides the stabilizing force for the shoulder. Continuing to play causes friction between the bone and tendon, which further deteriorates the tendon and leads to scar tissue formation, which further diminishes the healing ability of the area. Pain and mobility problems are the initial and most obvious signs of a rotator cuff problem. Other symptoms include an aching in the deltoid muscle area, impaired ability to lift, and throbbing "night pain," which may prevent sleep and cause weakness. The condition usually subsides with rest, but when the tear is severe, surgery is required. When tendons tear or are detached from the humerus, the lifting movement of overarm throwing is impaired. Surgical modifications to the cuff and tendon reattachment are needed to restore proper cuff functioning. A chronic rotator cuff injury, in which the ball of the humerus lifts farther and farther out of the shoulder because the rotator cuff is unable to hold the ball in place, may lead to an arthritic condition. For sports that apply maximum stress to the rotator cuff, healing may take up to a year or longer. Strengthening other muscles through exercise may help compensate for rotator cuff injury, so that surgery may be avoided.

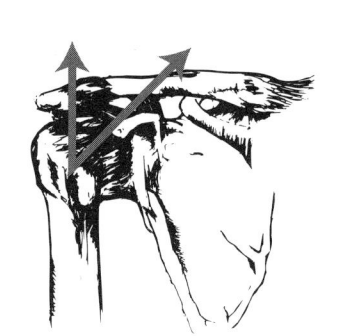

Shoulder separation. Although this can be a throwing-related injury, it usually occurs from a fall or a collision with another athlete or the ground. Injury occurs from a driving force of contact on the outside of the shoulder, which forces the collarbone (clavicle) up or back, and out of the joint it forms with the acromion. It results in severe pain and an inability to use the shoulder. Physicians classify shoulder separations in three groups: mild, moderate, or severe. Classifications are made by the degree of damage to the coracoclavicular ligament, with a severe case being a complete tear.

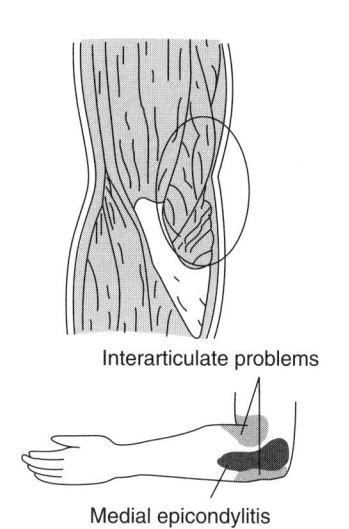

Interarticulate problems

Medial epicondylitis

Medial epicondylitis. Commonly called "bowler's elbow," it is only about 20 percent as common as lateral tennis elbow. It occurs most often among tennis players, baseball pitchers, swimmers, golfers, and bowlers. It is associated with repetitive throwing motions or striking (particularly among professional tennis players).

school pitcher becomes an avid golfer or tennis player in later life. An arm injury during youth might seriously restrict enjoyment of other sports later in life. Very few studies follow the careers of high school and college athletes in adulthood, zeroing in on the long-term effects of participation.

Nevertheless, there are several arm injuries that, if untreated or improperly rehabilitated, could cause future problems.

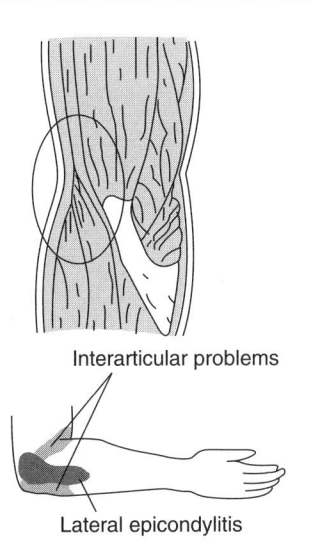

Lateral epicondylitis. Commonly called "tennis elbow," this is considered a form of overuse tendinitis. Degeneration of the tendon is the usual cause of pain. It occurs in athletes who repeatedly use the forearm muscle. In the case of the tennis player, energy that is not returned to the ball (e.g., from off-center hits) results in vibrational energy that gets dampened out by the elbow. It usually occurs on the outside of the elbow (lateral epicondyle) and is not as serious as Little League elbow. The condition heals well when the elbow is given the opportunity to rest. It has been estimated that 50 percent of all adult recreational tennis players will develop tennis elbow symptoms sometime during their playing careers (Nicholas, 1990). Since this injury rarely causes permanent damage, those affected can choose to play with the pain or rest.

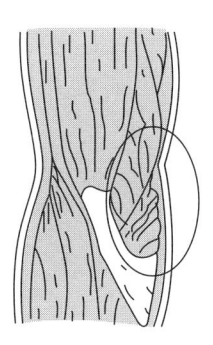

Little League elbow (osteochondritis). This is an overuse injury resulting from straining and tearing the muscles and ligaments that surround the elbow. Because the surface of the elbow joint is damaged, it can have serious long-term repercussions. It usually occurs along the inner side (medial), but can also occur along the outer side (lateral). Symptoms include pain with and without motion, some stiffness, and an occasional grinding or snapping sound. Early signs are pain and tenderness, but by continued use, the pain increases, and the elbow becomes stiffer and more difficult to straighten out. Continuing to throw or swing could permanently damage the elbow. Little League elbow is the primary reason coaches are advised to discourage youngsters from throwing curve balls.

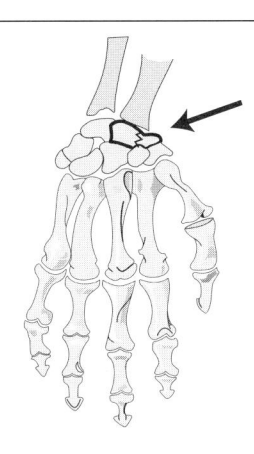

Wrist fracture. Like shoulder separations, wrist fractures usually occur from falls and not from throwing or swinging. The most common wrist injury is a fracture of the forearm bones, the radius and ulna. This injury usually heals well if the arm is treated immediately and kept in a cast until healed. The more troubling fracture is a fracture of the scaphoid bone in the wrist, which is sometimes misdiagnosed as a sprained wrist. A scaphoid fracture suffered during a fall during basketball season may go undetected until spring, when the athlete finds it too painful to swing a baseball bat. Like a sprain, a scaphoid fracture exhibits similar symptoms: pain, stiffness, and tenderness. Because this fracture is potentially so dangerous, many physicians recommend considering a wrist sprain a scaphoid fracture until proven otherwise. What makes this fracture so troublesome is the limited blood flow to this bone, which in some cases may require six months or more to heal.

Wrist Sprains

One of the most common wrist sprains among baseball hitters occurs when they "check" a swing. They try to pull back from swinging after the bat already has reached full velocity. The wrist gets caught in between, the unfortunate fulcrum (pivot point) of a high-velocity bat and forearm muscles that are straining to stop the swing.

Since then, some younger players, many of whom pattern their game after the U.S. tennis player Andre Agassi, now hit all their strokes with significant wrist snap. Using the wrist to generate additional torque generates much more power but also brings added stress to the tendons and ligaments in and around the wrist.

While wrist action is an unusual technique for tennis players, it always has been an important technique for badminton players. Because badminton players use an extremely light racket to hit an even lighter shuttlecock, the racket-shuttlecock impact force is minimal, and this in turn tends to make the force that the wrist must absorb minimal. Not surprisingly, then, wrist injuries never have been very prevalent in badminton.

Pathophysiology and Treatment

As more studies are published on the nature of sport-specific arm injuries, physicians continue to develop a more sophisticated understanding of the dynamics of arm injuries. Nevertheless, there is one fact they have always known with great certainty: the severity of a sports injury is related to the force involved. Arm injuries occur to either bone or soft tissue and vary in severity with three factors: direction of force, magnitude of force, and the velocity applied.

Minor strains and bruises to the shoulder complex usually heal quickly because a rich blood supply speeds healing. Ligaments and tendons in the arm are less vascularized—less blood flow is available—so the healing process takes longer. Often, improving the blood supply to the shoulder through exercise and by applying heat to the joint improves the nutrient flow, which in turn hastens healing, though it may increase swelling.

Because adults have greater mass and are able to generate greater velocity, most arm injuries occur more often to adults than to children. Adults generate greater linear momentum. The elasticity of the young body—bones, muscles, tendons, ligaments—helps limit the risk of serious injuries to youngsters. But as the body ages and loses some of its elasticity, the potential for injury increases. Most individuals' range of motion (flexibility) declines with age as well. The tight quarters of the shoulder complex make it one of the most common sites of range-of-motion impairment. Working near maximum stress, athletes are very susceptible to micro-tears in soft tissue such as the rotator cuff. When a soft tissue injury to the rotator cuff occurs, swelling and scarring of tissue surrounding the shoulder impinge on movement of the humerus; this is similar to the way a pencil stuck in a door hinge prevents the door from closing.

The impingement syndrome is a common shoulder problem among workers, recreational athletes, and world-class athletes. Athletic motions, and the differences in repetitive overuse from sport to sport and from person to person, are also important factors in the incidence of rotator cuff injury. Swimmers and tennis players are particularly prone to shoulder injury. Among elite athletes, over 80 percent of swimmers report shoulder pain, and over 50 percent of tennis players report problems with their rotator cuff and biceps tendons.

The natural arc of elevation in raising the arm is forward, not lateral—to the side. This means that impingement occurs predominantly against the anterior or front edge of the acromion and the coracoacromial ligament. Listed from mild to severe, the three progressive stages of impingement are as follows: first, edema, swelling and hemorrhage (clotting); second, thickening and fibrosis (build up of excessive connective tissue); and third, rotator cuff tears, biceps ruptures, and bone changes. However, the boundaries of these stages are not clearly defined, and symptoms often overlap.

The primary complaint of an athlete with a rotator cuff or biceps tendon problem is usually pain. The athlete may also complain of fatigue, functional "catching," stiffness, or weakness about the shoulder. These complaints are usually related to overhead activities, which are more prominent in athletes who throw. The characterization of the patient's pain varies depending on the amount of rest and rehabilitation.

Characterization of the nature and severity of pain is the most important diagnostic task in treatment. A painful athletic shoulder can fall into one of two categories: acute or macrotraumatic, which concentrates on the mechanism of injury; and chronic or microtraumatic, which concentrates on training patterns and the competitive arena. In either case, pain commonly radiates into the upper arm. For example, biceps pain is more anteriorly located and can radiate down the middle of the long head of the muscle. A throbbing night pain that radiates through the arm can awaken an athlete from a deep sleep, and is a common characteristic of rotator cuff tendinitis or a tear.

By focusing on the aggravating factors causing pain, and the specific timing of its occurrence during the throwing motion, it is possible to arrive at an accurate diagnosis. Nevertheless, a diagnosis based on pain alone is often erroneous. A pitcher who complains of pain during the cocking phase of throwing may well have an underlying forward instability problem that will lead to a rotator cuff problem.

The wide range of tolerance for pain also makes diagnosis difficult. Many athletes become accustomed to playing with considerable discomfort and pain as a simple fact of life. They can often play until they suffer from a loss of accuracy or endurance, that is, until pain interferes with performance. Only then are they ready to seek treatment. Most athletes with cuff problems notice distinct improvement with rest; however, rest is not a viable option for many competitive athletes.

Other symptoms include clicking in the shoulder, a feeling of instability, numbness, or radiating sharp pain down the arm into the hand, neck, or elbow. Such symptoms may suggest an alternate diagnosis, such as instability of the shoulder, rather than rotator cuff and biceps tendon anomalies. These complaints also may be present in shoulder cuff disorders. The vast majority (about 90 percent) of patients diagnosed with impingement are able to return to full activity with nonoperative treatment such as anti-inflammatory medication, ice, and therapy. If nonoperative treatment options fail, operative treatment through either traditional incision surgery or the latest arthroscopic techniques (small puncture incisions) is used to correct the problem.

Elbow surgery is far less prevalent. Most elbow injuries, particularly tennis elbow and bowler's elbow, subside with rest. However, when nerve entrapment or pinching occurs, it may cause elbow pain that requires surgery.

Until the 1970s, the options available to physicians for diagnosis and treatment were limited. Advances in technology and medical knowledge have greatly expanded the quality of medical treatment for arm injuries. Physicians can evaluate upper extremity injuries using CAT scans and magnetic resonance imaging (MRI) scanners. These diagnostic tests give physicians an intricate three-dimensional "road map" in and around the joint. The workings of the shoulder—the bony architecture and soft tissue structures such as ligaments and tendons—can be visualized by these examinations.

Arthroscopic treatment is one of the most common surgical techniques used to treat shoulder joint problems. An arthroscope resembles an extremely thin pen-flashlight and carries a camera that projects the internal workings of the joint onto a monitor. If a repair is necessary, another small incision is made to shave off and reshape the damaged area.

One of the major advantages of arthroscopic surgery is the potential for shorter recovery time. By avoiding open, large incision techniques less trauma impacts the joint, which makes it possible for some athletes to recover much more quickly than after open surgical intervention. Initially, arthroscopic techniques were used only on large joints, such as the knee. As techniques improved, and the surgical equipment became smaller and better, arthroscopic techniques became available for smaller joints, such as the shoulder, elbow, and wrist. Arthroscopic surgery has become one of the most frequently used treatments for impingement syndrome. To eliminate impingement, the front of the acromion bone is removed through the arthroscope.

Preventing Arm Injuries

A fuller understanding of the biomechanical and pathological causes of arm injuries may help athletes modify their behavior, by changing their habits or their mechanics. If arm injuries are ignored or mistreated, they may lead to more serious, persistent injuries. Knowing the signs of injury, as well as how to strengthen and stretch the shoulder, can significantly reduce the risk of injury and prevent chronic pain.

Proper conditioning is vital for preventing injuries to the arm. An athlete who may throw 100 fastballs in a game, 50 football passes a day, or play three sets of tennis must maintain leg and body strength as well as endurance. There are several preventive steps that athletes can take to preserve the health of the shoulder, elbow, and wrist.

Improving technique. One hundred serves by a tennis player with excellent technique may produce the equivalent strain of forty serves by a player with poor technique. An inability to follow through, or decelerate, smoothly and efficiently is the major cause of throwing and swinging arm injuries.

Year-round training. Trainers and coaches recommend year-round participation to keep the arm in shape. During the off-season, pitchers should throw three or four times a week to maintain strength and flexibility.

Weight lifting. Both off-season and in-season weight or resistance training is advised for endurance and, in particular, to work the rotator cuff muscles. Throwing will strengthen the "powering" shoulder muscles more than the interior stabilizing rotator cuff muscles. The activity increases the imbalance between muscle groups; therefore, the emphasis of weight or resistance training should be on strengthening the rotators—the muscles used to decelerate the arm. The slower, more powerful muscles in the legs and lower back benefit from a weight program that emphasizes both strength and endurance. The greater lower extremity strength makes a large contribution to throwing or striking velocity (*see also* STRENGTH TRAINING).

Physical fitness. Sprinting and distance running are important for strength, power, and endurance. Endurance is important, even for pitchers, because fatigue often adversely affects timing and technique, which causes some muscles and tendons to work harder to compensate for those that are fatigued.

Stretching. Before and after workouts and playing, a warm-up and stretching routine for both for upper and lower extremities is recommended.

Rehabilitation. Should an injury occur, proper rehabilitation and treatment are considered equally important. Regardless of how well treatment may have gone, returning to competition too soon, or improperly reconditioned, is likely to cause re-injury. Physical therapy focuses on restoring mobility and reducing pain as quickly as possible. Treatment begins with gentle stretching and gradually becomes more and more rigorous. Athletes suffering from shoulder impingement should start with isometric strength training—exercises that do not require shoulder movement, to avoid aggravating inflamed tissue (*see also* REHABILITATION).

John Zumerchik and David H. Janda, M.D.*

**The authors extend a special thanks to Don C. Hopkins for providing some of the physics examples.*

References

Adrian, M. and J. Cooper. *Biomechanics of Human Movement*. Dubuque, Iowa: Benchmark, 1989.

American Academy of Orthopaedic Surgeons. *Athletic Training and Sports Medicine*. Chicago, Illinois: American Academy of Orthopaedic Surgeons, 1984.

Bird, H. "When the body takes the strain." *New Scientist* 127, no. 1724 (7 July 1990): 49–52.

Hawkins, R., et al. "The athlete's shoulder." *Perspectives in Orthopedic Surgery* 1, no. 2 (1990): 1–26.

Jobe, F., et al. "An analysis of the shoulder in throwing and pitching." *American Journal of Sports Medicine* 11, no. 1 (1983): 3–5.

McLeod, W. "The pitching mechanism." In B. Zarins et al. (eds.), *Injuries to the Throwing Arm*. Philadelphia: Saunders, 1985.

Nicholas, J. *The Upper Extremity in Sports Medicine*. St. Louis: Mosby, 1990.

Rehnstrhom, A. *Sports Injuries: Basic Principles of Prevention and Care*. Boston: Blackwell, 1993.

Seireg, Ali. *Biomechanical Analysis of the Musculoskeletal Structure for Medicine and Sports*. New York: Hemisphere, 1989.

Southmayd, W. and M. Hoffman, *Sports Health*. New York: Putnam, 1981.

Skeletal Muscle

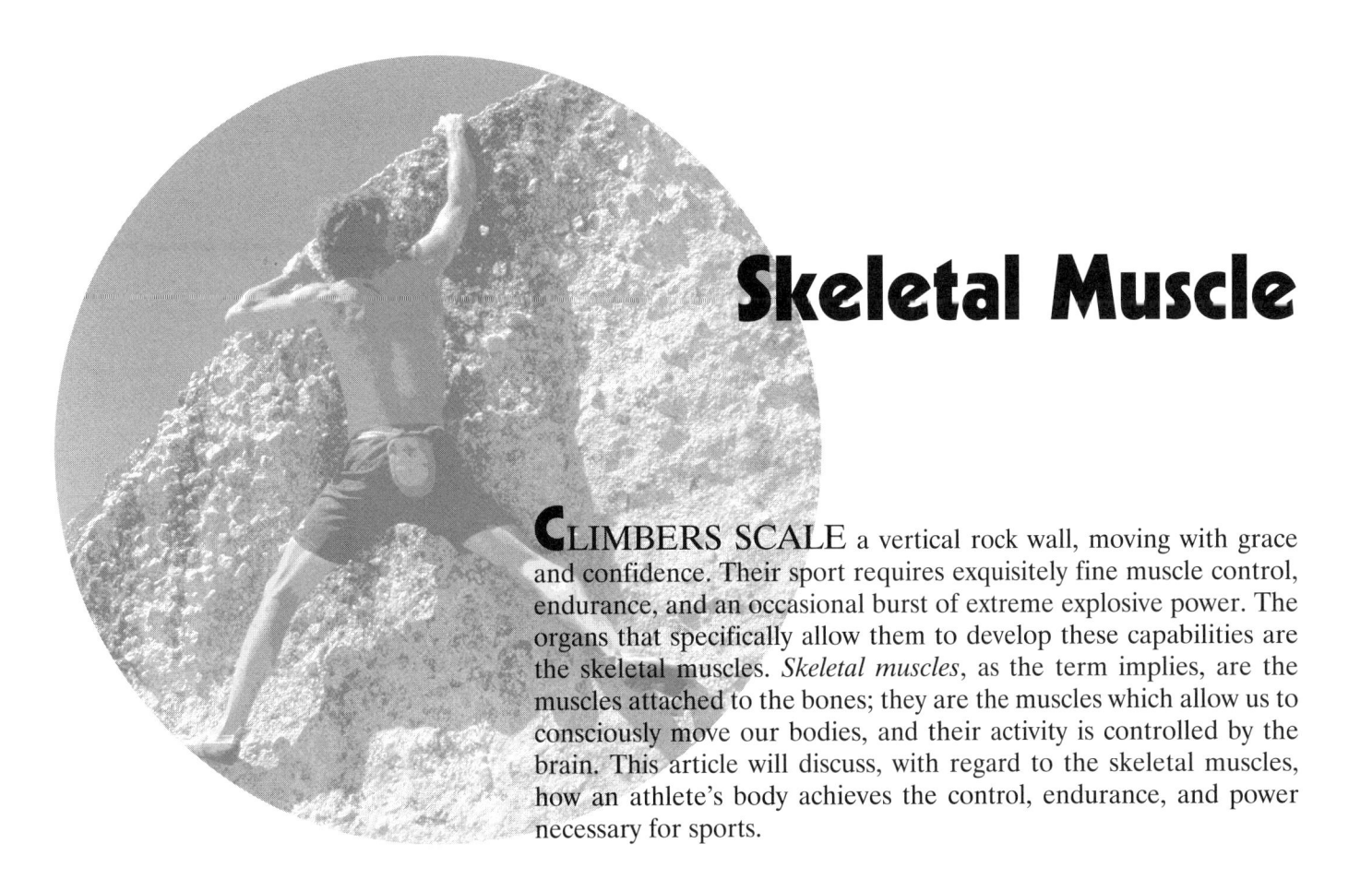

CLIMBERS SCALE a vertical rock wall, moving with grace and confidence. Their sport requires exquisitely fine muscle control, endurance, and an occasional burst of extreme explosive power. The organs that specifically allow them to develop these capabilities are the skeletal muscles. *Skeletal muscles*, as the term implies, are the muscles attached to the bones; they are the muscles which allow us to consciously move our bodies, and their activity is controlled by the brain. This article will discuss, with regard to the skeletal muscles, how an athlete's body achieves the control, endurance, and power necessary for sports.

Control of Contraction

This section will consider the role of the brain and nerves in controlling skeletal muscle, and what happens when that role is disrupted.

The Corticospinal Pathway

When the brain directs the skeletal muscles to move, the signal originates in the highest area of the brain, the cerebral cortex. The part of the cerebral cortex dedicated to conscious motion is the primary motor area, which is located in the frontal lobe of the brain just anterior to—that is, in front of—an indentation in the brain surface known as the central sulcus (*see Figure 1*).

In the primary motor area, there is a "map" of the body, so that different parts of this area control different parts of the body. However, this "map" is not anatomically accurate; that is, the size of a section devoted to a particular body part may be disproportionally large or small (*see Figure 2*). Body parts which require fine control, such as the hand and face, have a proportionally larger part of the primary motor area devoted to their control than parts which need less fine control, such as the trunk. This is one reason that, while our rock climbers can certainly adjust their trunk position, they have far more precise control over the position of their fingers.

Once an electrical nerve message, known as an action potential, begins in the primary motor area, it travels down through the brain

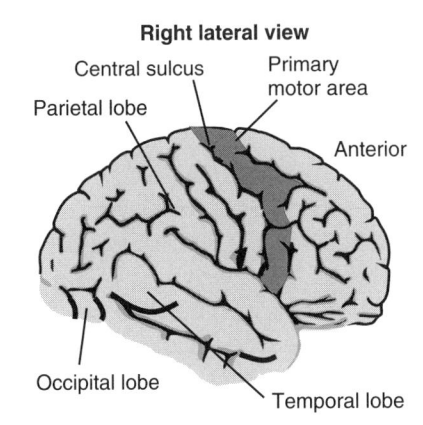

Figure 1: *Shown here is the exterior of the brain. The primary motor control area controls contractions of specific muscles or groups of muscles.*

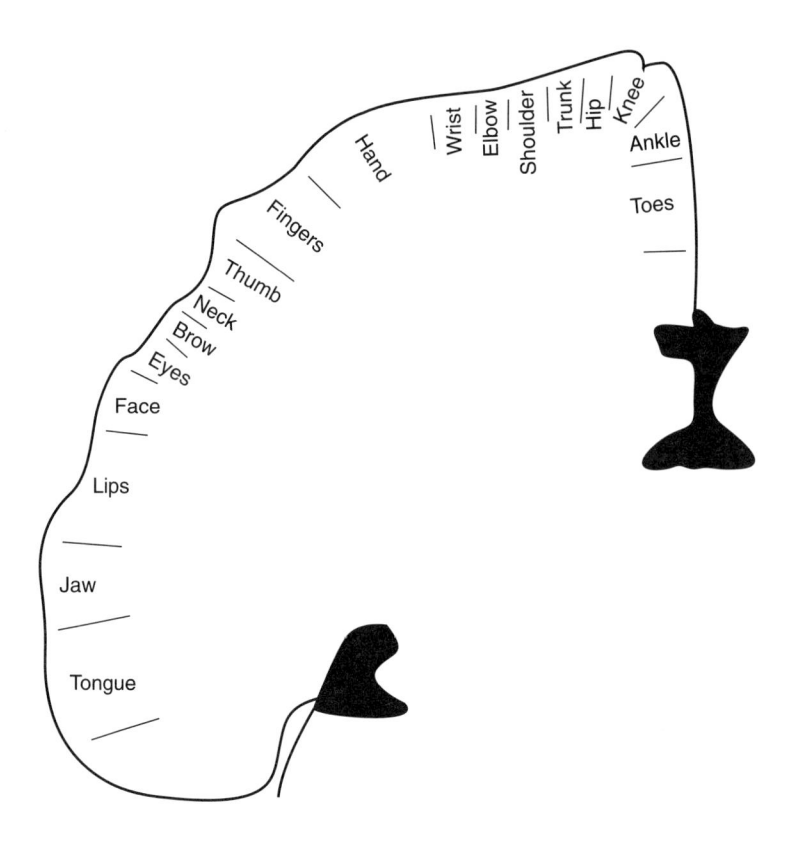

Figure 2. *Cutting a brain in coronal section (into front and back parts) reveals the right motor cortex. Note how much more of the motor cortex is devoted to moving the fingers and mouth than to moving the trunk.*

and spinal cord in a bundle of nerve fibers known as the corticospinal tract (*see Figure 3*). Some of these fibers cross to the opposite side of the brain from which they begin in a lower part of the brain, the medulla. Because of this "crossing over," the left side of the brain controls the right side of the body, and vice versa. This is the reason that a brain injury from a severe trauma or a stroke which destroys part of the right primary motor area can cause partial paralysis of the left half of the body.

The nerves of the corticospinal tract descend in the spinal cord until they reach approximately the level of the part of the body for which their message is intended. Thus, nerves that carry messages directing motion of the arms descend in the spinal cord only as far as the upper back (thoracic region of the spinal cord), whereas messages directing motion of the legs descend further in the spinal cord to the lower back (lumbar region of the spinal cord). It is interesting to note that the nerve fiber that begins in the primary motor area of the cerebral cortex and descends through the brain to the appropriate level of the spinal cord is a single cell. In a basketball player who is 7 feet (2.1 m) tall, then, the nerve cell which carries motor messages destined for the legs must be at least 3 feet (nearly 1 m) long.

Once it has descended to the appropriate level of the spinal cord, the nerve which originated in the primary motor cortex synapses with—that is, contacts—a second short nerve cell called an interneuron. The action potential which began in the brain passes to this interneuron and then to a third nerve cell known as a motor neuron.

This motor neuron begins in the spinal cord and sends an extension called an axon out of the spinal cord to contact the skeletal muscle. The motor neuron that sends messages to the muscles which move the big toe, for instance, begins in the back and ends in the foot; this is another very long cell, particularly in someone like the 7-foot basketball player. The axons of the motor neurons that extend from the spinal cord to the skeletal muscles run in bundles of nerve fibers called peripheral nerves.

Nerve Injuries and Muscle Function

The path of nerve messages through the spinal cord was dramatically—and sadly—illustrated in May 1995, when the actor Christopher Reeve was thrown from a horse during a jumping competition and hit his head, with the result that his neck was fractured and his spinal cord was damaged at a very high level: the cervical spinal cord. In cases like this, recovery is slow, and it is impossible to predict how much function a patient will eventually regain. With Reeve, however, there were some telling signs. After several months, he had no use of the arms or legs, and there was substantial weakness in the muscles that enable breathing: this indicated that the nerve messages needed to direct the motion of the limbs were failing to pass beyond the injured part of spinal cord in the neck.

A few years earlier, in November 1992, Dennis Byrd, who played defensive end for the New York Jets, fractured his neck during a game at Giants Stadium. Team physicians immediately immobilized Byrd's neck and transported him to a nearby hospital by ambulance. At the hospital he was given steroid medication to reduce the swelling of the injured spinal cord and underwent surgery to stabilize the fractured neck vertebra and to relieve pressure on the spinal cord. As a result of this prompt and appropriate treatment, Byrd, who might otherwise have been completely paralyzed, slowly regained some limited use of his arms and his legs.

Neck and back injuries leading to spinal cord damage and muscle paralysis are all too common in sports. In particular, these injuries can be caused by falls and by diving into shallow water. Since a partner or team member is often the first person on the scene when someone injures the back or neck, it is important that all athletes understand how vital it is to respond correctly to such emergencies:

1. Never move a person who may have injured the back or neck. Moving the patient can make a spinal cord injury worse.

2. Keep the injured person calm.

3. Summon trained medical help to the scene immediately.

4. Bear in mind that with possible spinal cord injuries, it is always best to err on the side of caution.

Coaches and referees can also help reduce the risk of spinal cord injuries in contact sports such as football. For instance, football players should be taught correct tackling technique, and rules

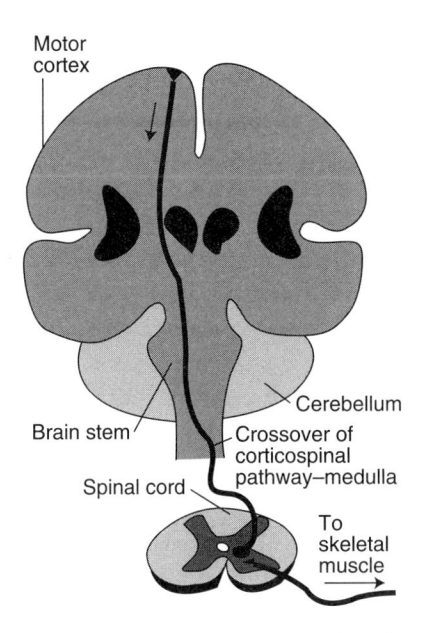

Figure 3. *The muscle signal pathway—the corticospinal pathway—goes from the motor cortex, passes through the brain stem and spinal cord, and then is relayed to the skeletal muscle.*

against spearing should be strictly enforced. Unfortunately, even with excellent training, good equipment, and proper technique, some risk of spinal cord injury will remain in contact sports. (For instance, medical experts who were present when Dennis Byrd was injured were convinced that he had not been spearing at the time of the accident.)

Peripheral nerves, the bundles of axons that carry messages from the spinal cord to the muscles, can also be injured either by compression from a specific trauma or by repeated overuse. Injury of a peripheral nerve does not have the devastating results that occur with spinal cord injury. However, peripheral nerve injuries should not be ignored and must be properly treated. One common example of peripheral nerve injury is "whiplash," damage to the spinal nerves in the neck. Whiplash can be caused by any traumatic bending of the head such as might occur in an automobile accident or in a collision during a contact sport. It can cause pain and muscle weakness of varying severity, depending on the exact peripheral nerves involved and the severity of the damage. Fortunately, this injury often responds well to rest.

Peripheral nerve injuries can also occur farther away from the spinal cord, in the extremities. Acute (that is, sudden) nerve injuries of the hands can occur in sports, such as rock climbing, that place abrupt, extreme stress on the hand. More chronic (slow-onset) peripheral nerve damage can occur in the wrists of weight lifters and rowers and in the elbows of participants in sports that involve throwing. This sort of nerve injury is usually the result of repetitive motions. Once again, pain and muscle weakness are the major symptoms, and a conservative course—resting the damaged nerve—is usually indicated.

Structure of Skeletal Muscle

Each skeletal muscle is attached to a bone by tough ropes of connective tissue called tendons (*see Figure 4*). Cutting the muscle across its widest point (belly) reveals its internal structure. Each muscle is composed of bundles of smaller structures called fasicles. Each fasicle, in turn, is made up of bundles of muscle fibers. Each muscle fiber is a single muscle cell—another impressively long cell—which can run the length of the muscle.

Because muscle fibers can run the length of a skeletal muscle, they can be over 30 centimeters (12 in.) long. However, each muscle fiber is only 10 to 80 micrometers (μm) in diameter (1 μm = 0.000001 m, or 0.001 mm). Thus a single muscle fiber is barely thick enough to see with the unaided eye. The cell membrane of a muscle fiber, the sarcolemma, has blind-ended tubes, called transverse tubules or T-tubules, which begin on the cell surface and dive deep into the interior of the muscle fiber. It is important to note that the wall of the

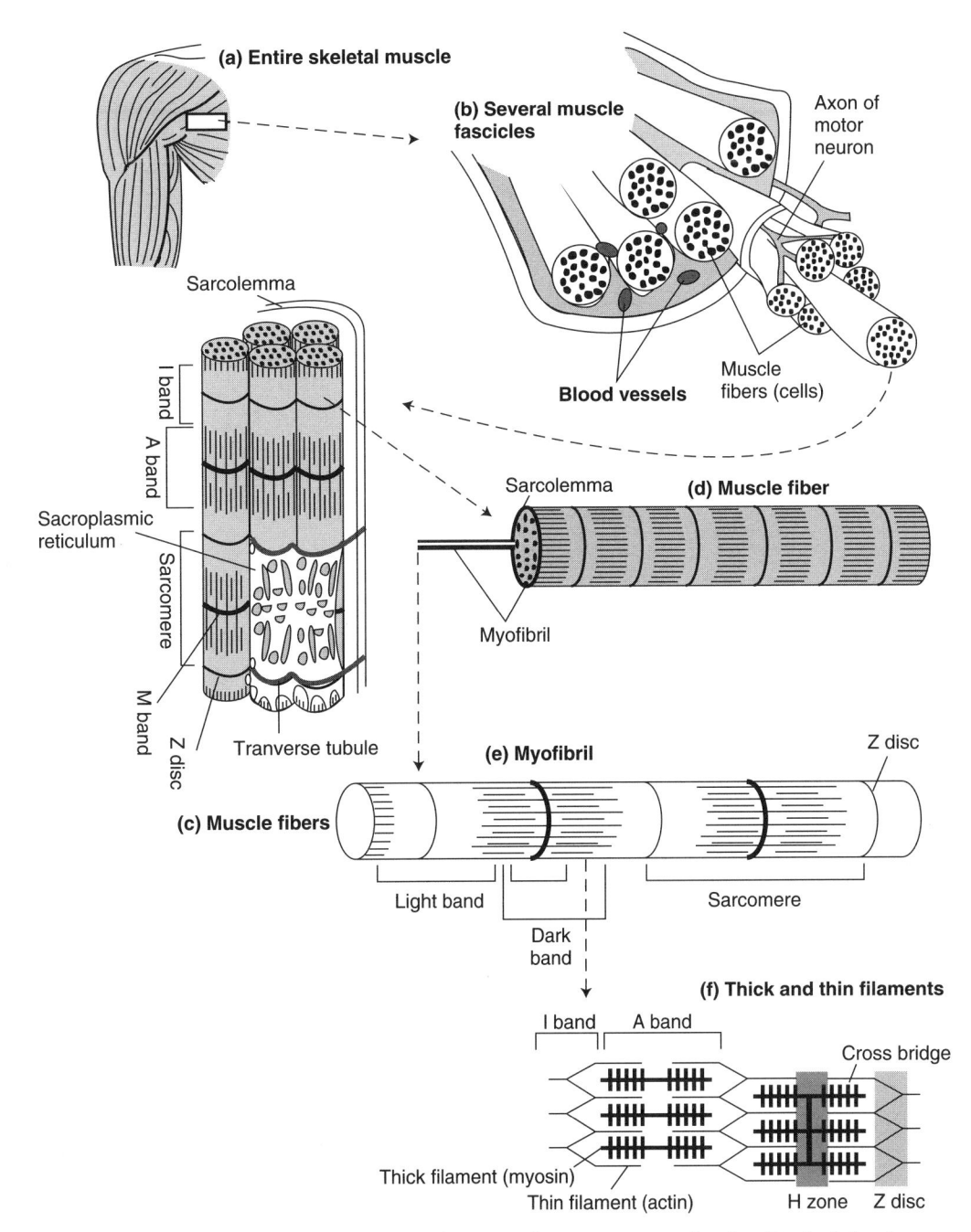

Figure 4. *Skeletal muscle ranges from gross to molecular. Each skeletal muscle contains numerous parallel myofibrils (shown in e).*

T-tubule is continuous with the sarcolemma of the exterior of the muscle fiber.

The interior of each muscle fiber is packed with still smaller units called myofibrils. The myofibrils are surrounded by an extensive system of sacs—the sarcoplasmic reticulum—containing a large amount of calcium. The inside of each myofibril is, in turn, packed with the smallest muscle structures, the muscle filaments. It is at the level of the muscle filament that muscle contraction takes place.

Stimulation of Skeletal Muscle

As noted above, a motor neuron is a nerve cell that begins in the spinal cord and sends an axon out to a skeletal muscle through a peripheral nerve. As the axon of a motor neuron approaches the skeletal muscle, it splits into multiple branches. Each branch ends on a different muscle fiber. A "motor unit" consists of a motor neuron and all of the muscle fibers to which it sends axon branches. An action potential (nerve signal) from a motor neuron will cause all the muscle fibers in its motor unit to contract. Action potentials are transmitted very rapidly along motor neurons. This is one reason that a hand can be withdrawn from a painful stimulus such as a hot stove in a few milliseconds (ms; 1 ms = 0.001 sec.). It is also part of the reason that a trained sprinter can "come off the blocks" so quickly when the starting gun fires.

Motor units vary considerably in size from one muscle to another. In muscles that require very fine motion, such as those which move the eyes or fingers, each motor neuron may send axon branches to only a few muscle fibers. However, in muscles in which such fine control is not needed, such as those responsible for posture (the back and stomach muscles), a single motor unit may contain over 100 muscle fibers. This difference in sizes of motor units, in conjunction with the unequal distribution of space in the primary motor cortex, works to allow very fine control of muscle motion where it is needed most.

The location at which the motor neuron reaches the skeletal muscle fiber is known as the neuromuscular junction (*see Figure 5*). The nerve terminal (end of the nerve) at the neuromuscular junction is filled with small sacs, called vesicles, which contain the chemical acetylcholine. When the action potential which began in the primary motor cortex reaches the nerve terminal of the motor neuron, it causes protein gates called channels in the cell membrane to open. When open, these gates allow calcium to enter the nerve terminal from the fluid surrounding the nerve. Through a process which is still poorly understood, the calcium causes the vesicles to fuse with the nerve membrane and to dump the acetylcholine out into the synaptic cleft, the small gap (about 0.03 μm wide) between the motor neuron and the muscle fiber.

Once it has entered the synaptic cleft, the acetylcholine diffuses across the short distance to the muscle fiber. The area of the muscle fiber opposite the nerve terminal is called the motor end plate. Each motor end plate contains special proteins in its cell membrane that are receptors for acetylcholine. The acetylcholine attaches to its receptor and begins an electrical signal (action potential) on the surface of the muscle fiber, the sarcolemma. As noted above, the surface of the T-tubules is continuous with the sarcolemma. Thus, when the action potential spreads along the sarcolemma, it also enters the T-tubules and dives deep into the muscle fiber. The T-tubules run into the interior of the muscle fiber, coming very close to the sarcoplasmic reticulum, the calcium-filled sac system which surrounds each

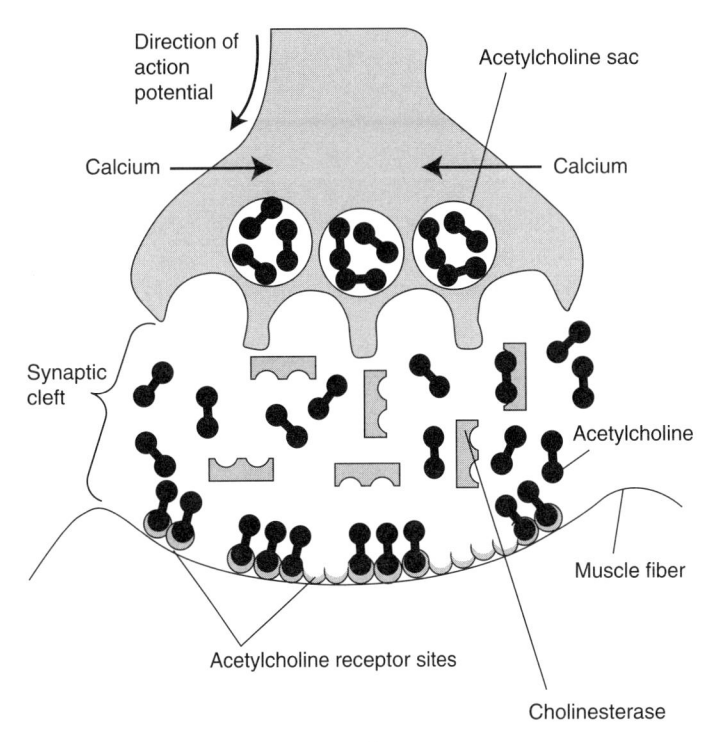

Figure 5. *Shown here is a neuromuscular junction.*

myofibril. The presence of the action potential in the T-tubules causes the sarcoplasmic reticulum to release its calcium into the interior of the muscle fiber. It is the presence of this calcium within the muscle fiber that is directly responsible for muscle contraction.

Contraction of Skeletal Muscle

To understand the process of muscle contraction, it is necessary to take a closer look at the interior structure of the myofibril. In each myofibril there are two types of filaments: thick and thin. Thick filaments are made up of the protein myosin, a huge protein shaped somewhat like a golf club with a long shaft and a globular head. In a thick filament, the shafts of many myosin molecules are twisted around each other to form the backbone of the filament; heads extend away from the filament backbone and are known as cross bridges (*see Figure 6*). Thin filaments are made up of two strands of the globular-shaped protein actin. These two strands are twisted around each other like two strands of pearls. Two other proteins, a long thin structure called tropomyosin and a smaller one called toponin, are also part of the thin filament. As will be seen below, the cross bridges are so called because they are the part of the myosin molecule that attaches to actin, forming a link or bridge which crosses between the thick and thin filaments.

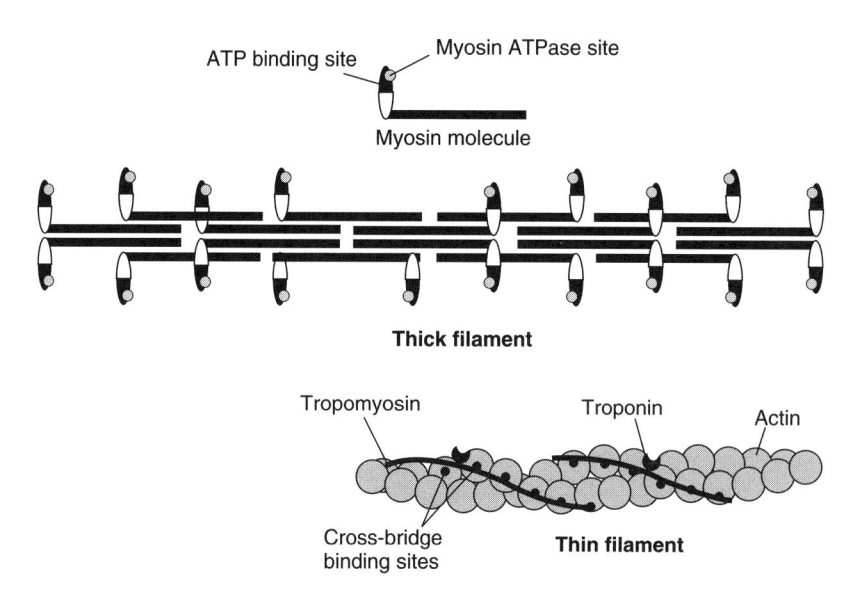

Figure 6. *Muscle consists of thick and thin filaments. Above: Orientation of myosin molecules in one thick muscle filament. Below: Binding and orientation of a thin muscle filament.*

The thick and thin filaments are arranged in a very regular parallel pattern in skeletal muscle. These two types of filaments partially overlap each other, giving skeletal muscle a striped or striated appearance of alternating light and dark bands when viewed under a microscope. The light bands contain only thin filaments; the dark bands contain the thick filaments and areas where the two types of filaments overlap. The ends of the thin filaments are embedded in another structure called the Z line. The area between two Z lines is called a sarcomere (*again, see Figure 4*).

The actin molecules of the thin filament contain specific sites at which the globular heads of the myosin from the thick filament (cross bridges) can attach. When a skeletal muscle is relaxed and the internal calcium level is low, the tropomyosin covers these myosin binding sites on the actin, preventing the cross bridges from attaching. However, when a skeletal muscle is stimulated and calcium is released from the sarcoplasmic reticulum, the calcium binds to the troponin of the thin filament and causes the tropomyosin to move and to uncover the myosin binding sites on the actin.

Once the myosin binding sites on actin are uncovered, the myosin cross bridges begin to interact with actin in a repetitive rowing motion that draws the thin filaments across the thick filaments much as the sections of a spyglass fold into each other (*see Figure 7*). First the myosin cross bridge attaches to actin, with the cross bridge at right angles to the thick filament backbone. Then the cross bridge undergoes a power stroke until it reaches a 45-degree angle relative to the thick filament backbone. During this power stroke, the thin filament is pulled across the thick filament. Then the cross bridge detaches from actin and recocks itself to a right angle.

As long as the internal calcium level of the muscle fiber remains high and the muscle remains activated, this process continues and the thin filaments are drawn farther and farther across the thick filaments. This is known as the "sliding filament" theory of muscle contraction. One of the major pieces of evidence for this theory is the fact that when a skeletal muscle shortens, the light bands become progressively smaller until they finally disappear, while the dark bands do not change in width.

As a muscle shortens against a load, work is being done and

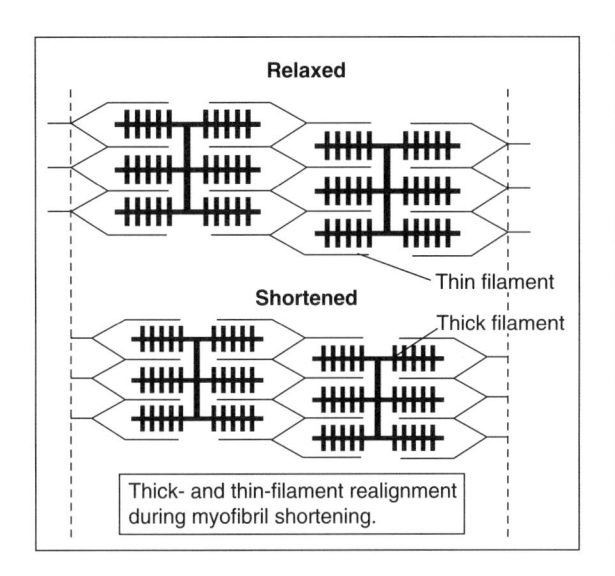

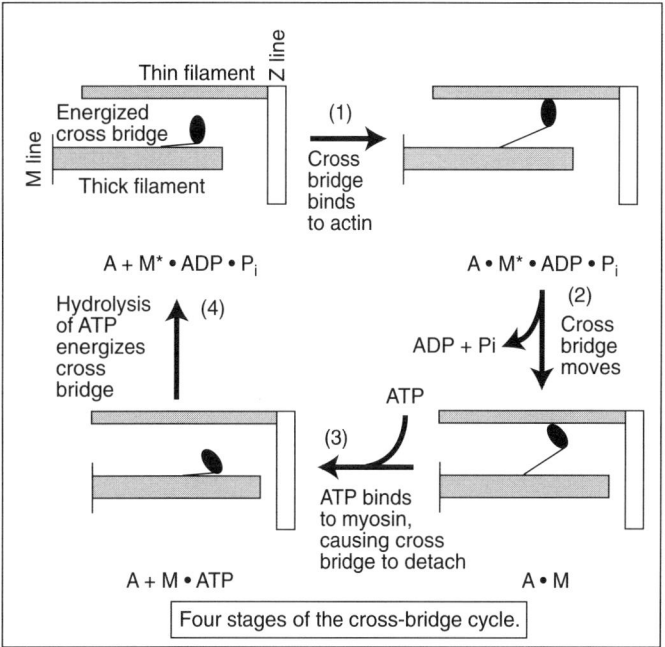

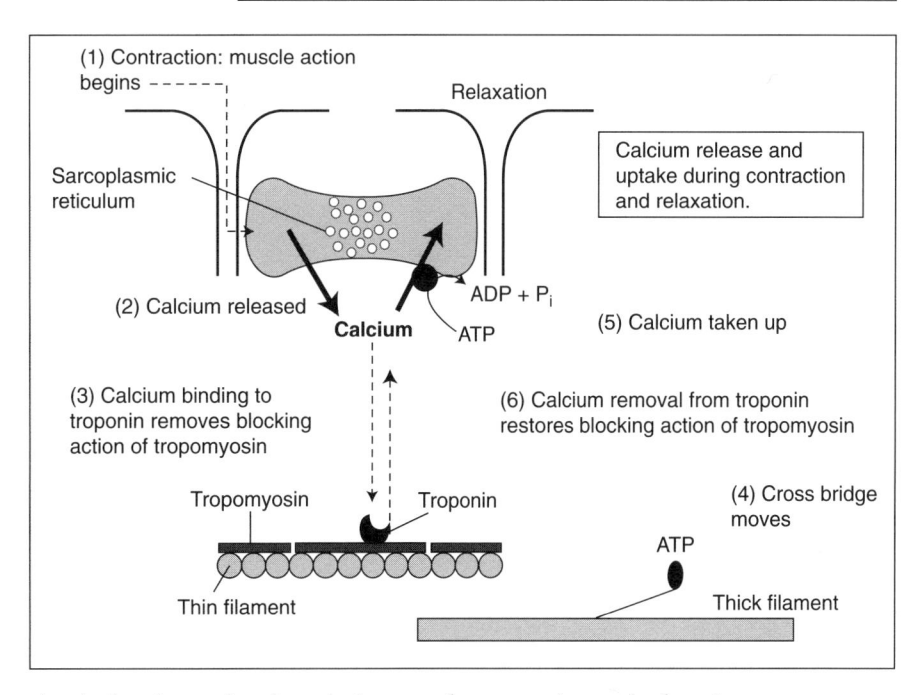

Figure 7. *These chemical and mechanical actions take place during muscle contraction and relaxation.*

energy is being consumed, though the exact relationship between energy and work in muscle can be a rather difficult concept. As with most cellular processes that require energy, the energy for muscle contraction comes from the breakdown of the high-energy compound adenosine triphosphate to adenosine diphosphate and inorganic phosphate (ATP $\rightarrow$ ADP + P_i + energy). The coupling of this reaction—a release of energy—to the work of muscle contraction would be easy to understand if the breakdown of ATP occurred simultaneously with the power stroke of the cross bridge that performs the work of muscle at the cellular level. However, this is not the case.

Let us begin with myosin and actin bound together after a myosin power stoke has been completed. The myosin cross bridge will be at a 45-degree angle. First ATP binds to myosin. This binding of ATP allows the myosin to detach from the actin. Next the ATP is split into ADP and inorganic phosphate with the release of energy. This energy is used to recock the myosin cross bridge to a 90-degree angle. The ADP and inorganic phosphate remain bound to the myosin. Now the myosin rebinds to actin, and the ADP and inorganic phosphate are released. During the release of the ADP and inorganic phosphate, the cross bridge undergoes its power stroke to 45 degrees. Finally, another ATP binds to the myosin, the cross bridge detaches from actin, and the process begins again.

One way to clarify that the binding of ATP to the myosin cross bridge causes myosin to detach from actin is to consider what happens to a body soon after death. A dead muscle can no longer make ATP. The muscle runs out of ATP, and all the myosin cross bridges are trapped in an attached state. The thick and thin filaments are firmly attached to each other, and the muscle resists stretching. This is what causes rigor mortis, the muscle stiffness characteristic of a dead body. (This state of the muscles, rigor mortis, gave rise to a slang term for a corpse—"stiff.")

Relaxation of Skeletal Muscle

Skeletal muscle contraction is turned off by a reverse of the process that turns it on. When the motor neuron stops sending action potentials to the muscle fibers, the release of acetylcholine stops. The acetylcholine, which is bound to the receptors in the motor end plate, detaches from its receptors and is broken down by an enzyme called cholinesterase in the synaptic space between the nerve and the muscle. With no acetylcholine bound to receptors, the muscle action potentials stop. This stops the process of calcium release from the sarcoplasmic reticulum. Pumps in the membrane of the sarcoplasmic reticulum pump the calcium back into the membranous sacs, and the calcium level within the myofibrils falls. As a result, the calcium bound to the troponin detaches, and the tropomyosin returns to its original position covering the myosin binding sites on the actin.

Myosin cross bridges can no longer attach to actin. The muscle is relaxed.

One interesting way in which the relaxation of skeletal muscle can be examined involves the drug curare. Curare was discovered by the native peoples of the Amazon rain forest of South America. They used it as an arrow-tip poison for hunting small animals. When curare enters the bloodstream of an animal (or a person), it makes its way to the neuromuscular junctions of the skeletal muscles, where it binds to the acetylcholine receptors of the motor end plates. With curare bound to these receptors, acetylcholine cannot bind and produce a skeletal muscle action potential. The skeletal muscles, including the muscles used for breathing—such as the diaphragm—cannot contract, and the victim is paralyzed. Death results from lack of oxygen, because the victim cannot breathe. In virtually all animals (including humans), curare is broken down and rendered harmless by the digestive system. For this reason, curare must be injected to be effective, and animals killed with curare are safe to eat. (It must have taken a brave person, though, to test this for the first time.) In modern medicine, curare and its chemical cousins are commonly administered to patients undergoing surgery with general anesthesia (*see also* RESPIRATION). These drugs are vital for such surgery because they produce the muscle relaxation the surgeon needs to work in the abdominal or chest cavity. Patients who have been given curare are placed on a respirator (ventilator) which breathes for them until the medication has worn off.

Individual skeletal muscles have no way to relengthen after they have shortened. For this reason, skeletal muscles are almost always arranged in antagonistic pairs in which one muscle is lengthened by the shortening of the other muscle. Even after a muscle is relaxed, it will remain shortened until it is restretched by the shortening of the other member of the pair, its antagonist. The muscles that move the forearm are a good example of this process. The muscle that flexes (bends) the forearm is the biceps muscle, located on the front of the upper arm between the shoulder and the elbow. The muscle that extends (straightens) the forearm is the triceps muscle, located on the back of the upper arm. If the biceps muscle is contracted with the triceps relaxed, the arm will flex. If gravity were not acting, the process could stop right there: the biceps could be allowed to relax and the arm would remain flexed. Only when the triceps muscle was contracted would the arm extend, restretching the relaxed biceps muscle.

Types of Skeletal Muscle Fibers

As already discussed, skeletal muscles are specialized for the tasks they perform in that muscles needed for fine control have small motor units, while muscles needed for coarse control have larger motor units. Skeletal muscles are specialized in another very important way at the level of the muscle fiber: some muscle fibers (fast-twitch fibers) are capable of producing rapid but short-lived motion, while others (slow-twitch fibers) can produce more sustained although slower motion.

Fast-twitch fibers are specialized to perform explosive activities, such as sprinting. They are stimulated by very rapidly conducting motor neurons and have an extensive sarcoplasmic reticulum that can release large amounts of calcium into the muscles fiber in a short time. Once stimulated, fast-twitch fibers are equipped with a type of myosin that goes though the steps of interaction with actin very rapidly. These features allow fast-twitch fibers to produce full tension in 1/20 (0.05) second and to shorten very rapidly when activated.

The quick response and rapid shortening capacity of fast-twitch muscle fibers comes at a price. Active fast-twitch muscle fibers use energy (ATP) more rapidly than they can replace it. The limiting factor for ATP production is oxygen supply. Fast-twitch muscle fibers do not have enough oxygen to keep up with the energy demands of their rapid activity. Fast-twitch fibers obtain the energy (ATP) they need from the partial breakdown of glucose to pyruvic acid (glycolysis), a process that can occur in the absence of oxygen (anaerobic metabolism). Some ATP is produced in this process, but only a fraction as much as would be produced if the glucose were broken down completely to carbon dioxide and water in the presence of oxygen (aerobic metabolism). Furthermore, the pyruvic acid is then converted to lactic acid, which builds up in the fast-twitch muscles during maximum exercise. The lactic acid causes the pH level of the muscle to drop (increased acidity). This low pH causes the muscle to fatigue. Thus, while fast-twitch muscles can perform rapid activity, they also fatigue and fail quickly when stimulated continuously. (For a more complete discussion of energy supply for muscle contraction, *see ENERGY AND METABOLISM*.)

By contrast, slow-twitch muscle fibers are specialized for prolonged activity. They have large numbers of mitochondria which produce the maximum amount of ATP from the full aerobic breakdown of glucose. They are also well supplied with the enzymes needed for aerobic metabolism. Slow-twitch muscle fibers even have their own internal oxygen supply, an oxygen binding protein called myoglobin, which is similar to the hemoglobin that binds oxygen in red blood cells. These features combine to allow slow-twitch muscle fibers to contract for long periods of time without fatigue. Slow-twitch muscle fibers are vital for prolonged activity, such as marathon running. However, they require 1/10 (0.1) second to reach full force, and they shorten more slowly than fast-twitch fibers.

Some muscles are predominantly composed of either fast- or slow-twitch fibers. This can be seen in carving a turkey. The slow-twitch fibers are darker because of their high myoglobin content; they are found in postural muscles and are often referred to as red muscle. In a turkey, they are found in the "dark meat" of the legs. Fast-twitch muscles are light in color and are called white muscle. In the turkey, these muscle fibers are found in the "white meat" of the turkey breast.

COMPARISON OF FAST-TWITCH AND SLOW-TWITCH MUSCLE FIBER

	Fast-twitch muscle fiber	Slow-twitch muscle fiber
Shortening velocity	rapid	slow
Metabolism	anaerobic	aerobic
Mitochondria	few	many
Nerve conduction	rapid	slow
Fatigue resistance	low	high
Sarcoplasmic reticulum	abundant	sparse
Activity	sprint	marathon
Myoglobin	scarce	abundant

Table 1.

In nonathletic people, most muscles are a more or less even mixture of fast- and slow-twitch muscle fibers. When a muscle is exercised at low intensity, the slow-twitch fibers are called on first. As the intensity of exercise increases, the muscle reaches a point where it can no longer perform the task with slow-twitch fibers alone. Then, fast-twitch fibers are called on as well. Since fast-twitch fibers can contract continuously for only short periods of time, the length of time that maximum muscle activity can be maintained is limited.

By contrast, the muscles of world-class athletes in some sports show a remarkable specialization of fiber types. For instance, world-class marathoners can have a slow-twitch muscle fiber content as high as 90 percent in the gastrocnemius muscle of the lower leg, whereas sprinters may have 25 percent slow-twitch fibers and 75 percent fast-twitch fibers in the same muscle. There is still some controversy over how much of this difference is innate and how much is acquired. On the one hand, it is known that for nonathletes, the relative proportions of the two types of muscle fibers are determined soon after birth and remain quite constant through life, though there is a tendency for slow-twitch fibers to increase in old age. However, it has also been found that if the nerves to a fast-twitch motor unit and a slow-twitch motor unit are switched in a laboratory, the muscle fibers will change to match themselves to the stimulation pattern of the new nerve. This raises the possibility that fiber content can be "trained" to meet the requirements of a particular sport. A number of studies of human athletes have found that muscle fiber type can be trained. For instance, sprint training increases the content of fast-twitch fibers, while heavy-resistance weight training tends to produce more slow-twitch fibers.

Effects of Exercise

Virtually all athletic activities require a combination of capabilities from the muscles, including strength, power, and endurance. Strength can be measured by determining the heaviest weight a person can lift once; it is best illustrated in a pure form by a weight lifting competition. *Power*, which is defined in physics as the product of force times velocity (power = force × velocity), is the explosive ability needed to hit a baseball or tennis ball hard; it can be determined by timing how fast a person lifts a heavy weight. *Endurance* is the ability to exercise at a high level for a long period of time; it can be measured by determining the maximum number of times a person can repeat an exercise requiring moderate strength.

Training

Training for sports is usually aimed at increasing muscular capacity in all three of these areas: strength, power, and endurance. Low-intensity aerobic training to improve endurance is excellent for the cardiovascular system, but it has little effect on muscle power or strength. To increase muscle power and strength, most athletes do some sort of high-resistance training such as weight training. Weight training increases muscle size predominantly by causing hypertrophy (making muscle fibers larger). It also may cause muscle fibers to split along their long axis so that a larger total number of muscle fibers results (hyperplasia).

Since the strength of a muscle correlates closely with its cross-sectional area, larger muscles are generally stronger muscles. Working out with weights and developing larger muscles, then, is usually a sign that strength is increasing. By the same token, when a limb is immobilized (as when a cast is used for a broken bone), the muscles become smaller (atrophy) and also become weaker. However, muscle size is not the only trainable factor with regard to muscular strength. The final "strength output" of a muscle results from the combined effect of the nervous system and the muscle itself. The neural factors include training, coordination, and some effects that are less well understood, such as the ability of the brain to call on more motor units and produce more muscle force under certain circumstances. Thus a variety of factors related more to the brain than directly to the muscle may affect strength and power. As athletes train, they should remember that they are training the entire body, not just the skeletal muscles.

Given this theoretical background, how should a training program be constructed to meet individual needs? Since different sports require different mixtures of strength, power, and endurance, it is certainly best to work with a coach or trainer to develop an exercise program tailored for a specific sport. However, some general rules probably apply to all people who exercise. Strength training can serve as an example (*see also STRENGTH TRAINING*).

To improve strength, it is necessary to practice strength training at least twice a week. The workouts should be well rounded, with a minimum of one set devoted to each muscle group. Each set should consist of 8 to 2 repetitions. A personal routine may vary considerably from this baseline minimum workout, though; much depends on individual goals, preferences, and lifestyles. In any routine, recovery time is vital for increases in strength; and the more intense the workout, the longer the recovery time must be. Regardless of details, a good strength workout regime will not only strengthen muscles but also thicken bones, strengthen tendons, decrease body fat, and increase muscle weight.

One attractive alternative to standard weight training is circuit resistance training (CRT). In CRT, 15 to 20 repetitions are performed on each of 8 to 12 exercises, using about 50 percent of the maximum weight the person can lift once for each exercise. The key to effective CRT is to allow only 15 seconds of rest between exercises. CRT can increase strength, particularly for people who have no previous weight training. It also increases aerobic fitness and endurance while burning a substantial number of calories. (It is important to note that no matter how much of a sweat is worked up in a weight room, standard weight training burns no more calories than walking on level ground.) In addition, in comparison with high-resistance weight training, the relatively low weights used in CRT put less stress on the muscles and tendons and thus may reduce the risk of injury. Finally, the compact nature of the workout is attractive to those with busy schedules.

Both women and men can benefit from strength training. The basic muscle tissue of women and men is identical, although on average women have smaller muscles and thus less muscle strength, particularly in the upper body. With weight training, women increase their muscle strength as much as men do. However, women do not develop the bulky muscles common in men who weight-train. One reason for this may be that the male sex hormone testosterone aids in muscle building and men have, on average, far higher testosterone levels than women do. The precise link between increased muscle mass with weight training and testosterone is somewhat obscured by the fact that the blood levels of this hormone vary over a fairly large range for both men and women. In general, women should not be discouraged if they do not show large increases in muscle size as a result of weight training. Some female athletes have doubled their strength through weight training programs with little effect on muscle size. This increased strength with little increased weight is particularly desirable in sports such as rock climbing and gymnastics where athletes lift their own body weight (*see also* FEMALE ATHLETES).

Exercise-Induced Pain

Virtually everyone who works out hard has experienced some soreness after exercise. The soreness felt during or immediately after exercise is known as acute muscle soreness. Acute muscle soreness is a result of an accumulation in the muscle of the products of glucose breakdown (such as lactic acid) and of an increase in acidity (decreased pH) within muscle cells. This type of muscle soreness usually decreases slowly over the course of several minutes.

Another type of muscle soreness is delayed-onset muscle soreness.

This is experienced 1 to 2 days after heavy exercise and may continue for several days. The cause of delayed-onset muscle soreness is not well understood, but structural damage to the muscle cell—including damage to the cell membrane and contractile filaments—may play a role. It is known that delayed-onset muscle soreness is most likely to occur after exercise in which the muscles lengthen under force, such as running downhill. Unfortunately, it is almost impossible to avoid this sort of activity completely during exercise. Delayed-onset muscle soreness can cause sufficient discomfort to force an athlete to curtail workouts until it resolves. To minimize delayed-onset muscle soreness, many athletes begin an exercise program with lower-intensity workouts and then gradually increase intensity.

Muscle cramps are uncomfortable involuntary contractions of skeletal muscles that can occur during intense exercise. Although cramps are usually not dangerous, they can force an athlete to drop out of an event. Muscle cramps are more common during hot weather than cool weather and may be related to blood imbalances of electrolytes (salts) caused by dehydration. Exhaustion and overheating can make a person more prone to cramps. Cramps can usually be relieved by rest, hydration, stretching the cramping muscle, massage, cold (in warm weather), or heat (in cold weather). Cramps can also occur at night, long after exercise is over. The calf muscles are notoriously susceptible to cramping at night. For reasons that are not well understood, some people seem to be more prone to cramps than others. If cramps persist, an athlete may need to analyze what specific activities bring on cramps and restructure workouts to avoid these situations. If the cramps continue, the athlete should consult a physician, since very stubborn cramps may be the sign of a more serious underlying medical problem.

A severe blow to a muscle can cause a muscle contusion, a bruise that leads to bleeding into the muscle tissue and muscle spasm. Muscle contusions can occur in any muscle and in many different sports. One of the more common sites for a muscle contusion is the quadriceps muscle on the front of the leg. Quadriceps contusions can occur during such sports as football and soccer, when one player's thigh strikes (or is struck by) another player. Quadriceps contusions can be quite painful, and a player may need to leave the game if the pain becomes so great that the muscle cannot be tightened. Prompt treatment by a skilled physician or trainer may include immobilizing the leg with the knee bent. The injured player may have to walk with crutches until light exercise can be performed without pain. Icing and passive exercise may be prescribed to speed the healing process. An athlete can safely return to play only when there is full range of motion in the leg and no residual pain or weakness.

David E. Harris, Ph.D.

References

Aronen, J., and R. Chronister, R. "Quadriceps Contusions." *Physician and Sportsmedicine* 20, no. 7 (1992).

McArdle, W., et al. *Exercise Physiology: Energy, Nutrition, and Human Performance*. Philadephia, Pennsylvania: Lea and Febiger, 1986.

McMahon, T. *Muscles, Reflexes, and Locomotion*. Princeton, New Jersey: Princeton University Press, 1984.

Stamford, B. "Muscle Cramps: Untying the Knots." *Physician and Sportsmedicine* 21, no. 3 (1993).

Vander, J., et al. *Human Physiology*. New York: McGraw-Hill, 1994.

Skeletal System

THE CONCERTED ACTION OF BONES, joints, and muscles directs all human movement; the three work together to operate a very efficient and effective system of motion and locomotion. This article will discuss the bones and joints; the associated musculature is covered in a separate article (*see SKELETAL MUSCLE*).

Any activity—running, jumping, throwing, lifting, swimming—requires its own variety of movements and creates its own stresses on the skeletal system. Over the short term and the long term, the skeletal system responds and adapts to these stresses. Adaptability has been designed into the human skeleton, so that structure affects function and function affects structure. In other words, the makeup of bone—its size, its strength, and its density—can affect and be affected by the tasks it has to perform. A good example of this adaptability was the legendary Australian tennis player Rod Laver in the 1960s: from years of playing tennis, the forearm bone and muscle were noticeably more massive and denser in Laver's racket arm than in his other arm. The same effect can often be observed in high jumpers: the takeoff leg is likely to be longer and stronger than the other leg. The skeletal system of a tennis player or a high jumper, subjected to continual stress, naturally adapts its structures to perform the necessary mechanical functions.

Many hereditary and environmental factors affect how the skeletal system responds and adapts to stresses in both the short term and the long term. One largely hereditary factor, for example, is physique: if parents and grandparents are "large-boned," children will probably be large-boned as well. One example of an environmental factor is, of course, gravity. In fact, gravity is the major determinant of a high jumper's adaptation. Every movement of the body is in some way influenced by gravitational forces, and the structural system develops in a way that will counter these forces. (Most people simply take gravity for granted, perhaps because they know only the environment of the earth, which exerts an attracting force of approximately 9.8 meters per second per second, m/s^2. Gravity would not be taken for granted if humans regularly made interplanetary trips: life would be much harder for humans on Jupiter, where body weight would be 2 1/2 times greater than it is on earth; and much easier on the earth's moon, where body weight is only about one-sixth what it is on earth. Also, a mature adult accustomed to the force of gravity would begin to grow again in zero-gravity space. Astronauts—at present the only space travelers—do come back from extended periods in zero-gravity space a few millimeters taller.)

Bone

The human skeleton consists of 206 bones, which serve many vital biomechanical and physiological functions. Although the 206 bones determine our dimensions, on average they account for only about 15 percent of total body weight. This section will examine several important aspects of bone, from its functions, anatomy, and physiology to bone fractures and their treatment.

Functions of Bone

The functions of bone are as follows:

1. Bone supports the body against loads imposed by gravity and by its own muscles.

2. Bone provides a framework for locomotion: levers for muscle to move.

3. The rib cage, skull, and spine protect the internal organs.

4. Bone serves as a reservoir for calcium, phosphate, and other vital minerals.

5. Bone marrow produces red blood cells.

As important as the mechanical and supportive functions of bone are, its physiological functions actually take precedence. The most important of these functions is to maintain the calcium levels in the blood. Bone, first and foremost, acts as a storage center for the nutritional needs of the body. As a camel's hump serves to store nutrients, human bones serve to store minerals. If the level of blood calcium falls, physiological demands will take over and calcium will be drawn from bone. Since calcium is an important structural component of bone, this depletion can be very detrimental to its mechanical and supporting functions. Bone is the last place to receive nutrients, but the first place the body goes to for replenishment.

Anatomy and Physiology of Bone

Skeletal composition: Bone and cartilage. The human skeleton lies beneath the soft tissues of the body. Two main tissues make up the skeleton itself: cartilage and bone. (The other tissues are joints and ligaments, both discussed later in this article.) Bone is rather hard and can withstand relatively little bending before it breaks. Cartilage, by contrast, is far more flexible, permitting a significant amount of bending. For example, costal cartilage is found at the ends of the ribs, which join onto the breastbone; and although it may seem insignificant, without it a gymnast would not have enough flexibility to perform deep arching back bends. In terms of both weight and volume, bone is much more prevalent than cartilage.

Bone consists of three materials: 40 percent (by weight) collagen, a rough matrix-like strengthening material; 30 percent mineral, predominantly calcium, but also phosphorus and salt; and the

BONE: STRUCTURE, LOCATION, AND FUNCTION

Type	Structure	Location	Function
Cancellous	Spongy porous matrix	Middle layers of flat bones and ends of long bones (e.g., pelvis and cranium)	Making blood
Cortical	Compact and dense	Outer layers of flat bones and shafts of long bones (e.g., leg and arm bones)	Supporting and protecting the body

Table 1.

remaining 30 percent water. It is primarily the mineral salts incorporated within bone that determine its hardness, and in turn its mechanical properties.

Cancellous and cortical bone. The human body has two types of bone: cancellous, or "spongy"; and cortical, or "compact" (*see Table 1*). Cancellous and cortical bones are made of the same materials; they differ in structure. Cancellous bone is spongelike and arranged in thin plates; cortical bone is denser and arranged in fiber bundles that generally run parallel to the long axis (loading direction) of the bone. The amount of these two tissues varies throughout the body and over the life span.

Cancellous bone is found in flat bones such as the pelvis (hip), vertebrae (backbone), and cranium (skull) and responds rapidly to changes in how we eat and burn energy. Although this less dense, spongy bone occupies a great deal of volume, it accounts for only about one-fifth of total bone mass. Cortical bone is designed to provide maximum strength and is found in the long bones of the leg and arm—the bones constantly under stress. A long bone (*see Figure 1*) has a hard outer layer consisting of cortical substance and a spongelike interior consisting of cancellous substance. Cortical bone evolved to withstand impacts, but cancellous bone did not; thus the body, especially as a person gets older, has more difficulty withstanding repeated heavy impacts (running, jumping, falling) to cancellous bone, such as the pelvis.

Growth and regeneration of bone. Unlike most other body tissues, bone is capable of growth and regeneration. As an example, consider a growing long—that is, cortical—bone (*see Figure 2*). Physiologists divide the long bone into two parts: the diaphysis is the main shaft, and the epiphysis lies at the ends. These sections are separated by the growth plate, which (as the term suggests) permits growth of the bone. The epiphysis serves two vital purposes: it is the location of the growth plate, and it acts as a cartilage cover, providing protection for the shocks and vibrations produced by movement (such as the movements that are common in sports). At the growth plate, the body actively generates cartilage. Cartilage is the firm but elastic connec-

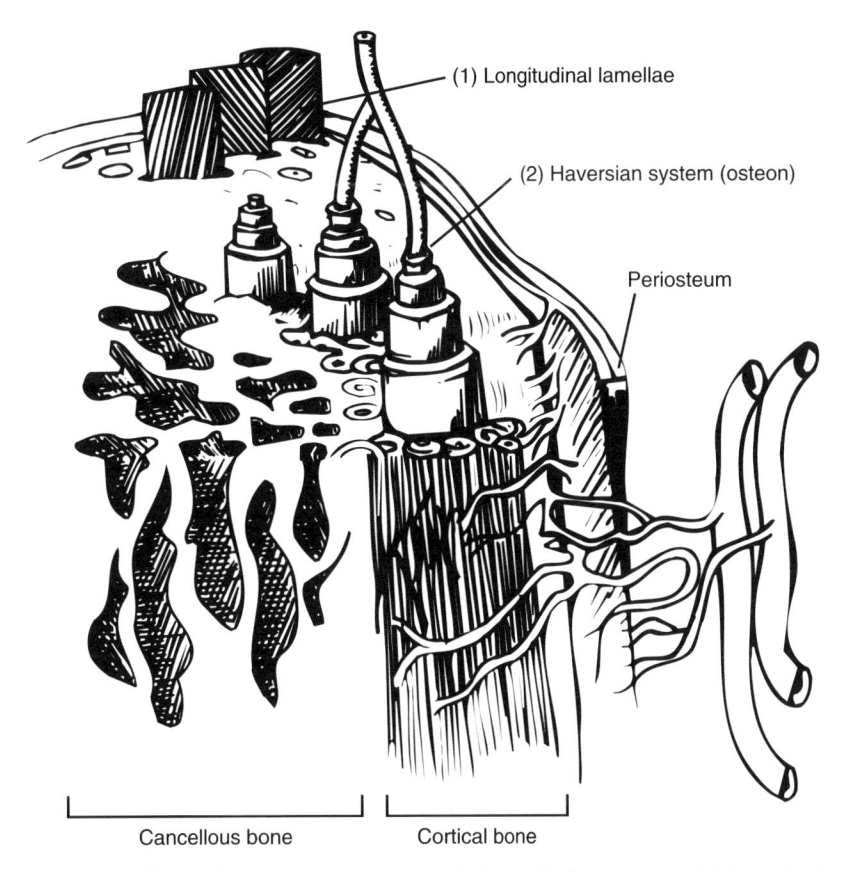

Figure 1. *Shown here is a cross-sectional view of a long bone. (1) Longitudinal lamellae. Tough collagenous fibers run in different directions in each layer, greatly strengthening bone. This pattern increases strength, much as a 2- by 2-inch laminated beam consisting of several strips of wood arranged in an overlapping pattern is stronger than a solid beam of the same size. The bone within the lamellae is made up of osteons. (2) Haversian system (osteon). Bone cells are arranged circularly in several layers around a haversian canal through which a small blood vessel runs to supply the layers with nourishment.*

tive tissue that develops into bone as cartilage-forming cells, called chondrocytes, are laid down in the interior of the growth plate.

The inner surface of bone is composed of porous tissue that becomes more and more compact (denser) as it matures; this maturation proceeds from the inside outward toward the surface. The periosteum, the special layer of connective tissue that surrounds the bone, carries blood to and from the bone. Similar internal tissue, called the endosteum, lines the inner surface of the bone. These tissues, vital in maintaining the strength and health of bone, provide a rich blood flow that brings nutrients to and removes wastes from the bone marrow. Both of these connective-tissue layers are fairly thick during childhood but slowly thin with age.

Regeneration of connective tissue—which consists of bone and cartilage—occurs in a special type of bone tissue that in turn consists of bone cells fixed in a matrix. Blood vessels transport nutrients to and from the bones in a continuous remodeling project, constantly forming new bone tissue as old bone is removed. The body effectively tears down and rebuilds the skeletal system roughly every 10 years. Because of this constant rebuilding, a nutrient-rich blood supply is vital.

Three "workhorse" cells are responsible for bone remodeling: (1) osteoclasts break down unneeded bone tissue; (2) osteocytes make up the healthy bone; (3) osteoblasts build new bone. Bone growth occurs when osteoblasts invade the cartilage matrix—a bone structure without calcium deposits (*see Figure 3*) Osteoblasts replace cartilage with bone cells starting in the center of the bone and spreading outward and toward the ends. New cartilage is laid down in the bone's interior by cells called chondrocytes. Replacement of cartilage with bone occurs by a process called ossification. (*Ossification* is the general term for the formation of new bone, both in the calcification of cartilage during the growth stage and in bone replacement during remodeling.) Bone and cartilage receive nourishment in different ways: bone receives its nourishment from blood vessels located within the bone; cartilage receives its nourishment from sources outside.

The growth plate, located near the end of each long bone, is the major determinant of the eventual length of the long bone (*again, see Figure 2*). The growth plate consists of layers of cartilage cells in different stages of maturity. The growth plate does not move; rather, it remains intact and gradually pushes outward from the bone shaft as it lengthens and widens. As bone cells mature, the bone continues to lengthen—until puberty, when the hormones signal the growth plate itself to convert to bone. The appearance of the growth plates, their closure (the point at which lengthening ceases), and the formation of bone vary, depending on a person's sex, hormonal state, and health, and on the person's history of bone injuries.

There are two periods of rapid bone growth: an initial spurt during the first 2 years of life, and then another spurt during puberty; this second spurt lasts several years for both sexes. Growth during puberty is greater for boys than girls; also, because boys begin puberty approximately 2 years later than girls, boys grow more before puberty. These two factors, in combination, account for the difference in average height between men and women.

Injuries to the growth plate during childhood and adolescence can result in significant problems. Because the growth plate is fragile during childhood, it can be prematurely closed by an injury, leading to deformity of the bone. If a child sustains an injury to the growth plate of the femur or tibia of one leg, premature closure may occur in that leg; potentially, then, one leg will be shorter than the other when the child reaches maturity. In that case, an unbalanced gait pattern (walking and running) results, which increases the risk of lower-body stress fractures and injuries to the knee and hip joints.

Bone grows not only in length but also in diameter. In fact, after the growth plate closes and a bone stops lengthening, it continues to expand in diameter until a person reaches the age of 25 to 30. For instance, the basketball superstar Karl ("The Mailman") Malone began as a skinny rookie in the NBA in 1984, at age 22, but became one of the league's biggest and strongest "wide-bodies" in the

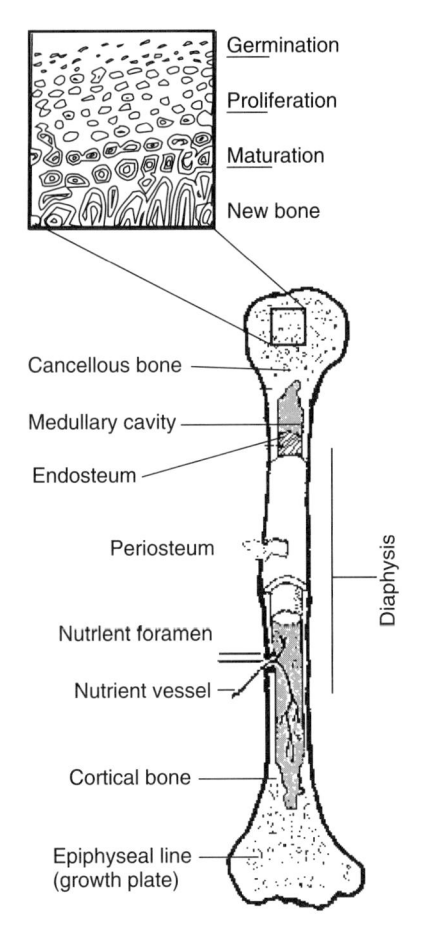

Figure 2. *Shown here is a long bone. The magnified view shows cell development from (top) embryonic cells to (bottom) mature cells.*

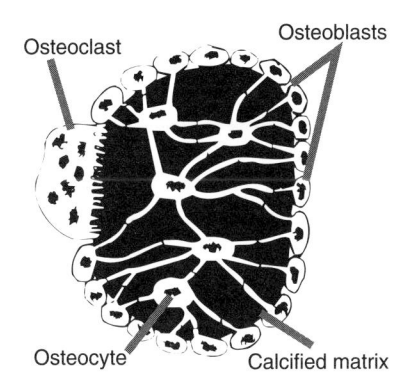

Figure 3. *Shown is a bone cross section. A continual process of remodeling takes place as osteoclasts "tear down" bone while osteoblasts "build" bone. Osteocytes connect with each other and osteoblasts through canals and form tight junctions.*

Hormonal Influences on Bone Mass

Increases: insulin, estrogen, testosterone, growth hormone.
Decreases: cortisol, parathyroid hormone, thyroid hormones.

1990s—a striking example of how much bone diameter can increase for athletes in their twenties.

The osteoclasts and osteoblasts work together to control bone thickness. As osteoblasts build new bone around the outside of the long bone, osteoclasts in the medullary cavity (marrow) break down and remove bony tissue. Bone becomes progressively thicker through adolescence. Once bone reaches its full size in late childhood to early adulthood, the growth plate closes, and a balance develops between bone formation (absorption) and destruction (resorption).

Hormones and bone. The endocrine system is one of two communication systems in the body (the nervous system is the other). Endocrine glands secrete a variety of chemicals called hormones. Hormones are chemical messengers that are released by internal and external stimuli, and they are carried by the blood from the endocrine glands to the cells on which they act. Several hormones affect bone growth: growth hormone, thyroid hormone, insulin, testosterone, and estrogen. These hormones promote bone lengthening by stimulating cell growth and division in the growth plate, which widens the plates for additional cartilage formation. For some reason (as yet unknown), the effects of hormones are not consistent over the course of a lifetime: a given hormone may stimulate growth at one stage in life but may have no affect at another stage. For instance, the thyroid hormone, estrogen (in females), testosterone (in males), and growth hormone stimulate growth in childhood and adolescence but are not a large factor in growth during infancy.

Excesses or deficiencies in growth hormone can create havoc. If the growing body does not produce enough pituitary growth hormone, which controls bone growth (among other things), dwarfism results. At the other extreme, an excess of pituitary growth hormone causes gigantism. Thyroid hormone is another hormone essential for normal bone growth throughout the life span. Decreased thyroid function limits the activity of osteoblasts and delays the closure of the growth plate. The sex hormones are also important in this regard: they affect growth and maturation and protect against the onset of osteoporosis (bone deterioration). Exactly how hormones affect bone is not completely understood. However, it is known that they serve two vital functions: first, at the molecular level hormones assist in the synthesis of collagen and other proteins; second, at the cellular and tissue level they help in bone matrix absorption and resorption.

Factors in the Health of Bones

Although the skeletal structure is primarily determined by genetics, it can, within limits, be modified by disease, nutrition, and exercise. The growth and health of bones are affected by hormones, adequacy of minerals (particularly calcium), vitamin D, protein supply, and activity. As noted above, bones store a tremendous amount of the body's minerals for use by the blood and muscles: 98 percent of the body's calcium, 40 percent of its sodium, and 30 percent of its potassium. From time to time, the body needs to draw on these stored nutrients, so it is important for the warehouse to remain amply supplied.

Genetics, bone density, and osteoporosis. Bone density usually follows a standard pattern over the life span. Bone mass continues to increase until age 25 and may even continue increasing well into the thirties before peaking. In children, the bones are supple and flexible, like young green twigs, but with age the internal architecture of bone changes. Aging (see *AGING AND PERFORMANCE*) brings on osteoporosis: a decrease in bone mineral content, increased porosity of the bone, and decreased resistance to fractures. Osteoporosis is a condition in which both bone matrix and minerals are being lost faster than they are being replaced. The activity of the osteoclasts outpaces that of the osteoblasts—in the end, eating away at bones as rust eats away at metals. As noted, the probability of fractures becomes greater, and healing of fractures becomes more difficult and lengthier. This is a major reason it becomes harder for top athletes to continue to compete at a very high level as they age, especially in contact sports like football and hockey. In general, significant osteoporosis is most often seen in the elderly, and it is much more common in women than men and in whites than blacks.

For years scientists have been searching for the cause of osteoporosis. In addition to environmental factors such as dietary calcium, exercise, and smoking, genetics plays a significant role. A team of Australian molecular biologists reported finding a genetic clue: two versions of a gene associated with varying bone density (Toufexis, 1994). The first version, called *b*, has been found in people with stronger skeletons; the second version, called *B*, has been found in people with weaker skeletons. The gene is not directly responsible for bone formation; rather, it provides blueprints for the construction of the receptors for a form of vitamin D that plays a crucial role in bone formation. Receptors are cell docking sites—highly specific points of attachment for certain molecules, in this case vitamin D (*see Figure 4*). Once vitamin D makes the connection, the receptors in a sense direct traffic by turning on and off other genes that regulate calcium absorption.

As had been suspected, whether a person develops osteoporosis depends on what version of the vitamin D receptor gene has been inherited. Inherited combinations can be *bb*, *Bb*, or *BB*. The combination *BB*—two genes for the trait—is worst: it represents a possible onset of osteoporosis as early as age 65. With one gene for the trait, *Bb*, onset will occur around age 69; with neither gene for the trait, *bb*, onset will occur at about age 76.

Individuals susceptible to osteoporosis can be identified through simple genetic screening and then treated (this is not the case with most genetic discoveries concerning incurable diseases). Changes in lifestyle, such as dietary changes, can be made to delay the onset of osteoporosis significantly. Moreover, the identification of this particular gene will speed the development of more effective treatments for the condition.

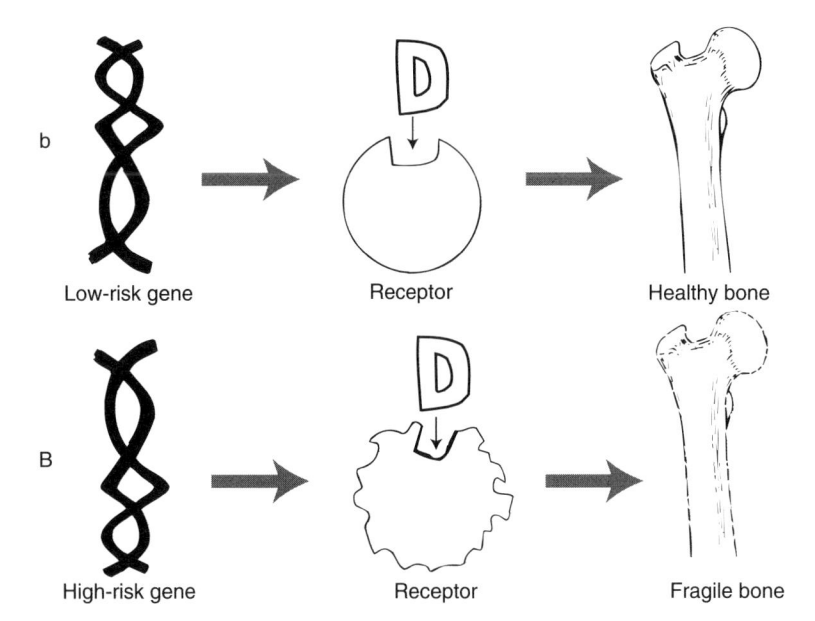

Figure 4. *Absorption of vitamin D is essential for the calcium absorption necessary to maintain healthy bones. People born with the gene mutation B are more likely to produce variant cell receptors—cells less capable of absorbing vitamin D. Inability to absorb vitamin D is a primary factor in the onset of osteoporosis.*

Older athletes who want to compete in contact sports, such as rugby, football, and ice hockey, should be made aware that bone mass and tensile strength begin to decline with age. Bone loss begins to exceed gains between ages 35 and 40. As the thickness of bone walls decreases, they are less able to withstand impacts. Therefore, it is important that coaches and trainers take age into consideration when they design sport training programs.

Diet. A good diet is the most important factor in maintaining healthy bones. And the most vital nutrient for bones is calcium. Consumption of calcium does not necessarily increase bone mass, but it has been found effective in slowing the loss of bone. Calcium provides bones with building material and serves as a calcium storage for the blood and muscle to draw on. If muscle tissues run low on calcium, the body draws calcium from the bones.

Other minerals can affect the body's use of calcium. For example, a diet including too much phosphorus—common among people who consume excessive amounts of high-phosphorus carbonated cola—can cause calcium loss. Even when a person ingests large amounts of calcium, it will not be absorbed if a high level of phosphorus is present. The reason for this remains unclear. However, scientists believe that phosphorus attaches to calcium as it circulates through the bloodstream. This can lead to an increased release of vitamin D and a subsequent increase in bone resorption.

Whereas phosphorus is detrimental to bones, vitamin D and sunshine are vital. Vitamin D is obtained in two ways: through the interaction between sunlight and a substance called 7-dehydrocholesterol that is found in the skin; and through ingestion of foods or supplements containing calcium. Because modern human beings wear clothing and spend less time outdoors, more and more people need to get vitamin D through their diet. The primary benefit of vitamin D is that it stimulates the intestine to actively absorb calcium ingested in food. A vitamin D deficiency decreases intestinal calcium absorption, which in turn results in lower levels of blood calcium. And, to repeat, when the body cannot get enough calcium from the blood, it will take calcium from the bones, compromising their mechanical and structural functions (*see also NUTRITION*).

Exercise. Activity, like genetics and diet, is an important factor in the health of bones, especially for the elderly. As a person ages, body fat usually increases, requiring the skeletal system to carry additional "dead" weight. At the same time, the body becomes more fragile as an increasingly smaller, more brittle skeleton must carry an ever greater weight.

Physical activity not only reduces fat but also helps the body retain skeletal mass. Like muscles, bones are made stronger as demands are placed on them. Exercise increases the stresses imposed on the bones by gravity and muscle tension; in turn, these forces stimulate greater osteoblastic activity. When a person who is out of condition begins to train strenuously, resorption might initially exceed absorption, causing overall bone loss. However, a gradual increase in training should result in a net calcium absorption after a few weeks, leading to bone building. Exercise also increases blood flow, and increased blood flow means that more nutrients—mainly minerals—arrive at the bone area that is experiencing the stress caused by exercise. Nutrients allow the osteoblasts to add needed mass and strength to that bone.

Total inactivity has the worst consequences for bone mass. In a sedentary person, the remodeling process of bone slows down, as the bone-demolishing osteoclasts outpace the bone-building osteoblasts. Studies of bedridden patients shows that bone loss begins shortly after immobilization. Patients experience a loss of nutrients and a decrease in the density of the outer wall of their bone, so that they are far more susceptible to injury. But if a patient begins rehabilitation therapy, bone mass increases almost immediately. Even people who are unable to exercise regularly should remember that mild exercise is better than none at all. Light activity may not increase bone mass, but at the very least it maintains bone mass. Movement through a full range of motion is also necessary to ensure that cartilage receives the nutrition necessary to remain healthy: cartilage depends on such movement for nourishment.

Many studies have shown that athletes who participate in running and jumping sports have greater bone density than both inactive people and people who participate in activities, like swimming, that place no weight load on the body (that is, little or no gravitational force). Impact from running and jumping helps increase the body's ability to absorb calcium. Scientists believe that rigorous running and jumping generate an electric potential in bone, which triggers a cellular response to increase bone remodeling. The skeletal system adapts to

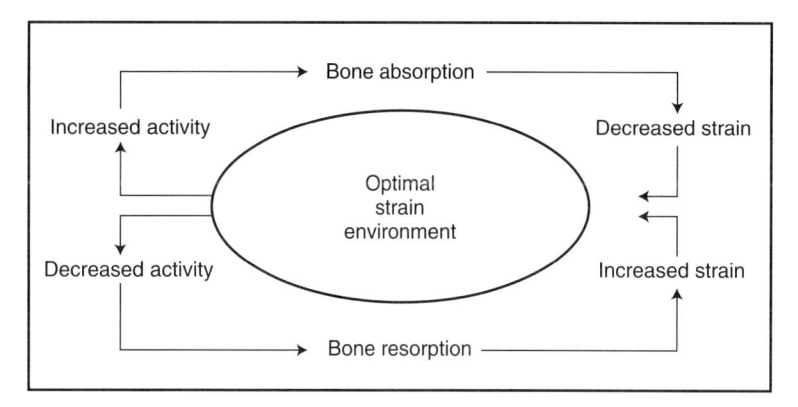

Figure 5. *Shown here is the process of bone absorption and resorption.*

gradually increasing loads without damage because bone remodels itself in response to the manner and magnitude of the loads imposed on it, just as the skin tans when exposed to small doses of sunlight but burns when exposed to strong sunlight for an extended period. Thus, bone remodeling is the body's natural way of matching structure to function (*see Figure 5*). Studies indicate not only the substantial benefits of exercise, but also the need to increase exercise gradually so that the skeletal system has time to adapt to new demands.

Bone Fractures

Of all sports, skiing is perhaps most often thought of in connection with broken bones. There is good reason for this. In a common scenario, a recreational skier, tired and sore by midafternoon after a day of strenuous skiing, decides to ski on anyway. This is when most accidents occur. Even if the skier decides on a very leisurely speed—say, 15 MPH (24 KPH)—a ski may jam against an immovable object like a mogul, twisting the skier's leg. The body pivots around the twisting leg and falls forward, in the direction of momentum, with great force. This twisting motion of the body around a planted foot can create tremendous force on the bones and joints of the lower body, often causing spiral fractures in the leg bones or severe damage to the knee joint.

Forces on bones. Skiing fractures, like most fractures, typically occur suddenly. Bone usually fractures when the dynamic impact of a fall is greater than the ability of the musculoskeletal system to cushion the impact. The dynamic forces involved (*see Figure 6*) come from gravity, from muscles, or from inertia—the tendency for a body in rest to stay at rest and for a body in motion to keep moving. Individually or in combination, these three forces are responsible for all sports-related stresses on bone.

The human body is an articulated system, a system of linked components. Muscles apply forces between these linked components; and because muscles act only in tension (rather than in compression and tension like bone), they always act in pairs to, say, rotate a knee joint

Bone Adaptation in Tennis Players

In a study of 35 tennis players who had active careers spanning several decades, a difference was discovered in the mineral content of their swinging and nonswinging arms (Huddleston, 1980). The mineral content of the radial (forearm) midshaft of the playing arm was, on average, 13 percent greater than that of the nonswinging arm. In an average adult male, the mineral content of bone in the dominant forearm is 6 to 9 percent higher than that of the nondominant forearm. Thus, these players' heavy use of the swinging arm had resulted in about twice the average difference in mineral content. Considering that a player makes thousands of impacts in one match, and that impact velocities exceed 100 MPH (160 KPH), this difference in mineral content would be expected.

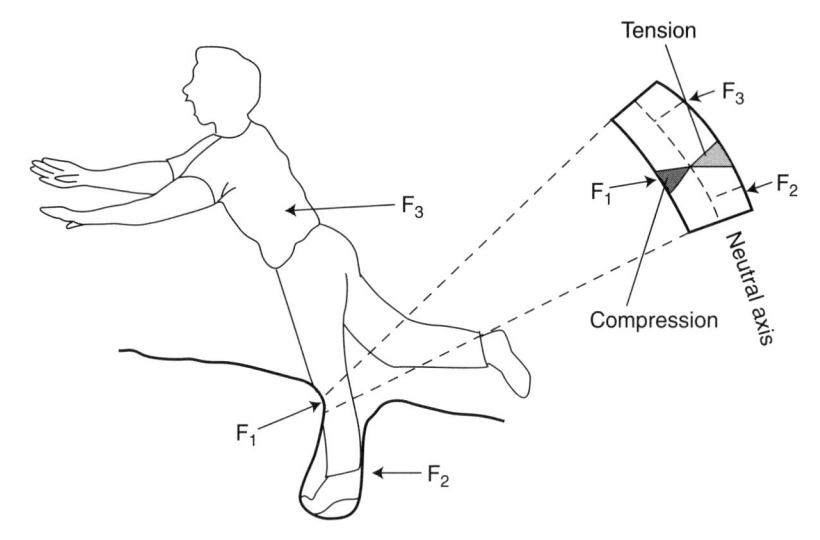

Figure 6. *Dynamics of a fracture are shown here. An accident bends a bone by creating tension on one side of it and compression on the other side. Because the tension strength of bone is 30 to 40 percent less than its compression strength (9×10^7 to 12×10^7 newton/meters versus 12×10^7 to 17×10^7 newton/meters), the fracture starts on the tension side and proceeds across to the compression side. The jogger in this illustration did not notice the hole; thus the autonomous reaction that might have prevented the fracture did not operate: the jogger did not contract the muscle of the lower leg to create a compression force to "pre-stress," or brace, for the oncoming tension force. (Adapted from Bachman, 1988)*

or an elbow joint. Gravity exerts an external force on each part of the body, proportional to the body's mass, resulting from its attraction by the earth. External forces caused by muscles and gravity are very straightforward; the external inertial forces involved are far more complicated.

To understand inertial forces, it is useful to consider the force caused by the wind. Wind can exert an external force on a body, a force no different from that of gravity or muscles. Any external force will cause a person to move unless movement is countered by some other external force—a floor that prevents further descent, for instance, or friction between shoes and floor that prevents linear motion. Wind is often not thought of as a force, because it is usually countered: the friction of a floor, say, will prevent a change in a person's state of motion. However, on a nearly frictionless surface, the force of wind becomes apparent; if an ice skater is standing still on a frozen pond, a strong enough wind will cause a change in state of motion: the skater will be whisked along in the direction of the wind.

Because the body has mass, it opposes changes in its state of motion by a dynamic or inertial force, which is equal and opposite to the net applied external force. In the case of wind, the force that the body exerts on a wind stream is balanced by the inertial force of the wind stream because the wind's state of motion is changed; here, then, two equal and opposite dynamic or inertial forces interact. In the case of one person pushing another across a floor, the inertial force of the person being pushed is equal to the external force applied by the person doing the pushing. What these two examples show is that the inertial force is just like any other force. According to D'Alembert's principle, the sum of all forces acting on a body, including the dynamic or inertial force, must always be zero. Thus if the sum of all identifiable external forces is zero, the inertial force must be zero and the state of motion of the body is unchanged. Because the direction of the inertial force is always opposite to that of the acceleration of the body, a dynamic (three-dimensional) problem is actually a static (two-dimensional) problem. How these external forces interact with muscles, tendons, and bones during athletic maneuvers has a great bearing on injury. Fractures become likely when forces are severe, or when bones and joints experience large external forces from multiple directions.

To take a specific example, the muscles, tendons, and bones in the arm are unlikely to fail when a gymnast hangs from a bar because hanging exerts a sustained gravitational and inertial force (nonabrupt loading) on the arm and shoulders. By contrast, the risk of a fracture increases substantially when the gymnast is performing fast-moving complex maneuvers, such as swinging around the higher uneven bar and then wrapping the lower body around the lower bar. The gravitational and inertial forces that accelerate the gymnast downward develop a great amount of linear momentum and necessitate a tremendous countering force on the arms and shoulders as the hips circle around the low bar. The gymnast experiences great inertial forces because the hips and upper body come to rest abruptly, yet the inertia of the lower body continues on as it wraps itself around the low bar. And the greater the mass of the lower body, the greater the force created at the shoulders and arms. Fortunately, the bars are designed with a fair amount of flexibility so that the impact force at the hips occurs over an extended period, thereby reducing the force the shoulders and arms must absorb.

Because athletic competition involves achieving optimal performance through mostly complex movements, athletes must continually contend with large forces that exceed the limits of safety set by nature. For various reasons—poor timing, bad footing, unexpected collisions—athletes incur a risk of fractured bones and dislocated joints every day. The breaking force, for the most part, correlates with the thickness of the bone. The thick femur (thighbone) can withstand a much greater force than the thinner fibula in the lower leg. At the same time, however, the fibula can withstand greater twisting forces (Evans, 1970).

Overall, the greater the body's bone and muscle mass, the greater its ability to absorb shock. Therefore, a larger person can better withstand impact and twisting and is less likely than a smaller person to fracture a bone.

Strength, stiffness, and fractures. As noted earlier, bone accounts for only 15 percent of total body weight—an amazingly small percent-

The Dynamics of Breaking a Bone

Up to its breaking point, bone will deform (bend) a measurable amount as stress is increased. A skier who falls can easily break a bone because the ski acts as a lever (much like a long pipe wrench). A force as small as 25 to 35 pounds (110 to 155 newtons) at the end of a ski creates between 100 and 150 pounds of force (445 to 665 newtons) at the tip of the boot. Torque of 25 pounds applied at 3 feet or 75 pounds at 1 foot is the same as 150 pounds of torque applied at the top of the boot (0.5 ft.).

age relative to the impact it is expected to absorb. Ounce for ounce, bone is stronger than steel or reinforced concrete; actually, since it is both light and strong, it is more like the "high tech" composite materials used in tennis rackets. But although bone is one of the strongest natural materials, fractures can occur when forces—usually a loading (compression) force and a twisting force—act on it in combination. The ability of bone to support weight or withstand strain depends on its mass and on the quality of the bone material itself.

Bone is a material with *viscoelastic* properties, a term meaning that the strain it can absorb depends on its elasticity as well as its strength. Bone does indeed possess the elastic properties of a spring and the absorbing properties of a sponge. Its tensile strength is like cast iron, yet under stress it exhibits plasticity: it can flex like the fiberglass battens in a boat sail that give the sail its characteristic stiff, bowed-out shape in a wind.

This combination of tensile strength and plasticity determines how much strain bone can absorb before fracturing. Structurally, the collagenous component of bone is responsible for resisting tensile (pulling) stresses, and the mineral component is responsible for resisting compression (pushing) stresses. The greater the mineral content of bone, the greater its hardness, compressive strength, and rigidity. However, a greater mineral content also makes bone more brittle. Brittle materials exhibit minimal elasticity, and thus they fracture under a relatively small strain. It should be noted that it is not the energy stored in the bone but rather the limiting value of strain that determines whether or not a bone will fracture. Although strength and strain are connected, the strain limit is more important because a large energy storage is a by-product—a consequence—of a larger strain limit. (Strong but brittle bones have little capacity to store energy.)

Calcium and phosphate are the minerals most responsible for giving bone its hardness; organic materials, like collagen, give bone its elasticity. The ratio between mineral and organic material in bone is 1:1 at birth but 7:1 at age 60 to 70. As a result, the bones are supple and flexible during youth but become more and more brittle with age. This in part explains why the twenties are the peak years for athletes in impact sports. A young athlete's skeletal system has the best balance of minerals and organic materials and thus is strong yet flexible.

The bones of a child are perfectly elastic in that they deform when subjected to a large strain and then return precisely to the original shape when the stress is removed; they are soft yet have an exceptional ability to strain (*see Figure 7*). The bones of an adult, by contrast, are stiff and yield a small strain for a large stress; moreover, they have a very small value of strain at which, when deformed, they will never return to their original shape. A useful analogy here is a steel rod. If stretched within limits, the rod always returns to its original shape. However, if stretched beyond a given limit, it exhibits a certain plasticity while sustaining the load, but now returns—at no load—to a new, stretched length. Stress fractures in bone occur sim-

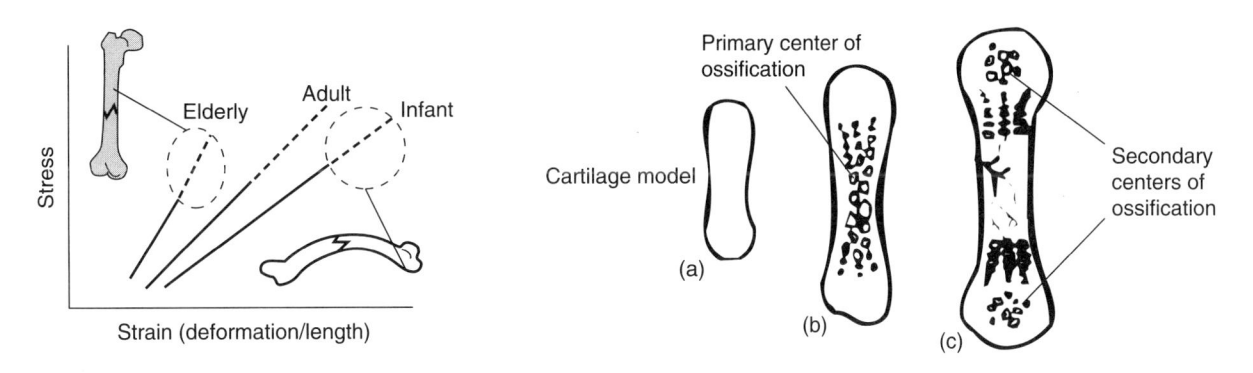

Figure 7. *Left: This yield curve shows the stress and strain characteristics of bone with age, in terms of the shape of bone at the point of fracture. Right: Shown here is bone formation during gestation and in the early years of life. Ossification begins (b) from the primary centers before birth, and (c) from the secondary centers during the first 5 years of life. The high organic content of a youngster's bones gives tremendous flexibility. With age, organic content is replaced by mineral content, so that the bones become progressively more brittle and can take less strain.*

ilarly when bone is damaged but there is not a complete fracture (*see below; see also ARCHERY and EQUIPMENT MATERIALS*).

In addition to the limits imposed by the material makeup of bone, there are limits imposed by tension strength and compression strength. Tension strength and compression strength are not the same. Bone, like concrete, is much stronger in compression than in tension. The compression force experienced by a 200-pound (91-kg) person jumping from a height of 3 feet (0.9 m) can usually be easily absorbed, but if a force of this same magnitude occurs as a tension force, the probability of a bone fracture is very high (*refer back to Figure 6*).

Muscles play a significant role in determining the amount of stress bone can absorb without fracturing (*see Figure 8*). As noted above, muscles always act in pairs because they contract but cannot elongate; for example, a contraction of the triceps must take place in association with a contraction of the biceps. All movement of the articulated body structure is predicated on muscles acting in pairs. These pairs also create pre-tension compression forces—interactions between muscle and bone that increase the stress bone can withstand. Muscles have a unique built-in function: an ability to "pre-stress" bone, bracing it for an oncoming impact (*again, refer back to Figure 6*). When muscle exerts compression stress on a part of the bone that is about to receive tension, the amount of tension absorbed by the bone increases proportionally. Great athletes are acutely aware of where a tension force will occur, and they instinctively create a compression force in that area. In essence, it is not primarily the bulk of muscle that prevents impact injuries, but the ability of muscle to create "pre-tension" compression forces. Still, muscle mass is also important: the greater the muscle bulk, the greater the potential to create pre-tension compression forces.

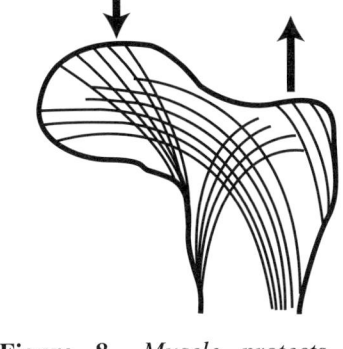

Figure 8. *Muscle protects the skeletal system by exerting a force opposite to the stress or load.*

Typical fractures. Doctors define a *fracture* as any break in a bone. Fractures range in severity from a simple crack to a shattering so

Bone Deformities

Researchers have found a common genetic mutation for almost all inborn abnormalities of the skeletal system, including Jackson-Weiss syndrome (in which the big toes point out toward each other like the thumbs), Crouzon syndrome (premature fusion of skull plates), and dwarfism. This common mutation causes a growth factor receptor to assume a very specific aberrant form (Angiers, 1994).

severe that it results in multiple fragments. Depending on the severity of the impact force, the fracture sight may be smooth (slow-loading) or rough (fast-loading).

Three major forces put stress on the bones and joints of the body (*see Figure 9*). (1) A *compression force* shortens (compacts) and widens bone. Compression is the force experienced in running or in landing from a jump. (2) A *tension force* is a force in the opposite direction that lengthens and narrows bone. Tension is the force experienced by a gymnast suspended from a high bar. (3) A *shear force* occurs when one part of the bone slides over another as a result of a blow. Often, bone is subjected to some combination of these forces.

Forces exerted on bone as a result of external loads generally are small in comparison with the compressive loads that occur in takeoffs and landings during jumping, or in comparison with bending loads from lateral impacts or external torque like that associated with skiing. In bending, there is increasing tension out to the bone filaments farthest from the neutral axis on the convex side, and similar compression on the concave side. Depending on the cross-sectional shape, there is a uniform shear too. Failure usually occurs in tension or on the convex side but may occur as shear—similar to the way a tree limb breaks off during a storm. Different fractures occur as a result of these different forces; the five major categories doctors use to describe fractures that result from different combinations of compression, tension, and shear forces are (1) transverse; (2) impact, (3) spiral or oblique, (4) greenstick, and (5) comminuted (*see the box "Different Types of Fractures Occur as a Result of Different Forces"*).

With fractures, as with most injuries, individuals heal at different rates. The rate of healing is determined primarily by age and heredity, but diet and environment are also factors. Healing begins as blood gathers around the break and forms a clot; this blood clot fills

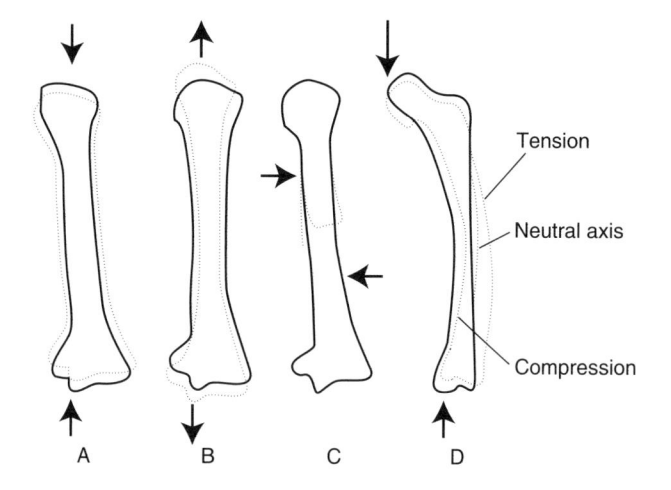

Figure 9. *The arrows indicate forces acting on the bone: A = compressive stress (shortening and widening). B = tensile stress (lengthening and narrowing). C = shearing stress (severe). D = bending where there is both tension (T) and compression (C). (Adapted from Adrian, 1989)*

the void in the bone and acts as the basis for new bone. Within a few hours, osteoclast and osteoblast cells start to move into the blood clot. While the osteoclasts break down (resorb) bone in the fractured area—dissolving jagged edges and preparing bone for rebuilding—the osteoblasts begin to form the matrix of future bony tissue in the clot. Calcification of the matrix follows, while the clot is slowly absorbed by the body. Calcification creates cartilage, which in time becomes bone.

In recent decades, doctors, trainers, scientists, and engineers have been developing new and better ways to treat bone trauma (injury), and they will surely continue to develop even better ways. These professionals are gradually gaining a more complete understanding of how injuries occur and are constantly refining treatment techniques. In addition to improved methods of diagnosing and treating typical fractures, advances will certainly be made in bone grafts and in artificial limbs and joints; eventually, new biotechnology (such as biomaterials, genetically engineered hormones) may further expand the range of treatment options. At present, two techniques of particular interest are electric stimulation and bone grafts.

Electric stimulation. There has been increasing use of electric stimulation to treat "nonunion" fractures—fractures that are not healing properly—and to speed healing in general. This therapy is useful for people prone to be slow healers, and for certain fractures that generally do not heal well, such as tibia fractures.

Electric stimulation is based partly on the fact that the ability of bone to heal itself depends directly on the adequacy of the blood supply to the injured area. A doctor or physical therapist can attach electrodes to a fractured bone and direct an electric current across the fracture, to try to stimulate increased blood flow. With an increased supply of nutrients, osteoblasts can work more effectively to build bone.

An electric current can also switch regional tissue from an "off," or dormant, state to an "on," or healing, state. The collagen in bone accounts for its negative and positive piezoelectric properties. Something that is piezoelectric responds to applied pressure by generating an electric potential. Electric potential is the kind of energy created by a battery—in this case, a very weak battery. It naturally increases and decreases with changes in the stress on bone. A common trait of nonunion fractures is a loss of electronegativity (polarity). Thus, implanting negative electrodes in the gap of a nonunion fracture may cause new bone to form near the negative electrode, where bone would otherwise remain dormant rather than growing.

A full understanding of what goes on during electric stimulation is still in the future, however. It is hoped that as more is understood about electric stimulation, supplemental biological and biochemical treatments designed for use in conjunction with such stimulation will produce improved results.

Bone grafts. Orthopedic surgeons sometimes have problems treating severe bone fractures because the patient's damaged bone tissue

Different Types of Fractures Occur as a Result of Different Forces

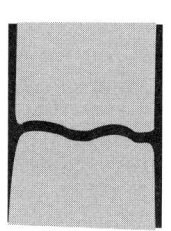

Transverse fractures. These usually occur at a right angle (perpendicular) to the length of the bone. A direct outside blow, such as a football helmet striking the humerus (long bone of the upper arm), often causes this injury. These fractures can result in internal damage to vital blood vessels and nerves.

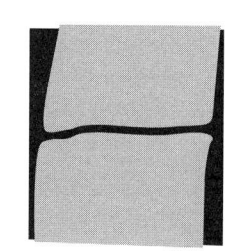

Impact fractures. These usually result from compression forces from a fall from a height. For example, when a gymnast comes off the high bar in an unbalanced position, a long bone like the femur can receive a force of such magnitude on landing that the tissue is compressed, so that one part of the bone hits the other.

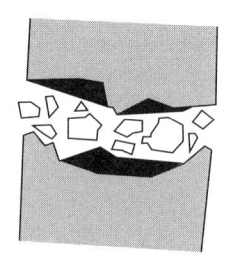

Comminuted fractures. In these, bone splinters or breaks into many pieces—usually three or more fragments. Hard blows or falls are the most common causes. Comminuted fractures can be very difficult to heal because the great compression forces displace bone fragments, and soft tissue can come between fragments, preventing them from knitting back together.

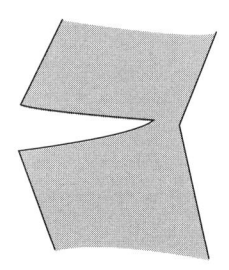

Greenstick fractures. These occur in the more flexible bones of young children, such as the collarbone. They are incomplete breaks in which a bone is partly broken and partly bent. Injured bone looks frayed.

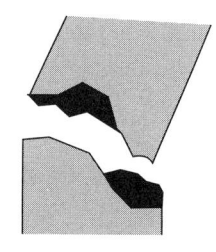

Spiral or oblique fractures. These have a curved or S-shape separation. They occur from torsion forces: when one end of the bone is fixed and the other receives a twisting motion. Often a skier or football player sustains this injury when a foot is fixed or planted and the body is suddenly rotated in another direction.

no longer retains its ability to repair itself. In these cases, surgeons must turn to bone grafts. Bone grafts are pieces of the patient's own healthy bone, usually segments from the pelvis, applied to major breaks to promote healing. Bone grafting usually begins by implanting fresh bone in the fracture to stimulate the osteoclasts to remove dead fragments, and the osteoblasts to deposit new matrix material. In essence, grafts "wake up" and "urge on" the healing process.

Survival of a bone graft depends on establishing blood flow from the surrounding tissue; and because adequate blood flow cannot be guaranteed, there is a high degree of uncertainty over whether a bone graft will "take." To improve the success of bone grafts, researchers have been attempting to increase blood flow into the bone substance by implanting blood vessels from other parts of the body into the fracture. This process, called vascularized bone grafting, has had some very promising results. Blood flow into bone may be introduced by implanting blood vessels with the bone graft in what is called a vascularized fibular graft.

Stress fractures. One universal tenet of exercise physiologists is that harder and harder training is the only way to improve the aerobic performance of distance runners. However, this continual pushing comes at considerable cost: it usually leads to severe muscle fatigue, and to an altered stride pattern. Distance runners with a high threshold of pain—and those caught up in the excitement of a race—are able to block out pain in the lower leg, even though the more they run, the more it hurts. Thus it is usually not until later that they discover the source of their pain: "bone fatigue" failure of the tibia. This scenario is common among runners, and the tibia is one of the most common sites of "bone fatigue"—more commonly called a *stress fracture*.

A stress fracture is a series of tiny microscopic cracks in bone. It can occur at any of various sites (*see Figure 10*), and it hurts only when forces from gravity or muscles create stress on the injured area. The exact causes of stress fractures are not yet known, but these fractures probably result from one or more of the following: rhythmically repetitive stress; change in ground reaction force (such as changing a running route from grass to concrete); increased bone stress due to muscle fatigue; an altered running pattern; and disregard of pain.

Muscle fatigue seems to be a particularly important factor; in this case, the process of bone remodeling is outpaced by the fatigue process. Fatigued muscles are less capable of storing energy and supporting bone against stress as the runner's feet pound the pavement. When tired muscles fail to carry their intended load, the skeletal system absorbs more of the shock, and this can lead to stress fractures.

Another apparently prevalent factor in stress fractures in the legs is an altered running pattern. For instance, fatigue or injury may cause a person to favor one leg over the other; before long, the constant abnormal loading on the favored leg leads to a stress fracture.

Ignoring pain is also a probable factor. Individuals have different "thresholds" of pain, and athletes with a high threshold—that is, a high tolerance of pain—are much more likely to suffer from stress fractures. Many world-class athletes hold such concepts as "No pain, no gain" and "If it doesn't hurt, you're not doing it right": that is, they believe that they are not training hard enough unless the training hurts. What often happens in such cases is that ignoring pain leads to an injury which forces the athlete to stop anyway.

A related phenomenon is overuse injuries. Like stress fractures, overuse injuries occur because of a gradual breakdown of the skeletal system. A good analogy is overstressed steel: as with steel, a cer-

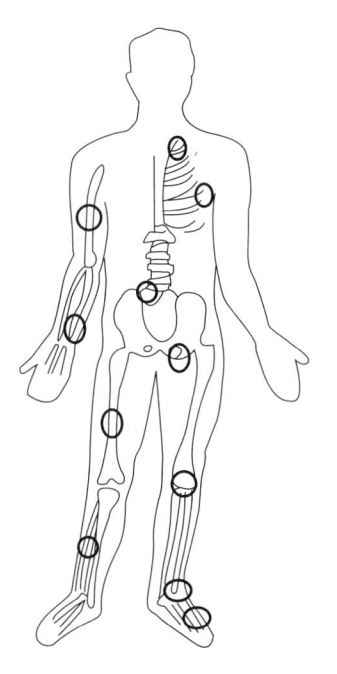

Figure 10. *Circles indicate common sites of stress fractures. Foot and shinbone are most common among runners; hips among dancers and gymnasts; and lower spine among weight lifters and field athletes.*

tain level of stress can be absorbed by the body, but an overload progressively weakens the tissues. The skeletal system can hold on for a while, but gradually it loses its ability to compensate for the overload. Finally, structural failure occurs, sidelining an athlete for several weeks.

Exercise physiologists have found that the first few weeks of training are critical with regard to bone (Stanitsky, 1978). During this time, weight-bearing bones undergo bone resorption and become weaker before they become stronger. Increased muscular forces and an increased rate of remodeling lead to greater bone resorption than absorption, producing progressively more severe stress fractures. It takes approximately 2 weeks of slowly increasing the rigor of training before bone starts to become stronger—that is, to reach the point where the process of absorption overtakes resorption. When an exercise training program begins, bodily self-regulation directs bone building, to ensure that the strains of increased exercise do not lead to fracture. This does not occur overnight, however; it may take a few weeks. For this reason, athletes should increase the length and intensity of workouts slowly and should closely monitor changing conditions and their own changing habits.

Coaches, of course, would like to know just how hard they can push their athletes without causing harm. Research has found one clue: hydroxyproline, an amino acid used in the digestion or decomposition of protein. By testing 104 Navy "Seals" who were undergoing a period of vigorous training, researchers found a link between high initial hydroxyproline levels and bone and joint injuries sustained later, during rigorous training (Marguia, 1988). They reported that among those who suffered bone or joint injuries (10 percent of the participants), the level of hydroxyproline was 29 percent greater at the onset of injury than it was among those who were not injured. Someday, athletes undergoing rigorous training may regularly have their hydroxyproline levels monitored and, if the level is high, may moderate their training programs to reduce the risk of injury. With some idea of what their limit is, athletes could push themselves to that limit without fearing injury.

Preventing Stress Fractures

1. Build up a workout schedule gradually and slowly. Do not overtrain.

2. Allow sufficient time to train properly for a second sport between seasons, such as moving from volleyball in the winter to track and field in the spring.

3. Remain aware of any changes in habits or conditions—such as new shoes, an altered running pattern from an injury like turf toe, or a different running surface—and adjust training to adapt to this change.

Joints

Activity—movement—occurs when muscles, working in pairs, contract and relax to pull various bones. But without joints, the skeletal system could not function; it would not be able to move. Effective functioning of the joints, in turn, depends on the coordinated action of many of them. This section considers how joints work.

Structure and Function of Joints

Joints give the skeletal system mobility. It is useful to think of bones as levers, and of joints as pivot points that control those levers:

Accelerating Bone Repair: Bone Morphogenetic Proteins

Bone morphogenetic proteins, or BMPs—proteins that promote bone growth—may be the next important medical innovation, allowing treatments that "turn on" the regenerative mechanism in bone, so that the bone can heal itself. BMP acts like a switch, activating surrounding cells and directing them to become chondrocytes: cartilage-forming cells. The cartilage formed will gradually harden into new bone tissue (*see the figure*). Some proponents of BMP call it a "bone graft in a bottle."

Eventually, there may be a multitude of uses for BMP, but its first application will probably be as a treatment for nonhealing ("nonunion") bone fractures. Treatment would proceed something like this. First, doctors would remove the shattered bone fragments, leaving a gap between the remaining parts of the bone. This gap would be treated with BMP, which switches regional tissue from an "off," or dormant, state to an "on," or healing, state. Cells from healthy bone around the fracture attract the bone proteins, which bind the receptors on the surface of these cells. Slowly the gap fills with cartilage. Even with severe fractures, the new bone—in time—takes on the same shape and structure as the original bone.

The most likely uses for BMP will be traumatic nonunions, delayed unions, spinal fusions, reconstructive surgery, and implant surgery. BMP could eventually replace cements for implant surgery, securing artificial joints to bone by growing bone around them. Beside the surgical use of BMP, doctors might inject BMP to speed the repair of simple breaks, prescribe a BMP pill to prevent osteoporosis, or even prescribe a pill for athletes preparing to start a rigorous training schedule. Another use may be to prevent stress fractures in fracture-prone athletes engaged in rigorous continuous-impact sports such as long-distance running.

Special BMP treatments may even be developed for collision sports like football. Studies have found that a disproportionate amount of bone trauma occurs in the first few weeks of practice. During this time, when bone absorption has not yet caught up to bone resorption, the skeletal system is particularly susceptible to injury. A BMP pill taken a few weeks before preseason training might prepare the skeletal system for the daily punishment that will be inflicted on it.

A BMP pill also might allow elderly athletes, especially women, to compete more effectively. BMPs may reduce an injured athlete's time on the "disabled list": BMP injections might possibly be used to speed up recovery time for a fracture from 2 months to 2 weeks. Perhaps the day is not far off when fans will be less concerned about a superstar quarterback's tibia (shinbone) fracture, midway through the NFL season, because they feel confident that he will be back in plenty of time for the playoffs.

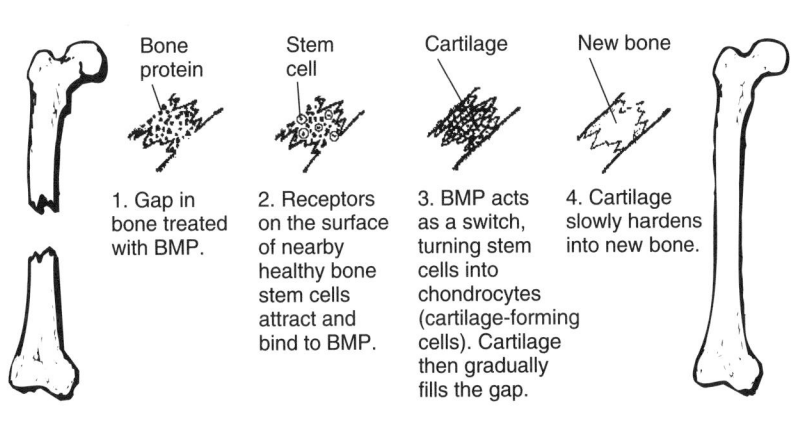

Bone morphogenic protiens (BMPs) repair bones following these steps: (1) gap in bone treated with BMP; (2) receptors on the surface of nearby healthy bone stem cells attract and bind to BMP; (3) BMP act as a switch, turning stem cells into chondrocytes (cartilage-forming cells) and cartilage then gradually fills the gap; (4) cartilage slowly hardens into new bone.

each joint in the human body is the pivot point of a particular lever. Joints also give the skeletal system stability; in fact, while some joints primarily provide mobility, others mainly provide stability. The greater the mobility—or range of motion—of a joint, the less its stability, or resistance to displacement. Because of their wide array of mobilizing and stabilizing functions, joints take many forms, evolved specifically to serve the attached limbs (*see the box "The Six Types of Joints"*).

Joint stability is chiefly determined by ligaments, tendons, the shape of the bone structure, and forces on the joint (muscle tension is an additional factor). Ligaments are the strong, flexible elastic tissues that attach ends of bones together and control limb movement within a normal range. Accessory ligaments, such as the cruciate ligaments in the knee, give added strength to a joint. Tendons, made of a similar elastic tissue, attach muscle to bone. The tendons of muscles that overlap joints serve the same purpose as the ligaments: any contractile force applied by the overlapping muscle generates a pulling force parallel to the long axis of the bone, thereby naturally increasing joint stability. One crucial objective of strength training is to increase the strength of the muscle tendons that pass over joints in order to increase joint stability and decrease the risk of joint sprains and dislocations (*see* STRENGTH TRAINING).

The main purpose of stretching before physical activity is to loosen up the tendons and ligaments. Loosening up tendons and ligaments increases range of motion, thus decreasing the risk of injury. However, ligaments can be overstretched. Like an overstretched rubber band, ligaments subjected to constant loads may undergo excessive lengthening and become unable to recoil to their original shape and size. (Cartilage too may become excessively deformed if it is subject to constant compressive forces.) Therefore, a ligament injury generally impairs athletic performance, even with the best treatment and rehabilitation. For example, an injury to the arm ligaments often means that a pitcher or a quarterback will not be able to throw as hard; and an injury to the knee ligaments usually means that a running back will not be able to run quite as fast. Ligaments, then, although they must be flexible enough for mobility, should also be strong enough for stability, to help prevent dislocation.

The structure of the joint itself also affects its stability. A negative pressure, or vacuum, exists within the joint that helps to hold the bones together (Steindler, 1970). The hip joint, for instance—even in a cadaver—cannot be pulled apart until a hole is drilled into the joint cavity to release the suction. Because of differences in shape and size, the stability of joints varies. For example, the deep socket at the hip joint gives it much greater inherent stability (due to suction) than the shallow socket at the shoulder joint. A narrow space, called a joint cavity, permits easy movement so that the muscles can move the joint while stability is still maintained.

Although the forces acting on joints are quite complex, especially when multiple segments are involved, there are two major types of forces: translational and rotational. Translational forces affect the ability of an object to move along the straight line of a force. Rotational forces tend to pivot a limb about the supporting joint and thus are a function of muscular strength available for moving or rotating the joint. Both kinds of forces can produce injuries. For instance, an action as

Muscle Can Cause Injury

World-class skiers sometimes sustain a little-understood joint injury while airborne with the knees flexed: the anterior cruciate ligament (ACL) in a knee tears. When a skier is moving a high speed and then is suddenly airborne, the autonomous "preemptive" muscle force on the bones and joints—generated to counter the effects of forces generated by gravity on the body—remains in effect. During flight, without the countering gravitational forces, muscles continue to create tremendous compression forces that can tear the ACL.

The Six Types of Joints

There are six major types of joints. Joints usually fit well together; and even when they do not, surface irregularities are usually evened out by extra layers of fibrocartilage. Muscles supply force, and bones are levers, but it is the joints that permit movement, usually as an axis of rotation.

The physics of levers explains why people with similar physical characteristics (such as size, weight, and age) have different abilities to generate power. If, for instance, one person has higher calf muscles than another, this in effect lengthens the lever that extends from the ankle, giving it more power-generating capacity. All else being equal, then, an athlete with higher calf muscles will probably be able to jump higher. This same principle explains why it is easier to turn a nut with long-handled wrench than a shorter one.

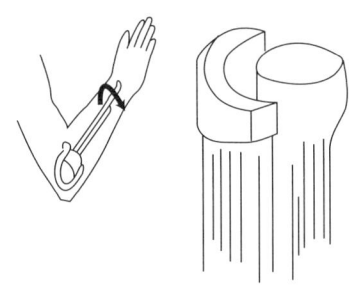

Pivot. Allows rotating movements in one plane—turning the head, for example.

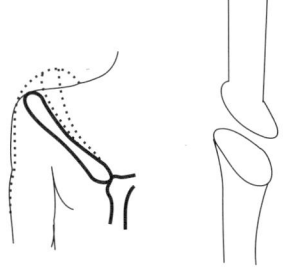

Gliding. Allows movements in one plane—when lifting the hands and feet, for example.

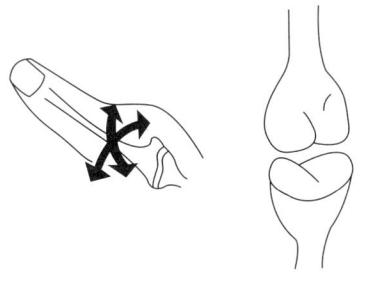

Saddle. Allows movements in two planes (biaxial)—the thumb is an example.

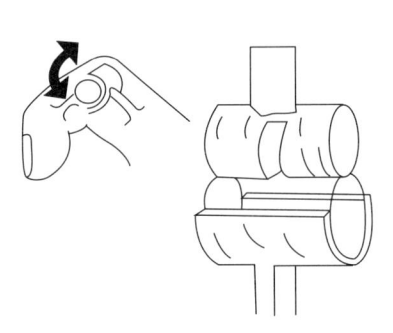

Hinge. Allows flexing movements in one plane (through one axis), characterized by bending and straightening—the elbow, knee, and ankle are examples.

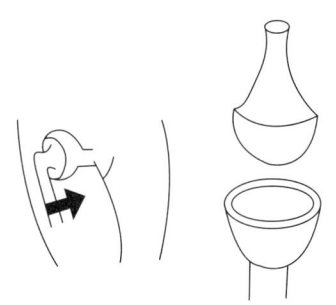

Ball and socket. Allows a full range of movements in three planes (triaxial)—the hip and shoulder are examples.

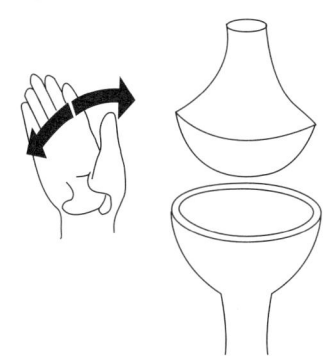

Condyloid. This is a modified ball-and-socket joint that allows a wide range of movement in two planes (biaxial)—the joints that join the fingers to the hands are examples.

simple as carrying a bowling bag can lead to an elbow injury because the tensile force—a translational force—at the elbow joint may cause microscopic tears in the connective tissues (*see also* SHOULDER, ELBOW, AND WRIST). Rotational forces, however, are a far more common cause of sports injuries than translational forces. In tennis, for example, the player's movement toward the ball, followed by impact with the ball, creates shearing—rotational—forces that can result in injury to tissues. That is, at contact with the ball the player's muscles are moving the racket, and at the same time the ligaments and tendons are reacting to the shearing forces created at impact.

Physiology of Joints: Synovial Fluid

A joint is surrounded by a joint capsule (*see Figure 11*), which protects the joint and holds synovial fluid, a lubricant that allows the joints to move smoothly, more or less as oil lubricates the moving parts of an engine.

Synovial fluid serves three basic functions. First, it lubricates areas of friction along the smooth-surfaced cartilage and areas of friction between tendons, ligaments, and bones. Second, it removes microorganisms and debris from tendons and ligaments. Third, it nourishes cartilage. In an adult, cartilage has no blood vessels or nerves, and so its nourishment must come solely from the back-and-forth flow of synovial fluid. The free flow of synovial fluid is vital, then, not only to reduce friction but also for the survival of cartilage. Immobilization of a joint, or intense, prolonged compressive forces (such as the forces that occur in rigorous distance running) will limit the nutrient flow to cartilage.

Near some joints are sacs of synovial fluid called bursae (*singular*, bursa). Their primary purpose is to prevent wear of the different structures that slide across them. The largest of the bursae is the suprapatellar bursa, which serves the knee and is located between the thighbone and the knee. When subjected to severe stress, the suprapatellar bursa produces additional quantities of synovial fluid, causing the knee to swell; an impact force received directly by the knee is a typical cause of such swelling. This condition, commonly called "water on the knee," usually goes away by itself but sometimes requires drainage. For an athlete with the condition, drainage may be needed before competition.

Factors in the Health of Joints

Physiologically, exercise benefits a joint. Exercise increases the pulse rate, which in turn increases the blood flow necessary for the distribution of nutrients throughout the body.

During the developmental years—childhood through adolescence—well-rounded, varied exercise is needed to ensure that the muscle and cartilage cells surrounding joints remain well nourished. Cartilage (unlike bone) is a tissue of low metabolism, with limited regenerative capacity. Suitable exercise thickens cartilage by increasing its metabolism (and the flow of nutrients it receives); also, exercise causes cartilage to increase its production of collagen (cells that provide flexibility) as it attempts to adapt to increased stress. Conversely, lack of exercise causes cartilage to thin out. Surrounding ligaments and tendons work in conjunction with cartilage, and they too require a certain amount of stress and strain in order to maintain and increase their strength.

Although the way a joint moves is primarily determined by its structure, its range of motion (ROM) is greatly influenced by several

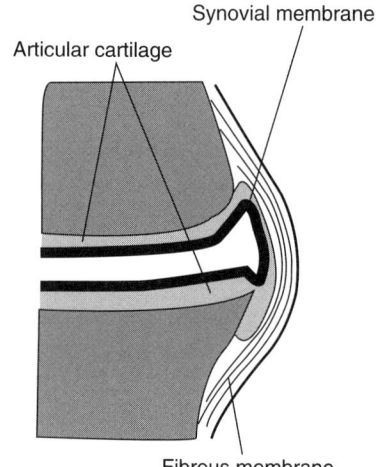

Figure 11. *In a typical joint, (1) cartilage covers the surface. (2) The joint is encased in a joint capsule. (3) Wherever cartilage is not found, a membrane lines the joint. (4) The synovial membrane secretes synovial fluid into the joint cavity to lubricate it. (5) Ligaments and tendons strengthen the joint—they may lie outside the joint or connect into it. (6) Nerves and blood vessels supply the joint.*

other factors, including use, disease, injury, and, in particular, the elasticity of muscles, tendons, and ligaments. Stretching and exercise lengthen the tissues of muscles, tendons, and ligaments, thereby increasing ROM in the direction of the lengthening. If a joint does not experience a full range of movements, imbalances in ROM occur. For instance, exercise that involves flexion (bending), but not extension (straightening), will—not surprisingly—result in an increase in flexion and a decrease in extension. Imbalances in mobility can often develop in sports, through repetitive movements; examples include the wrist flex of a pitcher, the hip flex of a hurdler, and the elbow hyperextension of a gymnast. For this reason, all in-season and off-season training programs try to achieve ROM balance by increasing ROM in the underused direction.

Thus not all exercise is good for joints. If exercise is extreme or creates uneven stress (as, for instance, with baseball pitchers), osteoarthritis develops: the cartilage deteriorates or wears down (*see Figure 12*). This seriously restricts movement at the affected joint. Most people start to feel some twinges of osteoarthritis around age 40, but a few are genetically predisposed to develop it earlier, often with debilitating pain. Joint cartilage acts as a shock absorber, so once it starts to wear down, bone will grind against bone. Few remedies are available: doctors can only prescribe pain relievers to be taken continuously or, in severe cases, resort to an artificial joint. Cartilage (again unlike bone) is a tissue that cannot naturally repair itself; however, some promising research is being done on the possibility of developing drugs that would not only repair defects but create new cartilage.

Joint Injuries

In sports, injuries to the joints usually occur from an unexpected or excessive force that the protective mechanism in a joint cannot

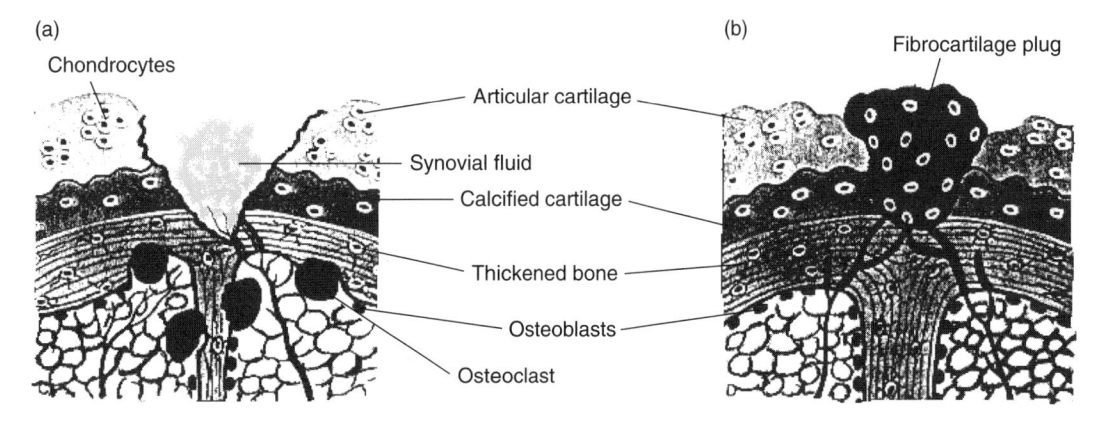

Figure 12. *In the development of osteoarthritis, (a) death of chondrocytes leads to a crack in the articular cartilage. An influx of synovial fluid follows, leading to a further loss and degeneration of cartilage. Cartilage gradually wears away. (b) New vessels grow in from the epiphysis, and new cartilage is deposited. This new cartilage, often mechanically insufficient to withstand loads, eventually wears away and exposes the bone plate.*

absorb or does not have time to absorb. Injury may also arise from overuse of an unconditioned joint or from faulty technique that results in repetitive stresses to a joint.

In gymnastics, joints and their supporting structures often fail because after one series of forces, they do not have time to recover their normal dimensions before being subjected to another series of forces. In other words, joints are subjected to a second force while still in an outstretched state from an initial force. For example, on the uneven bars a gymnast might experience a pulling force at the shoulder joint while executing a giant swing from the high bar, and then experience additional pulling as the hips wrap around the lower bar. A force from one angle is followed by a second force from a slightly different angle, before the gymnast has had a chance to adjust to the first force.

Physiologists once believed that strenuous, repetitive exercise was detrimental to joint tissue. However, recent studies do not support this belief; rather, they seem to indicate that most joint injuries in noncontact sports result from poor alignment of joint surfaces (which is often a hereditary condition), or from earlier injuries. If so, athletes need not worry about cumulative effects of everyday stresses on cartilage and joints. There seems to be no evidence that joint tissue will deteriorate or be damaged, as long as workouts are moderate and the athlete rests a joint that flares up with pain (as in conditions such as "jumper's knee").

Joint Braces
When an athlete can control excessive joint mobility with adequate bracing, strengthening of supporting muscles, or modification of training, there is no reason to stabilize the joint surgically.

Joint injuries are common at the elite levels of sports because athletes put tremendous demands on their bodies. Major joint injuries (such as torn knee ligaments) can sideline an athlete for months, although minor injuries (such as a sprained ankle), may heal by themselves, given a few days of rest. After an injury and a period of rest, an athlete attempting to resume a normal training schedule is likely to experience pain and difficulty of movement because of joint stiffness. This is usually caused by reduced blood circulation and waterlogged tissue in the underused joint. Over time, as training is gradually made more rigorous, the stiffness and swelling usually diminish (*see also* REHABILITATION).

Preventing Injury to the Bones and Joints

The durability of the musculoskeletal system is in great part determined by heredity. Consider, for example, the careers of two quarterbacks in the National Football League, Jim McMahon and John Elway, who both started in the league in 1983. McMahon spent the majority of his NFL career sidelined with injuries; when he did play, he did everything he could to avoid contact. Elway, in contrast, was never shy about contact, yet he rarely missed a game because of injury; undoubtedly, he was simply more durable. Many people, like McMahon, are prone to joint injuries because of their genetic

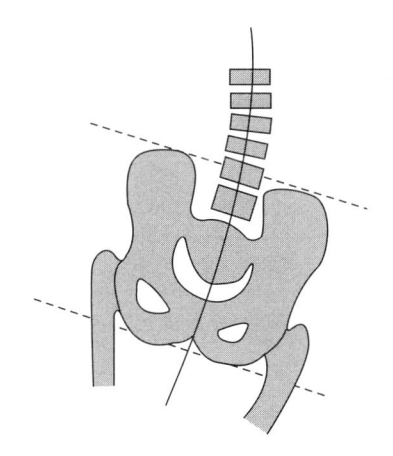

Figure 13. *Having legs of uneven length causes (1) pelvic tilt to the short side, (2) lumbar curvature to the tall side, and (3) uneven loading during walking, running, and lifting. Special shoes and shoe inserts can compensate for this unevenness and thus can prevent stress fractures, lower back pain, and osteoarthritis of the hip.*

makeup, but there are preventive measures that can greatly reduce risk: these include developing good posture, maintaining muscle tone and balance, improving joint mobility, and minimizing impacts.

Maintaining Good Posture

Good posture is an underappreciated factor in preventing injury, though it can be readily observed in athletes who manage to avoid injuries. To understand why posture is important, consider the fact that everyone is a few millimeters shorter at night, before going to bed, than in the morning. The reason has to do with gravity: subjected to the force of gravity over the course of a day, the skeletal system compresses slightly. For the same reason, astronauts who spend time in a gravity-free environment usually grow 1 or 2 inches (2.5–5 cm) taller; most of this growth comes from an expansion of the nucleus pulposus in the spine (and it sometimes results in mysterious back pain).

Bad posture exacerbates the compressive effect of gravity, and the constant pull of gravity makes bad posture even worse with age. Keeping the most erect posture possible, with shoulders back and head up, helps the musculoskeletal system maintain a position less susceptible to injury (*see also SPINE*).

Maintaining Muscle Tone and Balance

Muscles support the skeletal system. Thus, it is logical that the better muscle tone is, the better the chance of avoiding injury—and this is especially true with regard to preventing injuries to the spine and extremities. Thus athletes should try to develop muscular strength over and above what is required for a particular sport; developing additional strength provides significant protection by increasing the amount of muscle-generated compression to a joint or bone about to experience a tension force (*see also STRENGTH TRAINING*). The only way to accomplish this is through "overloading": that is, resistance or number of repetitions must be continually increased.

For most sports, athletes should concentrate on developing movements in which the larger, bulkier muscles do most the work, and the smaller, weaker muscles control the fine adjustments. Each time a person moves incorrectly, that creates a distortion of the proper movement—a distortion in which the weaker "fine-tuning" muscles are doing more work than they should or inessential muscles are being forced to contract. In other words, unnatural or incorrect movements or techniques represent excessive strain, and thus they usually lead to injury, though if they are reinforced through practice, they will become ingrained because they feel more comfortable. However, the body and brain are naturally lazy: given a choice, the brain will adopt the motion that strains the body least. Thus in correcting a poor technique, the athlete's goal is to get the brain to cancel an old image and replace it with a new image, a more effective way to move. It is important not simply to exercise but also to retrain the brain: in time, the retrained brain will make corrections, allowing the body in effect to protect and heal itself (*see also MOTOR CONTROL*).

Maintaining Joint Mobility

Joint mobility is very important in reducing the risk of injury. Inherent mobility—or range of motion (ROM)—and stability vary tremendously among individuals. Hereditary extremes include collagen defects, such as excessive levels of the enzyme lysyl oxidase, which causes extreme joint flexibility. At the other extreme is a condition such as arthrogryposes, which causes excessive joint stiffness and severely limited joint mobility. ROM and stability also vary from joint to joint. For example, the shoulder and hip are both ball-and-socket joints, yet the ROM of the shoulder is much greater than that of the hip. This explains, in part, why there are far more dislocated shoulders than dislocated hips.

ROM and stability do not need to be mutually exclusive goals. Gymnasts, divers, and hurdlers (and also dancers) prove that through flexibility training natural ROM can be increased. However, there is a fine line between the mobility that allows gymnasts to hyperextend and position their joints in almost unbelievable contortions and the excessive joint mobility that causes problems because of a lack of stability. A gymnast would never be able to perform acrobatic movements without both mobility and stability.

Minimizing Impact

The amount of shock the body must absorb has long been considered a major risk factor for athletes. These shock waves are "absorbed" by muscle stiffness, bone deformation, joint dislocation, and compression of cartilage. The foot-ground impact forces experienced during running are a typical example. When a person is standing still, the feet and legs need to support only the body weight. In walking, the feet and legs experience greater force as the feet strike the ground. Running imposes twice that force: when the forefoot strikes the ground, it is subjected to forces three to four times body weight. This means that running 20 miles (32 km) a week generates approximately 1.7 million additional shock waves for the body to absorb (Dickinson, 1985). Naturally, by reducing training and allowing the body to rest, an athlete can limit the shock waves the body must absorb. Most world-class professional athletes, however, do not have the luxury of reducing their training or taking much time to rest, and thus they are likely to return to action too soon.

Realistically, then, to avoid injury to the bones and joints an athlete should minimize impact forces. The more gradually the energy of the moving body gets absorbed, the less likely an impact will be to cause injury. Generally, most coaches do a very good job of teaching athletes execution skills, yet (with the exception of the martial arts) few coaches teach athletes how to minimize the effects of impact. In baseball, for instance, even in the major leagues, a great deal of downtime with injuries can be attributed to improper sliding technique.

In minimizing impact from a fall or a jump, four factors need to be considered: (1) height, (2) landing surface, (3) area of contact, and (4) flexing of the joints to gradually decrease velocity. For example, a

Improving Joint Mobility

1. Preseason training to condition a joint for a given sport.

2. Understanding the role of the joint in the sport.

3. Developing strength in muscles that control excessively stressed joints.

4. Attention to technique training.

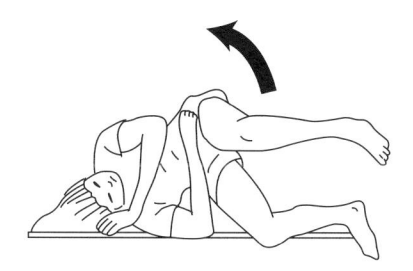

Figure 14. *The shoulder roll is an effective way to decrease horizontal momentum gradually in a fall. Impact is controlled by landing and rolling on the more heavily padded body parts. The roll also increases the surface area of impact, which decreases force per unit of surface area.*

person who falls 100 feet (about 30 m) from a helicopter, feet first, into 10 feet (3 m) of snow will probably land uninjured. The snow will decelerate the body gradually, helping the muscles and flexing joints absorb impact. However, if someone falls a mere 2 feet (60 cm) and lands on a hard floor with the knee joints locked, there is a high probability of injury. According to the laws of physics, something has to give. Under most circumstances, of the four factors affecting impact, only factor 4—how the joints absorb impact—can be controlled. Therefore, when falling or jumping, an athlete should attempt to land on the balls of the feet and immediately let the ankles, knees, and hip flex, deliberately controlling the contraction of the muscles associated with these joints. Ankle, knee, and hip joint can bend in concert to absorb the impact, spreading the impact force throughout the body and reducing the chance of injury. Another technique for minimizing impact during a fall is the shoulder roll (*see Figure 14*).

Using joints to minimize impact is also very important in collisions. In contact sports, collisions cause impacts at many different angles. In football, players develop a sense of how to absorb impacts by preparing for contact. Walter Payton, who as of the mid-1990s was the NFL's all-time leading rusher, missed only one game in a 14-year career. He claimed that he approached collisions with the idea of punishing the tackler before the tackler punished him. In effect, by taking a position with his knees bent and leaning forward, he could lower his center of gravity and keep it near the front edge of his base of support. Thus, when he drove into tacklers, he more easily controlled and absorbed the punishing impacts—and this in part explains his ability to avoid injury. It should be noted, though, that he was also an exceptional athlete, and exceptionally dedicated to keeping himself in top condition.

John Zumerchik*

The author would like to thank David A. Lind for providing much of the physics material, and David H. Janda for providing most of the medical material.

References

Adrian, M., and J. Cooper. *The Biomechanics of Human Movement*. Indianapolis, Indiana: Benchmark, 1989.

Alioia, A., et al. "Prevention of Involuntary Bone Loss by Exercise." *Annals of Internal Medicine* 89 (1978): 356ff.

Angiers, N. "Family of Errant Genes Is Found to Be Related to Variety of Skeletal Ills," *New York Times*, 1 November 1994, sec. C, pp. 1, 4.

Bachman, C. "Geometry." *Physics Teacher* 30, no. 6 (1988): 341–370.

Curry, J. *The Mechanical Adaptations of Bones*. Princeton, New Jersey: Princeton University Press, 1984.

Dickinson, J., S. Cook, and T. Leinhardt. "The Measurement of Shock Waves Following Heel Strikes While Running." *Journal of Biomechanics* 18 (1985): 415–419.

Evans, F. G. (ed.) *Strength of Biological Materials*. Baltimore, Maryland: Williams and Wilkins, 1970.

Gamble, J. *The Musculoskeletal System: Physiological Basics*. New York: Raven, 1988.

Hay, J., and J. Reid. *The Anatomical and Mechanical Bases of Human Motion*. Englewood Cliffs, New Jersey: Prentice-Hall, 1982.

Helminen, H., et al. (eds.) *Joint Loading: Biology and Health of Articulate Structures*. Bristol, England: Wright, 1987.

Huddleston, A., et al. "Bone Mass in Lifetime Tennis Players." *Journal of the American Medical Association* 244, no. 10 (1980): 1107–1109.

Kuo, C., et al. "Control of Torsion and Bending of the Lower Extremity during Skiing." *Ski Trauma and Safety: Fifth International Symposium*. American Society for Testing and Materials: ASTM STP 860 (1985).

Lawren, B. "Rebuilding Nature's Shock Absorbers." *Longevity* (July 1994).

Leung, P. *Current Trends in Bone Grafting*. New York: Springer Verlag, 1989.

Lind, D. *The Physics of Skiing*. New York: American Institute of Physics, 1996.

Maguia, R, "Elevated Plasma Hydroxyproline: A Possible Risk Factor Associated with Connective Tissue Injuries during Overuse." *American Journal of Sports Medicine* 16, no. 660 (1988).

Piscopo, J., and J. Bailey. *Kinesiology: The Science of Movement*. New York: Wiley, 1981.

Rubin, E., and J. Farber. *Essential Pathology*. Philadelphia, Philadelphia: Lippincott, 1990.

Simmons, D. *Nutrition and Bone Development*. New York: Oxford University Press, 1990.

Steindler, A. Kinesiology of the Human Body. Springfield, Illinois: Thomas, 1970.

Stanitski, C., et al. "On the Nature of Stress Fractures." *American Journal of Sports Medicine* 6, no. 391 (1978).

Sohn, R., and L. Micheli. "The Effects of Running on the Pathogenesis of Osteoarthritis." *Clinical Orthopedics* 198, no. 106 (1985).

Toufexis, Anastasia. "Why the Bones Break." *Time* (31 January 1994).

Tietz, C. *Scientific Foundations of Sports Medicine*. Toronto, Canada: Decker, 1989.

Vaughan, J. *The Physiology of Bone*. Oxford, England: Clarendon, 1975.

Williams, J., and P. Sperryn. *Sports Medicine*. Baltimore, Maryland: Williams and Wilkins, 1976.

Williams, K. "Muscle Sense." *Unlimited Health* 2, no. 8 (1992): 8ff.

Spine

ACCORDING TO DARWIN'S THEORY of evolution by natural selection, species adapt to their environment over time, in ways that increase the probability of surviving long enough to reproduce. During the long evolutionary process that led to the human species, one such adaptation was from walking on all fours to walking upright. Bipedalism—walking on two feet—offers obvious advantages for survival: for one thing, it allows a creature to see farther and thus to avoid many hazards; even more important, it frees the forelimbs for use as arms and hands. Ironically, though, while it was a crucial factor in the development of humanity, bipedalism has also been a factor in one of the most widespread of human ills: back problems. According to one popular belief, back disorders and back injuries occur primarily because the human spine was not originally designed for bipedalism (*see Figure 1*). But although it is true that the spine has unique structural and functional characteristics as a result of human beings' upright position, back problems are attributable far more to disuse, misuse, and abuse than to evolution.

For whatever reason, back problems are remarkably prevalent. In the United States, back pain ranks near the top of all disorders in incidence of complaints. According to one study, 8 out of 10 Americans can expect to seek treatment for back pain at some point during their lifetime (Lillegard, 1993). Back problems are less prevalent among high school and college athletes—who experience compara-

Figure 1. *There is debate over whether the evolution of the human spine—specifically, spinal curvature—is responsible for the high incidence of lower back pain. The spine of a newborn is straight, but a C-shaped curve develops as infants begin raising the head. At about age 1 year, the assumption of an upright position creates a forward curve in the lumbar region, which will eventually result in an S-shaped curve in adulthood. As a result, the center of gravity (shaded circle) drops. (Adapted from Adrian and Cooper, 1988)*

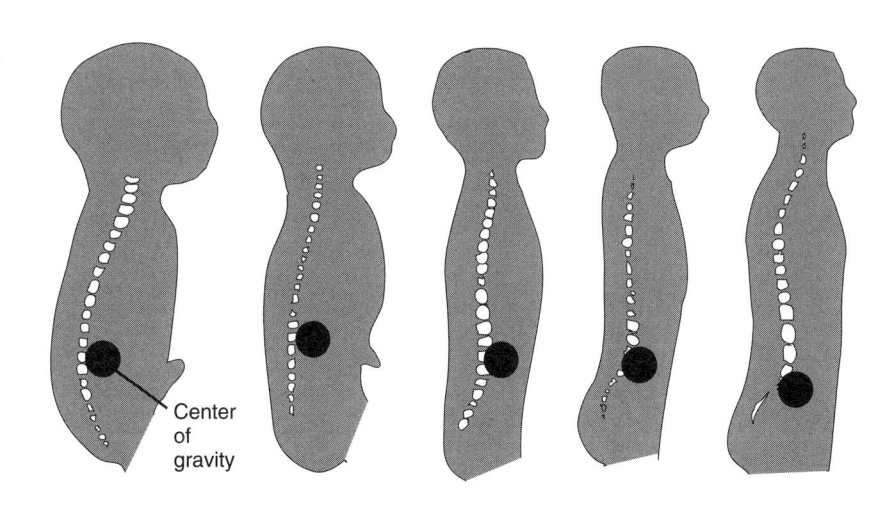

tively more injuries to the knee, ankle, and shoulder—but back injuries may have a more severe impact over time: a serious injury to the back can create a condition that will become a lifelong nuisance and cause chronic pain. Among professional athletes, back injuries are common and can have a devastating effect on a career; in the 1980s and 1990s, for instance, stars such as Larry Bird and Charles Barkley in basketball, and Don Mattingly and Dave Winfield in baseball, suffered back injuries. Many linemen in the National Football League have said that chronic back pain sidelined them and eventually brought their professional careers to a premature end.

Injuries to the spinal column can occur from a single incident or as a result of repetitive stress. Single incidents include collisions, falls, and strain from poor lifting technique. Repetitive stress usually arises from an exaggerated spinal motion. For example, tennis players hyperextend the spine while serving, in order to impart topspin (which makes the ball "kick up" after landing). According to a survey of 143 players on the men's professional tour, the repetitive stress of playing every day had caused 38 percent of players to miss at least one tournament, and 30 percent reported chronic lower back pain (Marks, 1988). Ivan Lendl, a tennis star of the 1980s, cited chronic back pain as the reason for the decline in the quality of his play and for his retirement in the early 1990s.

Severe spinal cord injuries—resulting in papaplegia, quadriplegia, and even death—are among the most traumatic of all injuries. However, sports-related spinal cord injuries account for only about 5 percent of such cases (most of which result from automobile accidents). Most back injuries resulting from repetitive stress are minor, involving a sprain or strain, and can be treated with rest and rehabilitation. Therefore, this article will focus not on catastrophic spinal events but rather on the biomechanics and physiology of the spine and on the causes and prevention of chronic lower back pain.

Anatomy and Function of the Spine

The spine is a portion of the skeleton that connects the head to the pelvis and controls the movement of the trunk. It must perform three basic functions: (1) allow motion of body parts, (2) carry weight, and (3) protect the spinal cord.

The spine consists of 32 vertebrae (*singular*, vertebra), of which 24 are movable. On the basis of differences in their size, curvature, and function, the movable vertebrae are grouped into three segments: *cervical*, consisting of the upper 7; *thoracic*, the middle 12; and *lumbar*, the lower 5. Their size increases from the first cervical vertebra to the last lumbar vertebra (*see Figure 2*). Unlike most bony structures in the body, the spine is not straight but has three curvatures. The cervical (upper) and lumbar (lower) vertebrae curve forward, creating two convex shapes. This makes it necessary for the thoracic

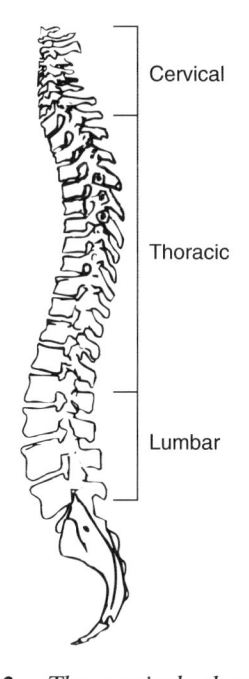

Figure 2. *The cervical, thoracic, and lumbar vertebrae make up the spine and attach to the pelvis at the sacrum. There are 24 movable vertebrae: 7 cervical, 12 thoracic, and 5 lumbar.*

(middle) vertebrae, which are connected to both ends, to curve in the opposite direction—backward—creating a concave shape. From its appearance alone, then, the spine looks incapable of supporting weight, even body weight: a tree with such a serpentine shape, for instance, could not remain standing very long. Why and how the spine works has to do with its chainlike mechanical structure, which makes it a system of significant complexity.

The spine acts much like a long series of short connected rods, allowing the body a tremendous range of motion (ROM). If the spine were a single stiff bone (like the long bones of the arms and legs), movement would be limited: even a person of medium height would have to kneel down to clear a low beam and would find it difficult or impossible to do something as simple as ducking to get into a car. Although no one vertebra provides a large ROM, collectively (in a physically fit person) the vertebrae provide the impressive total ROM. In large part, this is possible because of the intervertebral disks and the intervertebral foramen, which are located between the vertebral bodies (*see Figure 3*).

The intervertebral disks consist of a tough outer layer of fibrocartilage (annulus fibrosus) and a more pulpy elastic center (nucleus pulposus), which functions as a very effective shock absorber. (The spaces between disks also serve this shock-absorbing function; *see below*.) The nucleus pulposus is about 85 percent water. It takes on a round shape when the body is at rest; but when the spine experiences intense or extended stress, the nucleus pulposus shifts position and becomes flatter, as fluid is squeezed outward. The annulus fibrosus has a restraining effect, distributing the forces of bending, twisting, and turning. For example, when the back is arched the intervertebral disk responds to the gravitational load and muscle contraction by opening up in front and narrowing in back; meanwhile, the posteri-

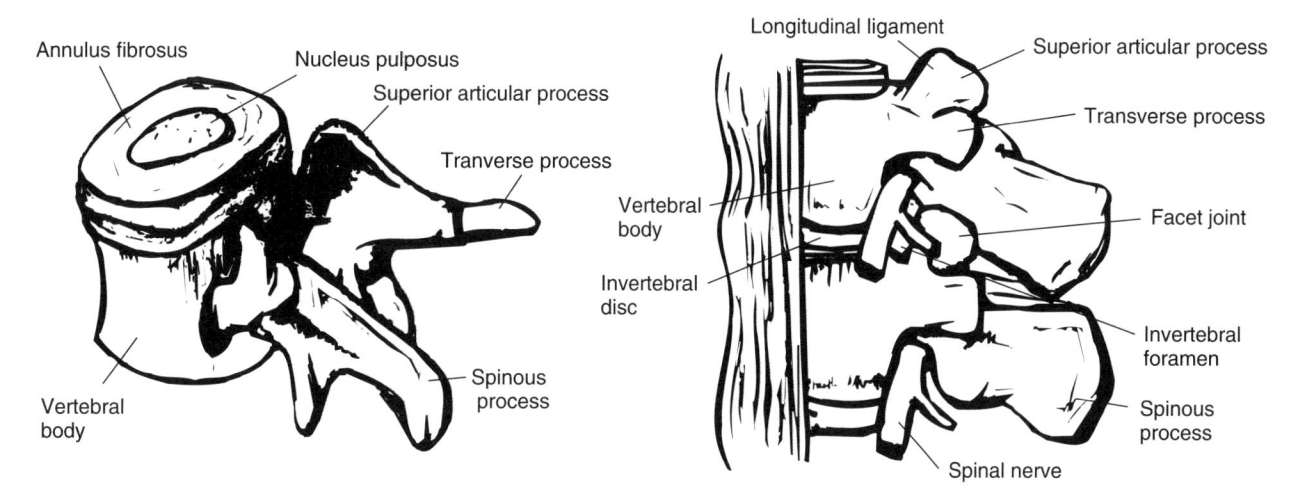

Figure 3. *Spinal anatomy. The intervertebral disk and foramen act as a shock absorber for compressive loads and as a ball bearing for loads requiring bending and twisting. Surrounding the nucleus pulposus is the annulus fibrosus, which provides stability and cushioning. The ligaments that run along the spine prevent hyperextension (arching) and hyperflexion (bending). The shape of the intervertebral disk can change to accommodate twisting and tilting of the vertebrae.*

Figure 4. *Dynamics of the nucleus pulposus. (a) When the body is arched back, the nucleus slides forward, and the intervertebral space opens up anteriorly as it closes posteriorly. (b) The opposite occurs in bending; the nucleus slides backward, and the intervertebral space opens posteriorly while closing anteriorly. (Adapted from Ghista, 1982)*

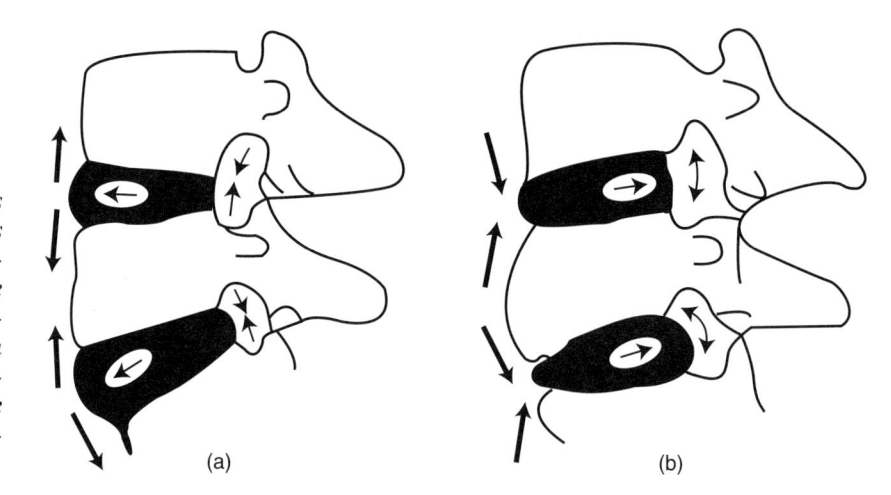

orly located nucleus moves toward the middle. The opposite occurs in bending down: the intervertebral disk closes down in front and opens up in back as the nucleus drifts backward. The back-and-forth movement of the nucleus plays a vital biomechanical function, allowing compressive forces to be distributed evenly throughout the nucleus and annulus of the intervertebral disk. Their interplay absorbs compressive loads that otherwise could injure the bony structure of the vertebrae (*see Figure 4*).

Besides acting as the primary shock absorber for compressive loads, the intervertebral disk also acts as a ball bearing for loads requiring bending and twisting. This is possible because only about one-third of the total height of the vertebral column consists of disks: the remaining two-thirds consists of space between the stalks of the vertebra, called the intervertebral foramen. Within this space, the nerves pass from the spinal cord, branching out to the different parts of the body. As noted above, this space acts as a shock absorber for compressive forces.

Compressive forces not only flatten the disks but also shrink the space between disks. Weight lifters are an extreme example of this effect: because of the great stress placed on the spine, the body may become a few centimeters shorter after a rigorous, heavy weight-training session. Also, x-ray studies of retired weight lifters have found that their disks are more tightly packed than is normal, as a result of the long-term repetitive stress of weight lifting (Granhed, 1988). It is worth noting, though, that this shrinkage is not confined to weight lifters: gravity itself has a sizable effect on anyone. Disk measurements show that an individual's disks are thicker after a night's rest than at midday or in the evening. Constant compressive pressure from sitting and standing all day pushes some of the fluid out; at night, while the body is in a recumbent position, water is absorbed back into the disks, expanding them.

The space between the disks, though it serves mainly as a shock absorber for compressive forces, also allows for greater ROM. It gives the spine enough mobility to bend and twist at a variety of extreme angles between the head and pelvis. The ROM is about 250 degrees in the sagittal plane (from touching toes to bending backward), 150 degrees side-to-side, and 180 degrees in rotation.

The lumbar region is capable only of bending and arching because its bony structure permits only up-and-down motion; side-to-side motion is made possible by the *lumbosacral joint*. This fifth lumbar junction to the sacrum is especially prone to injury because it is a "transitional" zone—a bony junction consisting of a mobile segment (last lumbar) and an immobile segment (sacrum). Faulty running style, excessive lifting, and abnormal loading from poor posture all contribute to the vulnerability of this transitional zone. Axial rotation and lateral rotation can, and often do, occur simultaneously, in a "coupling" motion. One of the most common examples of coupling occurs when a diver performs a somersaulting and twisting maneuver. Coupling is a strong characteristic of the cervical and lumbar spine, but a relatively weaker characteristic of the thoracic spine. Much of the reason for this is not design but location. The direction of the coupling motion in the lumbar region is opposite that of the cervical spine. The longitudinal rotation of the diver's cervical spine, for instance, must be countered, and an opposite reaction of the lumbar spine is necessary in the force-counterforce dynamics of airborne twisting. Like the center of a twisted rag, the thoracic spine twists in the opposite direction at the pivotal point of the movement. Strong abdominal muscles (such as gymnasts develop) provide enough stability to prevent an excessive amount of twisting, which may lead to injury. Understanding the coupling patterns of the spine is important not only in diagnosing the dynamics that cause injuries but also in improving acrobatic techniques in sports such as gymnastics, figure skating, and diving.

Back Injuries

This section considers the role of movement in injury to the back, and the pathophysiology of some common back injuries.

Factors in Injury

Some doctors believe that back pain results from a vertebra that fails, not from problems with the intervertebral disk. However, there is a causal relationship between the intervertebral disk and back pain. Even a structurally sound spine—one without any abnormalities—will weaken over time from the forces applied to it, if muscle tone is inaedquate, if the body is fatigued, or if body mechanics are poor. One or more defective disks can create a "domino effect," affecting adjacent disks and vertebrae. Eventually, the vertebrae compress, diminishing the intervertebral foramen and putting pressure on the exiting nerve. Moreover, the compressive strength of the vertebrae increases progressively from top (the first cervical vertebra) to bottom (the last lumbar vertebra).

The gravitational load on the lower spine of an average-size man in a standing position is considerable, estimated at about 800 to 900 newtons (180 to 202.25 lb.). Still, the spine's capacity to handle heavy loads is potentially far greater, approximately 10 to 15 times this amount (Schultz, 1982), and so a question arises: If the spine is physically capable of handling such tremendous loads, why are there so many back injuries?

The answer has to do with movement. There is no direct positive correlation between loads and injury, because measurements of load—such as those just cited—are for static work potential, and static work does not take into account the dynamics of human movement. For example, back injuries commonly result from shoveling snow; but contrary to popular opinion, the cause is usually not simply lifting too heavy a load. Instead, the injury is more directly a result of the combined bending, lifting, and twisting necessary to throw a shovelful of snow to the side.

Athletes' back problems usually fall into one or a combination of the following categories: excessive or uneven stress, sudden movements while in an awkward position, and weak or poorly trained back muscles.

To begin with the last of these categories, muscular weakness—or relative weakness—can be a particularly important factor. Significant alterations in the normal strength ratios of the trunk muscles (agonist versus antagonist) are often found to accompany lower back pain. This may be a result of unevenness in muscular strength. One example is a high ratio of extension (straightening) to flexion (bending) at the hip, which becomes evident in bending over: the pivoting hip joint is weak in flexion but very strong in extension. This type of asymmetry in muscular strength is not found exclusively among underconditioned athletes; equally abnormal ratios—and even more abnormal ratios—have been found in well-trained athletes. Still, this unevenness is not as great a hazard for well-trained athletes, because (as would be expected), other things being equal, they are much stronger than underconditioned athletes, and so the asymmetry becomes a matter of "very strong" versus "strong" rather than "strong" versus "weak."

In certain sports, specific positioning, movements, and training contribute to unevenness in muscle development. For example, fencing requires long periods of uneven loading, in which one foot is always in front and therefore carrying more load. This leads to a relative weakness of the lateral flexors (benders) on the nondominant side. During normal competition, the athlete may not experience any problems. But an athlete who makes a sudden off-balance movement—experiencing asymmetrical loading on the trunk—can sustain a lower back injury from the unbalanced strength between the agonist (contracting) and antagonist (extending) trunk muscles.

Excessive or uneven stress is a second category of causes of back problems. Sports that overload the right or the left side of the spine can have a cumulative effect, causing a gradual change in the alignment of the facet joint of the spine. One such recreational sport is bowling, which involves bending and twisting while swinging through the release of a 16-pound (7.3-kg) ball. A study at the Institute of Medicine in Washington, D.C., found that people involved in sports generally experienced comparatively few lower back injuries, with one exception—bowlers (Mundt, 1993).

Bowling creates stress on the lower back because of the bending and twisting motion involved, which is analogous to the motion of shoveling snow, lifting a child out of a crib, or turning a patient in bed. The bowler lifts the ball off the rack, which is about knee-high, and then holds it out in front of the chest or chin to aim it. During a typical three-game match, the bowler will repeat this lifting and holding motion about 70 times. Further, since a heavier ball produces better pin action, bowlers tend to choose a ball at the upper end of their strength limit. Without strong spinal support muscles, this repetitive bending and twisting with an extended weight reaches a point at which adjacent vertebrae no longer move rhythmically or smoothly in conjuction with each other. To minimize back problems, physical therapists recommend bending at the knees rather than the back to pick up a heavy object. Bowlers must of course lift the ball and aim it, but they can minimize unbalanced lower back tension by minimizing the time spent holding the ball up while aiming. Using a lighter ball would also limit back stress.

Sudden movements—another of the three categories of causes noted above—can also be illustrated in bowling. One cause of injury in bowling is a nonfluid delivery. If the smooth pendulum motion of the ball is interrupted, or if the bowler tries to "throw" the ball with a jerking motion, large stresses may be created. By adjusting their footwork and applying forces gradually to let the ball swing from the arm, bowlers can achieve a smooth delivery and reduce their risk of injury.

Many lower back problems also arise from accidents, such as uncoordinated lifting, or awkward landings in which a lateral buckling of the spine occurs. As the spine bows out when compressed from both ends, "buckling" is the point beyond which it can no longer bend without giving out. Spinal anatomy and muscle development allow for much greater bending without buckling in the forward-and-backward direction than the side-to-side direction. Side-to-side buckling is partly responsible for the large number of lower back injuries reported in the National Basketball Association each year. During the 1992–1993 season, for instance, there were 48 lower back injuries that necessitated sidelining, affecting about 15 percent of all players. The effect of awkward one-footed landings can be exacerbated by improper strength training, which results in unbalanced muscle mass. However, because most sports teams now have sophisticated strength and conditioning programs, asymmetry in muscle development has become less common than it once was.

Age is also a factor in back problems. The intervertebral disks

Some Causes of Sports-Related Back Injuries

Wrestling and football: Hyperextension and compression, especially for football linemen, who continually drive shoulder-to-shoulder into their opponents. Studies of retired wrestlers have found a high incidence of lower back pain, fractures, and impaired mobility.

Gymnastics, diving, and figure skating: Excessive stretching and twisting are required to perform acrobatics.

Basketball and volleyball: Unbalanced forces from landing in awkward positions. These sports require a great deal of jumping.

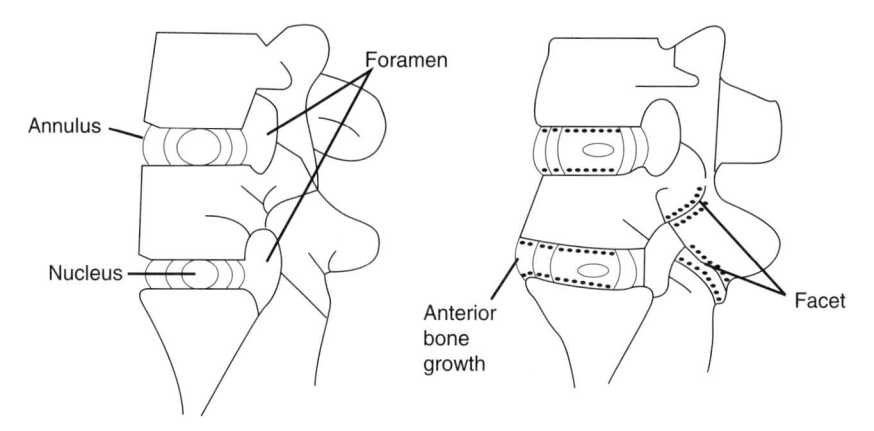

Figure 5. *Degenerative arthritis. Left: Normal lumbar disk; right: disk in which degenerative arthritis has developed. Bulging of the annulus causes excessive bone overgrowth; this overgrowth, which is extremely common among the elderly, results in a stiff lower back. Degenerative arthritis decreases flexibility, but the bony overgrowth has a positive side effect: it limits the movement of the nucleus. As a result, chronic back pain is a less common complaint among the elderly than among the young or the middle-aged. (Adapted from Ghista, 1982)*

and the ligaments and tendons that support the spine can all degenerate with age, as can the bony structure itself. This tissue degeneration can eventually restrict an athlete's ROM, and it explains in part why adults tend to lose height as they age.

Also, as the body ages, the water content in the nucleus of the disk begins to decrease: by the late twenties it has dropped about 15 percent; by age 40, about 30 percent. As a result, aging disks have less ability to withstand compressive forces and to rebound to their normal size after compression. As the water content of the nucleus pulposus decreases and becomes progressively more fibrous, the intervertebral space shrinks, reducing ROM. This narrowing of the disk space, which restricts ROM, is much more dramatic in rotation than in bending forward and backward.

Contrary to popular opinion, degenerative arthritis is not a cause of lower back pain (*see Figure 5*). When degenerative arthritis occurs, it usually involves the front or side portions of the vertebra; it rarely develops in the rear. This means that the stiffer disks found among the elderly are less likely to squeeze or push against the nerve root or pain receptors (*see also AGING AND PERFORMANCE*).

Finally, there are also some genetic factors involved in back pain. Some people have weaker disks than others, and some have a weaker skeletal or muscular structure. Furthermore, although the cause is unknown, some people are born with support struts made of soft fibrous ligaments instead of solid bone. In such people, normal flexion and extension of the spine can cause strains, sprains, and fractures.

Pathophysiology of Typical Injuries

Perhaps the main reason for the widespread fear of back injuries is chronic pain. Up to 50 percent of all adults experience back pain every year, and 5 to 10 percent suffer from chronic lower back pain (Lillegard, 1993). Back pain—unlike pain in many other parts of the body—cannot be escaped. For instance, a football player who injures a knee may not be able to play football again but can usually engage in a lifetime of other normal activities, including other sports. In contrast, a back injury can be totally debilitating because it involves long-term, nagging pain, not just during a certain activity but constantly.

There are many pathophysiological causes of back pain. The most common is a tear to the fibrous part of the disk, which pushes the disk nucleus backward and stretches the ligaments that run along the vertebral column toward the spinal canal. When these ligaments get stretched, pain is felt through the body's pain-sensitive cells. A popular misconception is that the injured disks are the only source of pain. However, the disks themselves have very few nerves, and so there is very little there that can perceive pain; the surrounding ligaments, muscles, and tendons all have far more pain-perceiving fibers and are therefore usually more responsible for the actual perception of pain.

Most back pain occurs initially, or worsens, when the disk nucleus bulges too far out—a condition called a slipped, herniated, or ruptured disk. The annulus fibrosus gives way to inner pressures, causing a portion of the nucleus pulposus to protrude, primarily backward and to the side. The nucleus creates a problem by pressing against the nerve root that passes through the intervertebral opening. Then muscles (nearby and farther away) that are supplied by the nerve experience pain. For example, pain in a shoulder muscle can be a result of injury to a cervical disk; and displacement of a lumbar disk usually results in a shooting pain in the irritated sciatic nerve down the leg.

Another factor contributing to pain is abnormal spinal curvature. Such a condition should be treated early on; otherwise, it usually worsens, leading to a decrease in ROM and pain from spinal deterioration. The normal curves of the spine can become exaggerated from poor posture, from injury, or from hereditary or acquired disease. A condition called kyphosis, or hunchback, occurs from excessive posterior curvature in the thoracic area; excessive anterior curvature in the lumbar region is called lordosis; rotation of vertebrae is called scoliosis. When curvature of the spine is mild, doctors usually recommend a regimen of exercises to prevent additional curvature. In more severe cases, doctors may recommend a back brace or surgery.

Medical science is still far from a complete understanding of lower back pain. Doctors from Hoag Memorial Hospital in Newport Beach, California, used magnetic resonance imaging (MRI) to examine the spines of 98 people who had never experienced back problems or back pain. On average, two-thirds of the group showed some sort of spinal abnormality, and one-third had more than one abnormal disk (Jensen, 1994). Among other problems, the spinal abnormalities found included herniated and degenerative disks. The study concluded that the assumed causal link between back pain and spinal abnormality may not exist: if the subjects in the study were typical, most people have abnormal spines but experience no pain. (Many

Whiplash
Whiplash, a common injury to the cervical spine and the neck, is poorly understood and poorly treated. An international team of experts reviewed more than 10,000 scientific articles published from 1980 to 1995 and found little justification for some existing therapies, such as traction, electric stimulation, ultrasound, laser, soft collars, muscle relaxants, and drug treatments (Altman, 1995). Although most whiplash injuries will heal on their own, a properly designed physical rehabilitation program can speed recovery from weeks to days, or in more severe cases, from months to weeks.

Of the 120,000 cases of whiplash each year in the United States, the majority occur from car accidents, but a fair number also occur from sports mishaps such as diving accidents and football collisions, in which the head is quickly thrust backward and then forward. The whiplash motion injures the muscles and soft tissue in the neck and upper spine, resulting in limited movement and neck pain. Strong neck muscles may prevent or limit the severity of whiplash injuries. The study cited above found that women were 50 percent more likely than men to suffer whiplash injuries, because men have thicker muscles in the upper back and the neck.

Spinal Injuries

Back pain ranks second to headaches as the most frequent type of pain. Back problems usually arise from trauma, from abnormal lifting, from muscle fatigue, or from a congenital problem.

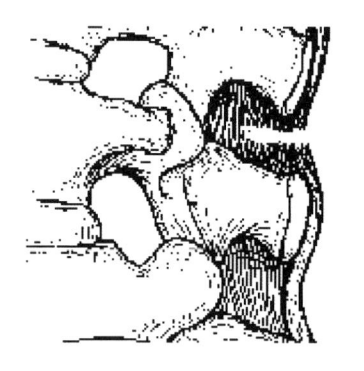

Back sprains. In a back sprain (*above*), the muscles and ligaments in the lower back are stretched and strained. Usually, back strains occur when the back is forcefully bent forward. Overstretching has been noted as a contributing factor. Doing too much stretching sometimes weakens the ligaments and joints in the back, making them particularly susceptible to injury. Minor sprains are like any other type of sprain; they heal well if treated properly. Sprains and strains are not a significant factor in the development of persistent pain or in the prevention of healing. Unless mechanical instability also exists, sprains and strains by themselves cannot be disabling.

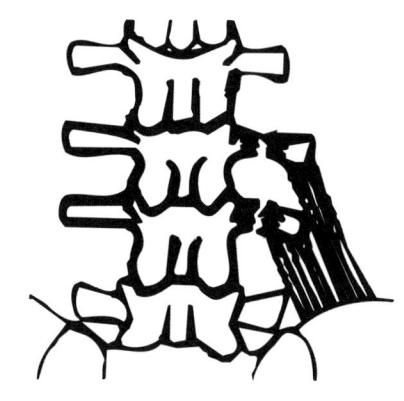

Lower spine fractures. Lower spine fractures are categorized as transverse process or compression. In a transverse fracture (*right*), the horizontal bony struts that support the back muscles snap or break. This usually occurs from a forceful and severe twisting motion. A compressive fracture is a bit different; it occurs when the lower back is flexed straight back with great force. Fractures can cause neurological damage if bony fragments become embedded in the spinal canal. Strength training improves the ability of the lower back muscles to absorb compressive forces capable of causing injury, but it cannot prevent injury altogether. This type of injury is common in football because the size and strength of the players and the forcefulness of impact increase the risk.

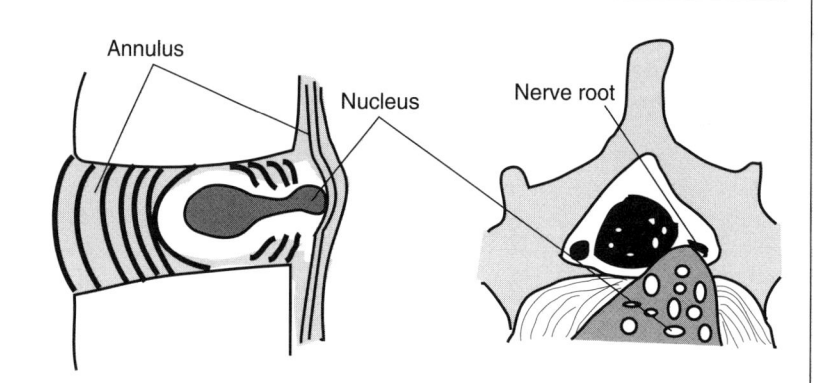

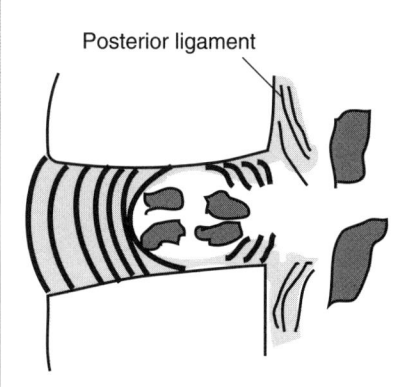

Disk injuries. A variety of different forces can cause a disk injury. Bending, coupled with rotation, creates a force capable of causing a dislocation, and sometimes neurological damage. Two common types of disk injuries are (*above left*) herniated and (*center*) protruding disk. Herniation causes a tear in the annulus and posterior ligament; protrusion causes a tear in the annulus and "pushes" against the posterior ligament. Both can create severe spasms and tremendous pain as (*right*) pressure is put on the nerve root.

physicians routinely use MRI to diagnose back pain in terms of spinal abnormalities. This study also suggests that many such MRI procedures are unnecessary.)

However, "markers" of back pain do continue to be uncovered among patients. One physiological marker may be a lower percentage of natural killer (NK) cells (Brennan, 1994). NK cells are a distinct class of lymphocytes, the white blood cells responsible for specific immune defenses. They circulate in the blood but are located primarily in the bone marrow, and the immune system calls on them to attack and kill targeted cells. Most scientists believe that there is some link between lower back pain and fewer NK cells, but the causal relationship remains a mystery: it is uncertain whether fewer NK cells lead to back problems and pain, or whether back problems and pain lower NK cell counts.

Finding a more conclusive cause of back pain could be important for many reasons. For one thing, the Department of Health and Human Services estimates that the United States economy loses billions of dollars each year because of medical bills, lost wages, and insurance claims for back troubles.

Prevention and Therapy

Once a back injury occurs, the range of treatment options is tremendous and quite varied. Today, many professionals treat back pain, including neurologists, orthopedists, chiropractors, acupuncturists, and physical therapists. Each group has advocates, but the virtues of any one of these treatment options over the others have been questioned in recent years.

Most back pain lessens over time. Regardless of the treatment sought out, 90 percent of people complaining of back pain recover after 2 or 3 months, according to the Department of Health and Human Services. Treatment undertaken during this time may then be credited for the improvement. No study has conclusively found that surgery produces better results than other forms of treatment—except for nerve root compression that does not respond to physical therapy (about 5 percent of all cases of back pain).

Of all treatments for back pain, inactivity and bed rest are usually worst: over a period of bed rest as short as 2 weeks, the body will lose 5 to 10 percent of bone calcium. The best course is usually gradual mobilization under the supervision of a physical therapist. Physical therapy can improve the strength and flexibility of the back so that normal activity can be resumed.

Regardless of the reason for back pain, it is usually still possible to improve the health of the back, and many common lower back troubles can be avoided with some simple preventive steps. In sports, for example, prevention begins with education of coaches and players. At an early age, players can be taught to modify their technique to prevent injuries. For instance, football players can learn how to keep the head up while tackling to avoid serious cervical spine injuries; they can also be fitted with the proper equipment and learn how to use it properly. Coaches can ensure that young athletes develop the correct technique and select the appropriate equipment for their size and strength. The following sections will consider basic factors important in prevention: first posture and weight, and then exercise.

Posture and Weight

Posture is extremely important to the health of the spine. Continuous sitting or standing in a misaligned position takes its toll on physical health. Bad posture leads to many kinds of chronic and recurring back pain, drains energy, and increases fatigue. In fact, slouching is a vicious circle. It compresses the diaphragm, and this in turn restricts the ability of the lungs to expand. Restricted breathing means that less oxygen is inhaled to supply the body's cells, hastening the onset of fatigue—and the greater the fatigue, the greater the slouching. The resulting worsened posture increases the load that the lumbar spine must support.

Maintaining the body in an upright position is accomplished by the brain and the reflex mechanisms "wired into" the spinal cord; the primary postural reflexes keep one's center of gravity over the base of support. Good posture relieves the pressure on the back by distributing the gravitational forces that act upon the spine over a greater area, thereby reducing the load—or pain—in any one region. Whether one is standing, sitting, or lying down, gravity exerts a force on the body. Most of the gravitational force on the spine is concentrated at the lower back, the lumbar region. The gravitational load on the lower back is greater in a prone or a sitting position than in a standing position, and this effect is increased by poor posture (*see Figure 6*).

Obesity has a tremendous effect on posture. Excess weight can make it more difficult to maintain an upright posture and may cause a stiff gait with a shorter stride. Weight concentrated in the abdominal area, in particular, can cause the body to lean slightly backward to balance the additional weight in front. This results in increased lumbar stress, as more weight is borne by the heels. Over time, this may cause the back to sway forward, increasing the lumbar curve and disk compression (*see Figure 7*).

Specialized strenuous athletic activity can also result in a change in posture. In gymnastics, for example, pommel-horse specialists are apt to develop overly rounded shoulders and curvature of the spine if they do not also engage in exercises that work the other muscles (contralateral muscles). Posture adaptations can be minimized or prevented by making a conscious effort to improve posture when not engaged in the sport or activity causing the problem.

Posture while lifting is also very important. Knees should be bent so that the arms remain level with the object, and one should try to push rather than pull any heavy object. Pushing is safer than pulling because pulling increases tension in the back muscles, whereas push-

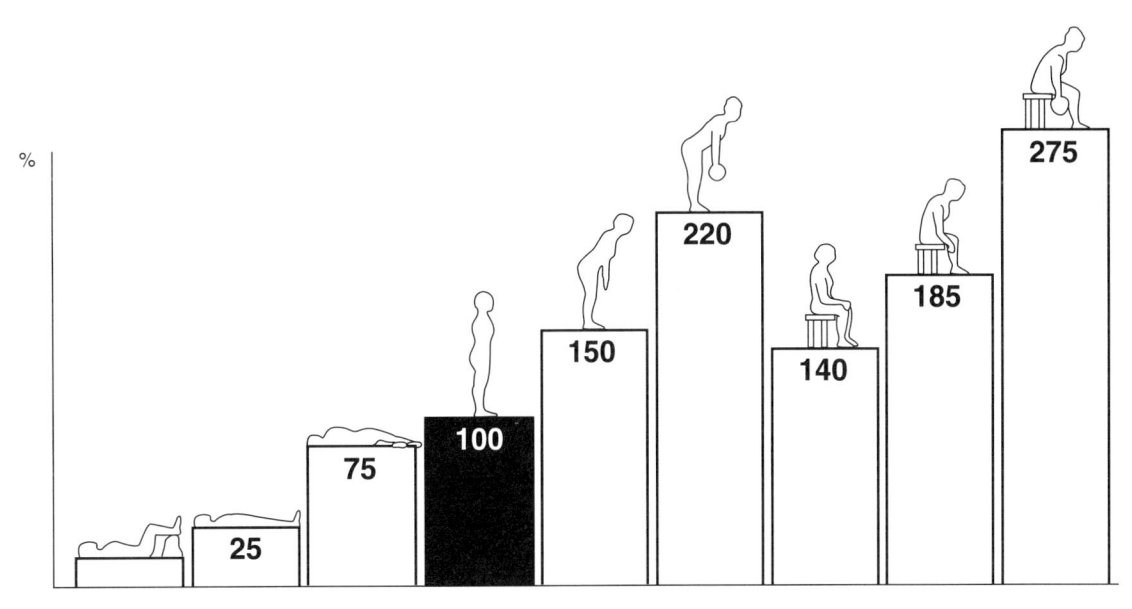

Figure 6. *Gravitational loads on the third lumbar disk during various postures and activities. The load on the spine for a slouched sitting position (185%) is almost twice that for the "benchmark" standing position (100%). (Adapted from Panjabi, 1985)*

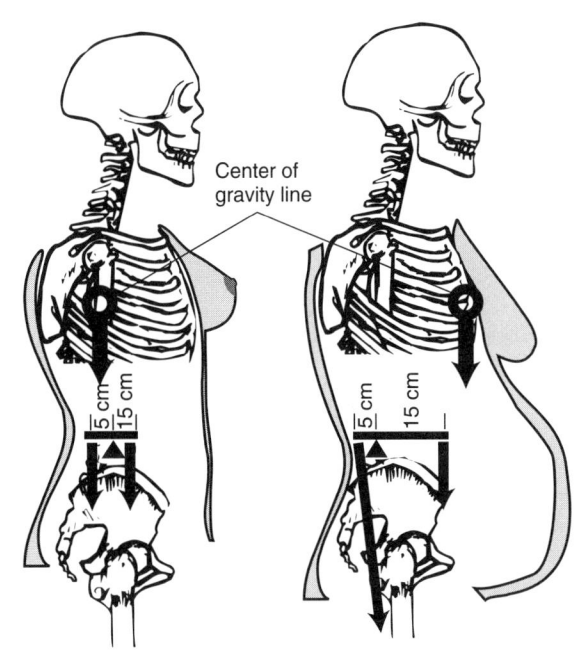

Figure 7. *Excess weight subjects the spine to a greater compressive force from gravity. In addition to the increase in force exerted on the spine, a wider girth shifts the line of the center of gravity farther away from the spine. For a typical standing woman (left), the center of gravity passes about 5 centimeters (2 in.) in front of the third lumbar disk, while the back muscles pass about 5 centimeters behind. To prevent the body from falling forward, the 300 newtons (67 lb.) of gravitational force must be balanced by a 300-newton force exerted by the back muscles; thus the total force acting on the disk is 600 newtons. The figure on the right has more weight and a longer lever arm (15 cm, or 6 in.). If the gravitational force were 400 newtons through the center of gravity line, the back muscles would need to generate a 1,200-newton force to remain erect (15/5 = 3; 400 ×3 = 1,200 N.) The force acting on the disk is 1,200 + 400 = 1,600 newtons (360 lb.).*

ing increases tension in the abdominal muscles—the primary support muscles for the spine.

It should be noted, though, that good posture cannot always compensate for a structural deformity. In fact, such deformities can cause postural compensations that may lead to lower back pain. For example, a discrepancy in length of legs—from a congenital flaw or a childhood injury—creates a potential for future back pain from uneven loading because of the asymmetrical stress on the lumbar spine. (For this reason, children who fracture a bone should be seen by an orthopedist to ensure that their skeletal structure is not creating asymmetrical stress on the spine.)

Nevertheless, in general good posture helps prevent back pain, just as poor posture will eventually result in pain. Over time, abnormal stresses caused by poor posture "wear down" the spinal structures. Then, even slight movements can trigger the onset of chronic lower back pain. Improving posture is a first step toward avoiding back pain.

Abdominal Muscles and Exercise

The spine cannot stand erect against the force of gravity without the action and support of muscles. The primary function of the muscles and ligamentous structures surrounding the spine is to contract, so that closure occurs, but they also stabilize other movements. An objective of most strength training programs is to "overstrengthen" the muscles surrounding the spine to overcome any instability of the joint.

Abdominal muscles work as the key benders and stabilizers of the spine. Well-functioning abdominal musculature "unloads" the back during lifting and stabilizes the spinal cord. The abdominal muscles (antagonists) create the counterforce to the back muscles (agonist). The spine tends naturally to sway forward, and this creates great stress

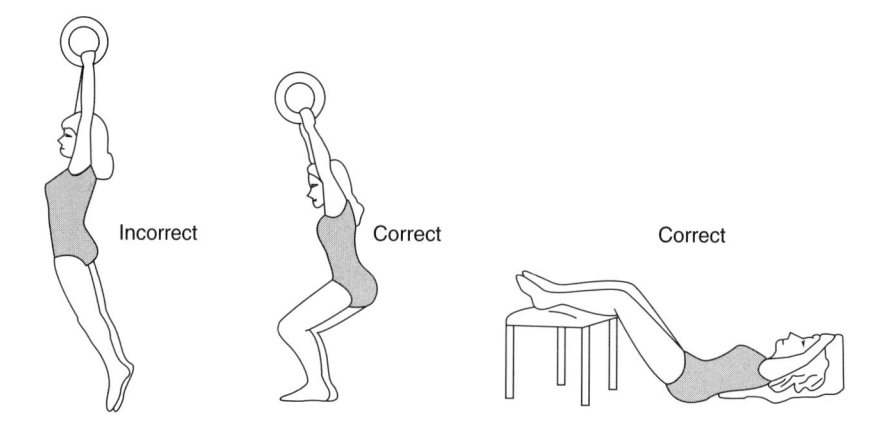

Figure 8. *Incorrect and correct ways to relieve stress to the spinal column. Maintaining a straight spine is a popular misconception. Instead, pressure is best relieved by maintaining the natural curve of the spine. Hanging from the bar reduces the pressure on disks, "unloading" the back, but it also unnecessarily stretches the back muscles; therefore the best hanging position for "unloading" is with bent hips and feet against the ground. When standing for a long period of time, it is best to put one foot on a step to tilt the pelvis and relieve stress on the lower back. (Adapted from Wirhed, 1984)*

Figure 9. *Abdominal muscles (left) at rest and (right) during lifting. The contraction (tensing) of strong abdominal muscles increases abdominal pressure, which widens the abdominal cavity. This helps "unload" the spine during lifting. Weak abdominal muscles are unable to unload the spine.*

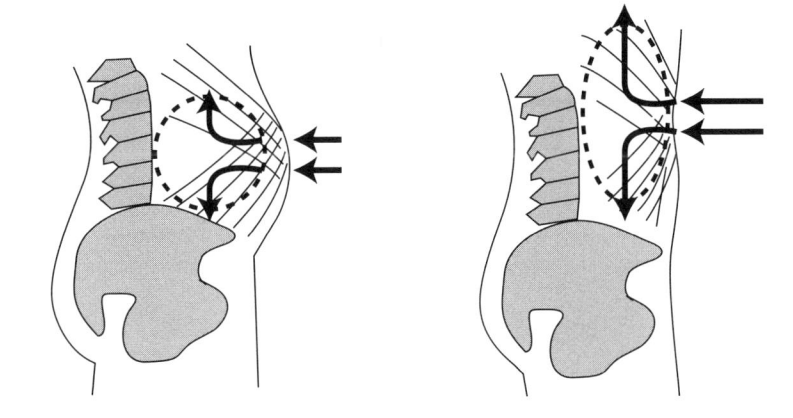

on the disks between the vertebrae. These disks are stabilized and "unloaded" when the abdominal muscles are contracted, or tensed, along with the diaphragm (*see Figure 9*).

Abdominal muscles are often weaker than the back muscles because the back muscles are forced into action during everyday activity while the abdominal muscles have no intrinsic function of support. It is common for the abdominal muscles to become weak from lack of exercise; for this reason, many experts recommend abdominal exercises to improve the overall health of the back.

Strong abdominal muscles are necessary to lower the probability of sustaining a back injury, but there is also some risk that the exercise itself may cause a back injury. To reduce the risk of injury during training, exercises should be undertaken only if the abdominal muscles are capable of stabilizing the spine during activity. To ensure that the abdominal muscles are getting the full effect, movement should take place only at the spine, not at the hips. By bending at the hips so that the pelvis muscles cannot contract forcefully, the abdominal muscles can be isolated. During exercises like sit-ups, bending at the hips and leaving the feet unsupported maximizes contraction of the abdominal muscles. Because only the first 45 degrees of bending and last 45 degrees of straightening work the abdominal muscles during full sit-ups, therapists recommend partial sit-ups or curl-ups, in which the knees are bent and the ankles remain unsupported. Full sit-ups put the back at risk with little added benefit to strengthening.

Besides strengthening abdominal muscles and the muscles surrounding the spine, a conditioning program also should include stretches for the hamstring and lumbodorsal leg muscles as well as pelvis tilt stretches. These stretches are necessary to keep tight hamstring muscles from creating additional force on the spine by "pulling down" on the posterior side of the pelvis and spine—an effect that can occur because shortened muscles at the back of the thigh prevent the pelvis from tilting forward. Runners compensate for tighter hamstrings by bending forward at the lumbar spine, but this can lead to back injuries from the effectively shortened hamstrings.

John Zumerchik[*]

[*]*The author would like to thank Bruce Hauger and Don C. Hopkins for their assistance in putting this article together.*

References

Adams, M. "The Effect of Posture on the Strength of the Lumbar Spine." *Engineering in Medicine* 10, no. 4 (1981): 199ff.

Adrian, M., and J. Cooper. *Biomechanics of Human Movement*. Dubuque, Iowa: Benchmark, 1989.

Altman, L. "New Findings in Whiplash Treatment: Most Don't Work." *New York Times* (2 May 1995).

Brennan, P., et al. "Lymphocyte Profiles in Patients with Chronic Low Back Pain Enrolled in a Clinical Trial." *Journal of Manipulative Physiological Therapies* 17, no. 4 (1994): 219–227.

Brinckmann, P., et al. "Sex Differences in the Skeletal Geometry of the Human Pelvis and Hip Joint." *Journal of Biomechanics* 14, no. 6 (1981): 427ff.

Ghista, D. *Human Body Dynamics: Impact, Occupational, and Athletic Aspects*. New York: Oxford University Press, 1982.

Gracovetsky, S. "An Hypothesis for the Role of the Spine in Human Locomotion: A Challenge to Current Theory." *Journal of Biomedical Engineering* 7, no. 3 (1985): 205ff.

Gracovetsky, S., et al. "The Abdominal Mechanism." *Spine* 10, no. 4 (1985): 317ff.

Granhed, H., and B. Morelli. "Low Back Pain Among Retired Wrestlers and Heavy Weight Lifters." *American Journal of Sports Medicine* 16 (1988): 417ff.

Hall, S. "Effect of Attempting Lifting Speed on Forces and Torques Exerted on the Lumbar Spine." *Medicine and Science in Sports and Exercise* 17, no. 4 (1985): 440ff.

Jensen, M., et al. "Magnetic Resonance Imaging of the Lumbar Spine in People without Back Pain." *New England Journal of Medicine* 331 (1994): 69–73.

Kolata, G. "Diagnostics in Doubt: Backache Not Necessarily Connected to Backbone." *New York Times* (17 July 1994).

Leskinen, T., et al. "The Inertial Factors on Spinal Stress When Lifting." *Engineering in Medicine* 12, no. 2 (1983): 87ff.

Lillegard, W., and K. Rucker (eds.). *Handbook of Sports Medicine*. Stoneham, Massachusetts: Andover Medical, 1993.

Marks, M., et al. "Low Back Pain in the Competitive Tennis Player." *Clinical Sports Medicine* 7 (1988): 277ff.

Mundt, D., et al. "An Epidemiological Study of Sports and Weight Lifting as Possible Risk Factors for Herniated and Cervical Discs." *American Journal of Sports Medicine* 21 (1993): 854ff.

Oonishi, H., et al. "Mechanical Analysis of the Human Pelvis and Its Application to the Artificial Hip Joint." *Journal of Biomechanics* 16, no. 6 (1983): 427–444.

Panjabi, M. "The Human Spine: Story of Its Biomechanical Functions." In D. Winter et al. (eds.), *Biomechanics IX-A*. Champaign, Illinois: Human Kinetics, 1985.

Root, L. *No More Aching Back*. New York: Villard, 1990.

Schultz, A., et al. "Analysis and Measurement of Lumbar Trunk Loads in Tasks Involving Bends and Twists." *Journal of Biomechanics* 15, no. 9 (1982): 669–675.

Viano, D., et al. "Injury Biomechanics Research: An Essential Element in the Prevention of Trauma." *Journal of Biomechanics* 22, no. 5 (1989): 403–417.

Wirhed, R. *Athletic Ability and the Anatomy of Motion*. New York: Wolf Medical, 1984.

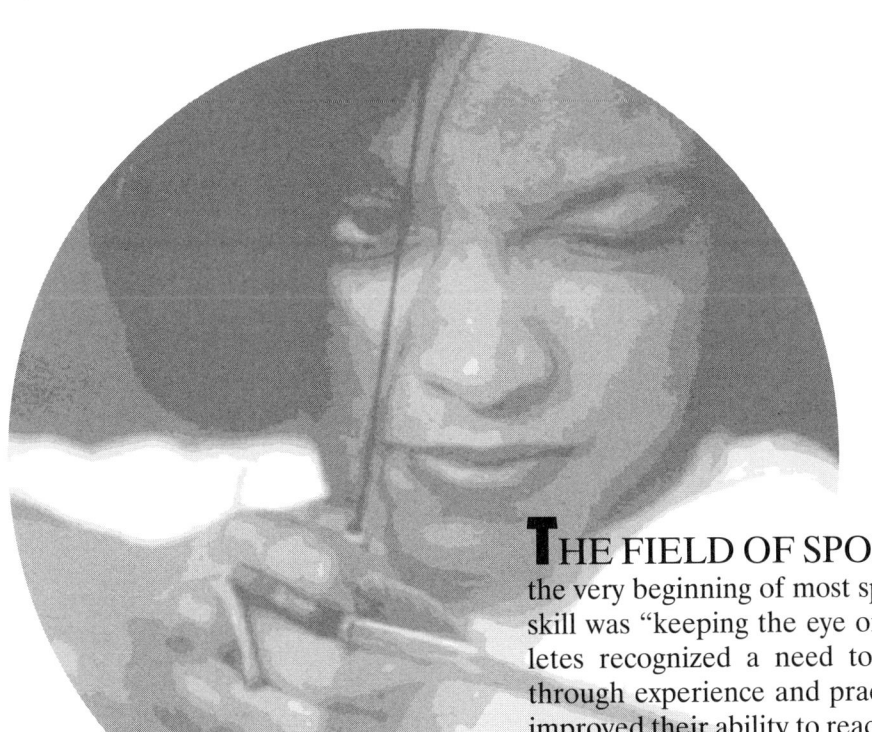

Vision

THE FIELD OF SPORTS VISION is not really new. From the very beginning of most sports, participants realized that a crucial skill was "keeping the eye on the ball"—or on something else. Athletes recognized a need to develop and refine their visual skills through experience and practice; and they realized that visual skills improved their ability to react to the environment around them. Even early humans—though their understanding of eyesight cannot have been more than rudimentary—must have known one basic fact: good eyesight helped them survive. It was not until the latter half of the nineteenth century that scientists began to understand the physiological and psychological workings of the visual system. And it was not until the twentieth century that scientists began to fully comprehend the possibility of enhancing visual performance through many different forms of visual therapy and visual training.

One of the first visual aids was developed by Native Americans for use in hunting. To reduce the glare from snow and ice, the ancient Inuit (Eskimos) cut a narrow slit in a small piece of bone or wood and banded it around the head and over the eyes. Whether this should be considered a sports aid or a survival aid is a matter of interpretation, but in either case it was innovative.

When commercial aids to vision were first being developed, frames and lenses were the primary concern. In 1896, Sears Roebuck carried an advertisement for "shooting and millers' spectacles"; this was one of the earliest attempts to design eyewear specifically for a sport. Around 1915, colored lenses were recommended for hunting, as a means of absorbing the rays of the sun, and various tints were promoted for different outdoor conditions.

Protective eyewear was also developed in the early twentieth century. Around 1900, a larger frame was developed for farmers and tennis players to eliminate potential interference with the field of sight from the frame itself. A few years later, in 1908, Robert J. Hallowell obtained a patent for "Eyeglass Protectors for Baseball Players" and gave the patent to Spaulding Brothers, one of the largest sporting goods manufacturers at that time. Since this device was similar in shape to a catcher's mask, it probably was designed for catchers. It failed in the marketplace, however, and it is not mentioned much in the baseball literature—nor does it seem to have been captured in old photos.

Medical concerns about the relationship between sports and

vision were relatively rare until the 1960s, though there were some forerunners. An article prescribing lenses for tennis and golf appeared in 1912. In the 1930s, there were articles dealing with visual imagery and sports skills. In the 1940s, there were four publications on sports vision. One article discussed how football and basketball affect vision; this article was consistent with a common belief of the time—that exercise could be dangerous to health. After the 1940s, research on sports vision began to expand; there were 18 publications in the 1950s, 74 in the 1960s, and more than 150 in the 1970s. As the number of publications continued to multiply in the 1980s and 1990s, sports vision consultants began to set up practices, delving into every area of sports and having considerable influence.

This article briefly outlines the physiology of vision and perception, the process of optical reception of stimuli, and the neural process that takes the visual image from the eye to the brain via nerve cells. Then, it discusses factors affecting vision in sports and some of the criteria and methods sports vision consultants use to improve the visual skills of athletes.

The Physiology of Vision

It is through the sense of sight that most experiences are first identified and interpreted. A widely accepted definition of vision is that it is a process through which data are received and integrated with other input into the brain, and with stored information, so that the meaning is abstracted and the organism institutes the appropriate output—movement, visualization, or projection. Vision triggers the chain-reaction motor system of the human body: it is a signal that causes a hitter in baseball to swing, a boxer to duck a punch, or a goalkeeper in soccer to dive for an oncoming ball. After the initial output, there is always some resultant input or feedback through sensory paths that enables the body to know whether or not the output satisfied the situation.

The visual process starts with light. Light is the stimulus outside of the body that produces vision. What registers as light is electromagnetic radiation waves that the body's visual apparatus is capable of sensing and responding to. This visible spectrum, as it is called, is actually a relatively small segment of the electromagnetic spectrum (*see Figure 1*). Measured in wavelengths (the distance between two successive wave peaks), the visual spectrum lies between 380 and 780 nanometers (billionths of a meter). Within this range, a variety of colors are visible. Waves at the short end of the spectrum appear violet, and waves at the long end appear red.

Although vision depends on light, most of the eye is concerned not with reacting directly to light but rather with shaping the incoming image into something that can be used by the neurons to formu-

Physiological Reasons for Sports Vision Training

1. Most visual skills are learned and thus can be relearned and enhanced through training.

2. Vision is the dominant sense in most sports.

3. The area of the brain (in the cortex) that relates to vision is as much as five times larger than the area related to all the other senses combined.

4. The eyes provide 80 percent of all the sensory information reaching the brain.

5. Twenty percent of the optic nerve fibers leaving the eyes "connect" to posture and balance centers in the brain. (Source: Sports Vision Guidebooks, 1984–1993)

late messages to send to the brain. Naturally, the more complex a visual image, the longer the shaping or processing time, which in turn affects reaction time. Whereas the human eye may to respond to a simple visual pattern quickly, in about 80 milliseconds, a complex visual pattern takes considerably longer, about 260 milliseconds (Griffing, 1987). This can affect performance. For example, almost all batters in major league baseball can react to the simple visual pattern of a fastball coming out of the pitcher's hand against a dark-green background (center field); but younger hitters often struggle to adjust to a curveball, a complex visual pattern involving rotation of the seams. Most major league managers have found at one time or another that a new player who reacted excellently to a simple fastball failed to live up to his promise because he was unable to hit a a curveball—a complex visual pattern.

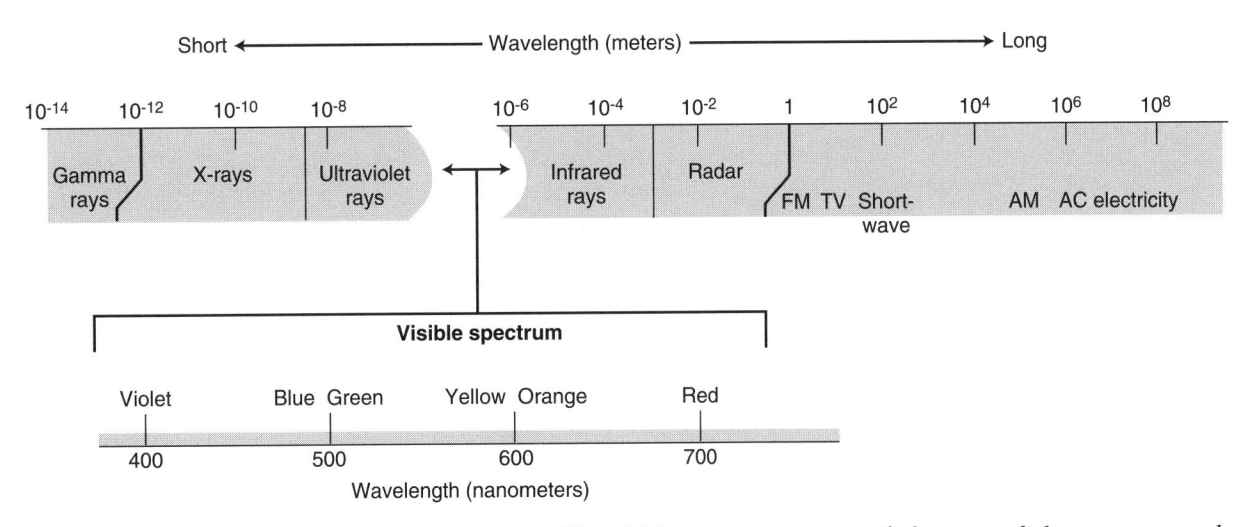

Figure 1. *The electromagnetic and visual spectra. The visible spectrum, commonly known as light, represents only a small fraction of all wavelengths.*

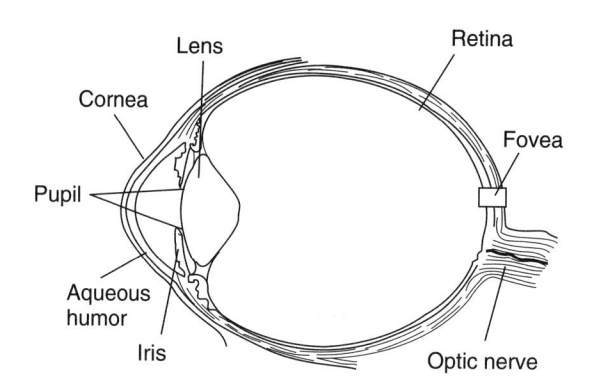

Figure 2. *Principal parts of the human eye.*

Eye Structure

Figure 2 shows the major parts of the eye. Light that reflects off an object (a soccer ball, say) first must travel through the cornea, the transparent outermost layer of the eye, which is lubricated and kept clean by tears. Light rays are refracted (bent) by the tears, then by the cornea, and then to a lesser extent by the lens. The result is a redirection of light rays. The curved cornea bends light rays by different amounts so that they converge at a point after passing through the lens.

After passing through the cornea, the bent light passes through the pupil. The pupil is the dark hole in the center of the iris (the ring-like colored muscle) that changes size as the amount of incoming light changes. In dim light, the pupil dilates (opens wide); in bright light, it constricts. When the pupil is small, it increases the range of distances in which objects stay in focus. On the other hand, a wide-open pupil limits the range of distances at which objects are in focus and makes it difficult to discern details. Without the ability to control the amount of light that passes into the eye, an athlete—or anyone else—is at a serious disadvantage.

Objects come into focus on the retina. This thin layer of neural tissue lines the back of the eyeball and converts electromagnetic energy—light—into useful information for the brain. Although the cornea does more of the total focusing of the visual image on the retina, it is the lens that makes all the adjustments for distance by changing its shape, a process called accommodation. In viewing distant objects, the muscles controlling the lens relax, allowing fluid within the eye to flatten the lens; in viewing close objects, these muscles contract so that the lens takes on a rounder shape.

Two types of light-sensitive receptor cells make up the retina: rods and cones (named for their rod- and cone-shaped light-sensitive tips). Rods and cones are distributed unevenly throughout the retina. The greatest concentration of cones is at the fovea, the part of the retina with greatest clarity, or visual acuity. Except for the blind spot (*see Figure 5 later in this article*), visual acuity is greatest at the fovea and gradually declines farther out toward the edge of the retina. Cones, which are primarily responsible for the perception of color,

**Fovea
(cone concentration):**

Reading
Detail reading
Color perception

**Away from fovea
(rod concentration):**

Night vision
Visual orientation
Fixating
Gazing at a moving object

are less sensitive to changes in incoming light, responding only to levels of illumination greater than twilight. Rods are extremely sensitive to changes in incoming light, respond to very low levels of illumination, and are relatively insensitive to colors and detail.

The rods are critical for peripheral vision (the ability to perceive objects outside the center of focus) as well as for night vision. If the lighting is dim enough, an athlete will perform better when the rods are stimulated while the cones remain inactive. In this situation, there is not enough light for the cones to discern color and detail, so the eye relies on the rods. For instance, if a tennis match is taking place at dusk, when daylight is rapidly turning to darkness, the players may actually see the ball better by looking slightly away from it as it approaches. Gazing slightly off-center means that the image from the lens does not fall on the relatively night-blind foveal cones but moves more toward the light-sensitive rods (Feldman, 1987).

Most tennis players, of course, prefer to finish an outdoor match well before dusk, and many complain if they have to play a game in a dimly lit gymnasium. However, some athletes find such situations more difficult than others do. This is because two athletes with very similar visual skills in bright daylight might have very different skills at dusk or in dim indoor lighting. A player with good night vision who performs better at dusk probably has more than the average number of rods (the average is about 125 million), or rods that are more sensitive. In this regard, though, the ability to play well in dim lighting may also be due to training: a player can learn to gaze slightly off-center at an oncoming tennis ball so that more rods, rather than cones, are stimulated. Another factor is the ability of the eye to adapt to light and darkness. Light and dark adaptation is a function of the rate at which changes occur in the chemical composition of the rods and cones. Cones reach their highest level of adaptation quickly, within 6 or 7 minutes, but rods need about 30 minutes to adapt (*see Figure 3*). Because of this need for adaptation, volleyball players coming out of a dimly lit locker room will have problems for the first few points of a match, until their eyes adapt.

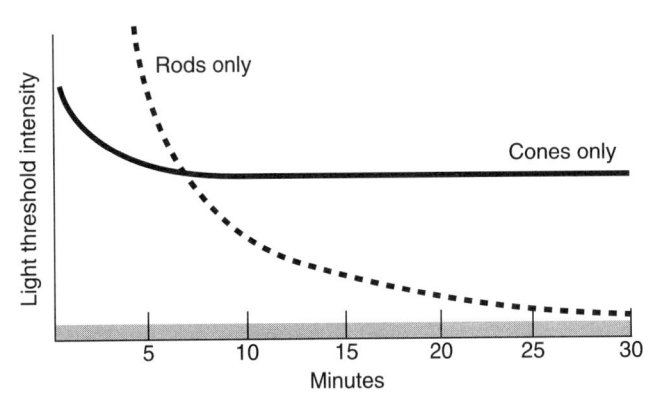

Figure 3. *Adaptation for night vision. The rate of adaptation is different for rods and cones. It take cones 6 or 7 minutes to adapt to dim light, while rods take about 30 minutes.*

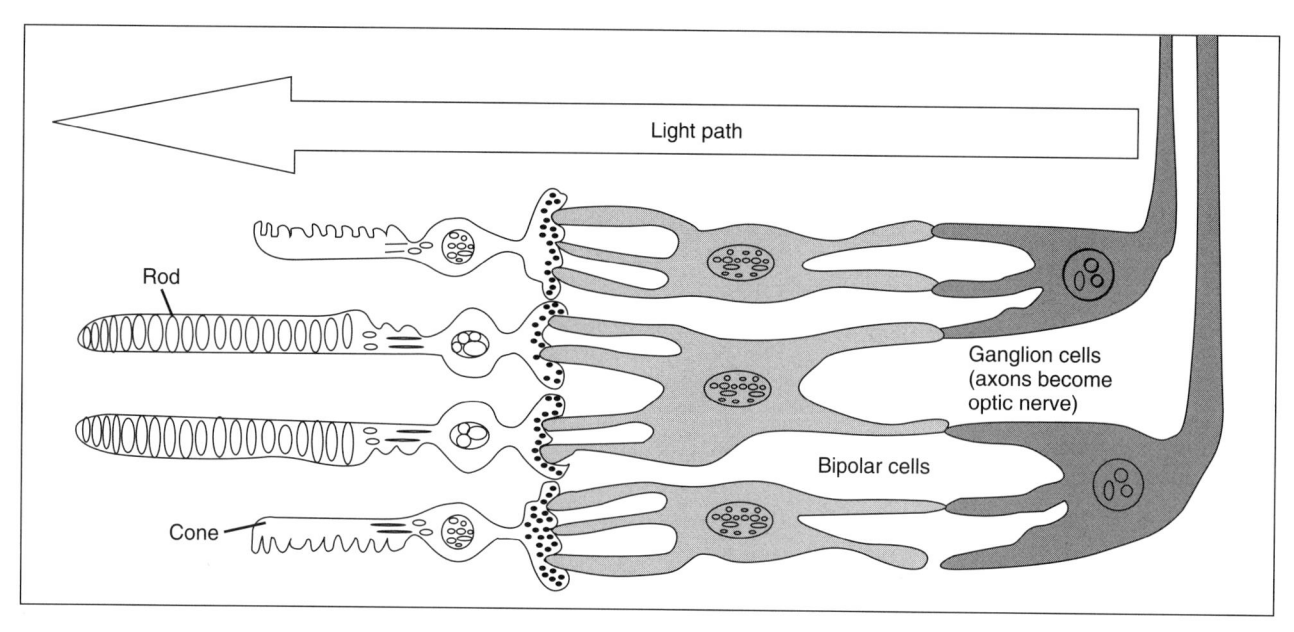

Figure 4. *Organization of the cells in the retina. The rods and cones lie on the side of the retina opposite to the entry of light; therefore, light must pass through all the retinal cells before reaching and stimulating the photoreceptors.*

Sending the Message: From the Eye to the Brain

When rods and cones are stimulated, they pass the information to bipolar cells. Bipolar cells pass information from one part of the retina to the other and on to the ganglion cells. The ganglion cells collect and summarize information coming from the rods and then move this information through the optic nerve (*see Figure 4*).

The point at which the optic nerve leaves the retina has no rods or cones; thus light that hits this area does not produce vision. This creates what is known as the eye's "blind spot" (*see Figure 5*). Everyone has two blind spots—one in each eye—but people are usually unaware of this because the eyes automatically use nearby objects to fill in the missing information and complete the field of vision, compensating for the blind spot.

The optic nerve leaving the eyeball does not take a direct route to the brain. Figure 6 shows the field of vision of the right and left eyes and the route that nerve impulses take to the brain. The optic

Figure 5. *The blind spot is an area with neither rods nor cones where the optic nerve leaves the eye. To find the blind spot: Close the left eye and focus on the X with the right eye. The man will still be visible, because of peripheral vision. Now slowly move the page closer to the eye; when it is within a few inches of the eye, the man should disappear. This happens because the light reflected from the image of the man is now falling on the blind spot. Usually, people are unaware of the blind spot, since the eye can use nearby objects to compensate for the missing information. However, athletes should know the location of their blind spot. When a quarterback allows an interception by throwing right at a defender, he is likely to claim afterward that he did not see the defender; if the defender was "hiding" in the quarterback's blind spot, this may be true.*

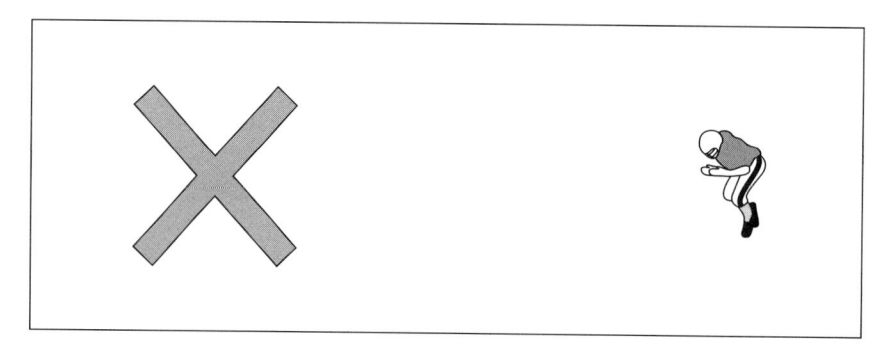

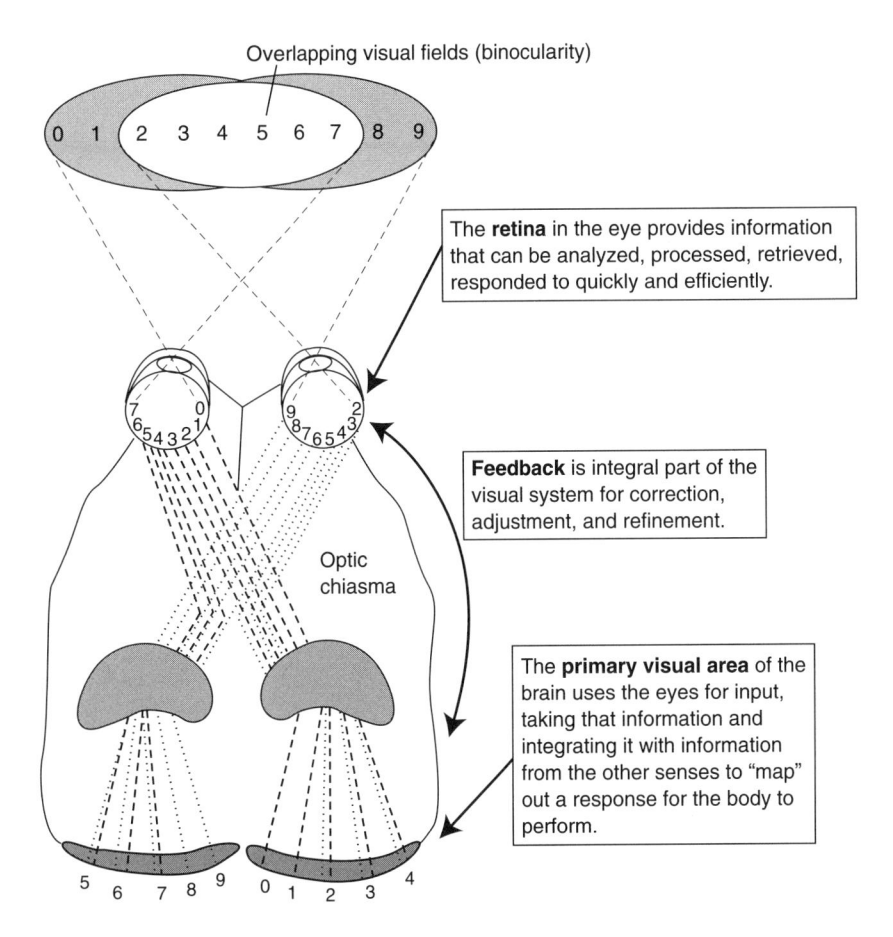

Figure 6. *The visual system. The optic nerves coming from the retina of each eye converge at the optic chiasma. Images coming from the right half of each retina are sent to the right side of the brain, and images coming from the left half of each retina are sent to the left side of the brain. The retina provides information that can be quickly analyzed, processed, retrieved, and responded to. The primary visual area of the brain uses the eyes for input, integrating that input with information from the other senses to "map" out a response. Feedback—for correction, adjustment, and refinement—is an integral part of the visual system. (Adapted from Feldman, 1987)*

The **retina** in the eye provides information that can be analyzed, processed, retrieved, responded to quickly and efficiently.

Feedback is integral part of the visual system for correction, adjustment, and refinement.

The **primary visual area** of the brain uses the eyes for input, taking that information and integrating it with information from the other senses to "map" out a response for the body to perform.

nerves actually split at the optic chiasma. Here the nerve impulses coming from the right half of each retina are sent to the right side of the brain, and the nerve impulses coming from the left side of each retina are sent to the left side of the brain.

Common Conditions That Impair Vision

Although everyone's eyes are different, a wide range of conditions are common in the general population. Over the course of a lifetime, most people will need treatment for at least one of the following conditions.

Presbyopia. As a normal part of aging, the lens of the eye becomes increasingly stiff, which makes accommodation for near vision increasingly difficult. As a result, at the age of 45 to 50, people often require reading glasses or bifocals. This condition is not a major concern of older athletes.

Cataracts. Cataracts—another change associated with aging—are one of the most common eye disorders, and surgery to remove cataracts is one of the most common of all surgical procedures. When a cataract develops, the lens of the eye becomes foggy or less transparent. This change in the lens is a slow process, and the early stages may be undetectable because they do not interfere with vision. Because the surgery entails removal of the lens, many doctors recommend waiting until a rather late stage of cataract formation: without the lens, the eye loses its ability to accommodate.

Myopia and hyperopia. Two eye disorders that affect many people are myopia, commonly called nearsightedness; and hyperopia, or farsightedness. The combination of the shape of the cornea and lens and the length of the eyeball determines where light rays converge (see Figure 7). If the eyeball is too long (myopic vision), the lens and cornea converge light rays so that images of close objects are in focus, but images of distant objects are focused at a point in front of the retina. If the eyeball is too short (hyperopic vision), the cornea and lens converge light rays so that images of distant objects are in focus on the retina, but near objects are focused behind it. Corrective eyewear, such as glasses or contact lenses, assists the cornea and lens in focusing light rays at the retina.

Astigmatism. In astigmatism, the lens or cornea has surface imperfections or does not have a smooth spherical shape. This condition usually can be corrected with glasses.

Glaucoma. High-pressure glaucoma affects 1 to 2 percent of the population of the United States. This disorder develops when the aqueous humor, a fluid occurring naturally in the eye, forms faster than it is removed, so that pressure builds up within the eye. In the initial stages, the nerve cells that communicate peripheral vision are constricted (tunnel vision). If no therapy is initiated, constriction continues and can eventually lead to total blindness.

Low-pressure glaucoma is believed to result from a deficient blood supply to the optic nerve. People with arteriosclerosis and diabetes are particularly at risk of developing low-pressure glaucoma.

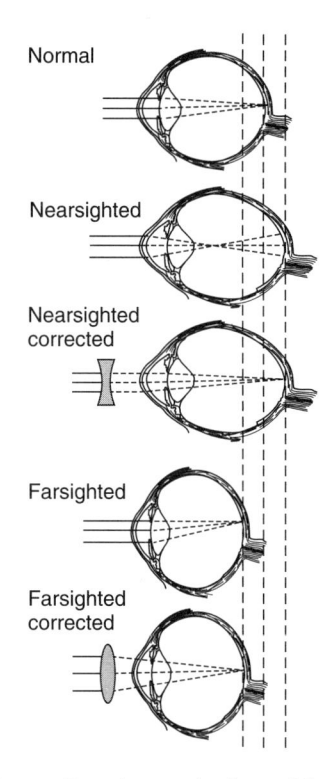

Figure 7. *A myopic (nearsighted) person needs a concave-shaped lens—that is, a lens curving inward—to bend light rays outward. A hyperopic (farsighted) person needs a convex lens—a lens bulging outward—to converge light rays inward.*

Processing Visual Information in Sports

"Vision" can have different meanings. In sports, for example, it can be passive, that is, reactive (the eyes tell the athlete what they see); but it can also be active, or initiatory (the athlete tells the eyes what to look for). Similarly, it can be thought of as innate or as learned.

There are considerable differences of opinion among experts about which visual skills are learned as opposed to innate; vision obviously has a large hereditary component, but research continues find a strong learning component as well. One instance is amblyopia ("lazy eye") in children. This condition must be treated by age 2: the child wears a patch over the normal eye so that the "lazy" eye will be forced to develop. If the condition is not treated, the retinal receptors of the affected eye will receive insufficient direct stimulation (light) and will not develop fully; a critical developmental stage will be lost.

Sports optometrists take advantage of the learned component of vision to teach athletes to better recognize what they see, as well as what their eyes should look for. Even the most anatomically strong and healthy eye must learn to perform. Thus optometrists have developed a number of criteria for performance skills. Vision can be improved by developing specific visual processing skills—through vision therapy, vision training, and establishment of the "visual environment."

The need for sports vision training is in some ways like the need for strength training. Participation in a sport, by itself, helps build muscle strength, yet muscle strength can pass a certain threshold only if the athlete engages in strength training. Similarly, through vision training, an athlete can pass the limiting developmental threshold—going beyond what can be achieved simply by participating in sports. That is, specific visual skills used in a sport can be enhanced by isolating and working on them individually.

To succeed in sports, athletes must be able to use their visual processing skills to extract information from objects, places, and events. When this vast information strikes the retina, an athlete must decipher and select the information that is most important to the task at hand.

The visual abilities needed for sports are much greater and more varied than those necessary to carry out normal visual functions. Active (initiatory) vision is critical for performance, yet at the same time all the various functions of the entire body must be able to react and operate instantaneously. To perform while in motion, athletes must have a clear understanding of the task at hand, must know where the opponents are in relation to themselves, what the different signs around them mean (such as the boundaries of a playing field), what state of balance they are in, and where the ground is located, especially if they are running, jumping, or moving in an unusual way. All of these visual decisions must be carried out, sometimes within hundredths of a second, as conditions of play change continuously.

With this in mind, sports vision professionals train the entire visual system to maximize athletic performance. In an environment that closely imitates the competitive environment, the primary approach is to isolate specific vision deficiencies and establish specific programs to enhance total visual skills.

Visual Skills

Acuity. The term *acuity* refers to the clarity or sharpness of a visual image, and to the ability to distinguish separate parts of a visual "target." Two aspects of acuity are vital in sports: static and dynamic. Static acuity is the ability to see while stationary; dynamic acuity is the ability to see while the athlete, or the perceived object, is moving. While static acuity is primarily determined by heredity, there is considerable potential to improve dynamic acuity.

Visual acuity aids a player's tracking ability and reaction time. In

Advantages and Risks of Corrective Vision Surgery

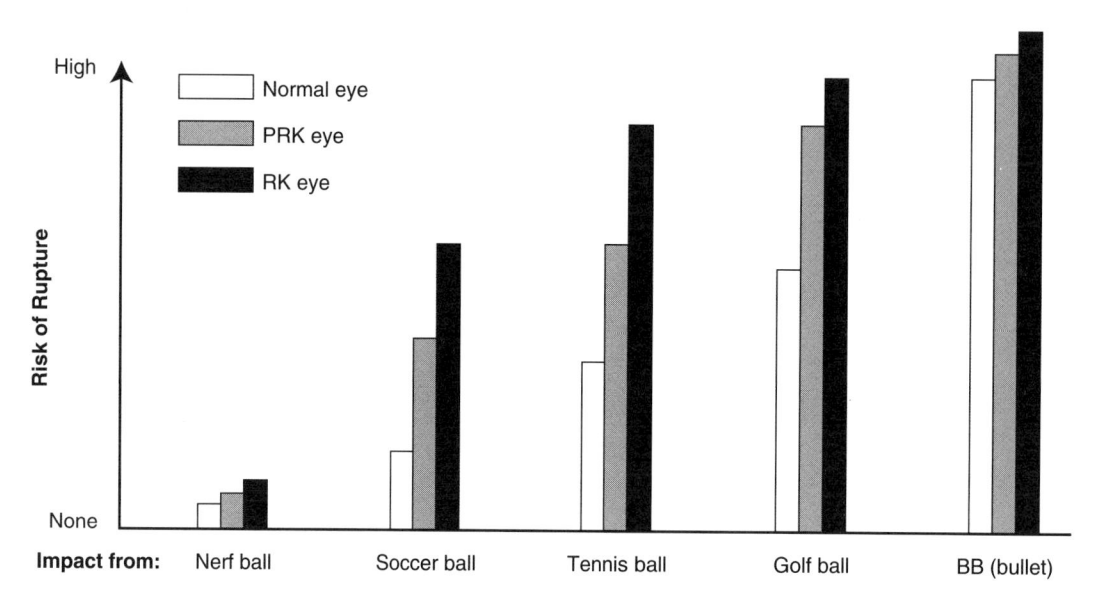

Relative risk of rupture. The RK and excimer laser procedures weaken the eye, and thus increase the risk of rupture. If athletes opt for surgery, it is important that they always wear eye protection while participating in "high risk" sports.

Many athletes who wear eyeglasses are resigned to the necessity of this burdensome nuisance, but they may long for the day when they can leave their spectacles on the sidelines.

Regardless of how good the prescription and the frame may be, eyeglasses usually cause some discomfort and inconvenience during play; and they may not be able to correct vision perfectly—for example, a prescription that gives excellent visual acuity may not provide the best peripheral vision or depth vision.

Eyeglasses have a number of disadvantages. For example, there is fit. Eyeglasses must be fitted so that they will lie squarely across the bridge of the nose, 14 millimeters away from the eyes. Many optometrists recommend that athletes wear support bands to keep the glasses in place. If the glasses bounce up and down off the bridge of the nose, visual abilities can be significantly impaired. For example, a ballplayer moving at a full sprint for an over-the-shoulder catch may drop the ball because of a sudden movement of the glasses and a consequent impairment of vision. Also, eyeglasses are an easy target. In sports like basketball, they can be easily knocked off and can cause considerable pain and discomfort when dislodged. Thus many athletes wear sports goggles. Because of their design, goggles are less likely to be dislodged and cause less pain if they are dislodged.

Contact lenses, which are worn directly on top of the cornea, avoid many of these problems, but some athletes find that contact lenses are uncomfortable and create a tendency to dryness and infection. Moreover, soft contact lenses cannot correct astigmatism.

Therefore, athletes are increasingly turning to another option: corrective eye surgery. Two procedures that gained popularity in the 1980s and 1990s are radial keratotomy (RK) and photorefractive keratectomy (PRK). RK began in the 1970s; PRK, using the eximer laser, was approved by the Food and Drug Administration in 1995.

The RK procedure entails cutting into the cornea. Using a diamond-bladed knife, the surgeon cuts slits in the cornea from the center of the eye outward. Some experts in sports vision believe that RK may be a risky, nonessential medical procedure for an athlete and fear that cutting into the eye may permanently weaken it. They fear that after the RK procedure, an athlete who is hit in the eye by a ball or fist is more susceptible to a rupture, which has the potential to cause blindness.

Because of these risks, PRK, or eximer laser surgery, was developed as an alternative procedure. *Eximer* is a short form of *excited dimer*; in an excited-dimer laser, molecules closely bound in a high-energy state are subjected to an electrical discharge in a laser cavity. The argon-fluoride eximer laser generates a beam of ultraviolet light that blasts apart the molecular bonds of corneal tissue through a mostly photochemical reaction. The eximer laser is useful as a surgical instrument because it can ablate (melt or dissipate) tissue without significantly heating adjacent tissue.

PRK requires the precise ablation of corneal tissue over approximately 6 millimeters of the visual axis. In PRK for myopia (nearsightedness), the central cornea is flattened to decrease refraction (that is, to make it "bend" light less; *refer back to Figure 7*). The conditions set by the FDA when it approved this procedure in 1995 limited the amount of ablation; Canada, however, does not impose such limits. The procedure takes about 35 minutes, including about 30 to 40 seconds of laser ablation.

Although some experts consider PRK very promising, it is usually not recommended for anyone who wears contact lenses and is satisfied with them. There are three major complications to consider:

1. *Corneal haze* is part of the normal healing process. It is variable, but in most patients it diminishes with time and treatment (topical anti-inflammatory drops).

2. *Pain* is extremely variable, but it is a possibility for all patients.

3. *Disturbances in night vision* have been reported. Complaints of nighttime glare and seeing halos and star bursts around lights are common among patients after RK surgery and can also be a problem after PRK. In one study, 38 percent of PRK patients complained of some impairment of night vision 1 year after surgery (Vinger, 1996). However, these effects decrease when the ablation area is larger, and because the FDA guidelines indicate a large ablation area, complications of this kind are likely to be fairly rare.

Other possibilities for people considering PRK surgery are second- and third-generation lasers that use a rotating mask, and the LASIK procedure (laser in-situ keratomileusis). In LASIK, which is considered less invasive than PRK, the outer epithelial corneal surface is "peeled" or lifted. Next, the doctor positions the laser to shoot pulses of ultraviolet light to ablate or reshape the inner stromal tissue. Finally, a soft contact lens is placed over the eye, protecting it until the epithelium is fully healed. LASIK allows for a more natural healing process and reduces the risk of postoperative complications. Nevertheless, doctors must closely monitor how the cornea grows back, and, if necessary, use medications to guide its formation.

Preliminary evaluations of PRK seem positive. In a clinical trial, reports taken 12 months after PRK showed that 99 percent of patients had 20/40 uncorrected vision or better and 80 percent had 20/20 or better. One percent lost two lines of best eyeglasses-corrected acuity (they had problems reading), and 2 percent experienced persistent corneal stromal haze.

However, as of 1996 there were no studies of the impact of laser surgery beyond a few years, so it was still too early to know what long-term side effects it might have. PRK leaves less scar tissue than RK, but whether scar

---

RISK FACTORS IN LASER SURGERY
The most important factor for optimal sports performance is visual acuity; but if a patient's visual acuity with contact lenses or eyeglasses is 20/20 or 20/15, refractive corneal surgery may not achieve that acuity. Thus to have 20/20 or 20/15 acuity, many patients will still need eyeglasses or contact lenses after surgery. In addition to this possibility, an athlete considering surgery should be aware of postsurgical complications. In other words, the athlete should weigh the risks against the rewards.

RISKS:
Greater chance of globular rupture.
Haziness.
Pain.
Poorer night vision; slower glare recovery.
Certain preexisting increase the risk of complications: diabetes, kerotaconus (cone-shaped cornea), dry eyes or eyelid pathology, cataracts, microvascular disease, and collagen-vascular disease.
Youth—the procedure is not recommended for athletes under 21 (refractive errors stabilize).
Possible continued need for corrective lenses.
No studies of side effects beyond a few years.

REWARDS:
Less dependence on vision correction.
Less regular personal eye care.

PRK ablation (flattening) of the cornea

Concaved lens

(continued)

Advantages and Risks of Corrective Vision Surgery (continued)

tissue from either procedure would interfere with vision after 20 or 30 years was still uncertain. One long-term side effect was already known: PRK and RK speed up the natural deterioration in close vision. This means that a 35-year-old person with myopia who would normally require bifocal reading glasses at age 45 may require them considerably earlier after the surgery. On the other hand, this might be of little concern to someone like a tennis player, who might reason that unencumbered vision today is worth needing bifocals a little earlier in life.

Another known disadvantage of both procedures is the possibility of follow-up surgery. About 30 percent of RK patients, and only a slightly smaller percentage of PRK patients, need secondary operations to "fine-tune" their vision. Secondary surgery creates additional long-term risk, since it creates additional cornea scar tissue.

There is also an age-related risk to consider. Here, the young assume a greater risk. In athletes under 25, the eyes may heal so quickly that they "resist" the correction and return to their original unfocused state. Therefore, the surgery is mostly recommended for people over 30.

Who are the best candidates for corrective eye surgery? Few. For those who absolutely, positively cannot tolerate either the interference of eyeglasses or the discomfort of contacts, surgery might be the best choice. For most people, eyeglasses and contacts remain a safe, effective way of correcting vision.

---

soccer, for instance, the player, the ball, the player's teammates, and the opponents are all in motion. It takes complex visual processing and well-developed dynamic acuity for the brain to make out details and respond quickly and accurately. An athlete with poor acuity usually needs more time to discern fine details and therefore is slower to react.

Optometrists measure acuity with the Snellen chart. An individual's ability to read the letters on this chart is expressed in relation to a standard, or norm. Thus if a patient can read the big letter "E" on the chart from a distance of no more than 20 feet (6.1 m), while a person with normal vision can read it at 200 feet (61 m), the patient's acuity is 20/200. For static acuity, 20/30 is average, 20/20 is good, and 20/10 is exceptional. Because static acuity is important in so many sports, athletes should have their acuity tested regularly. Many experts recommend that if visual acuity falls below 20/40, an athlete should consult an optometrist about corrective lenses.

There are many training techniques for improving dynamic acuity. One of the simpler drills is to write different letters about 3 centimeters high (slightly more than 1 in.) on several tennis balls. As a partner throws each ball so that it bounces off a wall, the athlete should call out its letter. This drill can be varied by varying the velocity and spin of the ball.

Accommodation. The ability to change focus quickly from one point in space to another is called accommodation. This is an important skill in sports like basketball, in which the athlete must simultaneously focus on the ball, opponents, teammates, and the basket.

Central field awareness. Central field awareness is the ability to see what is directly in front. This ability is primarily a function of the eye, of accommodation, and of another ability: fixation. In many sports, an athlete needs to quickly fixate and focus on a ball or some other object. A tennis player, for instance, must continually shift focus from near to far to intermediate distances within the central field. Similarly, the player must fixate on the ball to hit it; then quickly fixate on the spot in the opponent's court where the ball should land; and then remain fixated on that target until the ball does land. However, athletes should never stare, or remain fixated on the target for too long. Great basketball free-throw shooters know this from experience. They shoot as soon as they are balanced and make a "fine-focus" read. The shorter the fine-focus time on the target, the more intense the focusing ability. Fixation is also important for putting in golf.

Peripheral field awareness. Peripheral field awareness is the ability to see and recognize that which is not directly in front; it is commonly known as "seeing out of the corner of the eye." This is an essential skill in sports like basketball. It gives athletes a good sense of spatial localization—knowing their own position relative to other players, the boundaries of play, and the ball.

To improve peripheral vision, it is necessary to regularly concentrate on how much detail one can gather from the periphery without actually looking at details with central field vision. One common drill to improve peripheral vision is to walk down a street, looking straight ahead, and try to identify as many objects as possible in the store windows. Another drill is to sit down and focus on a single spot on the wall, with a ball hanging from the ceiling at about eye level. If the ball is swung in a circle around the head and shoulders, one should be able to detect it through the use of peripheral vision.

Eye tracking. The ability to follow the path of the ball or moving object, and to sustain this following, is called eye tracking. In tennis, quick accurate saccades (jerky or discontinuous eye movements) are necessary to follow balls served at more than 160 kilometers per hour (KPH; 100 MPH). During the flight of the ball, the player returning serve momentarily takes his or her eye off the ball, somewhere in the middle of its trajectory, shifting the field of vision closer, into the area of the swing. These are involuntary saccades; most athletes are not aware that such movements are occurring.

Depth perception. The ability to judge distance and spatial relationships, known as depth perception, is related to binocularity and eye teaming—the ability of the eyes to function in unison. The eyes perform a skill called triangulation: they are able to fix a moving target at the point of a triangle formed by the two lines of sight. As the target moves, the eyes adjust to keep the target in focus, at the point of this imaginary triangle. Triangulation is a particularly tricky skill for center-fielders in baseball, who must judge fly balls hit directly toward them. Because there is no background to provide context clues about the ball's movement, the fielders lose one of the dimensional perspectives that they have for a ground ball or, to a lesser extent, for a fly ball hit to their left or right (*see also* CATCHING SKILLS).

It is difficult to train for depth perception, but any drill that helps improve stereopsis awareness—three-dimensional clues from a two-dimensional environment—will help improve it. Many outfielders become adept at this skill through years of practice tracking fly balls slightly to the left and right of them.

A visual trait closely related to depth perception is spatial localization. A basketball player who misses a shot because he or she sees the basket somewhat to the right or left of its actual postion may mistakenly put the blame on poor technique. Also, players who consistently come up short on field goals may suffer from esophoria (objects tend to appear closer than they really are); and players who consistently shoot long may have exophoria (objects tend to appear farther away).

Eye-hand-foot coordination. The ability of the visual system to guide the motor system is known as eye-hand-foot coordination. Sometimes this guidance involves just eye-hand coordination, as in putting in golf; but it can be much more complex and sophisticated, as when a basketball player dribbles the ball and changes directions several times while moving quickly up the court.

Drills like tossing a beanbag under a strobe light may help improve eye-hand-foot coordination. This is because the strobe light forces the athlete to visually concentrate in response to greater "visual noise." Most experts believe that video games also improve eye-hand coordination.

Visualization and visual memory. The ability to imagine and memorize possible situations in order to react correctly is called visualization. This should not be confused with "talking to yourself." In fact, inner speech is not recommended in visualization, because it would be a distraction.

Visualization is a very important skill in golf (though it is of less concern in sports that are heavily dependent on reaction speed, such as ice hockey). In putting, a golfer first analyzes the situation: the "break of the green," the dampness of the surface, the length of the grass. Second, the golfer visualizes the path the ball will take to the hole. Third, the golfer selects a second "fine focus" spot (the first focus spot is the ball); this second spot is not the hole itself but rather is somewhere along this imaginary path. Fourth, after striking the ball, the golfer "locks on" the secondary fine-focus spot until the ball passes that spot on its way to the hole. Last is the playback or visual memory stage. This involves visualizing the complete sequence of making or missing the putt and reviewing all the visual images involved. This helps reinforce whatever lessons—positive or negative—are to be learned from the putt for future recall.

The potential usefulness of visual memory may be significant. Many professional basketball players, for example, are able to sink free throws blindfolded. This is a result of the motor memory they have developed through visualization practice. (At the time of this writing, the record for consecutive blindfolded free throws was 88.)

Visual reaction time. How rapidly an individual perceives and responds to visual stimulation is called visual reaction time. The speed of reaction to a visual cue depends on whether the signal is simple or complex. The fastest reaction time to a simple visual pattern is much quicker than the fastest reaction to a complex pattern. Sports like boxing, fencing, and tennis require exceptional visual reaction time.

Glare recovery. Glare recovery is the ability to adjust to various light conditions. In baseball, whenever an outfielder looks into the sun or into stadium lights, the eyes must "recover" from this sudden exposure to light in order to focus on and then catch a ball. Tennis and volleyball players face the same problem, and they must also learn to deal with distracting reflections from objects worn or held by spectators sitting nearby in the stands.

A visor or a broad-brimmed cap provides some protection from glare. Sunglasses are also becoming an increasingly popular option. However, it is important for sunglasses to be of good quality, absorbing both ultraviolet and infrared rays. Many cheaper sunglasses distort peripheral vision and may cause headaches. Some experts recommend antireflective lenses for outdoor sports in which glare is a problem, and Polaroid lenses are suitable for water sports. For some athletes, vitamin A and vitamin B2 therapy have increased the speed of glare recovery.

Instrument versus Free-Space Training

All the drills mentioned as examples in the preceding sections involve "free-space training"; that is, they take place in an environment that allows considerable movement, and the trainer can observe the athlete's eyes. Free-space training more closely approximates normal visual conditions than training using instruments. Instrument training uses techniques that require an athlete to look directly into an instrument. Such methods may restrict the athlete's ability to move and thus limit the trainer's ability to watch the reaction of the athlete's eyes. Furthermore, it may be difficult or impossible to mimic the visual skills needed in many sports through instruments. Instrument training is therefore considered a more artificial and less effective means of therapy than the other forms of training.

Visual Traits of Baseball Hitters

What makes a great hitter? This is a continuing controversy, centered mostly on technique, with one camp favoring "attack" and the other "read and react" (*see also* BASEBALL). But many observers believe that the secret of hitting lies elsewhere—that a good hitter is a good hitter regardless of technique, and so what really matters is not mechanics but visual ability. According to this argument, how long the stride should be, how long the head should stay down, and which hand should power the swing are certainly important; but no matter how these questions are answered, the ability to see the ball is crucial.

Once released, a fastball crosses the distance between mound and plate in about 0.4 second, so it is estimated that batters must make the decision to swing or not in about 0.2 second. This decision is based on an ocular split-second evaluation of the ball's seam rotation, the best cue available to batters for deciding when and where to swing.

More than 30 visual traits are involved in giving hitters the ability to spot the seams and determine rotation in less than 0.2 second. Of these traits, visual acuity is paramount. As noted in the text, 20/20 visual acuity is good, and 20/10 is exceptional. Most major league players have 20/20 visual acuity or better. Of people age 20 to 30, only 1 in 1,000 has 20/10 visual acuity. Ted Williams, often called the best hitter of all time, was one of those rare people. Williams actually claimed that his eyes were quick enough, and could track the ball well enough, to let him see the ball meet the bat.

One study conducted on Olympic-caliber baseball players showed that they had better static visual acuity and contrast sensitivity than nonathletes of a similar age (McHugh, 1985). Contrast sensitivity is measured by having the subject count and differentiate sine wave gratings (wide, widely spaced vertical bars that become thinner and more closely spaced). These two qualities are statistically significant because hitters need better visual acuity and contrast sensitivity to quickly judge the pitch by its speed and spin. The more quickly the batter makes these determinations, the larger the "window" of time to adjust the swing.

Dynamic acuity—that is, how clearly motion is seen—is also important in baseball. Although a player's visual acuity might be extremely sharp, it may deteriorate once motion is introduced. Curiously, the same batter who can read the label on a baseball from 63 feet away (19.2 m) may have great difficulty in judging speed, space, and spin once the baseball is set in motion.

Contrary to popular advice, and no matter how great their visual acuity and contrast sensitivity, hitters do take their eyes off the ball, especially a major league fastball. There are at least three reasons for this.

For one thing, the ball simply moves too fast for the eye to track.

Second, to prevent a hypnotized (or "lazy") focus, batters begin by watching the pitcher's windup with what is referred to as a "soft-centered focus." At first, they focus only loosely on the pitcher so that concentration will be particularly acute and will peak at the last moment, when the eyes are locked onto the pitcher's release point. If the eyes are locked into focus on the pitcher too soon, they lose some concentration as they focus on the moving ball, resulting in a slight decline in the very sharp focus needed to hit the ball.

Third, even the best hitters momentarily take their eyes off the ball somewhere in the middle of its trajectory and shift their field of vision closer to home plate. This eye movement, called a saccade, is usually involuntary. When a saccade is involuntary, it means that (as noted above) the ball is coming in faster than the eye can track. Saccades occur more frequently as the ball comes closer to the plate because the ball passes through the hitter's frame of vision more quickly. When the average

However, one advantage of instrument training is its accuracy. Instruments are useful in tracking improvements over time because testing can be performed with better consistency—variables can be kept to a minimum.

Eyewear: Correction and Protection

Although eye injuries are not the most prevalent sports-related injury, the long-term repercussions of an eye injury can be serious. Detached retina (*see* BOXING), eye ruptures, and corneal abrasions major league fastball is 5 feet (1.52 m) from the plate, it is moving three times faster than the human eye is able to track.

Still, major league hitters keep their eyes on the ball over as much of its flight as possible. In fact, although temporary involuntary saccades occur along the way, they are so quick (lasting just 1 millisecond) that the hitter is unaware of them. The player quickly judges the speed and spin, estimates the ball's point of arrival, and makes the appropriate adjustments in the swing. The eye is not actually able to see the ball at contact, but the athlete can maintain a line of vision on the path of the ball, anticipating its trajectory and its point of arrival.

Saccades may explain why a high fastball is more difficult to hit than a low one. A high fastball arrives along a flight path closer to the eyes, and the geometry of this situation indicates that each saccade will therefore shift the eye farther off the line of sight as the ball approaches the plate—which in turn means that the eye will take longer to get back on course after each saccade. This theory is supported by anecdotal comments from hitters: "I don't see the ball as well." "It's hard to follow the ball." "The ball seems to hop over my bat."

Because of the difficulty of keeping the eyes on the ball, hitters also rely on other perception skills. Instead of relying solely on sensory input from the oncoming ball, they also depend on visual memory and visualization techniques—on what they have learned to expect. Poor visualization may explain why the batting average of a hitter who has spent years in the National League often falls when he signs with an American League team. Unfamiliar with American League pitchers, he is less likely to know what to expect.

EYE DOMINANCE
Research indicates that a few sports favor athletes who are same-side eye-hand dominant while a few other sports favor cross-dominant athletes (either "left hand–right eye" or "right hand–left eye"). Baseball and golf, for example, favor cross-dominance while archery and riflery favor same-side dominance. A same-side-dominant hitter may be able to compensate for the fact that the dominant eye is farther away from the pitcher by "opening up" the stance more.

Another factor in hitting is eye dominance. Most people are right-handed (90%), some are left-handed (10%), and a few are ambidextrous. With regard to vision, most people (66%) are right-eyed, some are left-eyed (9%), and some (25%) are "ambi-eyed": central-ocular or non-dominant. The cause of eye dominance is unclear, but there are some patterns to its incidence. Though it is highly probable that a right-handed person will be right-eyed, there is not necessarily a correlation between eye and hand dominance: a small percentage of people are cross-dominant, and left-handed people more likely to be cross-dominant than right-handed people. One study found that cross-dominant batters have statistically higher batting averages than batters who are not cross-dominant, and central-ocular hitters have an even higher average (Portal, 1988). Since left-handed people are more likely to be cross-dominant than right-handed people, cross-dominance may partly explain why the number of left-handers in major league baseball is higher than their proportion in the general population. Many observers believe that with regard to hitting a baseball, it may be easier to train the eyes of young cross-dominant players; this would give these players a persistent advantage. However, much is still unknown about how the brain's hemispheres function in spatially tracking objects. (*See also the box "Are Left-Handers Inherently Superior Athletes?" in MOTOR CONTROL.*)

are three of the most common eye injuries that athletes are likely to experience. All three can have a drastic affect on vision, and in some cases may even result in permanent blindness.

The role of the optometrist is not only to correct vision and treat ocular conditions but also to enhance visual skills to improve athletic performance. Because of the variety of choices available to optometrists, corrective and protective prescriptions can be tailored to the needs of the individual athlete. Experimentation may allow every athlete to choose the most appropriate form of eyewear.

Principles of Eye Training

When developing a sports vision training program for an athlete or a team, try to follow a few general principles:

1. Establish an effective level of training. Setting a level at which the athlete can perform easily will minimize frustration.

2. Use positive reinforcement. This helps the athletes understand how visual system learning will improve performance.

3. Set specific (but flexible) goals, so that athletes know what level of performance they are working to attain.

4. To maintain the athletes' concentration, the training should provide continuous feedback.

IMPORTANCE OF VISUAL SKILLS IN VARIOUS SPORTS

Sport	Static acuity	Dynamic acuity	Eye tracking	Depth perception	Eye-hand coordination	Accommodation	Reaction time	Visualization	Glare recovery
Archery	4	1	3	5	5	3	1	3	1
Baseball (hitter)	4	5	5	5	5	5	5	5	2
Basketball	3	4	5	5	5	3	5	5	2
Bowling	2	1	3	3	5	2	1	5	1
Boxing	2	2	5	3	5	3	5	4	2
Football (quarterback)	4	5	5	5	5	3	5	5	4
Golf	3	1	2	5	5	3	1	5	1
Gymnastics	1	3	3	4	5	3	5	5	2
Hockey (goalie)	4	5	5	5	5	5	5	3	1
Pool	2	1	4	3	5	2	1	5	1
Racquetball	4	5	5	4	5	4	5	5	4
Running	1	1	1	1	1	1	3	4	1
Skiing	5	5	5	5	5	3	5	5	5
Soccer	3	4	5	4	5	3	5	5	3
Swimming	1	1	1	5	1	1	3	4	1
Tennis	4	5	5	5	5	5	5	5	5
Track (high jump)	1	3	3	3	4	3	4	4	2
Track (pole vault)	1	3	4	3	5	3	4	5	2
Wrestling	2	1	1	1	3	2	5	4	1
Volleyball	4	5	5	5	5	3	5	5	4

Key:
1 = Not important   2 = Marginally important   3 = Somewhat important   4 = Very important   5 = Extremely important

Table 1. *(Adapted from Sherman, 1990)*

Sunglasses

Sunglasses can provide significant protection for many sports (though some athletes find that they impair performance by causing distortion and problems with depth perception and peripheral vision). Sunglasses are especially important for playing conditions in which the sun's rays are the most intense: at high altitudes, or where sunlight reflects off water, snow, or sand. There are several guidelines for choosing the appropriate type of sunglasses:

Spectrum. Sunglasses should absorb ultraviolet light (290 to 400 nanometers), and a majority of blue light (400 to 510 nanometers; *refer back to Figure 1*). Glasses that conform to the American National Standard Institute (ANSI) standards for ultraviolet light (UV) absorption are labeled "Z-80.3."

Light reduction. Sunglasses should absorb at least 75 percent of visible light. Some brands have a "transmission factor" label. In addition to the transmission factor, they must fit properly, because the label assumes a good fit. Loose sunglasses that slip down the nose even a few millimeters can significantly increase transmission of sunlight.

Color. Gray, green, brown, and amber lenses are favored because they distort colors the least. Many athletes report that brown and amber lenses are better at enhancing contrasts in hazy and foggy conditions.

Overcast. Sunglasses are still useful even on cloudy days. Scattered clouds and water on the ground reflect radiation, which significantly increases exposure to UV and blue light.

Advice regarding eye correction and protection for athletes must include information about the safety of all types of ophthalmic lenses and frames and their value for their intended purpose. Some athletes find contact lenses irritating; others may have trouble with frames because of fogging and interference with peripheral vision. In some sports, options are limited; for example, soft contact lenses are generally considered the best option for boxers. In most sports, however, the choices are many: metal, carbon, or plastic frames; glass, plastic, or carbon-type lenses; gas-permeable or soft contact lenses; and standard, disposable, or extended-wear contact lenses. Corrective surgery is also becoming more and more popular (*see the box, "Advantages and Risks of Corrective Vision Surgery"*).

In many sports, whether or not an athlete's vision needs correction, some type of eye protection may be recommended to decrease the risk of injury. There are four basic types of protective eyewear: (1) face masks and shields; (2) lensless eyeguards with a narrow slit opening; (3) transparent bubble lenses and frames of uniform standard construction (goggles); and (4) eyeguards with lenses.

Polycarbonate lenses and frames are the most widely recommended for protective eyewear. These are the most durable and do not restrict vision as much as the other options.

Because eye injuries are usually preventable, many sports organizations advocate or mandate the use of eye protection. Amateur hockey players all wear face masks, most racquetball clubs mandate lensless eyeguards, and many basketball players use bubble-lens goggles to avoid inadvertent injuries to the eyes from other players.

If protective eyewear were universally mandated for sports, the number of eye injuries might decline significantly. However, protective eyewear does impair vision. Visual performance may decline by only, say, 1 percent with eyewear, but in highly competitive sports most athletes are reluctant to give an opponent even a 1 percent advantage. Thus mandating protective eyewear might affect outcomes because some athletes would be much better than others at adapting to such eyewear.

Research on protective eyewear and its effects on sports performance is still in its infancy. There are still many issues to be researched, such as how much eyeguards reduce the number of injuries, how they interact with players, and how they affect players' performance. Once such research is completed and protective eyewear is improved, it may find wider acceptance throughout the sports community.

John Zumerchik, Cheryl Zumerchik, O.D., and Harvey Schneider, O.D.

References

American Optometric Association. *Sports Vision Guidebooks*, vols. I–IV. St. Louis, Missouri: American Optometric Association, 1984–1993.

Feldman, R. *Understanding Psychology*, 4th ed. New York: McGraw-Hill, 1996.

Gregg, J. *Vision and Sports*. Boston: Butterworths, 1987.

Griffing, D. *The Dynamics of Sports*. Oxford, Ohio: Dalog, 1987.

Kirscher, D. "Sports Vision Training Procedures." *Optometry Clinics* 3, no. 1 (1993): 171–182.

Hitzeman, S., and S. Beckerman. "What the Literature Says about Sports Vision." *Optometry Clinics* 3, no. 1 (1993): 145ff.

Lucas, J., and H. Lorayne. *The Memory Book*. New York: Ballantine, 1975.

Lyons, R. "Take Your Eye Off the Ball." *New York Times* (12 October 1984), sec. C, p. 1.

McBeath, M. "The Rising Fast Ball: Baseball's Impossible Pitch." *Perception* 19 (1990): 545–552.

McHugh, D., and A. Bahill. "Learning to Track Predictable Target Wave Forms without a Time Delay." *Investigative Opthalmology and Visual Science* 26 (1987): 47ff.

Portal, J., and P. Romano. "Patterns of Eye-Hand Dominance in Baseball Players." *New England Journal of Medicine* 319, no. 10 (1988): 655–656.

Saunders, V. "How Visual Distortion Could Be Ruining Your Alignment." *Golf World* (December 1982): 54–56.

Sherman, A. "Sports Vision Testing and Enhancement: Implications for Winter Sports." In M. Casey, C. Foster, and E. Hixson (eds.), *Winter Sports Medicine*. Philadelphia, Pennsylvania: David, 1990.

Stock, J., and F. Cornell. "Prevention of Sports-Related Eye Injury." *American Family Physician* 44, no. 2 (1991): 515–520.

Vander, A., et al. *Human Physiology*, 6th ed. New York: McGraw-Hill, 1994.

Vinger, P. "Why I Don't Do Radial Keratotomy." *Journal of the American Optometric Association* 67, no. 2 (1996): 68–72.

Watts, R., and T. Bahill. *Keep Your Eye on the Ball: The Science and Folklore of Baseball*. New York: Freeman, 1990.

Zieman, B., et al. "Optometric Trends in Sports Vision: Knowledge, Utilization, and Practitioner Role Expansion Potential." *Journal of the American Optometric Association* 64, no. 7 (1993): 490–501.

Index

Page numbers in **boldface** refer to main articles on the subject.
Page numbers in *italics* refer to figures and figure captions.

A
Aaron, Hank, *56*
ABC. *See* American Bowling Congress
Abdomen
  in acrobatic maneuvers, 875
  back injuries and, 884–885
  boxing injuries and, 110–111
  weight-lifting belts and, 479–480
Abductor muscles, 310
Abdul-Jabbar, Kareem, 81
Absolute refractory period, 705
Absolute strength, 472
Acceleration
  acrobatics and, 21
  body size and, 24
  boxing punches and, 112–114, 115
  center of gravity and, 9, 57
  in cycling, 137
  dive starts in swimming and, 507–508
  in football, 234
  gravitational, 196–197, 198, 204, 209
  in hammer throw, 218, 219
  laws of motion and, 203
  sprinting and, 59–60, 346–347, 348, 350
  in throwing and pitching, 814–815
    baseball, 41–42, 43
    bowling, 95
  in volleyball spiking, 542–543
Accommodation, visual, 890, 893, 894, 898–899, *904*
Ace bandages, 768–769
Acetabulum. *See* Hips
Acetylcholine, 706, 830, 834, 835
Achilles tendon, 343, 362, 363, 607, 609, 611, 771
Acidity, of blood, 790–791, 795

ACL. *See* Anterior cruciate ligament
Acrobactics (gymnastics), **1–25**
  apparatuses, 3
  back injuries and, 877
  balancing skills, 4–6, 20–21
  body size and, 19–24
  competitive judging, 4, 7, 22
  eating disorder issues, 22, 656
  fluidity and summation of forces, 6–9
  inertia and angular momentum, 9–12, 14, 15–16, 17–18
  injury risks, 24, 853, 866, 877, 882
  linear momentum and, 7
  maneuvers
    back flips, *10*
    cartwheels, *12*
    flips, *12*
    giant swings and dismounts, 12, 16–18, *19*, 866
    handstands, 5, 6
    muscles used, 757
    somersaults, 3, 12–15, 18, 875
    spins, 11–12, *13*, 21, 392
    swinging, 12, 16–18, *19*, 22–24
    twists, 3, 12, 14–16, 23, 757, 875
  overcoming fear and, 4
  range of motion and, 868, 875
  sensory clues and, 18–19
  spinal coupling motion and, 875
  visual skills, *904*
Acromioclavicular joint, 812
Actin, 415, 550, 716, 831–835, 836
Action potential, 705, 825–826, 830–831, 834, 835
Action-reaction (Newton's laws of motion), 9, 102, 203, 498, 499, 537, 569
Action-reaction method, 15
Acuity, visual, 890, 895, 898, 902

Acute injury, 764
Acute mountain sickness, 796–800
Acute muscle soreness, 839
Adaptation
  to altitude, 800–801
  to light and darkness, 891
  skeletal and muscular, 842, 851
Adenosine diphosphate (ADP), 630–635, 834
Adenosine triphosphate (ATP)
  aerobic vs. anaerobic synthesis, 646–647, *648*
  cycling and, *149*
  energy and metabolism and, 629–639
  intermittent sports and, 446, 447
  muscle action and, 588, 834, 836
Adiabatic lapse rate, 262
Adipocytes, 636, 638
ADP. *See* Adenosine diphosphate
Adrenal glands, 706
Aerial skiing. *See* Freestyle skiing
Aerobic activity
  aging and, 591–593, 596, 599, 663
  blood pressure and, 680, 682
  body fat as factor, 622
  calories burned, *108*
  cycling and, 149
  effect on brain, 707
  energy and metabolism and, 646–647, 648–649
  fat energy and, 636
  ice hockey and, 307
  intermittent sports and, 446–447
  as rehabilitative treatment, 773–774
  running and, 354–355
Aerobie, 224
Aerodynamics
  Alpine skiing and, 430
  cycling and, 139–140, 141–146, 166

907

Volume 1: pp. 1–470; Volume 2: pp. 471–906

of football, 235
in golf, 50–51, 208, 284–288
of hockey pucks, 296, 297
of running, 344–346
of soccer ball, 442–443
speed skating and, 410–411
as throwing factor, 202, 207–208
    in discus event, 207, 219–220, 222
    in javelin event, 226–227
in volleyball, 535–539
Aesthetic movement, 4
Afferent nerves, 702
Agassi, Andre, 515, 522, 529, 820
Aggression, 118–119
Aging, **583–601**
athletes and, 597–600, 849
back problems, 877–878
biological theories, 584
body fat levels, 623
bone loss, 848, 850; *See also* Osteoporosis
dementia pugulistia and, 117
exercise and, 584–594, 597, 663
    circulatory system, 590–594, 596–598
    integumentary system, 584–585
    muscular system, 587–589, *593*, 596–597
    nervous system, 586–587, *593*, 707
    psychological effects, *593*, 594
    respiratory system, 589–590, *593*, 596–598
    sensory system, 585
    skeletal system, 363, 585–586, *593*, 596–597, 608, 850–851
hip replacement surgery, 758
inactivity and, 595–597
knee functionality, 691
life expectancy issues, 599–601
running injuries and, 363
strength training and, 487, 589, 596–597, 663
vision impairment, 585, 893–894
Agonist muscles, 449, 478, 605
Aiming
in archery, 29–30, 38
in bowling, 90
vs. sighting, 64
Air density
gliding and, 256, 267
sailing and, 372
as throwing factor, 220
Air embolism, 804
Air flight. *See* Gliding and hang gliding

Airfoil (glider), 255–256, 267, 268
Airfoil cross sections (bicycle wheels), 166–167
Air pressure, respiration and, 777–778, 780–781, 783–784, 794–807
Air resistance
cycling and, *135*, 136, 139–141, 345
football kicking and, 238–239, 241
in golf, 284–288
jumping ability and, 182, 188, 197, 198
running and, 344–346
shuttlecock flight and, 526
skiing and, 426–427, 429
in speed skating, 407–411
speed skiing vs. skydiving, 428–429
in tennis, 524, 526
as throwing factor
    in field events, 214, 220
    in football, 235
in volleyball, 535–536
See also Drag; Wind resistance
Alcoholism, 672
Alexeyev, Vasily, 558–560
Ali, Muhammad, 117
Allen, Phog, 80
Alley (bowling). *See* Lanes, bowling
Alpine skiing. *See under* Skiing
Altitude
acclimatization process, 800–801
acute mountain sickness, 796–800
air pressure and, 777–778, 790, 795–801
as environmental factor, 197, 204, 213–214
gliding and hang gliding, 253, 260, 264
pulmonary edema, 683–684
Aluminum equipment, 153
arrow construction, 35, 36, 175
baseball bats, 52–53, 153, 175, 303
bicycles, 132–133, 164–165, 166
composites, 159
paddle sports, 325
tennis rackets, 177, 514
vaulting poles, 156, 162, 192
Alveolar ventilation, 590
Alveoli, 783, 787–788, 792, 793, 794, 796, 804
Ambient pressure, 802, 803, 804–805
Amblyopia (lazy eye), 894–895
Amenorrhea, 654, 655, 656, 659–660
American Bowling Congress (ABC), 85, 87, 89, 92, 95, 96, 97, 101
American Heart Association, 731
American Institute of Nutrition, 720

American Medical Association, 118
America's Cup (yachting), 159, 177, 326, 384–385
Amino acids, 638–639, 642, 644, 724–726, 744; *See also specific acids*
Ammonia, 639, 670
Anabolism, 625
Anaerobic activity
cycling and, 149
energy and metabolism and, 643, 646–647, 649, 650
ice hockey and, 307
intermittent sports and, 446
running and, 354–355
starvation diet's impact on, 574
Analgesics, 771
Anchor point (archery), 28, 29–30
Anemia, 645, 655–656, 737
Angina, 682
Angle of attack
in Frisbee toss, 226
in gliding, *255*, 256, 267, 268
hockey shots and, 296
in sailing, 371, 378, 380
in swimming, 499, 500–502
in throwing events, 208, 220, 221, 224, 227–228
Angle of attitude
in gliding, 256–257
in throwing events, 208, 220, 221
Angle of elevation, baseball, 124, 125
Angle of launch
basketball, 69–72, 75–77
in football kicking, 237, 242–243
Angle of loft, 168, 169, 281
Angle of release, 188, 208, 210
in discus throw, 220, 221
in hammer throw, 217
in javelin throw, 227, 228
in shot put, 213, 214, *215*
Angle of takeoff, 188, 191
Angle of wrist-cock, 274–275
Angular acceleration. *See* Angular momentum
Angular frequency, 94
Angular momentum
acrobatics and, 9–12, 14, 15–16, 17–18, 21
baseball pitchers and, 809
bowling balls and, 97, 100
in boxing, 109, 112–114
conservation of, 10, 15, *217*, 219, 299
in Frisbee toss, 224, 225
golf swing and, 277, 278
in hurdling, 366

ice hockey shots and, 299, 301
throwing events and, 206–207, 217, 219, 223
zero, 15–16
Angular velocity
anatomical variation and, 809
in bowling, 94
of golf swing, 275
in gymnastics, 22
of soccer kick, 450, 451
in throwing, 206, 210–211
discus throw, 222
hammer throw, 217–218
shot put, 215
Animal speeds
aquatic, *494*
mammals, *341*
Ankle, foot, and lower leg, **603–615**
arch of foot, 172, 174–175, *604*
balance and, 605, 606
ball of foot, 713
baseball sliding and, 58
cycling and, 144
functional anatomy, 603–608
bones and joints, 604–605
ligaments, 603, 606
muscles, 605–606
tendons, 607–608
injury risks, prevention, and rehabilitation, 603–615, 767, 769, 866
running and, 342–343, 348, 868
soccer and, 448, 449
speed skating and, 414
wrestling and, 569–570
See also Athletic shoes
Annulus fibrosus, 873, 874, 879
Anorexia nervosa, 22, 616, 656, 664
Antagonist muscles, 449, 478, 605, 717, 835
Anterior cruciate ligament (ACL), 688, 689–690, 692, 694, 862
Antibodies, 725
Anticipation, handedness and, 711
Antifungal medications, 677
Antihistamines, 677
Anti–inflammatory drugs, 769, 771
Antioxidants, 737
Antireflective lenses, 901
Aorta, 668, *669*, 671, 675
Aortic valve, 671, 675
Apparent wind (sailing), 378–380
Approach
in soccer, 449
in volleyball, 541–542
Aqueous humor, 894
Arc. *See* Trajectory

Archer's paradox, 35
Archery, **26–38**
arrows
dynamics of, 35–36
fletching, 36
velocity, 28, 29, 31–32, 35, 36
basic technique, 28–30
bow and arrow energy, 30–32
bows
dynamics of, 32–35
shooting aids, 37–38
types and construction, 27–29, 30, 33–34, *34*, 36, *37*, 175
traditionalism in, 38
types, 27, 32, 36
vision and, 903, *904*
Archimedes, 491
Archimedes' principle, 620
Arch of foot, 172, 174–175, *604*
Area of cross-section
shuttlecock, 526
tennis racket strings, 518–519
Area to volume (A/V) ratio, jumping ability and, 182
Aristotle, 718
Arms. *See* Shoulder, elbow, wrist
Arrhythmia, heart, 677
Arrow rests (archery bows), 37
Arrows. *See under* Archery
Arteries, 668, 669, 677–682
blood pressure and, 678–679
cholesterol intake and, 732, 733
exercise and, 679–680, 682
hypertension and, 681–682
low oxygen levels and, 795–796
See also Arteriosclerosis; Atheriosclerosis
Arteriosclerosis, 894
Arthritis, 692, 818, 865, 878
Arthrogryposes, 868
Arthroscopic surgery, 692–693, 694, 822
Artificial turf, 247–250, 441
Artificial ventilation, 785–787
Aspect ratio (gliding), 259
Aspirin, 771
Asthma, 791–793
Astigmatism, 894, 896
Astrodome (Houston, Texas), 441
Astronauts, 15–16, 842, 867
Astroturf, 247–250
Atherosclerosis, 723, 731, 732, 733, 737, 746
Athletic amenorrhea, 659–660
Athletic shoes, 153, 172–175
cleated, 149, 250–251
for cycling, 149

for football, 176, 250–251
injury prevention and, 249, 363, 605, 613
orthotics, 363, 613
for running, 172, 173, 174, 363, 610
selection guidelines, 614
sneakers, 172, 613
treads of, 173
for volleyball, 545
Atmospheric lapse rate, 262
Atmospheric pressure, 777–778, 795, 799, *801*
Atomic bonding, 158
ATP. *See* Adenosine triphosphate
Atrioventricular (A-V) node, 673, 674
Atrioventricular (A-V) valves, 670–672, 675
Atrium. *See* Heart and circulatory system
Atrophy, 766, 838
Attack, angle of
in Frisbee toss, 226
in gliding, *255*, 256, 267, 268
hockey shots and, 296
in sailing, 371, 378, 380
in swimming, 499, 500–502
in throwing events, 208, 220, 221, 224, 227–228
Attack-the-ball hitting style, 54
Attitude, angle of
in gliding, 256–257
in throwing events, 208, 220, 221
Auditory system. *See* Ear; Hearing
Australia, 50
Autonomic nervous system
branches, 673
diencephalon and, 707
regulatory roles, 702–703
Average (statistics), 455–456
baseball batting, 456–461
A-V node. *See* Atrioventricular (A-V) node
A/V ratio. *See* Area to volume (A-V) ratio
A-V valves. *See* Atrioventricular (A-V) valves
Axis
horizontal, 15
longitudinal, 12, *13*, 15
medial, 12
transverse, 12, 15, 18
twisting and, 15
Axis of rotation
acrobatics and, 10–12, 15, 16, 22–23
soccer leg swing and, 450
tennis racket head size and, 512

weight distribution and, 383
wrestling throws and, 571
Axons, 116, 117, 703–704, 705, 827, 830
Aztecs, 292

B

Back (human body). *See* Back injuries and problems; Spinal cord; Spine
Backboard (basketball), 175
Back flips (acrobatics), *10*
Back flops (diving), 18
Backhand shot (tennis), 531–532
Backing winds, 386–387
Back injuries and problems, 871–885
    arm effects, 808–809
    prevalence of, 871–872
    spinal cord and, 827, 872, 875–882
    stress and, 876–877
Backspin
    in baseball, 45, 46, *47*, 55–56
    in basketball, 65, 69, 76, 81–82
    in bowling, 90–91, 93, 94
    as catch factor, 122
    as distance factor, 208
    in golf, 171, 271, 284, 288, 289–290
    in tennis, 69, 519
Backstroke (swimming), *503*, 504
Backswing (golf), 272–275
"Bad" cholesterol. *See* Low-density lipoprotein
Badminton, 526–527, 808, 820
Baggio, Roberto, 443, 444
Bailey, Donovan, 348
Balance
    ankle, foot, and lower leg function, 605, 606
    baseball pitching and, 40
    basketball shooting and, 66–67
    in ice skating, 401–404
    in karate, 312–313
    in paddle sports, 326, 337
    in wrestling, 569–570, 579
Balance beam (gymnastics), 18–19, 23
Balancing skills, 4–6
    body size and, 23
    center of gravity and, 4–5, 6
    response time and, 5–6
    vestibular system and, 20–21, 114, 125
Balata-covered golf balls, 282
Baldness, as soccer advantage, 451–452
Ball (of foot), 713
    in running, 342–343, 357–358
Ball-and-socket joint, 863

Ballast (sailing), 371, 382
Ball bearings, 294
Ballistic motion, *337*
Balls. *See specific sports*
Ball-to-heel running, 342–343, 357–358
Ball track (bowling), 98, 99, 100
Bamboo vaulting pole, 156, 157, 192
"Banana" kick (soccer), 442–443
Bandages, elastic, 768–769
Bandy (early field hockey form), 293
Banked curves (running tracks), 353
Bank shot (basketball), 64
Barbells. *See* Isotonic exercise; Strength training; Weight lifting
Baresi, Franco, 444
Barkley, Charles, 872
Barry, Rick, 73, 808
Basal metabolic rate (BMR), 626, 641, 655, 658, 748–749
Baseball, **39–60**, 62
    base running, 57–60
    bat and ball collision, 48–52, 53–54
        aluminum vs. wooden bats, 52–53, 153, 175, 303
        ball liveliness, 48–49
        bat weight, 49–52
        damping of energy, 162
        grip firmness, 53–54, 303
        illegally modified bats, 39, 54
    batting averages, 456–461
    catching skills, 122–125
    checked swings, 820
    fly balls, 46, 122–125, 288, 900
    hitting theories, 54–57
    home runs, 48, 49, 124
    injury risks, 40, 41, 42–43, 58–59, 60, 757, 819
    labor disputes, 455
    left-handed players, 710–711, 903
    pitch characteristics, *48*
    pitching, 808, 809, 810, 815
        compared to shot putting, 216
        cricket vs. baseball, 50–51
        dead arms, 43
        delivery angle, 41, 42–43
        longevity-enhancing techniques, 43
        motion phases, 40–42
        pitcher injuries, 816
        sidearm delivery, 43, 808
    pitch types, 43–48
        change-ups, 43
        curveballs, 44–45, 69, 208, 288, 815, 816, 889
        fastballs, 45–46, *47*, 51, *128*, 815, 816, 889, 902–903

        knuckleballs, 46–47, 297, 536–537
        sliders, 45–46, 815
        spitballs, 39, 47–48
    players' vision and, 305, 887, 889, 901, 902–903, *904*
    playoffs' length probability, 461–465
    random (statistical) nature of, 465
    softball, 52, 175, 808
    strategy factors, 39–40
Baseball pass (basketball), 81
Baseline shots (tennis), 523–524
Base of support (karate), 312–313
Bases, breakaway (baseball), 58–59
Base stealing, 57–60
Bash (volleyball), 538
Basketball, **61–83**
    backboards and rims, 175
    basket height, 79–80
    brain waves and "the zone," 68
    catching skills, 127
    defense, 82–83
    dribbling, 62, 63, 82–83
    footwear, 172
    hang time and shot blocking, 77–79
    injury risks, 66–67, 604, 697, 877
    jumping skill improvement, 540
    left-handed players, 712
    passing, 80–82
    playoffs' length probability, 461–465
    protective eyewear, 905
    shooting mechanics, 63–67
    shooting physics, 68–77
        backspin, 65, 69, 76, 81–82
        field shots, 69–72
        free throws, 72–77
        when moving, 77
    shot types
        bank, 64
        dunk, 62
        free throws, 64, 72–77
        hook, 66, 77
        jump, 62, 65–66, 67, 79
        layup, 62, 77
        set, 62, 65, 67
    visual skills, 64–65, 899, 900, 901, *904*
Bath (Mongol khan), 26
Bats
    baseball
        aluminum vs. wooden, 52–53, 153, 175, 303
        compared to cricket bats, 50
        damping of energy, 162
        diameter of, 45, 50
        dimpled, 50–51, 288

Index

grip firmness, 53–54
illegally modified, 39, 54
sweet spot, 49, 52
weight of, 49–52
cricket, 50
See also Sticks
Batter win average (BWA), 456
Batting averages (baseball), 456–461
Beamon, Bob, 142, 198–200
Beans (legumes), 729
Beating (sailing). *See* Tacking
Becker, Boris, 514, 515
Belly flops (diving), 18
Belts (strength training), 479–480
Bench press (weight lifting), 552, 555, 561, 564–565
Bends, the (decompression sickness), 672, 804–806
Beriberi, 732–733
Bernoulli, Daniel, 372
Bernoulli's principle
in gliding and hang gliding, 255
in golf, 286–287
in sailing, 287, 372
in volleyball, 536, 537
Beta-carotene, 735
Beta-endorphins, 359
Beta oxidation, 637
Biceps muscle, 42, 554–555, 814, 816, 821, 835
Bicycles
construction, 162–167
frame geometry, 131–132, 134, 163
frame materials, 132–133, 137, 163–166
stability, 132–135
tires, 238
wheels, 137, 138, 142–143, 163, 165–167
See also Cycling
Bile, 731, 733, 744, 746
Billiards, 82, 295, *904*
Bindings
ski, 58
snowboarding, 668
Bingeing and purging. *See* Bulimia nervosa
Binocular vision, 125
Bioelectrical impedance, 621
Biomechanical specificity, 475
Biomechanics
of baseball pitching, 40–43
of basketball shooting, 63–67
cycling and, 143–151
in discus throw, 222
footwear and, 172
muscle memory and, 6–7

in shot putting, 215
in soccer ball heading, 451
in tennis, 529–532
Biondi, Matt, 489
Bipedalism, 752–753, 871
Bipolar cells, 892
Bird, Larry, 71, 83, 872
Birdie. *See* Shuttlecock
Birth control pills, 659
Blade
hockey stick, 297, 306–307
ice skate, 390–391, 393, *394*, 398, *399*, *400*, 402, 404, 407
oars and paddles, 332–333
propeller, 499
Blair, Bonnie, 414
Bleeding and blood loss, 685–686
boxing injuries, 111, 116, 686
cold therapy, 767
Blindness
boxing injuries and, 116
vitamin A deficiency and, 734–735
Blind spot (human eye), 890, 892
Blocking
in basketball, 77–79
in football, 230
Blocks. *See* Starting blocks
Blood
acidity of, 790–791, 795
circulation pattern, 667–670
hemoglobin, 737, 788–789, 790, 795
plasma, 739, 778, 788–791, 804–805
skeletal system role, 845–846, 857, 858–859, 864
Blood clots
arterial plaque and, 681
from boxing, 116
in leg veins, 685
mountain climbers and, 798
Blood pressure
aging and, 590, 592
bleeding's effect on, 685, *686*
breathing and, 477
circulatory system and, 671, 675, 678–679
dehydration and, 740
during exercise, 679–680
hypertension, 681–682
isometric exercises and, 481
measurement of, 678–679
Blood sugar. *See* Glucose
Bloop hits, 124
BMPs. *See* Bone morphogenetic proteins
BMR. *See* Basal metabolic rate
Board breaking (karate), 316–320
Boats. *See* Canoeing; Kayaking; Paddle sports; Sailing; Shelling; Yachting

Bobsledding, 288, 398
Boccie, 85
Bodhidharma, 311
Body building, 473, 725; *See also* Strength training; Weight lifting
Body composition, **616–624**
density, 620
desirable weight determination, 623–624, 747
fat and nonfat components, 617–618, 747–750, 843
fat as performance predictor, 622
of female athletes, 652–655
flotation and, 492
measurement of, 618–623
bioelectrical impedance, 621
hydrostatic weighing, 619–621
skin-fold sum, 619
strength training and, 485
See also Body fat; Mass, body; Tissue, body; Weight (body)
Body fat, 617–618, 747–749
boxers and, 111
endocrine system functioning and, 575
energy and metabolism and, 642, 643
females and, 653, 654, 658
as flotation factor, 492, 494, 618, 747
gymnasts and, 24
heart disease and, 576, 658
measurement of, 618–623
obesity and, 616, 882
as performance predictor, 622
reduction vs. weight loss, 749–750
strength training and, 473, 485
sumo wrestlers and, 575–576
See also Weight
Body mass. *See* Mass, body
Body size and shape
acrobatics and, 19–24
badminton and, 527
competitive jumping and, 179–180, 182
cycling and, 140
eating disorders and, 22, 616, 656, 660, 663–665
football and, 233–235
genetics and, 842
as gymnastics injury factor, 24
as hurdling factor, 366–367
paddle sports and, 335

swimming and, 496
as tennis serve factor, 525
as throwing factor, 212
    Frisbee and Aerobie toss, 224
    hammer throw, 218
    javelin throw, *229*
    shot put, 216
weight lifting "sticking point" and, 556
wrestling and, 572
See also Female athletes; Height (body); Weight (body)
Body temperature, 740, 741
Body tissue. *See* Tissue, body
Body weight. *See* Weight
Boggs, Wade, 51, *461*, 711
Bonds, Barry, 710
Bonds, Bobby, 124
Bone density
    amenorrhea and, 660
    calcium and, 736
    genetics and, 848–849
    population variation in, 621
    running and jumping sports increasing, 850
    young women and, 653, 654–655
    See also Osteoporosis
Bone fatigue. *See* Stress fractures
Bone grafts, 857–859
Bone marrow, 843, 845, 847
Bone mass. *See* Bone density
Bone morphogenetic proteins (BMPs), 861
Bones, 843–860
    composition, 843–844
    functions, 843
    growth and regeneration of, 844–847, 861
    health factors, 847–851
    hormones and, 847
    See also Bone density; Fractures; *specific bones*
Boots (ice skate), *399*, 402
Boron, 159, 170
Borzov, Valery, 347
Bounce effect (weight lifting), 556–557
Bounce pass (basketball), 81–82
Boundary layer (paddle sports), 325, 330
Boundary-layer separation, 536–537
Boutiette, K. C., 409
Bow (boat), 325, 327
Bowler's elbow (medial epicondylitis), 818–19, 822
Bowling, **85–107**
    ball path, 91–99

ball weighting and, 97–99
    effects of spin, 93–97
ball specifications, 88, 95, 97, 98
ball throwing, 88–91, 808
game basics, 86–88
injury factors, 818–19, 822, 877
lane specifications, *87*, 92, 96–97
pin collisions, 100–107
    spares, 100, 105–107
    strikes, 87, 100, 102–105
visual skills, *904*
Bowling (cricket), 50–51
Bow recoil, 31, *34*
Bows. *See* Archery; *specific types*
Bow sights, 37, 38
Bow weight, 28–29
Boxing, **108–120**
    as aerobic activity, *108*
    amateur, 109, 117, 120
    footwear, 172
    gloves, 113, 117–120
    headgear, 113, 115, 117, 120
    head movement
        concussions and, 112–113, 114, *115*, 116–117
        forces on brain, 113–115
        recoil, 112, 115
    heavyweight fighters, 110–112, 113
    injury risks, 108–109, 110–111, 112–117, 120, 686
    knockouts, 114, 116, 117
    left-handed fighters, 711
    low blows, 110–111
    punching power, 109–112
    stance used, *112*
    visual skills, *904*
Braces, orthopedic. *See* Orthotics
Bracing (karate), 315
Brain
    aerobic activity effects on, 707
    aging and, 586–587
    boxing and damage to, 112–117
    cerebral edema, 796–797, 799
    football injuries and, 245–246
    function specialization, 708–709, 710
    glucose requirements, 724
    left-handedness and, 709, 710
    motor control and, 700, 702, 707–709
    parts of, 707–708
    skeletal muscle control and, 825–827, 838
    visual image processing and, 892–893
Brain stem, 707, 785, 795
Brain waves, 68

Braking force
    balls and, 294
    jumping and, 181, 185, 187–188, 190
    running and, 13, 334, 347, 348–349
Branch, Cliff, 243
Breaking Away (film), 130
Breaststroke (swimming), *503*, 504, 505–507
Breathing. *See* Respiration
Brett, George, 54, 711
Bronchi, 783, 792
Bronchodilator medications, 792
Brooklyn side (bowling), *96*, 104
Brown, Tim, 243
Bruises. *See* Contusions
Buckling (of spine), 877
Buckstaff, John, 377
Buddhism, 311
Bulimia nervosa, 22, 616, 656, 664
Bullwhip, 276–278
Bungee cord, 161, 556
Buoyancy
    of boats, 327
    center of, 381, 382, *383*
    swimming and, 491–494, 618
Bureau of Standards, U.S., 49
Burner (neck injury), 245
Bursae, 864
Butcher, Susan, 652
Butt end (hockey stick), 297
Butterfly stroke (swimming), *500*, 504
Buttocks, 151, 756
BWA. *See* Batter win average
Byrd, Dennis, 245, 827, 828

C

CAD. *See* Coronary artery disease
Caesar, Julius, 488
Calcaneofibular ligament, 606
Calcaneus, *604*, 605, 606, 607, 610
Calcification, 846, 857
Calcium
    bones and, 658, 660, 662, 736, 843, 847, 849–850, 854
    as mineral nutrient, 735, 736, 738
    muscle action and, 830–831, 832, 834, 836
    osteoporosis and, 585, 654, 737
Calcium channels, 415
Calf muscles. *See* Gastrocnemius muscle; Soleus muscle
Calisthenics, 485
Calories
    amenorrhea and, 660
    energy and metabolism and, 626, 641, 646, 748

Index

as nutritional energy measurement, 721
weight control tips, 576
Camber
  of sails, 374, *375*
  of skis, 432
Canada, 292, 293
Cancellous bone, 844, *845*
Cancer
  diet prevention, 723, 746, 737
  exercise prevention, 598, 653
  smoking as risk factor, 793
Canoeing, 322, *323*
  drag and, 495
  equipment materials, 176
  origins of, 321, 322
  paddles, *332*
  stroking motion, 334
Capillaries, 668–669, 683–684
  pulmonary, 787–788, 789, 796
Carbohydrate loading, 646, 725
Carbohydrates
  digestive system and, 744
  energy and metabolism and, 632–635, 642, 643, 646, 726
  mountain climbers' diet and, 797–798
  as nutrient, 720, 722–724, 741
  weight control and, 576
Carbon (element)
  compounds and chains, 628–629
  fatty acids and, 729
  metabolism, 725, 726
Carbon dioxide
  circulatory system and, 667–669
  respiration and, 779, 782, 785, 787, 788, 790–791, 795
Carbon fiber-reinforced polymers (CFRPs), 159, 160–161
Carbon fibers
  bicycle wheels, 143
  composites, 159, 160–161, 164, 165
  crew shells, 325
  gliders, 253
  golf clubs, 281
  vaulter's pole, 193
Cardiac output, 675–676, 678, 679–680
Cardiovascular fitness assessment, 680
Cardiovascular system. *See* Heart and circulatory system
Carew, Rod, 711
Carlton, Steve, 43, 710
Carpal bones, 817
Carry (golf), *284*
Cartilage
  knee, 690, 692–693, 694

osteoarthritis and, 865
skeletal system, 843, 844–845, 846, 850, 857, 861, 862, 864
Cartwheels (acrobatic), 12
Cash, Norm, 39, 54
Catabolism, 625, 630
Catalano, Patti, 664
Catamarans, 379
Cataracts, 116, 893–894
Catch (swimming), 504
Catches (acrobatic), 5
Catching skills, **122–129**
  basic technique, 126–127
  egg tossing and, 115, 126
  fly balls and, 122–125, 900
  in lacrosse, 126, 128–129
Catgut, 518
CAT scans, 822
Cat stance (karate), 312–313
Cavum septum pellucidum, 117
CE. *See* Center of effort
Cellular metabolism, 629–640, 646–647
Centerboard (sailboat), 374, 377
Center of buoyancy, 381, 382, *383*
Center of effort (CE), 381
Center of gravity (COG)
  acrobatics and, 4–5, 6, 8, 15, 16, 17, 18, *19*
    changes-in-motion forces, 9, 10
    rotational axis, 12, 13, 22–23
  aging's impact on, 587
  in Alpine skiing, 428–429, 432, 433–434
  back problems and, *871*, 882, *883*
  baseball and
    catching, 126
    hitting, 56–57
    sliding, 57, 59
  basketball and
    defense, 82–83
    shooting, 67, 78
  of bowling balls, 88, 97, 98, 99
  boxing and, 112–113, *112*
  competitive jumping and, 178–181
    high jump, 179–181, 183, 184–185
    long jump, 181, 187, 188, 189
    pole vaulting, 181, 195
  cycling and, 132, 133, 134, 135, 142
  in females, 179, 654, *883*
    during pregnancy, 661
  football and, 232, 756
  golf swing and, 271, 272, 273, 754
  human pelvis as, 752, 753–754, 756
  in hurdling, 361–362, 364–365
  karate and, 312–313

in males, 179
in paddle sports, 327
running and, 347, 349, 350, 352, 353, 756
sailing and, 133, 381–382, 383–385
in skating, 5, 401, 403, 404–405, 413
in snowboarding, 435
in swimming, 500, 508
in tennis, 530, 531
throwing events and, 205, 219, 223
in weight lifting, 560, 561
in wrestling, 568–570, 571, 572, 578, 579
Center of lateral resistance (CLR), 381
Center of mass. *See* Center of gravity
Center of percussion (COP), 515
Centers for Disease Control, 59
Central field awareness, 899
Central nervous system (CNS)
  fatigue and, 447, 645
  motor control and, 700, 702, 706–709
    brain, 700, 702, 707–709
    spinal cord, 702, 707, 717
  oxygen toxicity, 807
Centrifugal force
  in ice skating, 403, 406–407
  jumping and, 197
  throwing and, 204
Centripetal force
  acrobatics and, 16
  in Alpine skiing, 430, *431*
  cycling and, 134, 402
  hammer throw and, 217–218, 219
  in ice skating, 402, 403, 406
  in running, 351–353
  vs. centrifugal force, 204
Ceramic-matrix composites (CMCs), 159
Ceramics
  as equipment material, 153, *157*, 158, 162
    density, *160*
    elasticity modulus, *157*, 162
    for golf clubs, 171
    yield strength, *158*
  in hip replacement implants, 759
Cerebellum, 707
Cerebral cortex, 825
Cerebral edema, 796–797, 799
Cerebral hemispheres, 707–709, 710
Cervical vertebrae, 872, *873*, 875
CFRPs. *See* Carbon fiber-reinforced polymers
Chain sprocket (bicycle gear), 146
Chainwheel (bicycle gear), 147

Chamberlain, Wilt, 74
Changes-in-motion forces, 9
Change-up pitches, 43
Charlie Lau hitting style, 54
Chavez, Julio, 111, 112
Cheerleading, 5
Cheese, 728
Chermerkin, Andrey, 558
Chest pass (basketball), 81
Chest protectors, *293*
Chest shot (basketball), 73–77
Children
    amblyopia and, 894–895
    body fat levels of, 623
    motor skill development and, 715–718
    strength training and, 485
Chin, 114
China
    cycling, 130
    karate, 311
    soccer, 439
Chloride, 705
Choctaw (ice skating), 405, 406
"Choking" situations (muscle tension), 546
Cholesterol, 730–731, 733
    artery disease and, 732, 733
    estrogen and, 658
    exercise and, 597
    fiber and, 723
Cholinesterase, 834
Chondrocytes, 845, 846, 861, *865*
Chord line (airfoil), *255*
Christie, Linford, 589
Chrome-moly steel, 164
Chromium, 132, 164, 735
Chronic fatigue syndrome, 645
Chronic injury, 764
Chylomicrons, 733, 745
Chyme, 742–746
Cigarettes. *See* Smoking
Cilia, 787, 793, 794
Circuit resistance training (CRT), 839
Circular sprocket (bicycle), 147
Circulatory system. *See* Heart and circulatory system
Circus acrobatics, 3, 4
Clavicle (collar bone), 812, 818
Clay court (tennis), 510, 511, 528–529
Clean-and-jerk lift (weight lifting), 552, 556–557, 558, 560–561
Cleats
    cycling and, 149
    football and, 250–251
Cliff diving, 3

Clinical depression, 594, 596, 645, 653
Clothing
    cycling and, 137, 140
    neoprene material, 761
    skiing and, 427
    speed skating and, 408–410
    as sweating factor, 741
Clots. *See* Blood clots
Clouds
    gliding and, 263, 264
    as sailing factor, 386, 387–388
Cloud streets (gliding), 264
CLR. *See* Center of lateral resistance
Clubs. *See* Golf clubs
CMCs. *See* Ceramic-matrix composites
CNS. *See* Central nervous system
Coaches
    aggression control and, 119
    baseball, 53
    basketball, 72, 73, 77, 78–79
    gymnastics, 4, 18
    lacrosse, 128
    motor skill development and, 716–718
    swimming, 502
Cobalt, 159
Cobb, Ty, 39, 54, 456, 459, 460, 710
Cocaine, 677
Cochlea (ear), 20, 21
Cocking (baseball pitching), 40–41, 814
Coefficient of friction, 294, 295
    in ice skating, 393, 395, 396, 397–398
    in skiing, 423, 424
    in tennis, 528
Coefficient of restitution (COR)
    in baseball, 48–49, 52, 53, 54, 167
    in bowling, 100, 101, 102, 104
    equipment materials and, 167
    in golf, 283
    of soccer ball, 441–442, 451–452
    in tennis, 512, 515, 516–517, 518, 523, 529
    in volleyball, 544
Coenzymes, 627, 734
COG. *See* Center of gravity
Coiled tension, 273, 277
Cold therapy, 763–764, 767–768, 769–770
Collaborative reflex, 21
Collagen
    aging breakdown of, 585
    as bone component, 843, 854, 857
    connective tissue production of, 486

    exercise increasing, 865
    heredity and defects in, 868
    hormones and, 847
Collar bone (clavicle), 812, 818
Collateral ligaments (knee), 688, *689*, 690, 691, 695
Colle's fracture, 585
Collision theory (golf), 284
Columbia University, 230
Columbus, Christopher, 374
Comaneci, Nadia, 19
Comminuted fractures, 856, 858
Competitive judging, 4, 7, 22
Complex carbohydrates. *See* Carbohydrates
Composite materials, 153, 157–158, 159, 160–165
    Alpine skis, 433
    archery equipment, 175
    bicycles, 163, 166
    carbon fiber, 159, 160–161, 164, 165
    density, *160*
    elasticity modulus, *157*, 162
    golf clubs, 281
    hockey sticks, 176, 304
    tennis rackets, 177, 511, 513, 514, 520
    vaulting poles, 193
    yield strength, *158*
Composition court (tennis), 510, 528
Compound bows, *37*
Compression
    archery bows and, 33, *34*
    board breaking and karate, 317
    bone injuries and, 854, 855, 856, 862
    equipment materials and, *156*, 157, 158
    as rehabilitative treatment, 768–769, 770
    of snow, 423, 425–426
    of spine, 867, 874, 875–876, 877, 878
Computerized tomography, 622
Computer modeling, yacht design and, 385
Concentration (mental)
    basketball shooting and, 63, 68
    controlled aggression and, 119
Concentric contraction, 716, 717
    jumping and, 540
    skiing and, 433, *434*
Concrete, splitting of (karate), 318
Concussion (head injury)
    in boxing, 112–113, 114, *115*, 116–117
    in football, 246

Conduction (neuron), 704–705
Condyloid joint, 863
Cones (human eye), 890–892
Confidence, basketball shooting and, 63, 68
Connective tissue
 regeneration of, 845–846
 strength training and, 485–487
Conner, Dennis, 326, 385
Connors, Jimmy, 511, 512–513, 516, 531, 711
Conservation of angular momentum, 10, 15, *217*, 219, 299
Conservation of energy
 in archery, 31
 in bowling, 89
 equipment materials and, 161–162
 kinetic energy and, 8
 in pole vaulting, 195–196
 in skiing, 422
 in tennis, 516
Conservation of linear momentum, 505
Conservation of momentum
 in football, 231, 233, 241
 in golfing, 283
 in sumo wrestling, 578–579
 weight-aided jumping and, 186
Contact forces, 9–10
Contact lenses, 894, 896, 897, 905
Continuous timing (breaststroke), 506
Contractile proteins, 484, 638
Contrast sensitivity (visual), 902
Controlled mobility, 714, 715
Controlled skid stop (ice hockey), 400–401, 406
Contusions
 to muscles, 840
 to pelvic area, 757–758, 760
Convection
 thermal lift and, 261–263
 winds and, 386
Cool-down, 648
 stretching and, 363, 760, 772
Coordination
 fatigue and, 705
 rehabilitative treatment for, 774
COP. *See* Center of percussion
COR. *See* Coefficient of restitution
Corbett, James, 108, 119
Coriolis force, 204, 387
Corking (of baseball bats), 39, 54
Cornea, 890, 894, 896, 897
Corneal abrasions, 902
Corneal haze, 897
Corner kick (soccer), 443

Coroebus, 340
Coronary artery disease (CAD), 681–682
Corpus callosum, 709
Corrective lenses. *See* Eyewear
Cortical bone, 844, *845*
Corticospinal pathway, 825–827
Corticosteroids, 771
Cortisol, 847
Cortisone, 771
Costal cartilage, 843
Couples, Fred, 280
Coupling motion, spine and, 875
Course (ice skating), 401
Courts
 basketball, 697
 tennis, 510, 528–529
Court tennis, 510
Cousy, Bob, 80
Cradling (lacrosse), 128, 129
Cramps, muscle, 840
Crank length (cycling), 151
Creeping (archery), 28
Crew. *See* Paddle sports
Cricket, 50–51
Crossbows, 27, 175
Cross bridges, 831–832, 834, 835
Cross-country running. *See* Running and hurdling, distance running
Cross-country skiing. *See* Skiing, Nordic
Cross-dominance (vision), 903
Cross-handed putting, 280
Cross-section, area of
 shuttlecock, 526
 tennis racket strings, 518–519
Cross-sidedness, 711
Cross stroke (ice skating), 406, 416
Cross-training, 363, 447, 774, 776
Crosswinds
 football punting and, 239
 golf shots and, 289, *290*
 soccer ball kicking and, 443
Crouzon syndrome, 856
CRT. *See* Circuit resistance training
Cryotherapy. *See* Cold therapy
CT. *See* Computerized tomography
Cumberland wrestling style, 567
Cumulus clouds, gliding and, 263, 264
Cunningham, Randall, 250
Cups, protective, 110
Curare, 835
Curling, 295, 396, 808
Current pools, 492
Curveball (baseball), 44–45, 69, 208, 288, 815, 816, 889

Curves
 running track, 351–353
 in speed skating, 406, 411, 416–417
Cycling, **130–151**
 bicycle construction, 162–167
  frame geometry, 131–132, 134, 163
  frame material, 132–133, 137, 163–165
  handlebars, 141–142, 143–146, 144, 145, *151*
  saddles, 143–146, 151
  wheels, 137, 138, 142–143, 163, 165–167
 bicycle stability, 133–135
 biomechanics, 143–151
  alternative propulsion methods, 147–148
  crank length, 151
  floating pedals, 149–150
  gears, 146–147, 150
  muscle power, 151, 412
  pedaling stroke rate, 148–149
  saddle and handlebar adjustments, 143–146
 body positioning, 134, 139–140, 142, 143–146, 151
 dirt bikes, 130–131
 footwear, 149, 172
 forces at work, 135–143
  air resistance, *135*, 136, 139–141, 345
  gravity, 133, 134, *135*, 136–137
  hub friction, *135*
  inertia, 136–137, 149
  propulsion force, *135*
  rolling resistance, *135*, 136, 138
 helmets, 150
 injury prevention, 144–145, 150
 male sexual functioning and, 144–145
 mountain bikes, 131, 132, 138, 163, 165–166
 mountain sprint racing, 133
 road racing, 130–131, 137, *149*
 speed, 131, 133, 134, 136–137, 138, 139–141
 steering, 134, 135, 403
 Tour de France, 130, 141–142
 track racing, 130
 as transportation means, 130
 vibrational energy and, 132, 133
Cytoplasm, 634, 638

D
Dairy products, 728, 732, 738
D'Alembert's principle, 853

Daly, John, 271
Damping
　equipment materials and, 161–162, 167, 174
　in ice hockey, 304–305, 307
　soccer ball heading and, 452
　in tennis, 513, 518, 520–521, 523, 817, 819
　in volleyball, 545
Daniels, Terry, 240
Darts, 71
Davenport, Willie, 364
Davies, John, 286
Davis, Al, 243
Davis, Otis, 488
Davis, Wendell, 250
Davis Cup (tennis), 510–511
Dead lift (weight lifting), 552, 561, 562, 563
Deafness, age-related, 585
Death
　from anorexia nervosa, 656
　from bleeding, 686
　boxing-related, 108, 116, 686
　cardiac-related, 668, 676–677
　cycling-related, 150
　football-related, 230
　rigor mortis, 834
　snowboarding-related, 668
Deceleration
　in baseball pitching, 42, 814, 815
　in baseball sliding, 57, 58
　in cycling, 137
　in volleyball spiking, 543–544
Decompression sickness (the bends), 672, 804–806
Deformation
　of golf balls, 283
　in karate, 314, 315, 318
　of playing surfaces, 248–249
　of tennis racket strings, 516
　of volleyball, 537, 538–539
Deformation energy, 192
Degeneration, tissue, 765–766
Dehydration
　bioelectrical impedance measurements and, 621
　cardiac and circulatory problems from, 677, 685, 740
　cramping and, 840
　pregnancy and, 661–662
　water and, 739–740, 741
　weight loss and, 574, 750
Delayed-onset muscle soreness, 839–840
Delgarno, Pedro, 142
Delivery angle (baseball), 41, 42–43

Deltoid ligament, 606
Deltoid muscle, 813, 814
Dementia pugulistia, 117
Demers, Jacques, 306
Dendrites, 703, *704*, 705, 706
DeNiro, Robert, 118
Density. *See* Air density; Bone density; Equipment materials; Water, density of
Density, body, 620
Dependent variable (statistics), 467–468
Depression (clinical), 594, 596, 645, 653
Depth perception, 125, 899–900, *904*
Detached retina, 116, 902
Deviation (statistics), 459, 468
Devitt, John, 488
Dexamethasone, 800
Dexter-Hysol Cheetah (bicycle), 131
Dhow, 369, *370*
Diabetes, 644, 894
Diagonal stride (Nordic skiing), 436
Diamox, 798, 799
Diaphragm (muscle), 783, 784, 785, 835, 882, 885
Diaphysis, 844
Diastolic blood pressure, 590, *671*, 678–679
Diencephalon, 707
Diet. *See* Nutrition
Diet pills, 656
Diffusion of gases, 781–782, 793
Digestive system, 741–746
Dimpling
　of baseball bat, 50–51, 288
　of golf ball, 168, 208, 285, 286–288
Dirt bikes, 130–131
Disaccharides, 632, 723
Discobolos (statue), 202
Discus throw
　aerodynamics and, 207, 219–220, 222
　angle of attack and, 208, 220
　angle of attitude and, 208
　compared to Frisbee toss, 224, 225
　dynamics of, 219–222
　future performance prediction, 468
　international standards, *209*
　optimal conditions for, 209
　origins of, 201–202
　record throws, 219
　technique, 209–211, 222–223
Disks (spine). *See* Intervertebral disks
Dislocation, shoulder, 813
Dismounts (acrobatic), 16–18
Displacement of snow, 423, 425–426

Distance running, 353, 356–360
　body fat factor, 622, 747
　eating disorder issues, 656
　fatigue factor, 358–360
　fluid intake, 740
　glycogen depletion, 646
　hills and, 357–358
　joint action, 342
　muscles used, 342, 357, 757, 837
　performance improvement factors, 357
　strategies used, 356
　sweating and, 360
　technique, 342, 353, 357–360
　world records, 356, 457
Di Tullio, Jeffrey, 50, 288
Diuretics, 574, 656, 799, 800
Diving
　acrobatics and, 4, 7–8, 14, *16*, 875
　from cliffs, 3
　in competitive swimming, 507–508
　fluidity and summation of forces, 6–9
　horizontal momentum and, 7
　injury risks, 707, 877
　kinetic energy and, 8
　overcoming of fear, 4
　sensory clues and, 18–19
　springboard, 7–8, 10
　vertical momentum and, 7–9
　vestibular system and, 21
　See also Scuba diving
Dizziness, 676, 677, 740
Dog paddle (swimming stroke), 488
Dolphining (gliding), 264
Dolphin kick (swimming), *500*
Double-butted tubing (bicycle), 132
Double poling (Nordic skiing), 436
Downhill skiing. *See* Skiing, Alpine
Downsweep (swimming), 503, 504
Downswing (golf), 271, 272, 275–278
Down tube (bicycle), 131
Downwind sailing, 375
Draft
　of boat, 327, 383
　of sail, 374, *375*
Drafting
　cycling and, 140–141, 345
　running and, 345–346
Drag
　cycling and, 139–140, 166–167
　football kicking and, 241
　gliding and, 254–255, 256, 257–258, 259, 268
　in golf, 284, 286, 288, 289, *290*
　hockey pucks and, 295
　in paddle sports, 324–326, 330

running and, 344
  in sailing, 370–372, 374, 375, 377–378, 380
  in skiing, 423–425, 426–427
  on soccer ball, 443
  in speed skating, 407–411
  in speed skiing, 429
  in swimming, 494–498, *501*, 618
    breaststroke and, 506
    friction, 497–498
    water flow, 495–497
    waves, 497
  as throwing factor, 207, 208
    in discus throw, 219–220, 221
    in football, 235
    in Frisbee toss, 225–226
    in hammer throw, 217
    in shot put, 212, 214
  in volleyball, 535–537
Drawing (archery), 28, *29*, *30*, 35–36
Dribbling
  in basketball, 62, 63, 82–83
  in soccer, 448
Drive (golf shot), 271, *284*
Driver (golf club), 271, 288
Drop foot, 695
Drop shot (tennis), 522–523
Drop training drills, 540
Drugs
  antihistamines, 677
  anti–inflammatory, 769, 771
  for asthma, 792–793
  cardiac-related deaths and, 677
  corticosteroids, 771
  as hypertension factor, 681
  muscle relaxants, 786, 835
  steroids, 635, *636*, 771, 792
Dumbbells. *See* Isotonic exercise; Strength training; Weight lifting
Dunk shots (basketball), 62
Duodenum, 743–744
Dupont Corporation, 168
Dwarfism, 847, 856
Dwell time (tennis), 517, 520, 529, 531
Dynamic acuity, 895, 898, 902, *904*
Dynamic constant-resistance exercise, 481–482
Dynamic exercises. *See* Isotonic exercise; Isokinetic exercise; Variable-resistance exercise
Dynamic movement, 9
Dysmenorrhea, 659

E

EANx (oxygen-nitrogen mixture), 806

Ear
  scuba diving and, 802–803
  vestibular system, 20–21, 125
  See also Hearing
Eating disorders, 22, 616, 656, 660, 663–665
Eccentric contraction, 540, 716, 717
  skiing and, 433, *434*
Eckersley, Dennis, 42
Ecological theory (of motor control), 701
Edberg, Stefan, 531
Eddy currents (swimming), 495, 496, 502
Edema, pulmonary, 683–684, 796, 799, 800
Edge-ice interface, 398
Edging turn (Alpine skiing), 430, 432
Efferent nerves, 702
Eggs
  nutrition and, 728
  tossing of, 115, 126
Egypt, ancient, 26, 27, 85, 311
8–10 split (bowling), 105, 106, 107
EKG. *See* Electrocardiograph
Elastic bandages, 768–769
Elastic energy
  equipment materials and, 162, 174
  ice hockey shots and, *298*, 299–301, 304–305, 306
  plyometrics and, 716, 717
  in pole vaulting, 192, 193, 195, 196
  in running, 361
  strain potential, 31
  in weight lifting, 556–557, 564, *565*
Elasticity
  in archery, 32–33, 35, 36
  baseball pitching arms and, 43
  board and concrete breaking and, 318, 319
  damping vs., 161–162
  equipment materials and, 156–157, *157*, 161, 162, 167, 169, 171, 195
  of racket strings, 519
  See also Young's modulus of elasticity
Elasticity-to-density ratio, 159
Elastic strain potential energy (ESPE), 31
Elastin, 585
Elbow. *See* Shoulder, elbow, wrist
Electric stimulation, as bone trauma treatment, 857
Electrocardiograph (EKG), 673–674
Electrolytes, 574, 840
Elevation (geographic). *See* Altitude

Elevation (injury treatment), 769, 770
Elevation, angle of (baseball), 124, 125
Elizabethan era, 85–86
El Salvadoran-Honduran "Soccer" War (1969), 440
Elway, John, 235, 866
Embolism, pulmonary, 685, 798
Embolus, 798
Emphysema, 782, 787, 793–794, 804
Endocrine system, 574–575, 707, 708, 847
Endorphins, 359, 660, 706
Endosteum, 845
Endotracheal tubes, 786, 787
Endurance
  carbohydrate loading and, 646, 725
  cross-training and, 447
  in distance running, 357, 358–360
  glycogen stores as factor, 724, 727
  heart rate and, 446
  injury prevention and, 823
  lactate threshold and, 632
  measurement of, 838
  protein requirements, 727–728
  strength training and, 484
  water consumption and, 740, 741
Energy
  bow and arrow, 30–32
  conservation law. *See* Conservation of energy
  damping of, 162, 167, 174
  deformation of, 192
  gliding and, 260–265
  loss in cycling, 138
  transportation means and, *130*
  See also Elastic energy; Kinetic energy; Potential energy; Vibrational energy
Energy and metabolism, **625–650**
  aging and, 588, *593*
  body fat and, 575–576, 654, 658
  calories and, 721
  cellular, 629–640
    adenosine triphospate and, 629–639, 646–647
    carbohydrate energy, 632–635, *640*
    fat energy, 635–638, *640*
    oxidative phosphorylation, 631–632, 634, 637, 647
    protein energy, 638–639, *640*
  chemical basis of, 626–629
  dehydration's impact on, 574
  in distance running, 354–356, 358–360
  fatigue and, 446–447, 635, 645

gorging of food and, 575
movement efficiency and, 361
orgasm as performance factor, 118
in speed skating, 415
starvation's effect on, 684
strength training and, 485
whole-body, 641–650, 745
   absorptive and postabsorptive, 641–643
    body weight and, 641
    exercise and, 644–650
    insulin levels, 643–644, 645
See also Aerobic activity; Anaerobic activity; Nutrition
England
  archers, 26–27
  badminton, 526
  bowling, 85–86
  cricket, 50
  field hockey variant, 293
  shot put and hammer throw, 201
  soccer, 439
  Wimbledon tennis event, 510, 528
English, Alex, 71
English longbow, 27–28, 33, 34
Enriched Air (oxygen-nitrogen mixture), 806
Environmental factors
  altitude as, 197, 204, 213–214
  in ice skating, 395–398
  in jumping, 196–200
  latitude as, 204, 213–214
  Mexico City Olympic Games and, 198–200
  in sailing, 375, 386–388
  in skiing, 420–426
  in swimming, 490–498
  See also Water (liquid medium); Weather; Wind
Enzymes, 627, 638, 723, 724, 834
Epinephrine, 706
Epiphysis, 844
Equilibrium
  flotation and, 491
  in ice skating, 401–404
  vestibular system and, 20–21
  See also Balance; Balancing skills
Equipment materials, **153–177**
  Alpine skis, 433
  archery, 175
  baseball bats, 52–53, 162, 175, 303
  bicycles, 132–133, 137, 143, 162–167, 163, 166
  bows and arrows, 33–34, 36, 175
  boxing, 117, 120
  canoeing, kayaking, shelling, 176, 325

density of, 156, 159, *160*
elasticity modulus, *157*, 161
eyewear, 905
figure skating, 176, *399*
fishing, 176
football, 117, 176, 246–247
gliders and hang gliders, 253–254
golf, 153–154, 167–171, 281, 282
hockey, 176, 177, 304–305
lacrosse sticks, 128
landing pits, 192
material selection, 154–162
neoprene clothing, 761
paddle sports, 325
sailing, 159, 161, 176–177, 385
soccer ball, 440–441
tennis, 177, 510, 511, 513, 514, 518, 520, 523, 817
vaulting poles, 156, 160, 192–193, *194*
yield strengths, *158*
See also Athletic shoes; Playing surfaces; *specific materials*
Erythrocytes, 788–789, 796, 798, 800
Eskimos, 887
Esophagus, 742
Esophoria, 900
ESPE. *See* Elastic strain potential energy
Essential amino acids, 726, 728, 729
Essential fat, 617, 747
Essential fatty acids, 730
Essential nutrients, 720
Estradiol, 575
Estrogen, 730
  aggression and, 119
  bone density and, 654, 656, 660, 662, 736–737
  bone growth and, 847
  cholesterol and, 733
  menstruation and, 657–658, 662
EVA polymer (ethylene, vinyl, and acetate), 174
Eversion ankle sprain, 609
Evert, Chris, 511, 531
Exercise
  aging and, 584–601
  asthma attacks and, 792–793
  blood pressure changes, 679–680, 682
  bone mass loss prevention and, 586
  cancer prevention and, 598, 653
  during pregnancy, 660–662
  fatigue and, 645
  females and, 653, 659–660
  heart and, 675–677
  intensity vs. duration, 649

muscle soreness and pain, 839–840
osteoarthritis and, 865
osteoporosis and, 586, 596
respiratory rate during, 784–785
stress fractures and, 859–860
weight control and, 576, 641
Exercise dependency, 359
Exercises, strength-training, 480–483, 662
Eximer laser surgery, 896, 897
Exophoria, 900
Explosive muscles. *See* Fast-twitch muscles
Extracellular fluid, 739
Eye contact, 18, 19
Eye dominance, 711, 903
Eyeglasses. *See* Eyewear
Eyeguards, 905
Eye-hand and eye-hand-foot coordination, 900, *904*
  in ice hockey, 305
  in lacrosse, 128
Eyes. *See* Vision
Eye tracking, 898, 899, *904*
Eyewear, 894, 902–903, 905–906
  eyeglasses, 896, 897, 905
  sunglasses, 887, 901, 905

F

Fabric equipment material, 253, 254
Face masks, 905
  football, 176, 245
  ice hockey, *293*, 905
Face-offs (ice hockey), 305
FAI. *See* Federation Aeronautique International
Fainting, 676, 677, 740
Faldo, Nick, 280
Faraday, Michael, 394
Farsightedness (hyperopia), 894
Fasicles, 828
Fastball (baseball), 45–46, *47*, 51
  elbow effects of, 816
  shoulder effects of, 815
  speed, 51, *128*
  visual traits and, 889, 902–903
Fast-glycolytic muscles, 445
Fast-oxidative muscles, 445
Fast-twitch muscles, 836–837
  aging and, 588
  golf swing and, 270–271
  jumping ability and, 540
  sprinting and, 341–342, 348
  weight lifting and, 552
Fat (tissue). *See* Body fat
Fatigue
  causes of, 645, 734, 737, 740, 882

cycling and, 148, 150
distance running and, 358–360
energy and metabolism and, 446–447, 635, 836
injury prevention and, 612–613
intermittent sports and, 446–447
knee injuries and, 697
recovery time, 474, 477–478
in soccer, 446–447
speed skating and, 410
starvation dieting and, 574
stress fractures and, 859
volleyball spikes and, 543
Fats (compounds)
energy and metabolism and, 635–638, *640*, 658, 726
limiting of intake, 636, 731, 732
mountain climbers' diet and, 798
as nutrients, 720, 728–732
Fatty acids, 730, 731, 732, 733, 744, 745
Fear, overcoming of, 4, 492
Feathered (oars and paddles), 333
Featheries (golf), 282
Feathers
in arrows, 36
in shuttlecock, 526
Federation Aeronautique International (FAI), 265, 267
Feet-first slide, 59, *60*
Felt (billiards), 295
Female athletes, **651–665**
archers, 29
athletic shoes for, 613
basketball and, *69*, 80, 82
body fat
metabolism and, 654, 655, 658
speed skating and, 622
swimming and, 618, 747
tolerable limits of, 747–748
eating disorders and, 22, 656, 660, 663–665
future performance prediction, 468–469
gymnast body size, 19–24, 656
health and fitness findings, 653
metabolism and, 654, 655
reproduction function and, 657–663, 736, 737, 747
strength training, 839
Title IX impact on, 651–652
See also Osteoporosis
Female athlete triad, 656
Femur. *See* Thigh
Fencing, 711, 712, 876
Fiber, 633, 723, 739, 745, 746

Fiberglass materials, 159, 160, 161, 193, *194*, 253
Fibers, muscle, 828–831, 834, 835–837
Fibula, 604, 605
Fictitious forces, 203–204
Field archery, 27, 32
Field athletics, jumping, **178–200**
center of gravity, 178–181
high jump, 179–181, 183, 184–185
long jump, 181, 187, 188, 189
pole vaulting, 181, 195
environmental factors, 196–200
fluidity and summation of forces, 7–8
hang time, 78
takeoff speed, 178–181
high jump, 180, 181, 183–184
long jump, 185, 186–188
pole vaulting, 193–194
Field athletics, throwing, **201–229**
dynamics of, 208–223, 226–29
discus throw, 219–222
hammer throw, 217, *218*
javelin throw, 223, 226–228
shot put, 212–214, 220
environmental factors, 202–208, 213
aerodynamics, 202, 207–208, 219–220, 222
force of hand, 202, 205–207
gravity, 202–205, 207, 209
international standards, *209*
technique, 209–212, 808
in discus throw, 222–223
in hammer throw, 210–211, 217–219
in javelin throw, 210, 211, 228–229
muscle power, 211–212
release angle, 188, 208, 210, 213, 214, *215*, 217, 220, 221
release velocity, 205, 208, 210, 212, 213, *215*, 228
in shot put, 210, 215–216
throwing time, 210–211
See also Discus throw; Hammer throw; Javelin throw; Shot put
Field goals (football), 239–240, 242–243
Field hockey. *See* Hockey, field
Field shots (basketball), 69–72
Fignon, Laurent, 142
Figure skating
acrobatics, 4
center of gravity and, 5, 401
eating disorders and, 656

equipment and materials, 176, 391, *394*, *399*, 404
hockey and speed skating vs., 307, 308, 398–401, 402
inertia and angular momentum, 11–12
injury risks, 877
origins of, 391–392
pair skating, 398–399
skater endurance, 392
spinning, 11–12, *13*, 21, 392
twisting, 757
vestibular system and, 21
Fingers
baseball sliding and, 58, 60
basketball shooting and, 64, 65, 69
skiing injuries and, 430
in swimming, *501*
Fishing, 176
Fixation, vision and, 899
Flaim, Eric, 409
Flak jackets, 246–247
Flat dives (competitive swimming), 507
Flat feet. *See* Arch of foot
Fletching (feathers), 36
Flexibility
head injury prevention and, 245
knee injury prevention and, 694–696
rehabilitative treatment and, 772–773
strength training and, 472, 478
See also Stretching
Flexible shaft (golf clubs), 281
Flight distance (long jump), 188–189
Flight shooting (archery), 27
Flips (acrobatic), 12
Floater
Frisbee toss, 225–226
volleyball serve, 535–539
Floor exercises (gymnastics), 6, 22
Flotation (swimming), 491–494
Fluidity, acrobatics and, 6–9
Flutter kick (swimming), *500*
Flyaway dismounts, 16, 17
Fly balls (baseball), 46, 122–125, 288, 900
Flying. *See* Gliding and hang gliding
Flying Dutchman (sailboat class), 384
Flying rings (gymnastics apparatus), 3
Fly patterns (football), 244
Folic acid, 734
Follow-through
basketball shooting, 65, 66–67
golf swing, 278–279
soccer ball kicking, 450–451

tennis, 815
throwing, 814
volleyball, 538–539, 543–544
Fons, Valerie, 326
Food. *See* Nutrition
Food product labeling, 722
Foot. *See* Ankle, foot, and lower leg
Football, **230–251**
   catching skills, 122, 123, 126–127
   deaths resulting from, 230
   equipment
      flak jackets, 246–247
      footwear, 172, 176, 250–251
      helmets, 117, 176, 244–246
      hip and thigh pads, 761
      material composition, 176
      injury risks, 110, 244–251, 604, 707, 760, 827–828, 849, 877, 882
   kicking
      helium- vs. air-filled balls, 240–241
      placekicking, 239–243
      punting, 237–239
   origins of, 230
   passing, 230, 235–237, 808
   player testosterone levels, 118
   playing surfaces, 247–250
   receivers and running speed, 243–244
   tackling, 231–235, 445, 869
   visual skills, *904*
   See also Soccer
Foot-ground contact (running), 342–343, 348, 868
Foot race. *See* Running and hurdling
Footwear. *See* Athletic shoes
Force. *See specific types, e. g.,* Braking force; Centrifugal force; Gravity; Magnus force
Force couples, 10
Force generation
   basketball shooting and, 65–66
   in karate, 313–320
Forehand shot (tennis), 531
Foresail (jib), 373–374
Fork rake (bicycle), 134–135
Forward pass (football), 230
Fosbury, Dick, 181, 182
Fosbury flop, *180*, 181, 182–183, 184–185
Foul shots (basketball). *See* Free throws
4-6-7-10 split (bowling), 105, *106*
Fovea, 890, 891
Fractures (skeletal system), 848, 851–860
   bone strength as factor, 853–855

bone trauma treatments, 857–859, 861
   forces acting on bones, 851–853
   spinal, 880
   stress, 846, 854–855, 859–860
   of toes, 609
   types of, 855–857, 858
   of wrist, 585, 819
Free radicals, 737
Free-space training, visual, 901
Freestyle skiing, 4, *10*, 419
Freestyle stroke (swimming), *503*, 504
Freestyle wrestling, 567, 568
Free throws (basketball), 64, 72–77
Free-weight training. *See* Strength training
Freshwater, 495
Friction
   balls and, 294–295
   basketball passing and, 81–82
   bowling and, 92, 94, 95, 98, 99, 100, 102
   cycling and, 133–134, 140
   footwear and, 172, 250
   in golf, 284
   ice and, 392–395, 396, 397–398
   in-line skating and, 408, 409
   kinetic, 392
   in paddling sports, 324
   sideward force, 133–134
   skiing and, 423–424
   sliding and, 249
   speed skating and, 413
   swimming and, 497–498
   in throwing events, 212
   See also Coefficient of friction; Drag
Frictional heat, 394, 423–424
"Friendly roll" (basketball), 69, 76
Frisbee, 220, 224–226, 295, 296
Frontal drag
   in paddle sports, 325
   in running, 345
   in skiing, 427
Front crawl (swimming), *503*, 504
Front fork (bicycle), 134–135
Fructose, 632, 633, 722–723, 745
Fruits, 739, 746
Full rollers (bowling), 99, 100, 102, 104, 106
Full squats, 486
Functional braces, 697–698
Funk, Casimer, 732
Fútbol ("Soccer") War (1969), 440

G
Gait (running), 341
Galactose, 632, 633, 723, 745

Galleons, 321
Galton, Francis, 467
Gambling, 86, 510
Gamow tent, 799
Ganglion cells, 892
Gant, Lamar, 561–563
Garcia, Jimmy, 116, 686
Gardini, Raul, 384
Gases, respiratory, 777–782, 787–791
   exchange, 782, 787–788
   transport, 782, 788–791
Gastrocnemius muscle, 540, 605, 606, 607, 612, 713
Gastrointestinal system. *See* Digestive system
Gathers, Hank, 676
Gault, Willie, 243
Gears, bicycle, 146–147, 150
Gehrig, Lou, 710
Gender
   hormone levels and performance, 118–119
   See also Female athletes
Genetics
   back problems and, 878
   body fat and, 747–748
   cholesterol and, 733
   as jumping ability factor, 540
   left-handedness and, 710
   as running factor, 347–348
   skeletal system and, 842, 848–849, 856, 866–867, 868
   vision and, 895
Genghis Khan, 26
Geometry, catching skills and, 123–124
Germany, 3, 85, 192
Gervin, George, 71
G forces, 246
GFRPs. *See* Glass fiber-reinforced polymers
Giant slalom (Alpine skiing), 430
Giant swings. *See* Swinging
Gigantism, 847
Glare recovery, 901, *904*
Glass fiber-reinforced polymers (GFRPs), 159, 160, 161
Glaucoma, 894
Glenohumeral joint, 812, 813, 814
Glenoid cavity, 42
Glial cells, 703
Glide
   in Nordic skiing, 424–425
   in speed skating, 405, 413–416
Glide timing (breaststroke), 506
Gliding and hang gliding, 224, **252–268**
   energy sources, 253, 260–265

Index

flight physics, 254–259
origins of, 252–253
record flights, 253, 254, 261, 264
as sport, 265–267
Gliding joint, 863
Glima wrestling style, 567
Gloves
  baseball, 126
  boxing, 113, 117–120
  ice hockey, *293*
  weight-lifting, 480
Glucose
  abnormal levels of, *643*, 644
  alcoholism and, 672
  carbohydrate intake and, 723–724
  cellular metabolism and, 632, 633–635, 636, 638, 639, *640*, 836
  starvation dieting and, 574
  whole-body metabolism and, 642–645, 646, 745
Gluteus maximus (buttocks), 151, 756
Gluteus medius, 756–757
Gluteus minimus, 756–757
Glycerol, 636, 638, 644, 728, 733
Glycogen
  aging and, 588
  endurance and, 646, 725, 727
  energy and metabolism and, 635, 642, 644, 647–648, 724, 745
  fatigue and depletion of, 645
  insulin and, 575
  replenishment, 415, 447, 647–648
  running and stores of, 354, 356
  starvation dieting and, 574
  weight loss and, 749
Glycolysis, 633–635, 644, 646–647, 836
Goal posts (hockey), 58
Goaltending
  ice hockey, *293*, 298, 305, 307, 308, 905
  soccer, 443, 444–445, 712
Goggles, sports, 896, 905
Goitchel, Phillipe, 428
Golf, 269–290
  balls, 281–290
    aerodynamics of, 50–51, 208, 284–288
    club head and ball collision, 283–284
    coefficient of restitution, 283
    dimpling, 168, 208, 285, 287–288
    Polara design, 286–287
    effect of wind on, 289
    evolution of, 282, 285
    optimum position for, 272

    slices and hooks, 279, 286–287, 289–290
  clubs, 280–281
    drivers, 271, 288
    flexible shafts, 281
    inserts, 171
    irons, 168, 171, 271, 272, 288, 290
    perimeter weighting, 280–281
    sweet spot, 154, 169, 170, 171, 280
    woods, 168, 170, 171, 272
  equipment materials, 153–154, 167–171
    balls, 167–168, 282
    clubs, 168–171, 281
  origins of, 269
  playing surface, 279, 295, 900
  probability of scoring 80 or below, 465–466
  putting, 279–280, 899, 900–901
  sidehill lies, 279
  as stress reducer, 281
  swing power, 270–279, 754
    backswing, 272–275
    downswing, 271, 275–278
    follow-through, 278–279
    stance and weight distribution, 271–272
  visual skills, 899, 900–901, 903, *904*
Golgi tendon organs (GTOs), 713, 714, 717
"Good" cholesterol. *See* High-density lipoprotein
Gorging, 575
Grab start (competitive swimming), 507–508
Grady, Sam, 243
Grafts, bone, 857–859
Grains, 732, 737–738, 744
Graphite
  bicycle construction, 132–133
  as equipment material, 159, 160–161
  golf clubs, 170, 281
  hockey sticks, 304
  tennis rackets, 177, 511, 514
Grass playing surface
  football, 247–250
  golf, 279, 295, 900
  for indoor competitions, 441
  soccer, 441
  tennis, 510, 511, 528
Gravitational acceleration
  as jumping factor, 196–197, 198
  as throwing factor, 204, 209
Gravity
  baseball pitches and, 45, *47*

basketball shooting and, 71, 78
body size and, 24
bowling and, 88, 91, 95
center of. *See* Center of gravity
cycling and, 133, 134, *135*, 136–137
flotation and, 491–493
football punting and, 238
giant swings, dismounts, and, 16–17
as jumping factor, 196–197, 198
in paddle sports, 327–328
posture and, 867, 882, *883*
skeletal system and, 842, 851, 852, 867
skiing and, 421–422, *423*, 427–429
as throwing factor, 202–205, 207, 209, 213–214
in weight lifting, 550, 557
Great Britain. *See* England; Scotland
Greco-Roman wrestling style, 567
Greece, anciet
  boxing, 108
  discus throwing, 202
  foot race, 340
  hockey, 292
  paddle technology, 321
  wrestling, 567
  See also Olympics, ancient
Greens. *See* Grass
Greenstick fractures, 856, 858
Gretzky, Wayne, 301
Griffey, Ken, Jr., 122, 123, 710
Griffith, Darrell, 179
Grimmer, Gerhard, 434
Grinkov, Sergei, 676
Grip
  baseball hitting, 53–54, 303
  baseball pitching, 45
  ice hockey shooting, 303–304
  in Nordic skiing, 424–425
  pole vaulting, 193, 194–195
  in tennis, 303, 518, 520–521, 817
Groin muscles, 110, 111, 757, 760
Grove, Lefty, 710
Growth hormone, 847
Growth plate, 844–845, 846, 847
GTOs. *See* Golgi tendon organs
Gusts. *See under* Wind
Gutsu, Tatiana, 21
Gutta-percha golf balls, 282
Gutter balls (bowling), *87*
Gwynn, Tony, *461*
Gymnasiums, 3
Gymnastics. *See* Acrobatics
Gyration, radius of, 88, 95, 97, 99
Gyroscopic motion
  of bowling balls, 97
  cycling and, 134

of football passes, 236–237
in Frisbee toss, 224–225
Gyroscopic precession, 225

H

Haines, Jackson, 391–392
Hainstock, Janet, 188
Hair
   aging and, 585
   soccer ball heading and, 451–452
   as swimming drag factor, 497–498
Hair cells (vestibular system), 20, 21
Half nelson (wrestling hold), 573
Half-pipe slope, 419
Half squats, 486, 695, *696*
Hallowell, Robert J., 887
Halteres (jumpers' weights), 186
Hammer throw
   angular momentum and, 207
   dynamics of, 217, *218*
   international standards, *209*
   optimal conditions for, 209
   origins of, 201
   record throws, 217
   sidearm and underarm motion, 808
   technique, 210–211, 217–219
Hampton, Dan, 247, 249
Hamstring muscles, 757
   back injury prevention and, 885
   for bending knee, 690–691
   hurdling and, 760–761
   injury susceptibility, 757, 760–761
   soccer leg swing and, 450
   warm-up stretching of, 363
Handedness, 709, 710–712, 903
Hand-eye coordination. *See* Eye-hand and eye-hand-foot coordination
Handlebars, 141–142, 143–146, *151*
Hands
   baseball sliding and, 58
   basketball shooting and, 64, 65
   boxing and, 119–120
   catching technique and, 126, 127
   eye-hand coordination, 900, *901*
   golf putting and, 280
   golf swinging and, 272, 275, 277, 278–279
   ice hockey shots and, 302–303
   karate and, 314, 317, 319–320
   skiing injuries and, 430
   swimming and, 497, 498–499, 500–503, 504–505
   throwing and force of, 202, 205–207
   See also Fingers; Grip
Handstand, 5, 6
Hang (jumping technique), 188, 191

Hang gliding. *See* Gliding and hang gliding
Hang time
   acrobatics, 9
   basketball, 77–79
   football punting, 237
   high jump, 78
HAPE. *See* High altitude pulmonary edema
Harpastum (Roman soccer forerunner), 439
Harvard University
   football, 230
   Yale rowing competition, 321
Hashi (Okinawan king), 311
Haskell, Coburn, 282
Hayes, Charlie, 243
HCM. *See* Hypertrophic cardiomyopathy
HDL. *See* High-density lipoprotein
Head
   position as sensory clue, 19
   soccer and, 451–452
   wrestling and, 570
   See also Head injuries
Head (tennis racket), 511, 512
Head, Henry, 511
Headaches, 796, 800
Head-first slide, 57, 59, 60
Headgear
   boxing, 113, 115, 117, 120
   See also Face masks; Helmets
Heading
   in ice skating, 401
   as soccer maneuver, 443, 451–452
Head injuries, 708
   boxing and, 112–117
   cycling and, 150
   football and, 244–246
Headpin (bowling), 86–87, 104
Head tube (bicycle), 131, 132, *134*
Headwind
   football kicking and, 239, 241
   Frisbee tossing and, 226
   gliding and, 264
   running and, 344–345
   soccer ball kicking and, 443
   as throwing event factor, 209, 220, 221, 222
Hearing
   aging and, 585
   catching skills and, 125
   sensory clues, 19, *234*
Heart and circulatory system, **667–686**
   aging and, 586, 590–594, 596–597
   anemia, 645, 655–656, 737

arteries, 668, 669, 677–682
   blood pressure and, 678–679
   cholesterol intake and, 732, 733
   exercise and, 679–680, 682
   hypertension, 681–682
   low oxygen levels and, 795–796
bleeding and blood loss, 685–686
   boxing injuries, 111, 116, 686
   cold therapy, 767
blood
   acidity of, 790–791, 795
   circulation pattern, 667–670
   hemoglobin, 737, 788–789, 790, 795
   plasma, 739, 778, 788–791, 804–805
   skeletal system role, 845–846, 857, 858–859, 864
body fat and, 576
capillaries, 668–669, 683–684
cardiovascular fitness assessment, 680
deaths related to, 668, 676–677
dehydration effects on, 574, 677, 740
endorphin release and, 359
fat intake and, 731–732
females and, 656, 660, 662
heart's role and functioning, 670–677
   basic structure and design, 667, 668
   cardiac cycle, 674–675
   during exercise, 675–677
   electrical activity, 672–674
   valve operation, 670–672, 675
intermittent sports and, 446
veins, 668, 669, 684–685
water's role, 739
water therapy and, 493
See also Blood clots; Blood pressure
Heart attacks, 682, 731
Heart murmur, 672
Heat
   energy and metabolism and, 626
   frictional, 394, 423–424
   thermal lift, 253, 260, 261–264
Heat therapy, 763, 764, 767–768, 770–771, 820
Heavyweight fighters, 110–112, 113
Heel (sailing), 372, 374, 380, 381–382
Heel cleats, 250–251
Heel counters (athletic shoes), 174–175, 363
Heel spurs, 609
Heel-to-toe running, 342, 343, 362
Heiden, Eric, 412, 414–415

Height (body)
  of basketball players, 79–80, 83
  of gymnasts, 20–24
  hormone imbalances and, 847
  male vs. female, 846
Height (vertical distance)
  in jumping events, 178–181, 182
  in pole vaulting, 192, 193–194, 195–196
  in throwing events, 205, 213, 214, *215*, 220, 221
  See also Altitude
Helicopter (snowboard manuever), *10*
Helium, 240–241
Helmets
  cycling, 150
  football, 117, 176, 244–246
Hematomas. *See* Blood clots
Hemoglobin, 737, 788–789, 790, 795
Henderson, Rickey, 58
Henie, Sonja, 392
Henrich, Christy, 22
Heredity. *See* Genetics
Herniated disk, 879, 880
High altitude pulmonary edema (HAPE), 683–684
High bar. *See* Horizontal bar
High blood pressure. *See* Hypertension
High-density lipoprotein (HDL), 597, 658
High jump, 178, 182–185
  body size and, 179–180
  center of gravity, 179–181, 183, 184–185
  environmental factors, 200
  future performance prediction, 468
  hang time, 78
  measurement of, 184
  record jumps, 183
  styles, *180*, 181, 182–184
  takeoff leg adaptation, 842
  takeoff speed, 180, 181, 183–184
  technique, 184–185
  visual skills, *904*
High set (volleyball), 541, 542
High-tensile steel, 164
High-top sneakers, 613
Hinge joint, 863
Hip flexor muscles, 757, 760–761
Hip pointer, 760
Hip replacement surgery, 758–759
Hips, 752–761
  aging and, 585
  in baseball pitching, 40–41
  in cycling, 151
  in golf swing, 271, 273, 274, 278
  in hurdling, 365, 366

  in karate kicks, 316
  in soccer, 449, 450, 451
  in swimming, 504
  in weight lifting, 555, 556, 560, 564
  width-inertia relationship, 23
Hip throw (wrestling), 571, 572
Hitch kick (jumping technique), 188–189, 191
Hitting
  in baseball, 54–57, 162, 303
    batting averages, 456–461
    checked swings, 820
    vision factor, 305, 889, 902–903, *904*
  in cricket, 50–51
Hockey, field, 176, *249*, 292, 294, 808
Hockey, ice, **292–310**
  aggression levels and, 119
  equipment
    for goalies, *293*, 905
    goal posts, 58
    pucks, 293–297
    sticks, 176, 297, 298, 304–307
  goaltending, *293*, 298, 305, 307, 308
  older player injury factors, 849
  origins of, 292–293
  player skills, 305
  shooting, 297–304
    grip firmness, 303–304
    puck trajectories, 296–297, 303
    slap shots, *128*, 298–301
    wrist shots, 301–303, 304
  skating and, 307–310, 398–401, 402, 405, 406
  visual skills and, 297, 305, *904*
Hockey, roller, 292
Hockey, street, 177, 292, *294*
Hockey stop, 400
Holland, cycling in, 230
Hollow (of waves), 328
Holmstrom, Fred, 286, 287
Holyfield, Evander, 677
Homer, 26, 108
Home runs, 48, 49, 124
Honduran-El Salvadoran "Soccer" War (1969), 440
Hook (boxing punch), 109
Hook (bowling), 87, 89, 91, 94, 95–96, 97–99, 104, 106
Hook bounce pass, 82
Hooke's law, 32, 33
Hook shot
  basketball, 66, 77
  golf, 287, 289–290
Hook slide, 57, 58
Hook spin (bowling), 91, 95, 96, 99
Hop, step, and jump. *See* Triple jump

Horizontal axis, 15
Horizontal bar (gymnastics apparatus), 3, 12, 16–17, 22–23
Horizontal friction force. *See* Sideward friction force
Horizontal momentum
  diving and, 7
  in golf, 283
  jumping and, 184, 188, 191
Hormones, 724–725, 730
  cholesterol and, 733
  digestive system and, 744
  hip replacement surgery and, 759
  levels-performance relationship, 118–119
  male infertility and, 145
  menopause and, 662–663, 736
  muscle mass and, 839
  skeletal system and, 736–737, 847
  starvation diet effects, 574–575
  See also specific hormones
Hornsby, Rogers, 457
Horse stance (karate), 312–313
Hrudey, Kelley, 306
Huang-Ti (Chinese emperor), 439
Hub friction, *135*
Hull
  paddle sport boats, 325, 326, 327, 328
  sailboats, 369, 370, 377–378, 380, 381–382
Hull, Bobby, 301
Humeral epicondyles, 816
Humeral head, 42, 813, 814
Humerus, 812, 813, 815, 816, 818, 820
Humidity
  ice conditions and, 397–398
  as sweating factor, 741
Hump (of waves), 328
Hunchback (kyphosis), 879
Huns, 26
Hunting, 27, 32
Hurdling. *See under* Running and hurdling
Hurley (early field hockey form), 293
Hurling (sport), 126
Hydrochloric acid, 742
Hydrodynamics (swimming), 496–497
Hydrogen, 631–632, 634, 725, 726, 729, 791
Hydrogenation, 729
Hydrostatic pressure, 491, 493
Hydrostatic weighing, 619–621
Hydroxyproline, 860
Hyman, Flo, 676
Hyperbaric chamber, 806
Hyperextension, 816, 865, 868, 877

Hyperglycemia, *643*, 644
Hyperopia (farsightedness), 894
Hyperplasia, 484, 838
Hypertension, 681–682
Hypertrophic cardiomyopathy (HCM), 676–677
Hypertrophy, 838
Hypoglycemia, *643*, 644
Hypothalamus, 659
Hypothyroidism, 645, 660
Hypoxia, 795–796, 797, 799, 800

I

IACC. *See* International America's Cup Class
Ibuprofen, 771
Ice and skating, 392–398
   friction factor, 392–395
   indoor rink conditions, 396–398
   temperature factor, 395–396
Ice boats, 378, 379
Ice dancing, 399
Ice-edge interface, 398
Ice hockey. *See* Hockey, ice
Icelandic wrestling style, 567
Ice skating. *See* Skating
Icing of injuries. *See* Cold therapy
Ileum, 744, 746
Iliad (Homer), 108
Iliofemoral ligament, 756
Iliopsoas muscle, 761
Ilium, 754, 756
Immune system, 574, 759
Impact (soccer), 450–451
Impact, minimization of, 868–869
Impact fractures, 856, 858
Impact wave (running), 173
Impingement syndrome, 820–822
Impotence, 144–145, 681
Impulse (boxing), 111
Independent variable (statistics), 467–468
Indians. *See* Native Americans
Indoor ice rinks, 396–398
Indoor natural grass, 441
Induced drag, 257–258, 259
Indurain, Miguel, 149
Inertia
   acrobatics and, 9–12, 14–15, 16, 18, 22, 23
   in archery, *37*, 38
   in baseball hitting, 55
   in basketball shooting, 77
   in bowling, 88, 94–95, 98, 100
   in boxing, 112
   cycling and, 136–137, 149
   in Frisbee toss, 225
   in ice hockey, 308, 400, 404
   in paddle sports, 323–324
   in running, 352
   in sailing, 383–385
   in skating, 404
   skeletal system and, 851, 852–853
   in skiing, 424, 430, *431*
   in tennis, 512, 513, 531
   in throwing events, 202–203, 205
   in weight lifting, 550, 553, 555, 565
Inertial forces, 203–204
Inertia matrix (golf clubs), 169
Infertility, 145
Infield pop-ups, 124
Inflammation, 765, 766, 767, 769
Inflation panel (volleyball), 537–538
Infraspinatus muscle, 813, 814
Inhalers, asthma drug, 792
Injury risks and prevention
   acute vs. chronic injury, 764, *765*
   aggression and, 119
   ankle, foot, and lower leg, 603, 604–605, 606, 607–615, 866
   back and spine, 871–872, 875–885
      spinal cord, 244–246, 707, 827–828, 872
   during pregnancy, 661–662
   equipment use and selection, 613–615, 776
      athletic shoes, 249, 363, 605, 613, 614
   eyes and vision, 116, 797, 902–903
   head, 112–117, 150, 244–246, 708
   knee, 688, 691–698
   pelvis, hip, and thigh, 757–761
   shoulder, elbow, and wrist, 814–815, 816–820, 863
   skeletal system, 585, 609, 819, 846, 848, 851–860, 861, 866–869, 880
   skill improvement and, 612–613, 823
   strength training and, 245, 363, 485–487, 612, 761, 823
   stretching and, 363, 611, *612*, 696, 759–761, 823
   See also Pain; Rehabilitation; *specific body parts; injuries, and sports*
Injury threshold, 608
In-line hockey. *See* Hockey, roller
In-line skating, 4, 408–409
Inner ear, 20–21, 114, 125
Inoue, Junichi, 396
Insole (athletic shoes), 173–174
Instrument training, visual, 901–902
Insulin, 575, 643–644, 645, 847

Insweep (swimming), 503, 504
Inswinger (soccer kick), 443
Integumentary system, 584–585
Intermittent (stop-and-go) sports, 446–447, 649
International America's Cup Class (IACC), 384
International Cycling Union, *139*
Interneurons, 826
Interval training, 649, 776
Intervertebral disks, 873–876, 877–878, 879, 880
Intervertebral foramen, 873, 874, 875
Intracellular fluid, 739
Inversion (temperature), 262
Inversion ankle sprain, 609
Ireland
   field hockey variant, 293
   shot put and hammer throw, 201
   wrestling style, 567
Iris (human eye), 890
Iron (dietary), 737
   anemia and, 655, 656, 737
   Recommended Dietary Allowance, 722
Iron (metal), 390, *399*
Iron lung (ventilator), 785–786
Iron man competitions, 355–356
Irons (golf clubs), 168, 171, 271, 272, 288, 290
Ischium, 754
Ismail, Rocket, 243
Isokinetic exercise, 482–483
Isometric exercise, 480–481, 612, 662
Isometric muscle activity, 433, *434*
Isotonic exercise, 481–482
Ivanisevic, Goran, 514, 515

J

Jab (boxing punch), 109
Jackson, Bo, 758
Jackson, Joe, 39, 459
Jackson-Weiss syndrome, 856
Jacobs, Franklin, 184
Jahn, Friedrich Ludwig, 3
Jai alai, *128*
James II (king of Scotland), 269
James IV (king of Scotland), 269
Jansen, Dan, 395–396, 407
Japan
   archers, 27, 34
   golf popularity, 269
   volleyball popularity, 534
   wrestling, 567–568, 573, 576–579
Javelin throw
   aerodynamics and, 226–227
   design change impact, *227*, 228

dynamics of, 223, 226–228
international standards, 209
linear momentum and, 207
origins of, 202
record throws, 223
running launch, 90, 223, 228–229
technique, 210, 211, 228–229
Jejunum, 744, 746
Jerk lift. *See* Clean-and-jerk lift
Jett, James, 243
Jib. *See* Foresail
Jogging, 597, 695, 712
John, Yvon, 188
Johnson, Ben, 348
Johnson, Earvin (Magic), 81
Johnson, Michael, 347
Johnson, Randy, 711
Joint capsule, 864
Joint cavity, 862
Joints, 604–604, 860–866
    basketball shooting and, 64
    health factors, 864–865
    injuries to, 865–866
    strength training and, 485–487, 867
    structure and function, 860–864
    types of, 863
    water therapy and, 493
    See also specific joints
Jordan, Michael, 68, 78, 79
Joyce, Joan, 808
Joyner, Seth, 250
Judging, competitive, 4, 7, 22
Judo, 568, 571
Ju-jitsu, 568
Jumper's knee (patellar tendinitis), 545, 697, 866
Jumping
    acrobatics and, 7–8
    of barrels, 188
    bone density and, 850
    change-in-motion forces and, 9–10
    by early man, 178
    environmental factors, 196–200
    fluidity and summation of forces, 7–8
    human vs. animal, 182
    muscle forces and, 179, 181–182
    skill improvement, 540
    in volleyball, 541–542, 545
    weight-aided, 186
    See also Field athletics, jumping; Running and hurdling, hurdling; *specific jump types*
Jump serve (volleyball), 536, 539
Jump shot (basketball), 62, 65–66, 67, 79

K
Karate, **311–320**
    balance and base of support, 312–313
    generation of force, 313–320, 539
    origins of, 311
Kayaking, 321, 322, *323*
    equipment design, 324, 326–327
    equipment materials, 176
    paddles, 332–333
    rower's physique and, 335
    technique, 337–339
Keel (sailing boat), 374, 377, 381–382, 384–385
Keglers, 85
Ketoacidosis, *643*, 644
Keto acids, 639
Kevlar, 143, 176, 177
Kick double poling (Nordic skiing), 436
Kicking
    in football
        placekicking, 239–243
        punting, 237–239
    in karate, 313, 314, 316, *320*
    in soccer
        ball velocities, *450*
        "banana" kicks, 442–443
        coefficient of restitution, 441–442
        corner kicks, 443
        penalty kicks, 443–445
        player technique, 448–451
        side volleys, 443
    in swimming, *500*, 506
Kickoffs (football), 239
Kick returns (football), 242
Kick serve (tennis), 530–531
Kidneys
    boxing injuries to, 111
    circulatory system role, 670
    dehydration's impact on, 574
    football injuries to, 111
    hypertension and, 681
    hypoxia and, 796, 800
    metabolism role, 639, 725
Kim, Du Ku, 108
Kinesthetic memory. *See* Muscle memory
Kinetic (tennis racket), 521
Kinetic chain, 773
Kinetic energy
    acrobatic swinging and, 17
    airborne trajectory and, 8
    in archery, 30–31, 32
    in baseball, 41, 58
    board breaking and, 318
    in bowling, 88, 89, 99, 100, 101, 102

in boxing, 110
catching skills and, 126, 127
in cycling, 133
in diving, 8
in football, 232–233
in karate, 315
in lacrosse, 128–129
in pole vaulting, 192, 193–195, 196
in skiing, 422, *423*, 427
soccer ball kicking and, 449–450
in tennis, 516
in throwing events, 205–206
two-rod and multilever models of, 271, 276–277
in volleyball, 541
in weight lifting, 551, 556–557
Kinetic friction, 392
King, Bernard, 66–67
King, Billie Jean, 651
Kite, Tom, 280
Knee, **688–698**
    baseball sliding and, 58
    cycling and, 144, 149–150, 151
    functional anatomy, 688–691
    ice hockey skating and, 309
    injuries, 688, 691–698, 866
        females and, 654
        jumper's knee, 545, 697, 866
        orthopedic braces, 696–698
        prevention of, 693–698
        treatment for, 691–693, 768
        water on the knee, 693, 864
        water therapy and, 493
    running and, 173
    soccer ball kicking and, 450
    speed skating and, 404–405, 411, 413
    strength training and, 479, 694–696
    volleyball and, 545
    in weight lifting, 486, 555, 556, 560, 561, 564
Knee-bend exercises, 694–695, *696*
Knee-bend squats. *See* Squat lift
Knockouts (boxing), 114, 116, 117
Knuckleball, 46–47, 297, 536–537
Knuckles, 119–120
Koch, Bill (Nordic skier), 437
Koch, Bill (yacht racer), 384, 385
Konishiki (sumo wrestler), 577, 578–579
Korbut, Olga, 19
Kotogaume (sumo wrestler), 577
Koufax, Sandy, 45, 710
Krebs cycle, 634, 635, 636, 637, 639, 643
Krone, Julie, 652
Kruk, John, 54

Kuroiwa, Toshiyuki, 396
Kushimaumi (sumo wrestler), 577
Kwashiorkor (deficiency disease), 684
Kyphosis (hunchback), 879

L

Labeling, food product, 722
Labor disputes, 454–456
Lacrosse, 126, 128–129
Lactate threshold, 632, 649
Lactic acid
    anaerobic activity and, 649
    energy and metabolism and, 354, 632, 635, 644, 647, 836
    fatigue and, 447, 645, 648
Lactose, 632, 723
Lambeer, Bill, 74
Laminar water flow, 324, 495
LaMotta, Jake, 118
Landetta, Sean, 239
Landing mats, 3
Landing pits, 192
Landing technique
    impact minimization, 868–869
    in long jump, 189
    in running, 347
    in volleyball, 544
Lanes
    bowling, *87*, 92, 96–97
    in sprinting, 351–353
Large intestine, 745–746
Laser surgery, for eyes, 896, 897
LASIK eye surgery, 897
Lateen rigging, 369, *370*
Late hit (golf shot), 274
Lateral collateral ligament (LCL), 688, 690, 695
Lateral epicondylitis (tennis elbow), 520–521, 697, 766, 817, 819, 822
Lateral humeral epicondyle, 816
Latissimus dorsi muscle, 42, 813, 814
Latitude, as environmental factor, 204, 213–214
Lau, Charlie, 54
Launch angle
    in basketball, 69–72, 75–77
    in football kicking, 237, 242–243
    See also Angle of release
Launch speed
    in basketball, 69–72, 75–77
    See also Release, speed and throwing
Laver, Rod, 711, 842
Lawn bowls, 85
Lawn tennis, 510

Laxatives, 574, 656
Layout (position), 14
Layup shot (basketball), 62, 77
Lazy eye. *See* Amblyopia
LCL. *See* Lateral collateral ligament
LDL. *See* Low-density lipoprotein
Lean
    in Alpine skiing, 430
    in cycling, 402, 403
    in hurdling, 366
    in ice skating, 393, 403–404, 405, 406–407, 417
    in running, 352
Least-square curve (statistics), 468
Lee helm (sailing), 381
Lee-wave lift (gliding), 260, 264–265
Left-handedness, 709, 710–712, 903
Legs
    in Alpine skiing, 433–434
    baseball pitching and, 41
    basketball and, 65, 83
    bone type, 844
    circulatory problems and, 684–685
    distance running and, 357
    in golf swing, 270, 271, 278
    in hurdling, 363, 364, 365–366
    in ice hockey skating, 309
    jumping ability and, 179–180, 181–182, 540
    in soccer ball kicking, 449–451
    in speed skating, 411–412, 414–415
    sprinting and, 349
    strength testing of, 696
    in swimming, *500*, 506
    as throwing event factor, 211–212
    See also Ankle, foot, and lower leg; Knee; Pelvis, hip, and thigh
Legumes, 729, 737–738, 746
Le Mond, Greg, 132, 141–142
Lendl, Ivan, 515–516, 872
Lennon, Boone, 141
Lens (human eye), 890, 893, 894
Lenticular clouds, 264
Leonard, Ray (Sugar Ray), 116
Leonardo da Vinci, 252
Leverage
    in weight lifting, 554–556
    in wrestling, 571–573
Lever propulsion (cycling), 147–148
Lever system (bones and joints), 314, 554–556, 860–862, 863
Levitt, Bunny, 73–74
Lewis, Carl, 185–186, *187*, 348
Lewis, Reggie, 676, 677
Lies, sidehill (golf), 279
Lift
    football punting and, 239

    gliding and, 254–255, 256, 257, 268
        lee-wave lift, 260, 264–265
        slope lift, 260–261
        thermal lift, 253, 260, 261–264
    in golf, 287, 288, 289
    of hockey shots, 296–297
    in sailing, 370–373, 374, 375, 376–378
    in swimming, 498–499, 501–502
    as throwing factor, 207, 208
        in discus event, 219–220, 221
        in Frisbee toss, 224, 226
        in javelin events, 226–227, 228
Lifting force, 287, 288
Lifting speed (strength training), 477
Lift-off (speed skating), 414
Lifts
    acrobatic, 5
    bench press, 552, 555, 561, 564–565
    clean-and-jerk, 552, 556–557, 558, 560–561
    dead, 552, 561, 562, 563
    snatch, 552, 557–558, 560
    squat, 144–145, 486, 552, 555, 556, 557, 561, 564, *565*
Ligaments
    ankle, foot, and lower leg, 603, 606
    hip, 755–756
    knee, 688, 689–690, 862
    shoulder, elbow, and wrist, 820
    skeletal system, 862, 864
    spine, 879, 880
    sprains and tears, 691–692, 694–695, 866
Light, vision and, 888, *889*, 890–891, 901, 905
Lilienthal, Otto, 252, 260
Line (boat), 325
Linear momentum
    angular movement and, 10
    in bowling, 100, 103
    in boxing, 109, 112
    in football, 231, 232–233
    injury potential, 820
    in swimming, 505
    in tennis, 512, 513
    throwing events and, 206–207, 228–229
    velocity factor, 7
    in weight lifting, 555
Line drives (baseball), 124
Linemen (football), 233–235, 445, 576, 747, 877
Lipids. *See* Fats
Lipoproteins, 658, 733
"Little 500, The" (cycling race), 130
Little League baseball, 51–52, 58

Little League elbow (osteochondritis), 819
Liver
   alcoholism effects, 672
   circulatory system role, 669–670
   digestive system role, 744, 745
   lipoproteins and, 733
   metabolism and, 635, 639, 642, 644, 724, 725, 729, 731, 732
Load (golf club), 281
Lob (tennis shot), 522, 527, 528
Locked-arm blocking (football), 230
Loft angle, 168, 169, 281
Lombardi, Vince, 231
Longbows, 27–28, 33–34
Longitudinal axis, 12, *13*, 15
Long jump, 178, 185–189
   braking force, 185, 187–188
   center of gravity, 181, 187, 188, 189
   records, 142, 187, 198–200
   takeoff speed, 185, 186–188
   techniques, 185–188
   weight-aided, 186
Long-track speed skating, 391, 406, 412
Lordosis, 879
Louganis, Greg, 14
Louis X (king of France), 510
Low blows (boxing), 110–111
Low-density lipoprotein (LDL), 658, 733
Luge, 398
Lug rig, 370
Lulls. *See under* Wind
Lumbar vertebrae, 872, *873*, 875, 882
Lumbosacral joint, 875
Lung cancer, 793
Lungs
   aging and, 589–590
   asthma effects on, 792
   circulatory system and, 667, 668
   primary functions, 782
   scuba diving and, 802–804
   See also Pulmonary *headings*; Respiration
Luteinizing hormone, 575
Luther, Martin, 86
Lymphocytes, 881
Lynn, Fred, 456
Lysyl oxidase, 868

M

Macrophages, 765
Magnetic resonance imaging (MRI), 822, 881
Magnum, Jenifer, 664
Magnus force
   baseball hitting and, 46
   baseball pitching and, 44, 45, 48, 51, 208, 288
   basketball shooting and, 69
   in golf, 287, 288, 290
   soccer ball and, 443
   throwing and, 207–208
Main sail, 373–374
Malone, Karl, 846–847
Maltose, 632–633, 723
Mancini, Ray (Boom Boom), 108
Mantle, Mickey, *56*, 672
Marathon running. *See* Distance running
Marathon skating (Nordic skiing), 437
Marie, Thierry, 142
Marino, Dan, 236
Marquis of Queensberry rules, 108
Marrow, bone, 843, 845, 847
Martial arts. *See* Karate; Judo; Ju-jitsu
Masks. *See* Face masks
Mass, body
   composition of, 747
   football players, 231–232, 234, 241, 747
   gymnasts, 22, 23, 24
   inertia and, 11
   sumo wrestlers, 577
Mass, bone. *See* Bone density
Mass, center of. *See* Center of gravity
Mass, head, 113, 114
Mass weight (archery), 28–29
Mattingly, Don, 872
Mawashi belt (sumo wrestling), 573, 577, 579
Maximum-energy-transfer (MET) point, 52
McEnroe, John, 119, 511, 523, 711
MCL. *See* Medial collateral ligament
McMahon, Jim, 235, 866
MCP joint. *See* Metacarpophalangeal joint
McSorley, Marty, 306
Mean (statistics), 455
Mean square (statistics), 459
Meat, 728, 732
Medial axis, 12
Medial collateral ligament (MCL), 688, 690, 695
Medial epicondylitis (bowler's elbow), 818–19, 822
Medial humeral epicondyle, 816
Median (statistics), 455
Mediastinal emphysema, 804
Medications. *See* Drugs
Melting (of ice), 393–395

Memory. *See* Motor memory; Muscle memory; Visual memory
Meniscus, 688, 690, 692–693, 694
Menopause, 662–663, 736
Menstruation, 654–655, 656, 657–660, *737*
Metabolic rate, 626, 641, 655
Metabolism. *See* Energy and metabolism
Metacarpophalangeal (MCP) joint, 430
Metal equipment materials, 153, 158
   density, 159, *160*
   elasticity modulus, *157*
   yield strength, *158*
   See also specific metals
Metal-matrix composites (MMCs), 159, 171
Metatarsophalangeal joints, 605
MET point, 52
Mexico City Olympic Games (1968), environmental factors, 198–200
Mey, Uwe-Jens, 396
Middle ear, 802–803
Midsole (athletic shoes), 174, 614
Milk, 728
Miller, Shannon, 20, 21
Milon of Croton, 473, 549, 567
Mineral nutrients, 720, 735–739
   skeletal system and, 843, 847, 848, 854
Minoan culture, 108
Minute ventilation, 784, 785
Miscarriage, 661
Mitchell, Scott, 250
Mitochondria
   aerobic energy production, 446, 592–593, 637, 648
   ATP formation, 631–632, 634
   in slow-twitch muscle fibers, 836
MMCs. *See* Metal-matrix composites
Mobility
   in karate, 312
   motor control development and, 714, 715
Mode (statistics), 455
Modulus of elasticity. *See* Young's modulus of elasticity
Modulus of rupture, 317, 320
Mogul skiing. *See* Freestyle skiing
Mohawk (ice skating), 405, 406
Molitor, Paul, 54
Molybdenum, 132, 164
Moment of inertia. *See* Inertia
Momentum
   basketball shooting and, 63

bowling pin action and, 101–102, 103
catching technique and, 126, 127
changes in, 14
conservation of. *See* Conservation of momentum
gliding and, 255, 267
in golf, 170, 271, 278
in karate, 314, 315, 316, 319
in skating, 405, 406
in soccer, 449–450, 451
in wrestling, 570, 578–579
See also Angular momentum; Horizontal momentum; Linear momentum; Vertical momentum
Monoglycerides, 744
Monosaccharides, 632, 633, 722–723, 744
Monounsaturated fat, 729, 731–732
Montana, Joe, 127
Moore, Doug, 396
Morceli, Noureddine, 457
Morgan, William, 534
Morrison, Fred, 224
Moser, Francesco, 137
Moses, Edwin, 367
Motion. *See* Changes-in-motion forces; Gyroscopic motion; Range of motion
Motion, Newton's laws of
action-reaction, 9, 102, 203, 498, 499, 537, 569
and bowling, 91
hockey pucks and, *295*
sailing and, *377*
and swimming, 498, 499
and throwing, 202–204, 210, 212, 224
Motion sickness, 21, 125
Motor control, **700–719**
basketball shooting and, 64–65
brain waves and "the zone," 68
cavum septum pellucidum and, 117
central nervous system and, 700, 702, 706–709
brain, 700, 702, 707–709
spinal cord, 702, 707, 717
concussions and loss of, 117
eye-hand-foot coordination, 128, 305, 900, *904*
fatigue and, 447
ice hockey goaltending and, 298
injury-movement relationship, 876–877
injury prevention and, 612–613, 867
as jumping ability factor, 540

nervous system and, 700, 701–706
sensory system and, 700, 702, 703, 707, 709, 712–714
skill development issues, 714–718
theories of, 701
in throwing events, 211
volleyball and, 546
Motor end plate, 830, 834
Motor memory
curling and, 295
golf swing and, 270, 280
shuffleboard and, 295
skill development and, 715, 716
tennis swing and, 515
visualization and, 900–901, 903
Motor neurons, 826–827, 830, 834, 836
Mountain bikes, 131, 132, 138, 163, 165–166
Mountain climbing, 636, 668, 685, 777, 794–801
Mountain sickness, 796–800
Mountain sprint racing (cycling), 133
Movement
as back injury factor, 876, 877
See also Motor control
MRI. *See* Magnetic resonance imaging
Mucus, respiratory, 787, 793
Multilever model (of kinetic energy), 276–277
Muscle. *See* Skeletal muscle
Muscle cramps, 840
Muscle fibers, 828–829, 830–831, 834, 835–837
Muscle filaments, 830
Muscle forces
acrobatics and, 9–10, 16, 17, 24
jumping ability and, 179, 181–182
in paddle sports, 337
in speed skating, 411–412
throwing and, 211–212
Muscle hypertrophy, 484
Muscle memory
in acrobatics, 7
in archery, 30
basketball shooting and, 65, 66–67, 68, 272
in cycling, 145–146
golf swing and, 272
injury prevention and, 612–613
in weight lifting, 553–554
Muscle power, 552
Muscle relaxant drugs, 786, 835
Muscle spindles, 713, 714, 716–717
Muscle strength, 472, 588
Muscle tension, 546

Musial, Stan, *56*
Myelin, 586, 703–704, 705
Myofibrils, 830, 831–834
Myoglobin, 836
Myopia (nearsightedness), 894, 897
Myosin, 415, 550, 716, 831–835, 836
Myositis ossification, 760
Myron (Greek sculptor), 202

N
Naismith, James, 62, 69, 80, 534
Naproxen, 771
National Hockey League (NHL), 304, 306, 455–456
National Strength and Conditioning Association, 486
Native Americans, 292, 322, 887
Natural killer (NK) cells, 881
Navratilova, Martina, 711
Nearsightedness (myopia), 894, 897
Neck
aging and, 587
boxing and, 115, 117
injuries to, 244–246, 827
Negative pressure ventilation, 784
Nehamiah, Renaldo, 243
Neoprene clothing, 761
Nepela, Daniel, 286, 287
Nervous system
aging and, 586–587, *593*
balance and, 20–21
catching skills and, 125
divisions of, 702–703
fatigue and, 447, 645
motor control and, 700, 701–706
nerve impulses, 704–705
neuron anatomy, 703–704
neuron communication, 706
skeletal muscle functioning, 827–828
plasticity and, 715
running and, 348
See also Autonomic nervous system; Sympathetic nervous system
Netherlands, cycling in, 130
Neuromuscular junction, 830
Neurons
aging and, 586
anatomy of, 703–704
boxing injuries and, 116
communication between, 706
electrical impulses, 704–706
vision and, 64, 888–889
Neurotransmitters, 645, 706, 715
Never-exceed speed (redline speed), 258

Newby-Fraser, Paula, 652
Newcombe, John, 514, 531
Newell, Pete, 80
Newton, Isaac, 86
Newton's laws of motion. *See* Motion, Newton's laws of
NHL. *See* National Hockey League
Nicklaus, Jack, 271, 279
Nifedipine, 800
Night vision, 891, 897
Ninepins, 85, 86
Niramiai (sumo wrestling), 576, 577
Nitrogen
   energy and metabolism and, 638–639, 725, 726
   respiration and, 778, 779–780, 791, 804–807
Nitrogen narcosis, 806–807
Nitrox (oxygen-nitrogen mixture), 806
Nixon, Richard, 651
NK cells. *See* Natural killer cells
NMR. *See* Nuclear magnetic resonance
Nocking (archery), 28, *29*
Nodes of Ranvier, 704, 705
Nomographs, 266
Nonequilibrium falling technique (ice skating), 405
Nonessential nutrients, 720
Nonsteroidal anti–inflammatory (NSAI) medication, 769, 771
No-pole skating (Nordic skiing), 436–437
Nordic skiing. *See under* Skiing
Norepinephrine, 706
Norway, 420
NSAI medication. *See* Nonsteroidal anti–inflammatory (NSAI) medication
Nuclear magnetic resonance (NMR), 622
Nucleus pulposus, 873–874, 878, 879
Nunchaku sticks, 276, *277*
Nutation, bicycle-wheel, 237
Nutrition, **720–751**
   calorie definition, 721
   carbohydrate loading, 646, 725
   diabetes and, 644
   digestive system and, 741–746
   eating disorders and, 22, 616, 656, 660, 663–665
   food product labeling, 722
   nutrients, 720–746
      carbohydrates, 722–724, 741
      defined, 720–721
      fats, 728–732
      proteins, 724–728
      vitamins and minerals, 732–739
      water, 739–746
   Recommended Dietary Allowances, 721–722, 726, 727–728, 737
   skeletal system and
      bone health, 847–848, 849–850
      bone loss, 654–655, 736–737, 850
      bone regeneration, 845–846
   vegetarianism and, 729
   weight control and, 576, 641, 746–751
   weight fluctuation hazards, 574–576
   See also Energy and metabolism; Starvation; *specific nutrients*
Nylon, 518

O

Oars. *See* Paddle sports
Obesity, 616, 882
Oblique (spiral) fractures, 856, 858
Obree, Graeme, 139
Offset skate blades, 391
Ogodai (Mongol khan), 26
Oiling (of bowling lanes), 92, 96–97
Oils (cooking), 732
Okinawa, 311
Olajuwon, Hakeem, 718
Oligomenorrhea, 654, 656
Olson, Billy, 492
Olympics, ancient
   jumping events, 185, 186
   running events, 340
   throwing events, 202
Olympics, modern
   archery, 27
   gymnastics, 20–21
   Mexico City environmental factors, 198–200
   running events, 348
   swimming vs. running records, 488
   weight lifting events, 551–552
O'Neal, Shaquille, 65, 74
One-set (volleyball), 542
1-3 pocket (bowling), 87, 100, 102–105
Open stroke (ice skating), 406
Opiate receptors, 706
Optic chiasma, 893
Optic nerve, 892–893
Oral contraceptives, 659
Orbit (ice skating), 401
Orgasm, as performance factor, 118, 119
Orientation (of sail), 371
Orthopedic shoes and inserts, 867
Orthotics, 363
   ankle, foot, and lower leg, 613–615
   joint, 866
   knee, 696–698
Oshidashi (sumo wrestling), 579
Osseointegration, 759
Ossification, 846
Osteoblasts, 846, 847, 848, 850, 857, 858
Osteochondritis (Little League elbow), 819
Osteoclasts, 846, 847, 848, 850, 857, 858
Osteocytes, 487, 846
Osteoporosis
   aging and, 585–586, 596, 849
   exercise lack and, 596
   female athletes and, 656, 736–737
   genetics and, 848–849
   hormones and, 662, 736, 847
   weight-bearing exercise benefits, 586
   young women's preventive measures, 653, 654–655, 736
Ott, Mel, 54
Outgassing, ice making and, 397
Outsole (athletic shoes), 173
Outsweep (swimming), 503, 504
Outswinger (soccer kick), 443
Ovaries, 736–737
Overhand shot (basketball), 73–77
Overlap timing (breaststroke), 506
Owens, Jesse, 188, 361
Oxidative phosphorylation, 631–632, 634, 637, 647
Oxygen
   circulatory system and, 667–670, 681–682, 683–684, 739
   consumption of
      aging and, 591–593, 597–599
      body fat as factor, 622
      exercise and, 675–676, 680
      females and, 655, 656
   cycling and, 140–141, 146
   death from deprivation of, 668
   distance running and, 354–355, 358
   endurance vs. intermittent sports, 446–447
   energy and metabolism and, 631–632, 635, 648, 726, 737, 836
   respiration and, 778–782, 785, 787, 788–790
   in high altitudes, 795, 799, 800
   under water, 802, 807
Oxygen debt, 354, 355, 358
Oxygen-nitrogen mixtures (as bends preventive), 806
Oxygen toxicity, 807

P

Pace, running
  in distance races, 358
  optimization of, 354–356
PACT 95 (yachting syndicate), 385
Padding, protective, *293*, 761
Paddle sports, **321–339**
  equipment, 176
  footwear, 172
  injury factors, 337, 828
  oar and paddle dynamics, 330–334
  origins of, 321, 322
  rower's physique, 335
  technique, 335–339
    kayaking, 337–339
    sculling and rowing, 336–337
  watercraft basics, 323–330
    boat stability, 326–327
    gravity and wave dynamics, 327–328
    shallow-water effects, 329–330
    surface resistance, 325–326, 330
    water flow and resistance, 324–325
  See also Canoeing; Kayaking; Shelling
Pain
  back problems and, 878–879, 881
  distance running and, 360, 362
  endorphins and, 706
  eye laser surgery and, 897
  injury and, 765, 768, 775, 821
  skeletal muscle and, 839–840
  stress fractures and, 859
Pain threshold, 859
Pair skating, 398–399
Palmer, Arnold, 279
Palmer, Jim, 42, 43
Pancreas, 643, 744, 746
Parallel bars (gymnastics apparatus), 3
Parallel squats. *See* Half squats
Parasympathetic nervous system, 673, 703
Parathyroid hormone, 847
Parkinson's disease, 117
Partial pressure (of gases), 778–782, 789, 790
  mountain climbing and, 795, 799
  scuba diving and, 804–805, 806, 807
Passing
  in basketball, 80–82
  in football, 230, 235–237, 808
  in volleyball, 544–546
Pastorini, Dan, 246
Patellar tendinitis (jumper's knee), 545, 697, 866

Patent foramen ovale, 805
Path (ice skating), 401
Payton, Walter, 869
PBA. *See* Professional Bowlers Association
PC. *See* Phosphocreatine
PCL. *See* Posterior cruciate ligament
Pectoralis major muscle, 42, 813, 814
Pedaling. *See* Cycling
Pedals, floating, 149–150
Pedestrianism, 340
Pelé, 448
Pelota, *128*
Pelvis, hip, and thigh, **752–761**
  bone type, 844
  functional anatomy, 754–757
    male vs. female, 654, 754–755
  hip replacement surgery, 758–759
  human evolution and, 752–753
  injury prevention and rehabilitation, 757–761, 768
  role in athletics, 753–754
  See also Hips; Thigh
Penalty kick (soccer), 443–445
Pendulum motion, in bowling, 88–91
Penis, 144
Pepsin, 742
Perec, Marie-Jose, 488
Perfect game (bowling), 87, 104
Performance
  body fat as indicator, 622
  hormone levels as factor, 118–119
  prediction of, 467–469
Perimeter weighting
  of golf clubs, 280–281
  of tennis rackets, 512–513
Perineum, 144, 145
Periosteum, 845
Peripheral nervous system (PNS), 702–703, 828; *See also* Autonomic nervous system
Peripheral vision, 891, 899
Peroneus longus and brevis tendons, 607–608
Perry, Gaylord, 39, 47
Phosphate, inorganic, 834, 854
Phosphocreatine (PC), *149*, 588
Phospholipids, 635, *636*, 730
Phosphorus, 843, 849
Photorefractive keratectomy (PRK), 896, 897–898
Physical therapy. *See* Rehabilitation
Physics
  of acrobatics, 9
  of basketball shooting, 68–77
  of bowling, 88–107

  of skating, 401–407
  of skiing, 421–426
Physique. *See* Body size
Phytochemicals, 737, 739
Pike (position)
  in acrobatics, 14
  high jump and, 183, 184
  in racing dives, 507
Pin action (bowling), 86–87, 89, 100, 101, 103, 105
Pitching (baseball), 808, 809, 810
  angular momentum and, 809
  compared to shot putting, 216
  cricket vs. baseball, 50–51
  dead arms, 43
  delivery angle, 41, 42–43
  longevity-enhancing techniques, 43
  motion phases, 40–42
  pitch characteristics, *48*
  pitcher injuries, 816
  pitch types, 43–48
    change-ups, 43
    curveballs, 44–45, 69, 208, 288, 815, 816, 889
    fastballs, 45–46, *47*, 51, *128*, 815, 816, 889, 902–903
    knuckleballs, 46–47, 297, 536–537
    sliders, 45–46, 815
    spitballs, 39, 47–48
  sidearm delivery, 43, 808
  strike zone, 50–51
Pitching (cricket), 50–51
Pitching (sailing), 383
Pituitary gland, 359, 657, 660
Pituitary growth hormone, 847
Pivot joint, 863
Placekicking (football), 239–243
Planform (javelin), 226, 228
Plant (in soccer), 449
Plantar fasciitis, 609
Plaque, arterial, 681–682, 732
Plasma, 739, 778, 788–791
Plasticity, 33, 34, 715–718
Plastics. *See* Polymers
Playing surfaces
  artificial turf, 247–248
  basketball, 697
  billiards, 295
  deformation of, 248–249
  football, 247–250
  golf, 279, 295, 900
  grass for indoor competitions, 441
  as injury factor, *249*, 697
  softness of, 248–249
  tennis, 510–511, 528–529
  See also specific types
Pluto Platter. *See* Frisbee

Plyometric training, 540, 716–717, 774
PMS. *See* Premenstrual syndrome
Pneumothorax, 804
PNS. *See* Peripheral nervous system
Point of aim, 29, 30
Polar (gliding), 258–259
Polara golf ball, 286–287
Polarization, 705
Polaroid lenses, 901
Poles
    Alpine skiing and, 430, 433
    Nordic skiing and, 436–437
Pole vault, 178, 191–196
    center of gravity, 181, 195
    environmental factors, 200
    equipment material impact, 153, *154*, 156–157, 159, 160, 161, 193
    future performance prediction, 468
    record jumps, 192
    technique in, 193–195
    visual skills, *904*
    water training and, 492
Polycarbonate eyewear, 905
Polyethelene foam, 440
Polymer materials, 153, 158–159, 160, 175, 177
    for athletic shoes, 173–174, 175
    density, *160*
    elasticity modulus, *157*
    for golf clubs, 171
    in paddle sports, 176, 325
    for tennis rackets, 511
    yield strength, *158*
Polypeptides, 638
Polysaccharides, 633, 723
Polyunsaturated fat, 729, 732
Polyurethane, 408, 440
Polyurethane elastomers, 174
Pommel horse (gymnastics), 882
Pool. *See* Billiards
Pools, swimming, 492–493, 497
Poona (badminton variant), 526
Popov, Alexandre, 488
Pop-ups, infield, 124
Positioning (basketball shooting), 63–64
Positive-pressure ventilators, 786–787
Posterior cruciate ligament (PCL), 688, 689–690, 695
Posture, 586, 587, 588, 867, 882–884
Potassium, 447, 704–705, 847
Potential energy
    in archery, 30–31, 33, 34
    in baseball, 40–41
    in bowling, 88, 89

    in pole vaulting, 192, 193, 195, 196
    in skiing, 421–422, 427
    in weight lifting, 551
Powell, Mike, 185–186, *187*, 198
Power
    body weight as factor, *622*
    of golf swing, 270–279
    of ice hockey skaters, 307–309
    in karate, 312
    measurement of, 838
    paddling sports and, 323–324
    strength training and, 484
    in tennis, 514–515, 517
    throwing events and, 206, 211–212
    in weight lifting, 551–554
Power lifting, 473, 551, 552–554, 561–565
Power takeoff (high jump), 184
Precession, gyroscopic, 225
Precision, motor control and, 700
Pregnancy, 660–662
Premenstrual syndrome (PMS), 658–659
Presbyopia, 893
Press pin (wrestling), 573
Pressure drag
    in speed skating, 409–410
    in swimming, 495, 496
    in volleyball, 536
Pressure melting (ice skating), 393–395
Presteering, 403
Price, Mark, 73
Primary motor area, 825, 830
Prince (tennis racket), 511
Princeton University, 230
Prizefighting. *See* Boxing
PRK. *See* Photorefractive keratectomy
Probability (statistics), 461–466
ProCap, 117, 246
Professional Bowlers Association (PBA), 87
Profile drag
    cycling and, 139–140
    gliding and, 257, 258, 259
    speed skating and, 410
Progesterone, 656, 657–658
Progressive resistance training, 473, 474–475, 476, 549
Prolactin, 575
Pronation, 172, 174–175, 610
Prophylactic braces, 696, *698*
Proprioceptive exercises, 612
Propulsion force
    in cycling, *135*
    in ice skating, 393, 413
    in swimming, 490, 491, 496–503, 507

Prostate gland, 144–145
Protective cups, 110
Proteins, 720, 724–728
    circulatory system and, 683, 684, 739
    contractile, 484, 638
    digestive system and, 742, 744
    energy and metabolism and, 638–639, *640*, 642, 646
    fatigue and, 415
    mountain climbers' diet and, 798
    muscle contraction and, 831–834
    skeletal system and, 847, 861
    starvation dieting and, 574
    vegetarianism and, 729
    See also specific proteins
Protruding disk, 880
Psychological effects of aging, *593*, 594
Puberty, 652–653, 846
Pubiofemoral ligament, 756
Pubis, 754
Pucks (ice hockey), 293–297, 306
Pugilism. *See* Boxing
Pulling force, 141
Pulmonary artery, 668, 669, 671, 796
Pulmonary capillaries, 787–788, 789, 796
Pulmonary edema, 683–684, 796, 799, 800
Pulmonary embolism, 685, 798
Pulmonary oxygen toxicity, 807
Pulmonary system. *See* Respiration
Pulmonary valve, 670–671
Pulmonary vein, 668, 669
Pumping
    acrobatic swinging and, 17
    in speed skating, 410–411
Punch drunk syndrome, 117
Punching force, 111–112, 115
Punch through, 112, 113
Punting (football), 237–239, 240–241
Pupil (human eye), 890
Purging. *See* Bulimia nervosa
Pursuit racing (cycling), 130
Push-off
    in ice hockey skating, 308–309
    in Nordic skiing, 436
    in speed skating, 413–414, 415, 416, 417
    in sprinting, 348–349
Putting (golf), 279–280, 899, 900–901
PW-5 (glider), 267
Pygmy tribes, 27
Pyruvic acid, 632, 633, 634–635, 636, 638, 644, 836

Q

Quadricep muscles
  cycling and, 146, 149, 150, 151
  injuries to, 760, 840
  jumping and, 179
  knee and, 690–691
  running and, 363
  soccer ball kicking and, 450
Quarterbacks (football), 235–237, 246–247
Quartering wind, 222
Questra (soccer ball), 440
Quickness, jumping ability and, 540
Quick set (volleyball), 542
Quisenberry, Dan, 42

R

Racket. *See* Badminton; *under* Tennis
Racquetball, 44, 808, *904*, 905
Radial keratotomy (RK), 896–898
Radians per second (rad./sec.) (bowling), 93, 99
Radius (bone), 815, 816, 817
Radius of gyration, 88, 95, 97, 99
Rake (bicycle), 134–135
Random (statistics), 461
Range of motion (ROM)
  acrobatics and, 4
  aging and, 587–588, 820, 877–878
  of foot, *604*
  injuries and, 611, 615
  joints and, 864–865, 868
  soccer and, 449, 451
  spine and, 873, 874–875, 877–878
  strength training and, 478, 482
  stretching and, 760
Ranvier nodes, 704, 705
RDAs. *See* Recommended Dietary Allowances
Reach sailing, 375–378
Reaction time
  aging and, 586, 587
  balance and, 5–6
  ball of foot and, 713
  in football, 445
  handedness as factor, 711, 712
  in ice hockey, 305
  soccer goaltending and, 445
  visual, 889, 898, 901, *904*
Rear sprocket (bicycle gear), 146
Rebound
  in tennis, 528
  in volleyball, 544–545
Recognition time, 5
Recoil
  archery, 31, *34*
  boxing, 112, 115
  karate, 315, 316
  lacrosse, 128, 129
Recommended Dietary Allowances (RDAs), 721–722, 726, 727–728, 737
Recompression chamber, 806
Recovery time
  exercise, metabolism, and, 647–648
  strength training and, 474, 477–478, 839
Recurves, *27*, 33, 34–35
Redline speed, 258
Redundancy, bodily, 794
Reeve, Christopher, 707, 827
Reflexes
  collaborative, 21
  of ice hockey goalies, 305
  in karate, 312–313
  motor control and, 709
  vestibular system and, 21
Refractory periods, 705
Regelation (ice skating), 393–395
Regeneration
  of bone, 844–847
  of tissue, 765
Regression analysis (statistics), 467–469
Rehabilitation, **763–776**
  back problem therapy, 881
  orthopedic braces and, 696
  phases and treatment, 766–776
    aerobic training, 773–774
    cold and heat therapy, 767–768, 769–771, 820
    compression, 768–769, 770
    coordination restoration, 774
    drug therapy, 769, 771
    elevation of injured area, 769, 770
    flexibility and stretching, 772–773
    rest as, 766–767, 770
    strength training, 764, 773
  proprioceptive exercises, 612
  running injuries and, 363
  shoulder, elbow, and wrist injuries, 823
  tennis elbow and, 521
  tissue injuries and, 764–766
  water therapy, 492–493
  See also Strength training; Stretching
Rehabilitative braces, 696, *698*
Relative strength, 472
Release
  angle of, 188, 208, 210
    discus throw, 220, 221
    hammer throw, 217
    javelin throw, 227, 228
    shot put, 213, 214, *215*
  in archery, 28, *29*, 30, 31, 35
  in baseball pitching, 42
  in basketball, 74–75, 77, 78–79
  in football passing, 235–236
  height of, 213, 214, *215*, 220, 221
  speed and throwing, 205, 208, 210, 212, 213, *215*, 228
Repetitions maximum (RM), 472
Reproduction function
  female athletes and, 657–663, 736, 737, 747
  male cyclists and, 145
Resistance
  rolling, *135*, 136, 138
  "sticking point" in weight lifting, 555
  surface, 325–326, 330
  vascular, 678, 679–680, 682
  See also Air resistance; Water resistance; Wind resistance
Resistance exercises, 472–473, 476, 485, 596, 679, 839
Respiration, **777–807**
  aging and, 589–590, *593*, 596–597
  air pressure environment and, 777–778, 780–781, 783–784, 794–807
  cycling and, 140–141, 146
  diseases related to, 791–794
  distance running and, 354–355, 358
  physiology of, 782–791, 795
  respiratory gas physics, 777–782
  rowing and, 335
  strength training and, 477
  as throwing factor, 214
  water therapy and, 493
  See also Oxygen
Respirators, 785, 835
Respiratory membrane, 788
Respiratory rate, 784
Response time, balance and, 5–6
Rest, as rehabilitative treatment, 766–767, 770
Retina, 890, *892*, *893*
  detached, 116, 902
  hemorrhaging of, 797
Retton, Mary Lou, 20
Return (speed skating), 414–415
Reuther board (gymnastics apparatus), 3, 7, 16
Reverse block injury, 803
Revolutions per minute (RPM)
  baseball pitching and, 44
  bicycle pedaling and, 148

bowling and, 93, 99
of golf ball, 288
Reynolds number, 536
Rhythmic motor patterns, 709, 712
Rice, 729
Rice, Jerry, 127
Ridge lift. *See* Slope lift
Rigby, Cathy, 664
Riggings, 369, 370
Riggs, Bobby, 651
Rigor mortis, 834
Rim (basketball), 175
Rings (gymnastics apparatus), 3, 24
Rinks, ice skating, 396–398
Riot club, 276, *277*
RK. *See* Radial keratotomy
RM. *See* Repetitions maximum
Road racing (cycling), 130–131, 137, *149*
Robertson, Oscar, 81
Rock climbing, 828
Rocker (boat design), 327
Rocker profile (in-line skates), 408
Rods (fishing), 176
Rods (human eye), 890–892
Rogallo wing, 254
Rogers, Kenny, 718
"Roll with punches" (boxing), 112, 115
Roller blading (in-line skating), 4, 408–409
Roller hockey, 292
Rolling resistance, *135*, 136, 138
ROM. *See* Range of motion
Rome, ancient
　soccer-like game, 439
　wrestling style, 567
Roosevelt, Theodore, 230
Rose, Pete, 51, 57, 711
Rotation
　angular momentum and, 10, 14, 15–16
　axis of. *See* Axis of rotation
　of baseball pitches, 44, 46
　of bicycle wheels, 137
　of bowling balls, 93–94
　of earth, 196–197
　giant swings and dismounts, 12, 16–18, *19*
　in golf swing, 273, 276
　mass as factor, 10, 11, 22
　somersaulting and twisting, 12–15, 875
　takeoff as factor, 8–9, 13, 15
　in throwing events, 206, 218, 219, 222–223
　See also Torque

Rotational forces, bone injuries and, 862, 863–864
Rotator cuff
　baseball pitching and, 42, 809
　injuries to, 773, 814–815, 818, 820–821
　shoulder, 773, 811, 813–814
　tennis elbow and, 766
　ultrasound treatment, 768
Rowing. *See* Paddle sports
RPM. *See* Revolutions per minute
Rubber-core golf balls, 282
Rubber equipment material
　athletic shoes, 173
　bungee cord, 161
　golf balls, 282
　hockey puck, *294*, 295
　soccer ball, 440
　tennis balls, 510
Rugby, 246, 849
Run (golf), *284*
Runner's high, 359, 706
Runner's knee, 695
Running and hurdling, **340–367**
　aerodynamics of, 344–346
　basic mechanics, 341–343, 348, 868
　bone density increase and, 850
　braking force, 13, 334, 347, 348–349
　exercise dependency and, 359
　in football, 243–244, 756
　footwear for, 172, 173, 174, 363, 610
　future performance prediction, 468–469
　hurdling, 244, 361–367, 691
　　muscle stretching, 760–761
　　physique as factor, 366–367
　　stride, 363–364, 366–367
　　technique, 365–366
　　world records, 362
　injury risks, prevention, and rehabilitation, 362–363, 608, 609–611, 613, 695, 760, 767, 776, 859, 885
　rhythmic motor pattern, 712
　speeds of mammals, *341*
　track design and composition, 360–361
　visual skills, *904*
　water training and, 492
　See also Distance running; Sprinting
Run-up
　air resistance and, 197, *198*
　hammer throw, 201
　high jump, 184

javelin throw, 90, 223, 228–229
long jump, 186–187
pole vault, 193–194, 196
triple jump, 190
in volleyball, 541–542
Rupture, modulus of, 317, 320
Ruptured disk, 879
Rutgers University, 230
Ruth, Babe, 39, 710
Ryan, Nolan, 40, 43

S
Saccades, 899, 902–903
Sacculus, 20, 21
Sacking (of football quarterback), 236
Saddle joint, 863
Saddles, bicycle, 143–146, 151
Sail (jumping technique), 188, 191
Sailing, **369–388**
　air forces and, 370–374
　Bernoulli's principle and, 287, 372
　center of gravity and, 133, 381–382, 383–385
　directional, 374–381
　　downwind, 375
　　reaching, 375–378
　　windward, 378–381
　drag reduction methods, 498
　equipment materials, 159, 161, 176–177
　fastest recorded speed, 377
　hull design, 381–382
　origins of, 369–370
　weight distribution importance, 383–386
　wind and weather factors, 375, 386–388
　See also Yachting
Sailplanes. *See* Gliding and hang gliding
St. Andrews (Scotland) golf site, 269
St. Martin, Ted, 74, 77
Saliva, 742
Salt (dietary), 741
Salts (bodily), 739, 843
Salt water, 495
Same-side-dominance (vision), 903
Sampras, Pete, 155, 514, 522
Sanchez Vicario, Arantxa, 155
Saneyev, Viktor, 190–191
SA node. *See* Sinoatrial node
Sarcolemma, 828, 829, 830
Sarcoplasmic reticulum, 830, 831, 834, 836
Saturated fat, 729, 731, 732
Scaphoid bone, 819

Scapula, 812, 813
Scar formation, 765
Schayes, Dolph, 73
School figures (ice skating), 401, 402
Schweitzer schwingen wrestling style, 567
Sciatica, 586
Scoliosis, 562–563, 879
Scotland
　field hockey varient, 293
　golf, 269
　shot put and hammer throw, 201
Scott, Dave, 355–356
Scows, 382
Scrotum, 145
Scuba diving, 672, 777, 781, 791, 801–807
Sculling, 321–322, 336–337
Sea kayaking. *See* Kayaking
Sears Roebuck, 887
Seasickness. *See* Motion sickness
Seats, sliding (rowing), 321
Seat tube (bicycle), 131, 132, 144
Seaver, Tom, 41, 43
Seles, Monica, 711
Self-esteem
　aging and, 585, 589, 594, 596
　female exercise and, 653
Semicircular canals (ear), 21
Semirollers (bowling), 98–99, 100, 102, 106
Semitight spirals (football), 237
Sensory clues
　acrobatics and, 18–19
　catching skills and, 123–124, 125
　in football, *234*
Sensory system
　aging and, 585, 587
　motor control and, 700, 702, 703, 707, 709, 712–714
　See also specific senses
Separation, shoulder, 818
Serratus anterior muscle, 42, 814
Serve
　in tennis, *128*, 525–527, 529–531
　in volleyball, 535–539
Set-point theory (body weight), 749
Set shot
　basketball, 62, 65, 67
　volleyball, 546–547
7–9 split (bowling), 106–107
7–10 split (bowling), 104, 105, 106, 107
Sexual activity
　cycling's impact on, 144–145
　as performance factor, 118, 119
Shadow boxing, *108*

Shaft
　flexible golf club, 281
　hockey stick, 297, 298
　of paddles and oars, 331–332
Shaolin monestary (Buddhist), 311
Sharman, Bill, 73
Shear force, bone injuries and, 856, 863–864
Shearing, equipment materials and, 158
Shelling, 176, 322, 324
Sherrill, Jackie, 240
Shin bone. *See* Tibia
Shin pads, *293*
Shin splints, 363, 608, 767
Shinty (early field hockey form), 293
Shoes, orthopedic, 867; *See also* Athletic shoes
Shooting aids (archery), 37–38
Shoot-out (soccer), 444
Short-track speed skating, 391, 406
Shot clock (basketball), 67
Shot put
　dynamics of, 212–214, 220
　future performance prediction, 468
　international standards, *209*
　muscle power and, 484
　optimal throwing conditions, 209
　origins of, 201
　record throws, 213
　technique, 210, 215–216, 808
Shoulder, elbow, and wrist, **808–823**
　aging and, 585, 588
　in baseball
　　hitting, 55, 56
　　pitching, 41–42, 43, 47–48, 808, 809, 810
　　sliding, 58, 60
　basketball shooting and, 65–66, 69, 76
　bone type, 844
　catching skills and, 127
　football passing and, 235–236, 237, 808
　functional anatomy
　　elbow, 815–816
　　shoulder, 811–814
　　wrist, 817
　golf swing and, 273–278
　　swing signature, 270
　ice hockey shots and, 302–303
　injury risks, prevention, and rehabilitation, 814–823
　　bowler's elbow, 818–819, 822
　　impingement syndrome, 820–822
　　Little League elbow, 819

　　rotator cuff problems, 773, 814–815, 818, 820–821
　　shoulder dislocation, 813
　　shoulder separation, 818
　　tennis elbow, 520–521, 697, 766, 817, 819, 822
　　wrist fractures and sprains, 585, 819, 820
　in karate, 319–320
　in skating, 402, 410–411, 412
　strength training and, 479
　in swimming, 498–499, 502–505, 506
　in tennis, 520–521, 524–525, 766, 808–811
　throwing and swinging mechanics, 808–811
　in volleyball, 542–543, 544–546
　in weight lifting, 554–555, 560–561
　in wrestling, 573
　See also Wrist snap
Shoulder roll (landing technique), 869
Shuffleboard, 295
Shuttlecock (badminton), 526–527
Sidearm pitchers, 42, 808
Sidearm throw (discus throw), 222
Side cut (Alpine ski), 432, 433
Sidehill lies (golf), 279
Sideslipping (Alpine skiing), 431
Sidespin
　in basketball, 66, 82
　in golf, 289–290
　in tennis, 519
Side volley (soccer kick), 443
Sideward friction force, 133–134
Sight. *See* Vision
Sighting (basketball shooting), 64–65
Sight windows (archery bows), 37, 38
Sikma, Jack, 74
Silverdome (Ponitac, Michigan), 441
Sinking, 491, 493–494
Sinking speed (gliding), 258–259
Sinoatrial (SA) node, 673–674
Sinuses, 802–803
6-9-10 split (bowling), 106
Skating, **390–417**
　barrel jumping, 188
　blades and boots, 390–391, 393, *394*, 398, *399*, *400*, 402, 404, 407
　comparison of types, 398–401, 402
　ice conditions and, 392–398
　origins of, 390
　physics of, 401–407
　　center of gravity, 5, 401, 403, 404–405

directional change transitions, 405–406
dynamic steering, 404–405
equilibrium, balance, passive steering, 401–404
momentum maintenance, 405
stroking and turns, 393, 406–407, 415–417
See also Figure skating; Hockey, ice; In-line skating; Skiing, Nordic; Speed skating
Skeletal muscle, **825–840**
aging and, 587–589, *593*, 596–597, 641
Alpine skiing and, 433–434
ankle, foot, and lower leg, 605–606
back injuries and, 876, 877, 880, 884–885
baseball pitching and, 41, 42
body composition and, *617*, 618, 748
"choking" situations, 546
circulatory system and, 684
contraction control, 825–828
contraction process, 831–834
cycling and, 146, 148, 150, 151, 412
exercise and, 837–840
blood flow, 679–680
pain and soreness, 839–840
training strategies, 838–839
fast-twitch muscles, 836–837
fatigue and, 415, 447
fibers, 828–831, 834, 835–837
football and, 235
glucose and, 724
golf swing and, 270–271, 274, 278
injury prevention, 363
jumping ability and, 540
karate and, 313–314
knee, 690–691
mass and, 24, 140, 653
motor control and, 702, 713–714
neck, 115, 117, 827
nerve injuries and, 827–828
pelvis, hip, and thigh, 756–757
plyometric training and, 540, 716–717
relaxation of, 834–835
running and, 341–343, 346–348, 354, 361, 605, 606
shoulder, elbow, and wrist, 809, 813–814, 816
skeletal system and, 851–852, 855, 859, 862, 867
skiing and, 433–434
slow-twitch muscles, 342, 836–837
soccer and, 445, 449–450, 451

speed skating and, 411–412
sprinting and, 341–342, 348
starvation dieting and, 574
stimulation of, 830–831
structure of, 828–829
summation of forces and, 7
volleyball and, 541, 544–546, 713
water therapy and, 493
See also Muscle memory; Strength training; Stretching; Weight lifting; *specific muscles*
Skeletal system, **842–869**
aging and, 363, 585–586, *593*, 596–597, 608, 848, 850–851
body composition and, *617*, 618, 843
bones, 843–860
calcium and, 658, 660, 662, 736, 843, 847, 849–850, 854
genetic factor, 842, 848–849, 856, 866–867, 868
injury treatment and prevention, 857–859, 861, 866–869
joints, 604–605
lever system, 314, 554–556, 860–862, 863
running and, 341, 342, 859
of women, 654–655, 660, 662, 736–737
See also specific components
Skid stop (ice hockey), 400–401
Skiing, **419–438**
air drag, 426–427, 429
Alpine, 427–434
motor control and, 715
muscle action required, 433–434
potential vs. kinetic energy, 422, *423*, 427
ski design, 432–433
turning in, 430–433
equipment
bindings, 58
skis, 421, 433
freestyle, 4, *10*, 419
gravity and, 421–422, *423*, 427–429
injury factors, 430, 604, 851, 862
Nordic, 398, 420, 434–438
diagonal stride, 436
double poling, 436
eating disorder issues, 656
kick double poling, 436
marathon skating, 437
no-pole skating, 436–437
skier heart rate, 446
V1 technique, 437
V2 technique, 437–438
waxing of skis, 424–425, 438

origins of, 419–420
snow physics and, 420–426, 429
speed, 428–429
visual skills, *904*
See also Snowboarding
Ski jumping, 419
Skill, motor control development and, 714–715
Skin
aging's effects on, 584–585
exercise and blood flow, 680
as swimming drag factor, 497–498
Skin-fold sum measurement, 619
Skin suit (speed skating), 408–410
Skittles, 85
Skull, 113, 150, 844
Skydiving, 4, 15–16, 428–429
Slalom (Alpine skiing), 430
Slap shot (ice hockey), *128*, 298–301
Sledding, 288, 398
Sleep disturbances, as fatigue factor, 645
Slice
golf shot, 279, 286–287, 289–290
in tennis, 519, 528
Slider (baseball pitch), 45–46, 815
Sliding
in baseball, 57–60
friction and, 294–295
of golf shot, 290
of hockey puck, 294, 295
Sliding filament theory, 833
Sliding seats (rowing), 321
Slingshots, 26
Slipped disk, 879
Slipping, in bowling, 93–95, 98, 99
Slope lift (gliding), 260–261
Slope soaring (gliding), 260–261
Slot effect (sailing), 373
Slouching, 882
Slow-oxidative muscles, 445
Slow-twitch muscles, 342, 836–837
Small intestine, 743–745
Smoker's cough, 793
Smoking, 733, 787, 791, 793–794
Snatch lift (weight lifting), 552, 557–558, 560
Sneakers, 172, 613
Snellen chart, 898
Snow
deaths related to, 668
skiing and, 420–426, 429
Snowboarding, 419, 420, 435
acrobatics and, 4, *10*, 11
deaths related to, 668
Soaring. *See* Gliding and hang gliding

Soccer, **439–452**
 ball aerodynamics and construction, 440–445
 dribbling and trapping, 448
 fatigue factor, 446–447
 goaltending, 443, 444–445, 712
 headers, 443, 451–452
 injury risks, *249*
 kicks
  ball velocities, *450*
  "banana," 442–443
  corner, 443
  muscles used, 757
  penalty, 443–445
  player technique, 448–451
  side volleys, 443
 origins of, 439
 visual skills, 898, *904*
"Soccer" War (1969), 440
Sodium
 neuron conduction, 704–705
 skeletal system and, 847
 See also Salt (dietary); Salts (bodily)
Softball, 52, 175, 808
Soft-centered focus, 902
"Soft hands"
 football, 127
 lacrosse, 128
Softness (of playing surfaces), 248–249
Soleus muscle, 540, 605, 607
Solubility (of gases), 779–780
Somatic nervous system, 702
Somatosensory system, 712–714
Somersaults, 3, 12–15, 18, 875
Sommer, Roland, 521
Sotomayor, Javier, 184
Sound. *See* Ear; Hearing
South American soccer fervor, 440
Spalding (company), 49, 887
Spare (bowling), 100, 105–107
Spatial localization, 899, 900
Spearing (football), 245, 828
Spears, 26, 30, 202
Specific elasticity, 159
Specific gravity, 491–493
Specific strength, 159
Spectra (equipment material), 176, 177
Spectrum, visible, 888, *889*
Speed
 of animals, *341*, *494*
 cycling, 131, 133, 134, 136–137, 138, 139–141
 football
  receivers and, 243–244
  tackling skills and, 232–233
  gliding, 255–259, 263–264

hurdling, 363–364
motor control and, 700
paddle sports, 333–334, 336
running, 342, *344*, 346, 348, 349–351, 354
sailing, 377, 378, 379–380, 382, 383
skiing, 423, 427
speed skating, 401, 410
speed skiing vs. skydiving, 428–429
swimming, 494–498
takeoff
 high jump, 178–181, 183–184
 long jump, 186–188
 pole vault, 193–194
in throwing release, 205, 208, 210, 212, 213, *215*, 228
See also Acceleration
Speed skating, 407–417
 air resistance and, 407–411
 body fat as factor, 622
 curves and turns, 406, 411, 416–417
 elite skater attributes, 416
 figure and hockey skating vs., 307, 309, 310, 398–401, 402
 as fitness exercise, 390
 ice conditions and, 395–396
 importance of start, 412–413
 long-track vs. short-track, 391
 muscle power required, 411–412
 origins of, 390–391
 skater's physique and, 413
 straightaway skating, 413–416, 417
Speed skiing, 428–429
Speed takeoff (high jump), 184
Sperm development, 145
Spike (volleyball), 541–544
Spin
 baseball pitching, 41, 44–46, 47, *47*, 815, 816
 basketball passing, 81–82
 in billiards, 82
 in bowling, 90–91, 93–97, 100
 as catch factor, 127
 cricket pitching, 51
 of hockey puck, 297, 303
 of soccer ball, 442–443
 in tennis, 519–522
 as throwing factor, 207–208
  discus, 220–221
  Frisbee toss, 225
  hammer throw, 201
  shot put, 213
 See also Backspin; Sidespin; Topspin
Spinal cord
 motor control and, 702, 707, 717
 skeletal muscle and, 826–827

Spinal cord injuries, 244–246, 707, 827–828, 872
Spine, **871–885**
 aging and, 586, 587, 588, 877–878
 anatomy and function, 872–875
 back injuries and, 827, 872, 875–882
 curvature of, 562–563, 879
 pelvis and, 756
 posture, 586, 587, 588, 867, 882–884
Spine (of arrow), 35–36
Spinnaker sail, 375, *376*
Spinners (bowling), 99, 100, 104, 107
Spins (acrobatic), 11–12, *13*, 21, 392
Spiral (oblique) fractures, 856, 858
Spiral passes. *See* Football, passing
Spitball, 39, 47–48
Spitz, Mark, 415, 489–490
Split (bowling), 104, 105–107
Split-finger fastball, 45–46, *47*
Spokes (bicycle), 142–143, 165–167
Sports anemia, 655–656
Sports goggles, 896, 905
Sports Illustrated magazine, 240
Sports vision. *See* Vision
Sprains
 ankle, 609, 769, 866
 back, 880
 cold therapy, 767
 knee, 691
 wrist, 820
Springboard (gymnastics). *See* Reuther board
Springboard diving, 7–8, 10
Sprinting, 346–353
 age as factor, 589
 air resistance effects, 344–345
 block starts, 349–351
 coordination fatigue, 705
 in football, 243–244, 756
 joint action, 342
 lanes as factor, 351–353
 muscles used, 341–342, 346, 605, 757, 837
 record performances, 346, 488, *489*
 runner attributes, 349
 stride, 346, 348–349, 416
 technique, 342, 343
Sprint racing (cycling), 130
Sprockets (bicycle gears), 146–147
Squat lift (weight lifting), 144–145, 486, 552, 555, 556, 557, 561, 564, *565*
Stability
 of bicycles, 133–135
 motor control and, 714, 715

Volume 1: pp. 1–470; Volume 2: pp. 471–906

of sailboats, 381–382
  wrestling throws and, 571–572
Stabilizers (archery), 28, 37–38
Stadion (ancient Greek footrace), 340
Stadiums
  astroturf, 247–250
  baseball, 39
  indoor natural grass, 441
Stalling speed (gliding), 258
Stance
  of football linemen, 234
  in golf, 271–272, 279–280
  in karate, 312–313
  in volleyball, 542
  in wrestling, 569–570
Standard deviation (statistics), 458–459
Standing vertical jump, 178–180
Stannard, Henry, 340
Starches, 633, 723
Starting blocks
  in sprinting, 349–351
  in swimming, 507–508
Starvation
  basal metabolic rate and, 749
  as diet method, 574, 656
  effect on circulatory system, 684
Static acuity, 895, 898, 902, *904*
Static exercises. *See* Isometric exercise
Statistics, **453–469**
  baseball batting averages, 456–461
  basketball free throw percentages, 72–73
  bowling of perfect games, 87, 104
  future performance prediction, 467–469
  in labor disputes, 454–456
  probability, 461–466
Steel equipment, 153
  bicycle construction, 132, 133, 163, 164, 166
  figure skates, 176, *399*
  golf clubs, 170, 281
Steering
  in cycling, 134, 135, 403
  in skating, 403, 404–405
Steinborn, Heinrich, 486
Stenerud, Jan, 242
Stengel, Casey, 118
Stereopsis awareness, 900
Stern (boat), 325
Steroids, 635, *636*, 771, 792
Sterols, 730–731
Stevens, John Cox, 340
Stewart, Payne, 280
"Sticking point" (weight lifting), 554–556, 563

Sticks
  field hockey, 176
  ice hockey, 176, 297, 298, 304–307
  lacrosse, 128
  See also Bats
Stiffness
  of bones and joints, 853–855, 868
  golf clubs and, 167, 169, 170
Stinger (neck injury), 245, 707
Stockton, John, 80
Stolen bases, 57–60
Stomach, 742
Stop-and-go (intermittent) sports, 446–447, 649
Storage fat, 618, 622, 636, 728
Straddle technique (high jump), *180*, 181, 183
Straightaways (speed skating), 413–416, 417
Straight-gauge tubing (bicycle), 132
Straight-in slide, 57, 59–60
Straight punch (boxing), 109
Strain
  in archery, 32, 33–34
  as bone fracture factor, 854–855
  equipment materials and, 156, 157
  in karate board breaking, 317
  running injuries and, 362
Straps (strength training), 479
Streamlines (sailing), 372–373, 374
Street hockey. *See* Hockey, street
Strength
  in archery, 29, 30
  body size and, 24
  of bones, 853–855
  equipment materials and, 156–157, 159
  of female athletes, 652–655
  measurement of, 472, 837–838
  in weight lifting, 551–554
Strength-to-weight ratio, 159
Strength training, **471–487**
  aging process and, 487, 589, 596–597, 663
  aids for, 478–480
  basketball shooting and, 74
  children and, 485
  exercise types, 480–483
  guidelines, 476–478
  injury prevention and, 245, 363, 485–487, 612, 694–696, 761, 823, 880
  knee-bend squats and, 486
  muscle functions, 472
  myths about, 472, 473
  physical fitness and, 484–485
  plyometric training vs., 540, 716

  principles of, 473–476, 482
  protein requirements, 727
  rehabilitation and, 764, 773
  running and, 363
  shot putting and, 216
  skeletal system health and, 867
  strategies for, 838–839
  volleyball and, 543
  women and, 839
  See also Weight lifting
Stress
  back injuries and, 876–877
  body fat and, 747
  equipment materials and, 156, 157–158
  golfing and, 281
  Hooke's law, 32, 33
  skeletal and musculature adaptation to, 842, 851
  in strength training, 473–474
  tennis injuries and, 520, 872
Stress fractures, 846, 854–855, 859–860
Stretching
  as injury prevention and rehabilitation, 363, 611, *612*, 696, 759–761, 763, 764, 772–773, 823, 862, 885
  in plyometric training, 540, 716–717
  strength training and, 478
Stride
  in baseball hitting, 54–55
  in hurdling, 363–364, 366–367
  in ice hockey skating, 309–310
  in running, 341, 342–343
    distance races, 357, 360
    sprinting, 346, 348–349, 416
Strike (bowling), 87, 100, 102–105
Strike zone
  in baseball and cricket, 50–51
  in bowling, 87, 100, 102–105
String dampeners (tennis), 132, 520
Strings (tennis racket), 516–519
  dampeners, 132, 520
  tension, 516–518
  thickness, 518–519
Stroke (cerebral), 681
Strokes. *See* Golf; Paddle sports; Skating; Swimming; Tennis
Subcutaneous emphysema, 804
Sublimation, 397
Subscapularis muscle, 42, 813, 814
Subtalar joint, 605, 606
Sucrose, 632, 723
Sugars, 632–633; *See also* specific types
Suinin (Japanese emperor), 567

Sukune (sumo wrestler), 567
Sullivan, John L., 108, 119
Summation of forces (acrobatics), 6–9
Sumo wrestling, 567–568, 573, 575–579
Sunfish (sailboat), 369
Sunglasses, 887, 901, 905
Sunlight, vitamin D and, 849–850
Superflight, Inc., 224
Super G (Alpine skiing), 430
Supination, 610
Suprapatellar bursa, 864
Supraspinatus muscle, 813, 814
Surface drag, 408–409, 410
Surface melting, 394–395
Surface resistance, 325–326, 330
Surgery
    arthroscopic, 692–693, 694, 822
    hip replacement, 758–759
    laser, for eyes, 896, 897
Surlyn (polymer), 168, 282
Sverre (king of Sweden), 419
Sweating
    dehydration and, 574, 739–740
    distance running and, 360
    water intake and, 740
Sweden, 419
Sweep rowing, 321–322
Sweet spot
    baseball bat, 49, 52
    golf club, 154, 169, 170, 171, 280
    hockey stick, 297
    tennis racket, 512, 514–516, 520, 544
Swelling, treatment of, 767–768
Swimming, **488–508**
    body fat advantages, 618, 747
    dive starts, 507–508
    injury factors, 820–821
    long-distance, 495
    propulsion and, 490, 491, 496–497, 498–503, 507
        arm speed, 502–503
        kicking, *500*, 506
        lift, 498–499, 501–502
        propellerlike mechanics, 499–500
    record performances, 488–490
    strokes
        backstroke, *503*, 504
        breaststroke, *503*, 504, 505–507
        butterfly, *500*, 504
        dog paddle, 488
        front crawl, *503*, 504
        function of hands, 497, 498–499, 500–503, 504

        functions of shoulder, elbow, and wrist, 811
        sweep actions, 503–505
    swimsuits and caps, 498
    visual skills, *904*
    water and, 490–491
        buoyancy and flotation, 491–494
        drag, 494–498
    See also Water therapy
Swing
    in baseball, 55–56
    in golf, 270–279, 754
    in tennis, 524–525, 809
Swinging (acrobatic), 12, 16–18, *19*, 22–24, 866
Swing signature (golf), 270
Swing weight (oars and paddles), 332
Swiss wrestling style, 567
Swivel-heel cleats, 251
Sympathetic nervous system, 673, 678, 679, 703, 706
Synapses
    basketball shooting and, 64–65
    motor control and, *704*, 706, 715
Synaptic cleft, 830
Synaptic transmission, 704, 706
Synchronization, in paddle sports, 333, 336–337
Synovial fluid, 864–866
Synovium, 693
Systems theory (of motor control), 701
Systolic blood pressure, 590, 592, *671*, 678–679

T

Tacking (sailing), 375, *376*, 378, 387, 388
Tackling (football), 231–235
    impact avoidance, 869
    lineman's role, 233–235, 445
Tailwind
    football kicking and, 239, 241
    in Frisbee toss, 226
    as jumping factor, 199–200
    as running factor, 344–345
    soccer ball kicking and, 443
    as throwing factor, 209, 220, 221, 222
Takeaway point (golf swing), 274
Takeoff
    angle of, 188, 191
    in volleyball spiking, 542
Takeoff board (long jump), 185, 186
Takeoff point (hurdling), 363–364
Takeoff speed
    in competitive jumping, 178–181

    high jump, 180, 181, 183–184
    long jump, 185, 186–188
    pole vaulting, 193–194
Talofibular ligaments, 606
Talus, 604, 605, 606
Tanner, Roscoe, 514
Taping
    of ice hockey sticks, 306–307
    injury prevention and, 613–615
    as rehabilitative treatment, 768–769
Target archery, 27, 32, 36
Target width (bowling), 105–106
Tarkenton, Fran, 235
Tartars, 33
Taylor-Smith, Shelley, 652
Tee (football), 240
Telegraphing, in football, 236
Telemarking, 420
Temperature
    of human body, 740, 741
    ice skating conditions and, 395–396, 397–398
    skiing conditions and, 423–424
    tennis balls and, 523
    as viscosity factor, 326, 330, 497
Tempered glass, 175
Tendons
    ankle, foot, and lower leg, 607–608
    Achilles, 343, 362, 363, 607, 609, 611, 771
    knee, 697
    rehabilitative treatment for, 764–766
    shoulder, elbow, and wrist, 813, 816, 817, 818, 820
    skeletal muscle and, 828
    skeletal system and, 862, 864
Tennis, **510–532**
    arm adaptation to stress, 842, 851
    ball temperature, 523
    footwear, 172
    grip firmness, 303, 518, 520–521, 817
    injury risks and rehabilitation, 775, 863–864
        chronic back pain, 872
        tennis elbow, 520–521, 697, 766, 817, 822
    left-handed players, 711
    origins of, 510
    player testosterone levels, 119
    playing surfaces, 510–511, 528–529
    rackets, 155, 177, 511–19, 809
        evolution of, 514
        frame, 512–513
        head size, 511, 512
        "spaghetti," 522

string dampeners, 132, 520
strings, 516–519
sweet spot, 512, 514–516, 520, 544
scoring system, 510
serves, 525–527
   biomechanics of, 529–531
   power of, 514–515
   velocity of, *128*, 810–811
shoulder, elbow, and wrist action, 808–809, 815, 817, 820–821
strokes, 519–525
   backhand, 531–532
   with backspin, 69, 519
   baseline shots, 523–524
   forehand, 531
   with slice, 519, 528
   spin principles, 519–521
   swing and accuracy, 524–525
   with topspin, 519, 521, 522, *523*, 525
   touch shots, 522–523
vibrational energy and, 132, 515, 518, 520–521, 817, 819
visual skills, 899, 901, *904*
volleyball compared with, 544, 546
Tennis elbow, 520–521, 697, 766, 817, 819, 822
Tenocytes, 765
Tension
   archery bows and, 33, *34*
   board breaking and karate, 317
   as bone fracture factor, 854, 855, 856
   equipment materials and, *156*, 157
   golf swing and, 273, 277
   motor control and, 713
   of tennis racket strings, 516–518
Teres minor muscle, 813, 814
Terminal velocity, 428, 526
Testicles, 145
Testosterone, 730
   aging and, 662
   bone density and, 736
   bone growth and, 847
   cholesterol and, 733
   cycling and, 145
   muscle mass and, 839
   as performance factor, 118–119
   starvation dieting and, 575
Theodosius, 340
Therapy. *See* Rehabilitation; *specific types*
Thermal (air mass), 253, 262–264, 266
Thermal lift (gliding), 253, 260, 261–264

Thermodynamics, 626
Theseus, 108
Thiamine, 734
Thigh (femur), 752–761
   childhood injuries to, 846
   cycling and, 144, 146, 149, 150, 151
   ice skating and, *405*
   jumping ability and, 540
   knee and, 690
   male vs. female, 754–755
   soccer ball kicking and, 449, 450, 451
Thirst, 740
Thomas, Frank, 54
Thoracic vertebrae, 872–873, 875
300 game (bowling), 87, 104
Thrombi. *See* Blood clots
Throwing. *See* Field athletics, throwing; Pitching
Throwing time, 210–211
Throws
   acrobatic, 5
   wrestling, 571–572
Thumb, 430
Thyroid gland, 645
Thyroid hormone, 847
Thyroxine, 575
Tiant, Luis, 41
Tibialis posterior tendon, 607
Tibia (shin bone), 604, 605, 857
   childhood injuries to, 846
   cycling and, 144
   knee and, 690
Tidal volume, 590, 784
Tiebreakers (soccer), 444
Tight spirals (football), 237
Tilt, cycling and, 134
Time, as momentum factor, 231
Time trials (cycling), 130
Timing
   basketball shooting and, 66–67
   in wrestling, 572
Tires, bicycle, 138
Tissue, body
   circulatory system and, 667, 668–669
   connective, 485–487, 845–846
   lean vs. fat, 617, 621, 641
   nitrogen and, 804–805, 806
   rehabilitative treatment for, 764–766
   strength training and, 485–487
   See also Ligaments; Tendons
Titanium
   as equipment material, 159, 165, 166
   in hip replacement implants, 759
Title IX (legislation), 651

Tobacco. *See* Smoking
Toe clips (bicycle), 148–149
Toe-hook slide, 57, 58–59
Toejam power (Frisbee toss), 226
Toe pick (ice skates), *399*
Toes
   fractures to, 609
   heel-to-toe running, 342, 343, 362
Toltec culture, 62
Toon, Al, 246
Topflight, Shirley, 105
Topspin
   baseball pitching, 46, *47*
   basketball passing, 82
   in bowling, 91, 98–99, 104
   as distance factor, 208
   in golf, 171, 208
   in tennis, 519, 521, 522, *523*, 525
   in volleyball, 539, 543
Top tube (bicycle), 131
Torque
   in acrobatics, 10, 11, 13
   in archery, 28
   balls and, 294
   in baseball pitching, 40, 809, 816
   in baseball sliding, 58
   in basketball shooting, 67
   in bowling, 94–95, 97, 98
   in cycling, 134, 135, 146, 149–150
   in golf, 170, 278, 280
   ice hockey shots and, 298
   In Frisbee toss, 224–225
   as throwing event factor, 205, 209–210, 211, 218
   in weight lifting, 555, 556
   in wrestling, 568–569, 571, 572
   wrist and, 817, 820
Torsion, 158
Touch
   basketball shooting and, 64, 65
   sensory clues and, 19
Touchbacks (football), 242
Touch shots (tennis), 522–523
Tour de France, 130, 141–142
Tracheostomy tubes, 787
Track and field. *See* Field athletics, jumping; Field athletics, throwing; Running and hurdling; *specific events*
Track grab start (competitive swimming), 508
Tracking ability, vision and, 898, 899
Track racing (cycling), 130
Trail length (bicycle), *134*, 135
Trainers (boxing), 118
Trajectory
   acrobatics and, 7, 8

in archery, 36
of badminton shots, 527
baseball hitting and, 55–56
basketball shooting and, 69–72, 73, 74, 75, 80
in bowling, 99
fly balls and, 122–123
of hockey pucks, 296–297, 303
of tennis shots, 624
Trampolines, 14, 16
Transfatty acids, 731, 732
Translational forces, and bone injuries, 862–863
Transon, Ann, 652
Transportation energy requirements, 130
Transverse axis, 12, 15, 18
Transverse fractures, 856, 858
Transverse tubules (T-tubules), 828, 829, 830–831
Trapeze (gymnastics apparatus), 3
Trapeze artists, 3
Trapezius muscle, 587, 588, 813
Trapping (soccer), 448
Treadmill pools, 492
Treads (athletic shoes), 173
Triangulation, visual, 899–900
Triceps muscle, 814, 816, 835
Triglcyerides, 635, 636–637, 638, 728–729, 733, 744, 745
Trimming (of sail), 372–374
Triple-butted tubing (bicycle), 132
Triple jump, 178, 189–191
  records, 191, 198
  technique, 191
Trochanteric bursitis, 760
Tropomyosin, 415, 831, 832, 834
Troponin, 415, 831, 832, 834
True wind (sailing), 378–379
Tsu-chu (early soccer variant), 439
Tsukioshi (sumo wrestling), 579
Tsukioshi-zumo (sumo wrestling), 577–578
T-tubules. *See* Transverse tubules
Tubing (bicycle), 132–133, 163–165
Tuck (position), 14
Tumbling, 3
Tuned tracks (running), 360–361
Tungsten carbide, 159
Tunnel vision, 894
Turbulence
  baseball pitching and, 44, 45, 46
  as drag factor
    in gliding, 259
    in golf, 285, 287–288
    in paddle sports, 324–325
    in speed skating, 409–410

in swimming, 495–496, 497, 502, 507
Turks, 33, 34
Turnplatz (gymnastics place), 3
Turns
  in Alpine skiing, 430–433
  in cycling, 134
  in skating, 406–407, 411
  in snowboarding, 435
  See also Curves
Turnverien (gymnastic association), 3
Twists (acrobatic), 3, 12, 14–16, 23, 757, 875
Two-rod model (of kinetic energy), 271, 276
Tylers, Robert John, 408
Tyson, Mike, 111, 112

U
Ulna, 815, 816, 817
Ulnar collateral ligament, 430
Ultrasound electromagnetic waves, 622–623
Ultrasound therapy, 764, 768, 771
Underhand shot (basketball), 73–77
Underwater weighing. *See* Hydrostatic weighing
Uneven bars (gymnastics apparatus), 23–24, 866
United States Golf Association (USGA), 171, 281, 283, 287
Unsaturated fat, 729, 732
Unweighting (Alpine skiing), 431–432
Uppercut (boxing punch), 109
Upsweep (swimming), 503, 504–505
Urea, 639, 670, 725
Urine, 670, 725, 739
Ursinus, Oscar, 252
USGA. *See* United States Golf Association
USRDA (U.S. recommended daily allowances), 722
Utriculus, 20, 21

V
Valsalva maneuver, 477, 662
Van Dyken, Amy, 504
Variable (statistics), 467–468
Variable-resistance exercise, 482, *483*
Variance (statistics), 459
Varicose veins, 684–685
Vascularized bone grafting, 859
Vascular resistance, 678, 679–680, 682
Vasoconstriction, 767
Vasodilation, 768
Vasquez, Juan, 3

Vasquez, Miguel, 3
Vaulting horse (apparatus), 3
Vaulting pole. *See* Pole vaulting
Veering winds, 386–387
Vegetables, 729, 732, 737, 739, 746
Vegetarianism, 729
Veins, 668, 669, 684–685
Velocity
  of arrows, 28, 29, 31–32, 35, 36
  baseball hitting and, 49, 50, *52*, 53–54
  baseball pitching and, 44, *128*, 810, 816
  base running and, 58
  basketball shooting and, 77–78, 79
  as bowling factor, 89, 92, 103
  breaststroke and fluctuations in, 505–507
  catching skills and, 127
  cycling and, 139
  golf balls and, 167
  of golf-club head, 271, 274, 275, 278, 281, 283–284
  of ice hockey shots, *128*, 299–301, 302, 306
  inertia and, 10–11
  in jai alai, *128*
  in karate, 313–314, 319–320
  of kicked football, 241
  in lacrosse, 128
  in long jump, 187–188
  of release, 205, 208, 210, 212, 213, *215*, 228
  rotational, 6, 16–17
  summation of forces and, 7
  of tennis serves and strokes, *128*, 810–811
  terminal, 428, 526
  in throwing events, 206, 215, 217–218, 219, 222, 228
  in triple jump, 190
  of volleyball spike, 542–543
  of wind, 260, 261, 267, 289
  See also Angular velocity; Linear momentum
Ventilation, respiratory, 782, 783–787, 795
Ventilators, 785, 835
Ventricle. *See* Heart and circulatory system
Vertebrae, 844, 872–876, 877–878
Vertical jumps, 178–180, 184
Vertical momentum
  acrobatics and, 7–9
  jumping and, 184, 188
Very low density lipoprotein (VLDL), 733

Vestibular-ocular tracking, 64–65
Vestibular system
  balance and, 20–21, 114, 125
  catching skills and, 125
  knockout punches and, 114
Vibrational energy
  baseball bats and, 53–54, 303
  board breaking and, 318
  cycling and, 132, 133
  tennis and, 132, 515, 518, 520–521, 817, 819
Vikings, 369
Villi, 744
Violence in sports
  aggression and, 119
  football and, 230
  ice hockey and, 293
Viscoelastic (material property), 174
Viscosity, as drag factor, 326, 330, 497
Visible spectrum, 888, *889*
Vision, **887–906**
  acute mountain sickness and, 796, 797
  aging and, 585, 893–894
  of baseball hitters, 305, 889, 902–903, *904*
  binocular, 125
  blind spots, 890, 892
  brain waves and, 68
  catching skills and, 123–124, 125, 128
  corrective surgery, 893–894, 896–898, 905
  eye dominance, 711, 903
  eyewear, 887, 894, 896, 897, 901, 902–903, 905–906
  injury risks, 116, 797, 902–903
  at night, 891, 897
  physiology of, 888–894
    eye structure, 890–891
    information processing, 892–893
  sensory clues
    in acrobatics, 18, 19
    in football, *234*
  sight impairment, 893–894
    astigmatism, 894, 896
    blindness, 116, 734–735
    cataracts, 116, 893–894
    glaucoma, 894
    myopia and hyperopia, 894, 897
    presbyopia, 893
    tunnel vision, 894
  vestibular system role, 21
  visual skills and training, 889, 894–906

accommodation, 890, 893, 894, 898–899
acuity, 890, 895, 898, 902
aiming, 29–30, 38, 64
basic training principles, 904
central field awareness, 899
contrast sensitivity, 902
depth perception, 125, 899–900
eye-hand-foot coordination, 128, 305, 900
eye tracking, 898, 899
glare recovery, 901
instrument vs. free-space training, 901–902
peripheral vision, 891, 899
sighting, 64–65
spatial localization, 899, 900
stereopsis awareness, 900
visualization and visual memory, 900–901, 903, *904*
visual reaction time, 901
Visual cortex, 64
Visualization, 900–901, 903, *904*
Visual memory, 901, 903
Visual skills and training. *See under* Vision
Vital capacity, 589
Vitamin A, 734–735, 737, 901
Vitamin B, 734
Vitamin B1, 733
Vitamin B2, 901
Vitamin B6, 722
Vitamin B12, 738
Vitamin C, 720, 721, 737
Vitamin D, 654, 737, 847, 848, 849–850
Vitamin E, 737
Vitamin K, 746
Vitamins
  absorption of, 731
  disease prevention and, 737
  as nutrients, 720, 732–735, *736*, 737, 739
  See also specific vitamins
VLDL. *See* Very low density lipoprotein
Volito, 408
Volleyball, **534–547**
  ball aerodynamics, 535–539
  injury factors, 543–544, 604, 760, 877
  jumper's knee, 545, 697, 866
  jumping skill improvement, 540
  muscle spindles and, 713
  origin of, 534
  passing, 544–546
  protective padding, 761

serves, 535–539
setting of shots, 546–547
shoe selection, 545
spike shots, 541–544
visual skills, 901, *904*
Voluntary movement, 709
V1 technique (Nordic skiing), 437
V2 technique (Nordic skiing), 437–438

W
Wagner, Honus, 456–457
Wait-and-react hitting style, 54
Wake
  of golf ball, 286, 288
  of water, 328
Walking
  as aerobic activity, 596, 597
  braking force, 13
  compared to running, 608
  transportation energy requirements, *130*
Warm-up exercises, 363, 696, 760, 772–773
Wasserkuppe (Germany), 252, 260
Water (liquid medium)
  density of, 159, 490, 492, 494, 815
  hydrostatic weighing technique, 619–620
  paddle sports and, 324–326, 327–330, 334
  pressure of, 778
  sailing and, 382
  scuba diving and, 672, 777, 781, 791, 801–807
  swimming and, 490–491
    buoyancy and flotation, 491–494, 618
    drag, 494–498, 618
  training and rehabilitation utilization, 492–493, 774
  See also Ice and skating; Snow; Water resistance
Water (nutrient), 720, 739–746
  body weight control and, 576
  as bone component, 844
  mountain climbers and, 798
  See also Dehydration
Watercraft. *See* Paddle sports; Sailing; Yachting; *specific types*
Waterline (of boat), 382
Water on the knee, 693, 864
Water polo, 127, 815
Water resistance
  paddle sports and, 324–325, 328, 329, 334
  physical therapy and, 492–493

sailing and, 382
swimming and, 490–491, 494–498
Water therapy, 492–493, 774
Watson, Tom, 279
Waves
  paddle sports and, 327–330
  sailing and, 382
  swimming and, 497
Waxing (of skis), 421, 424–425, 438
Weather
  ice skating and, 396
  mountain climbing and, 798, 799
  sailing and, 386–388
  as tennis ball factor, 528–529
  as water consumption factor, 740–741
Weather helm (sailing), 380–381
Wedges (golf clubs). *See* Irons
Weight (body)
  as back problem factor, 882, *883*
  control, 576, 746–751
  cycling and, 136–137, 140
  desirable weight determination, 623–624
  golf stance and, 271–272, 273, 278
  gravity and, 204
  jumping ability and, 182
  knee injuries and, 694
  loss and gain hazards, 574–576, 656, 750
  metabolism and, 641–650, 748
  obesity, 616, 882
  reaction time and, 713
  running injuries and, 362–363
  skating and, *400*
  strength training and, 485
  wrestlers and, 574–576, 656, 750, 751
  See also Body composition; Body fat; Body size and shape; Eating disorders
Weight-aided jumping, 186
Weighted golf clubs, 280–281
Weight lifting, **549–565**
  basic principles, 550–557
    bounce effect, 556–557
    "sticking point," 554–556, 563
    strength vs. power, 139, 551–554
    work and energy, 550–551
  children and, 485
  injury risks, 828
  lifts
    clean-and-jerk, 552, 556–557, 558, 560–561
    dead, 552, 561, 562, 563
    snatch, 552, 557–558, 560

squat, 144–145, 486, 552, 555, 556, 557, 561, 564, *565*
  Olympic-style, 551–554, 557–561
  power lifting, 473, 551, 552–554, 561–565
  record lifts, 558, 561
  as resistance exercise, 472, 549, 679
  spine compression and, 874
  See also Strength training
Weight-lifting belts, 479–480
Weight training. *See* Strength training; Weight lifting
Wetteland, John, 292
Wham-O (toy company), 224
Wheelbase (bicycle), 132
Wheels
  bicycle, 137, 138, 142–143, 163, 165–167
  in-line skates, 408
Whiplash, 245–246, 828, 879
Whitewater kayaking. *See* Kayaking
Whole-body metabolism, 641–650, 745
  absorptive and postabsorptive, 641–643
  body weight and, 641
  exercise and, 644–650
  insulin levels, 643–644
Wicket, 51
Williams, Ted, *56*, 456, 710, 902
Wimbledon (tennis tournament), 510, 528
Wind
  apparent vs. true, 378–380
  gusts
    football punting and, 239
    golf shots and, 289
    sailing and, 380, 386–388
  lulls, 380, 387, 388
  quartering, 222
  veering vs. backing, 386–387
  velocity of
    gliding and, 260, 261, 267
    and golf shots, 289
  See also Headwind; Sailing
Wind resistance
  on bowling ball, 92–93
  as catch factor, 124–125
  cycling and, 139, 141, 143
  in discus throw, 220, 221–222
  in football passing, 236
  in Frisbee toss, 226
  in ice hockey, 295–296, 297, 303
  in javelin throw, 228
  jumping ability and, 182
  running and, *344*
  See also Crosswinds; Headwind; Tailwind

Windsurfers, 379, 382
Windup
  baseball pitching, 40
  speed skating, 413
  throwing, 814
Windward sailing, 378–381
Winfield, Dave, 54, 872
Wing loading (gliding), 259
Wobble
  in cycling, 402
  of hockey puck, 297
  in ice skating, 402
Wobbly spirals (football), 237
Wohlers, Mark, 700
Wolff-Parkinson-White (WPW) syndrome, 674
Women. *See* Female athletes
Wood, 153, 159
  baseball bats, 52–53, 54, 162, 175, 303
  basketball courts, 697
  bows and arrows, 33–34, 36, 175
  gliders, 253
  golf clubs, 281
  hockey sticks, 176, 304–305
  karate board breaking, 317–318
  paddles, 325
  tennis rackets, 513, 514, 523
  vaulting poles, 156, 192
Woods (golf clubs), 168, 170, 171, 272
Woosnam, Ian, 270, 271
Work
  as defined in athletics, 205–206, 216
  energy and metabolism and, 626
  intermittent, 446
  weight lifting and, 550–551, 552, 553, 557
World Cup (soccer), 440, 443–444
Wound (golf) ball, 168
"Wounded ducks" (football), 237
WPW syndrome. *See* Wolff-Parkinson-White syndrome
Wraps (strength training), 479
Wrestling, **567–579**
  back injuries and, 877
  basic principles, 568–573
    balance and motion, 569–570, 579
    leverage, 571–573
    torque and center of gravity, 568–569
  freestyle, 567, 568
  moves and holds
    half nelson, 573
    press pin, 573
    throws, 571–572

origins of, 567–568
sumo, 567–568, 573, 575–579
testosterone levels and, 119, 575
visual skills, *904*
weight extreme fluctuation hazards, 574–576, 656, 750–751
Wright, Alexander, 243
Wright brothers, 252, 254, 260
Wrigley Field (Chicago), 39
Wrist. *See* Shoulder, elbow, and wrist
Wrist-cock angle, 274–275
Wrist shot (ice hockey), 301–303, 304
Wrist snap
baseball pitching and, 42, 47–48
basketball passing and, 81
ice hockey shots and, 302

in tennis, 525, 529, 530, 820
torque and, 817, 820
in volleyball, 543

Y

Yachting
boat and sail design, 374, 378, 384–385
center of gravity and, 133
equipment materials, 153, 159, 385
See also America's Cup; Sailing
Yale University
early gymnasium, 3
football, 230
Harvard rowing competition, 321
Yankee Stadium (New York), 39

Yield strength, 157, *158*, 164, 165
Yokozuna (top sumo wrestlers), 576–577
Yotsu-zumo (sumo wrestling), 577, 578
Young, Steve, 127
Young's modulus of elasticity
in archery, 32–33, 35, 36
equipment materials and, 156, *157*, 161, 162, 167, 169, 171

Z

Zelezny, Jan, *229*
Zero angular momentum, 15–16
Zirconia, 171
"Zone, the" (basketball), 68

WITHDRAWN
CARROLL UNIVERSITY LIBRARY